Nursing Theories & Nursing Practice

third edition

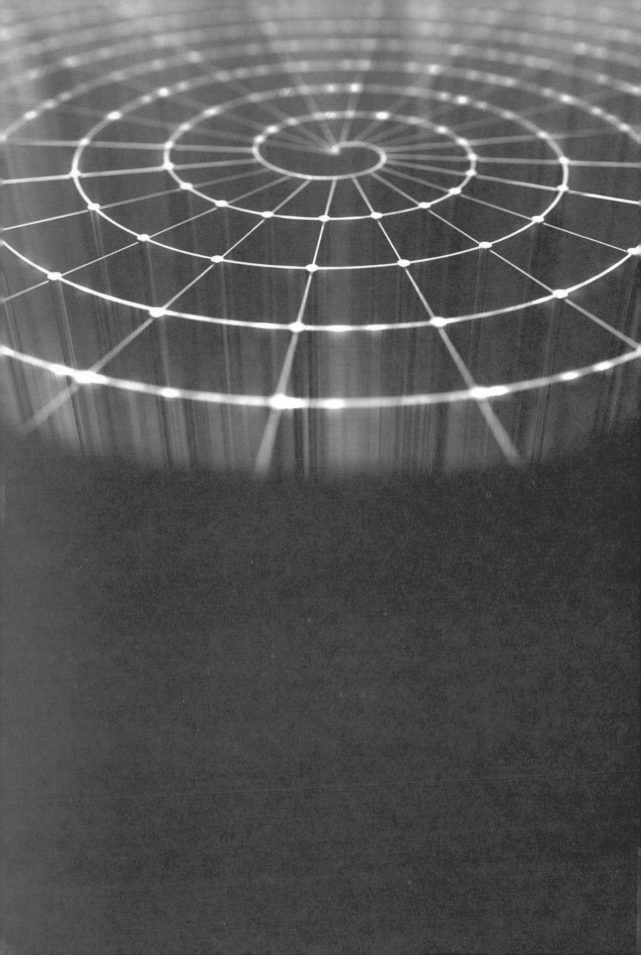

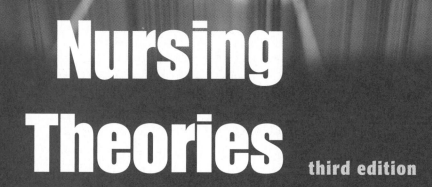

Nursing
Theories

third edition

& Nursing
Practice

Marilyn E. Parker, PhD, RN, FAAN
Marlaine C. Smith, PhD, RN, AHN-BC, FAAN

F. A. Davis Company • Philadelphia

F. A. Davis Company
1915 Arch Street
Philadelphia, PA 19103
www.fadavis.com

Printed in the United States of America

Last digit indicates print number: 10 9 8 7 6 5 4 3 2

Publisher, Nursing: Joanne Patzek DaCunha, RN, MSN
Director of Content Development: Darlene D. Pedersen
Assistant Editor: Maria Z. Price
Art and Design Manager: Carolyn O'Brien

As new scientific information becomes available through basic and clinical research, recommended treatments and drug therapies undergo changes. The author(s) and publisher have done everything possible to make this book accurate, up to date, and in accord with accepted standards at the time of publication. The author(s), editors, and publisher are not responsible for errors or omissions or for consequences from application of the book, and make no warranty, expressed or implied, in regard to the contents of the book. Any practice described in this book should be applied by the reader in accordance with professional standards of care used in regard to the unique circumstances that may apply in each situation. The reader is advised always to check product information (package inserts) for changes and new information regarding dose and contraindications before administering any drug. Caution is especially urged when using new or infrequently ordered drugs.

Library of Congress Cataloging-in-Publication Data

Nursing theories and nursing practice / [edited by] Marilyn E. Parker, Marlaine Cappelli Smith. — 3rd ed.
  p. ; cm.
 Includes bibliographical references and index.
 ISBN-13: 978-0-8036-2168-8
 ISBN-10: 0-8036-2168-X
1. Nursing—Philosophy. 2. Nursing. I. Parker, Marilyn E. II. Smith, Marlaine Cappelli.
 [DNLM: 1. Nursing Theory—Biography. 2. Nurses—Biography. WY 86 N9737 2010]
 RT84.5.N8793 2010
 610.7301—dc22   2010005930

Preface to the Third Edition

This book offers the perspective that nursing is a professional discipline with a body of knowledge that guides its practice. Nursing theories are an important part of this body of knowledge, and regardless of complexity or abstraction, reflect nursing and should be used by nurses to frame their thinking, action, and being in the world. As guides, nursing theories are practical in nature and facilitate communication with those we serve as well as with colleagues, students, and others practicing in health-related services. Our hope is that this book illuminates for the reader the interrelationship between nursing theories and nursing practice, and that this will focus practice more meaningfully and make a difference in the health and quality of life of people who are recipients of nursing care.

This very special book is intended to honor the work of nursing theorists and nurses who use these theories in their day-to-day practice, by reflecting and presenting the unique contributions of eminent nursing thinkers. Our foremost nursing theorists have written for this book, or their work has been described by nurses who have thorough knowledge of the theorist's work and who have a deep respect for the theorist as person, nurse, and scholar. Indeed, to the extent possible, contributing authors have been selected by theorists to write about their work. Seven additional grand or middle range theories and the conceptualizations of an early nursing scholar have been added to this edition of the book. This expansion reflects the growth in nursing theory development especially at the middle range; it was not possible to include all existing middle range theories in this volume.

This book is intended to assist nursing students in undergraduate, masters, and doctoral nursing programs to explore and appreciate nursing theories and their use in nursing practice and scholarship. In addition, and in response to calls from practicing nurses, this book is intended for use by those who desire to enrich their practice by the study of nursing theories and related illustrations of nursing practice. The contributing authors describe development processes and perspectives on the work, giving us a variety of views for the twenty-first century and beyond. Each chapter of the book includes both descriptions of a particular theory and an illustration of use of the theory in nursing practice. Each chapter offers a glimpse into the theory and how it might be used in practice. We anticipate that this will lead to deeper study of the theory by consulting published books and articles by the theorists and those working closely with the theory in practice or research.

The first section of the book provides an overview of nursing theory and a focus for thinking about evaluating and choosing nursing theory for use in nursing practice. Section II introduces the work of early nursing scholars whose ideas provided a foundation for theory development. The nursing conceptual models and grand theories were clustered into three sections. Section III includes those that have been classified within the interactive-integrative paradigm, while the fourth section includes those in the unitary-transformative paradigm. We separated the grand theories that focus on caring within Section V. The final section includes a selection of middle range theories.

An outline at the beginning of each chapter provides a map for the contents. Major points are highlighted in each chapter. Since this book focuses on the relationship of nursing theory to nursing practice we invited the authors to share a practice exemplar. The research methods and key research findings related to the theories have been placed on the book's website under "Additional Chapter Content" at http://davisplus.fadavis.com. We recognize the value of research in expanding nursing theory and in serving as a foundation for theory; however, this decision allowed us to focus the book more explicitly on theory and its relationship to practice. Having said this, readers will notice that not all the theorists chose to provide a practice exemplar, and some authors insisted on including research related to the theory in their chapters. Two chapters, 8 and 18, were not updated from the second edition.

The book's website features materials that will enrich the teaching and learning of these nursing theories. Materials that will be helpful for teaching and learning about nursing theories are included as online resources. For example, there are case studies and activities that facilitate student learning; powerpoint presentations are included in both instructor and student websites. We have cited online resources, more extensive bibliographies and have included biographies of chapter contributors. The ancillary materials for students and faculty have been prepared for this book by Dr. Shirley Gordon and a group of doctoral students from Florida Atlantic University. We are so grateful to Dr. Gordon for her creativity and leadership and to the doctoral students for their thoughtful contributions to this project.

For the latest and best thinking of some of nursing's finest scholars, all nurses who read and use this book will be grateful. For the continuing commitment of these scholars to our discipline and practice of nursing, we are all thankful. Continuing to learn and share what you love keeps the work and the love alive, nurtures the commitment, and offers both fun and frustration along the way. This has been illustrated in the enthusiasm for this book shared by many nursing theorists and contributing authors who have worked to create this book and by those who have added their efforts to make it live. For us, it is a joy to renew friendships with colleagues who have joined in preparing this book and to find new friends and colleagues as contributing authors.

Nursing Theories and Nursing Practice, now in the third edition, has roots in a series of nursing theory conferences held in South Florida beginning in 1989 and ending when efforts to cope with the aftermath of Hurricane Andrew interrupted the energy and resources needed for planning and offering the Fifth South Florida Nursing Theory Conference. Many of the theorists in this book addressed audiences of mostly practicing nurses at these conferences. Two books stimulated by those conferences and published by the National League for Nursing are *Nursing Theories in Practice* (1990) and *Patterns of Nursing Theories in Practice* (1993).

For me (Marilyn), even deeper roots of this book are found early in my nursing career, when I seriously considered leaving nursing for the study of pharmacy. In my fatigue and frustration, mixed with youthful hope and desire for more education, I could not answer the question "What is nursing?" and could not distinguish the work of nursing from other tasks I did every day. Why should I continue this work? Why should I seek degrees in a field that I could not define? After reflecting on these questions and using them to examine my nursing, I could find no one who would consider the questions with me. I remember being asked, "Why would you ask that question? You are a nurse; you must surely know what nursing is." Such responses, along with a drive for serious consideration of my questions, led me to the library. I clearly remember reading several descriptions of nursing that, I thought, could have just as well have been about social work or physical therapy. I then found nursing defined and explained in a book about education of practical nurses written by Dorothea Orem. During the weeks that followed, as I did my work of nursing in the hospital, I explored Orem's ideas about why people need nursing, nursing's purposes, and what nurses do. I found a fit of her ideas, as I understood them, with my practice, and

I learned that I could go even further to explain and design nursing according to these ways of thinking about nursing. I discovered that nursing shared some knowledge and practices with other services, such as pharmacy and medicine, and I began to distinguish nursing from these related fields of practice. I decided to stay in nursing and made plans to study and work with Dorothea Orem. In addition to learning about nursing theory and its meaning in all we do, I learned from Dorothea that nursing is a unique discipline of knowledge and professional practice. In many ways, my earliest questions about nursing have guided my subsequent study and work. Most of what I have done in nursing has been a continuation of my initial experience of the interrelations of all aspects of nursing scholarship, including the scholarship that is nursing practice. Over the years, I have been privileged to work with many nursing scholars, some of whom are featured in this book. My love for nursing and my respect for our discipline and practice have deepened, and knowing now that these values are so often shared is a singular joy.

Marlaine's interest in nursing theory had similar origins to Marilyn's. As a nurse pursuing an interdisciplinary master's degree in public health I recognized that while all the other public health disciplines had some unique perspective to share, public health nursing seemed to lack a clear identity. In search of the identity of nursing I pursued a second master's in nursing. At that time nursing theory was beginning to garner attention, and I learned about it from my teachers and mentors Sr. Rosemary Donley, Dr. Rosemarie Parse and Dr. Mary Jane Smith. This discovery was the answer I was seeking, and it both expanded and focused my thinking about nursing. The question of "What is nursing?" was answered for me by these theories and I couldn't get enough! It led to my decision to pursue my PhD in Nursing at New York University where I studied with Martha Rogers. During this same time I taught at Duquesne University with Rosemarie Parse and learned more about Man-Living-Health,

which is now humanbecoming. I conducted several studies based on Rogers' conceptual system and Parse's theory. At theory conferences I was fortunate to dialogue with Virginia Henderson, Hildegard Peplau, Imogene King and Madeleine Leininger. In 1988 I accepted a faculty position at the University of Colorado when Jean Watson was Dean. The School of Nursing was guided by a caring philosophy and framework and I embraced caring as a central focus of the discipline of nursing. I had studied Newman's theory of Health as Expanding Consciousness and was intrigued by it, so for my sabbatical I decided to study it further as well as learn more about the unitary appreciative inquiry process that Richard Cowling was developing.

We both have been fortunate to hold faculty appointments in universities where nursing theory has been valued, and we are fortunate today to hold positions at the Christine E. Lynn College of Nursing at Florida Atlantic University where faculty and students ground their teaching scholarship and practice on caring theories, including Nursing as Caring, developed by Dean Anne Boykin and a previous faculty member at the College, Savina Schoenhofer. Many faculty colleagues and students continue to help us study nursing and have contributed to this book in ways we would never have adequate words to acknowledge. We are grateful to our knowledgeable colleagues who reviewed and offered helpful suggestions for chapters of this book, and we sincerely thank those who contributed to the book as chapter authors. It is also our good fortune that many nursing theorists and other nursing scholars live in or willingly visit our lovely state of Florida. Since the first edition of this book was published we have lost several nursing theorists. Their work continues through those refining, modifying, testing and expanding the theories. The discipline of nursing is expanding with more research and practice in existing theories and the introduction of new theories. This is especially important at a time when nursing theory can provide what is missing and needed most in health care today.

All three editions of this book have been nurtured by Joanne DaCunha, an expert nurse and editor for F. A. Davis Company, who has shepherded this project and others because of her love of nursing. We are both grateful for her wisdom, kindness, patience and understanding of nursing. We give special thanks to Kimberly DePaul and Maria Price of F. A. Davis, for their gentle and wise editorial assistance, attention to detail, and creative ideas during the development of the project and to Berta Steiner who so carefully directed the book's production. Marilyn thanks her husband, Terry Worden, for his abiding love and for always being willing to help, and her niece, Cherie Parker, who represents many nurses who love nursing practice and scholarship and thus inspire the work of this book. Marlaine acknowledges her husband Brian for his love and support, and her children Kirsten, Alicia and Brady for their understanding, and gives special recognition to her parents, Deno and Rose Cappelli, for instilling in her the love of learning, the value of hard work, and the importance of caring for others.

MARILYN E. PARKER
WEST PALM BEACH, FLORIDA

MARLAINE C. SMITH
BOCA RATON, FLORIDA

Nursing Theorists

Charlotte D. Barry, PhD, RN, NCSN
Associate Professor of Nursing
Florida Atlantic University
Boca Raton, Florida

Anne Boykin, PhD, RN
Dean and Professor
Florida Atlantic University
Boca Raton, Florida

Barbara Montgomery Dossey,
PhD, RN, AHN-BC, FAAN
International Co-Director
Nightingale Initiative for Global Health
Santa Fe, New Mexico

Joanne R. Duffy, PhD, RN, FAAN
Professor
Indiana University
Indianapolis, Indiana

Helen L. Erickson*

Lydia Hall†

Virginia Henderson†

Dorothy Johnson†

Imogene King†

Katharine Kolcaba, PhD, RN
Associate Professor Emeritus
The University of Akron
Akron, Ohio

Madeleine M. Leininger*

Myra Levine†

Patricia Liehr, PhD, RN
*Professor and Associate Dean for Nursing Research
and Scholarship*
Florida Atlantic University
Boca Raton, Florida

Rozzano C. Locsin, PhD, RN
Professor
Florida Atlantic University
Boca Raton, Florida

Betty Neuman, PhD, RN, PLC, FAAN
Beverly, Ohio

Margaret Newman*

Dorothea E. Orem†

Ida Jean Orlando (Pelletier)*

Marilyn E. Parker, PhD, RN, FAAN
Clinical Professor
University of Kansas
Kansas City, Kansas

Rosemarie Rizzo Parse, PhD, FAAN
Distinguished Professor Emeritus
Loyola University Chicago
Chicago, Illinois

Josephine Paterson*

Hildegard Peplau†

Marilyn Anne Ray, PhD, RN, CTN
Professor Emeritus
Florida Atlantic University
Boca Raton, Florida

Pamela G. Reed, PhD, RN, FAAN
Professor
University of Arizona
Tucson, Arizona

Martha E. Rogers†

Sister Callista Roy, PhD, RN, FAAN
Professor and Nurse Theorist
Boston College
Chestnut Hill, Massachusetts

Savina O. Schoenhofer, PhD, RN
Professor of Nursing
Alcorn State University
Natchez, Mississippi

Marlaine C. Smith, PhD, RN, AHN-BC, FAAN
Helen K. Persson Eminent Scholar and Associate Dean
Florida Atlantic University
Boca Raton, Florida

Mary Jane Smith, PhD, RN
Professor and Associate Dean
West Virginia University
Morgantown, West Virginia

Mary Ann Swain, PhD
Provost and Vice President for Academic Affairs
Binghamton University
Binghamton, New York

Kristen M. Swanson, PhD, RN, FAAN
Professor and Dean
University of North Carolina
Chapel Hill, North Carolina

Evelyn Tomlin*

Joyce Travelbee†

Jean Watson, PhD, RN, AHN-BC, FAAN
Distinguished Professor of Nursing
University of Colorado at Denver–Anschutz Campus
Aurora, Colorado

Ernestine Wiedenbach†

Loretta Zderad*

*Retired
†Deceased

Contributors

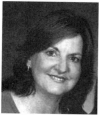

Patricia Deal Aylward, MSN, RN, CNS
Assistant Professor
Santa Fe Community College
Gainesville, Florida

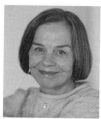

Elizabeth Ann Manhart Barrett, PhD, RN, FAAN
Professor
City University of New York
New York, New York

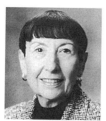

Nettie Birnbach†

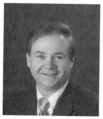

Howard Karl Butcher, PhD, RN, PMHCNS-BC
Associate Professor
University of Iowa
Iowa City, Iowa

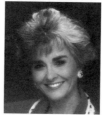

Marcia Dombro, EdD, RN
Chairperson
Miami-Dade College
Miami, Florida

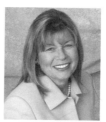

Lynne M. Dunphy, PhD, APRN-BC
Professor
Routhier Endowed Chair for Practice
University of Rhode Island
Kingston, Rhode Island

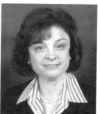

Laureen M. Fleck, DNS, FNP-BC, CDE
Family Nurse Practitioner
Florida Atlantic University
Boca Raton, Florida

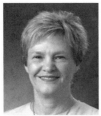

Maureen A. Frey, PhD, RN
Research Associate
Wayne State University
Detroit, Michigan

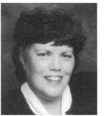

Bonnie Holaday, RN, DNS
Professor
Clemson University
Clemson, South Carolina

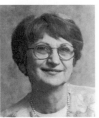

Theresa Gesse, PhD, RN
Professor
University of Miami
Miami, Florida

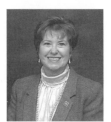

Mary B. Killeen, PhD, RN, NEA-BC
Consultant
Evidence Based Practice Nurse Consultants, LLC
Howell, Michigan

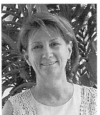

Shirley C. Gordon, PhD, RN
Associate Professor
Florida Atlantic University
Boca Raton, Florida

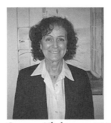

Susan Kleiman, PhD, RN, CS, NPP
Founder
International Institute for Human Centered Caring
Riverdale, New York

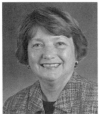

Donna L. Hartweg, PhD, RN
Director
Illinois Wesleyan University
Bloomington, Illinois

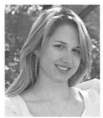

Kaitlin A. Laubham
Nursing Student
University of Kentucky
Lexington, Kentucky

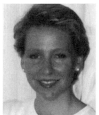

Danielle Linden, MSN, ARNP-BC, ARNP
Nurse Practitioner
Coral Springs, Florida

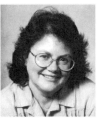

Violet M. Malinski, PhD, RN
Associate Professor
Hunter-Bellevue School of Nursing
New York, New York

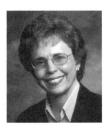

Marilyn R. McFarland,
PhD, RN, CTN, FNP-BC
Associate Professor
University of Michigan at Flint
Flint, Michigan

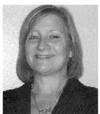

Linda G. Payne, MSN, RN, BC, CARN-AP
PhD Student and Teaching Assistant
Florida Atlantic University
Boca Raton, Florida

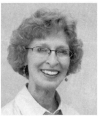

Ann R. Peden, ARNP, CS, DSN
Professor
University of Kentucky
Lexington, Kentucky

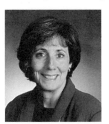

Margaret Dexheimer Pharris,
PhD, RN, MPH, FAAN
Associate Professor
College of St. Catherine
St. Paul, Minnesota

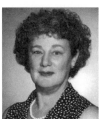

Maude Rittman, PhD, RN
Associate Chief of Nursing Service for Research
Gainesville Veteran's Administration Medical Center
Gainesville, Florida

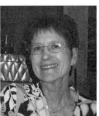

Karen Moore Schaefer, PhD, RN
Associate Chair
Temple University
Philadelphia, Pennsylvania

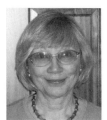

Christina L. Sieloff, PhD, RN, CNA-BC
Associate Professor
Montana State University
Billings, Montana

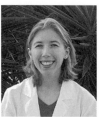

Jacqueline Staal, MSN, ARNP, FNP-BC
PhD Student
Florida Atlantic University
Boca Raton, Florida

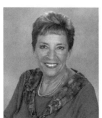

Theris A. Touhy, DNP, GCNS-BC
Professor
Florida Atlantic University
Boca Raton, Florida

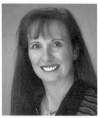

Marian C. Turkel, PhD, RN
Director of Professional Nursing Practice
Albert Einstein Healthcare Network
Philadelphia, Pennsylvania

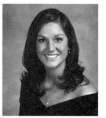

Autumn Wells
Nurse Research Intern
University of Kentucky
Lexington, Kentucky

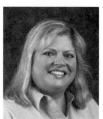

Kelly N. White, MSN, FNP-BC
PhD Student
Florida Atlantic University
Boca Raton, Florida

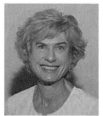

Terri Kaye Woodward,
MSN, RN, CNS, AHN-BC, HTCP
Founder
Cocreative Wellness
Denver, Colorado

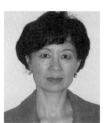

Lin Zhan, PhD, RN, FAAN
Dean and Professor
Massachusetts College of Pharmacy and Health
    Sciences
Boston, Massachusetts

Reviewers

Geraldine Allen, RN, DSN, FNP
MSN Program Director
Troy University
Selma, Alabama

Cathryn J. Baack, PhD, RN, CPNP
Assistant Professor
MedCentral College of Nursing
Mansfield, Ohio

Mary Baumberger-Henry, PhD, RN
Associate Professor
Widener University School of Nursing
Chester, Pennsylvania

Beverly M. Brown, EdD, MSN, APRN/GCNS, BC
Assistant Professor
Tennessee State University
Nashville, Tennessee

Nancy Hinzman, MSN, RN
Associate Professor of Nursing
College of Mount St. Joseph
Cincinnati, Ohio

Marlene Huff, PhD, MSN
Associate Professor
University of Akron
Akron, Ohio

Kathleen Ann Kalb, PhD, RN
Associate Professor of Nursing
The College of St. Catherine
St. Paul, Minnesota

Barbara Kearney, PhD, RN
Assistant Professor
Murray State University
Murray, Kentucky

Norma Krumwiede, EdD, RN
Professor
Minnesota State University
Mankato, Minnesota

Judy Kuhns-Hastings, PhD, APRN-BC, FNP
Associate Professor of Nursing
University of Maine
Orono, Maine

Carole-Lynne Le Navenec, PhD, RN
Associate Professor
University of Calgary
Calgary, Alberta, Canada

Margherite Matteis, PhD, RN, PMHCNS-BC
Associate Professor
Regis College
Weston, Massachusetts

Victoria Menzies, PhD, APRN-BC
Assistant Professor
Florida International University
Miami, Florida

Carel Mountain, MSN, RN
Nursing Faculty
Shasta College
Redding, California

Carla Mueller, PhD, RN
Professor
University of St. Francis
Fort Wayne, Indiana

Barbara R. Norwood, MSN, EdD, RN
Associate Professor
University of Tennessee at Chattanooga
Chattanooga, Tennessee

Lauren E. O'Hare, EdD, RN
Chair
Wagner College
Staten Island, New York

Nelma B. Shearer, PhD, RN
Associate Professor
Arizona State University
Phoenix, Arizona

Christina L. Sieloff, PhD, RN, CNA-BC
Associate Professor
Montana State University
Billings, Montana

Pamela Wessling, MSN, ARNP, NP-C
Assistant Professor
Barry University
Miami Shores, Florida

Contents

An Introduction to Nursing Theory

An Introduction to Nursing Theory

In this first section of the book we, the editors, have written three chapters that will introduce the reader to the purpose of nursing theory and how to study, analyze, and evaluate it for use in nursing practice. If you are new to the idea of theory in nursing, the chapters in this section will orient you to what theory is, how it fits into the context of nursing as a professional discipline, and how to approach its study and evaluation. If you have studied nursing theory in the past, we hope the chapters will provide you with additional knowledge and insight as you continue your study. We assert that nursing is a professional discipline focused on the study of human health and healing through caring. Nursing practice is based on the knowledge of nursing, which consists of its philosophies, theories, concepts, principles, research findings, and practice wisdom. Theories are patterns that guide the thinking about being, and doing of nursing. All nurses are guided by some implicit or explicit theory, or pattern of thinking, as they care for their patients. Too often, this pattern of thinking is implicit, and is colored by the lens of diseases, diagnoses, and treatments. This does not reflect practice from the disciplinary perspective of nursing. The major reason for nursing theory is to improve nursing practice, and therefore the health and quality of life of those we serve. The first chapter in this section focuses on nursing theory and how it fits within the context of nursing as a professional discipline. We examine the relationship of nursing theory to the characteristics of a discipline. You'll learn new words that describe parts of the knowledge structure of the discipline of nursing, and we'll speculate about the future of nursing theory as nursing, health care, and our global society change. Chapter 2 is a guide to help you study the theories in this book. We hope you'll use this guide as you read and think about nursing theory for use in practice. Nurses embrace theories because they fit with their values and ways of thinking. They choose theories to guide their practice when the theories help them to create a practice that is meaningful to them. Chapter 3 focuses on the selection, evaluation, and implementation of theory for practice. Students often get the assignment of evaluating or critiquing a nursing theory. Evaluation is coming to some judgment about value or worth based on criteria. Various sets of criteria exist for you to use in theory evaluation. We introduce some that you can explore further. Finally, we offer reflections on the process of implementing theory-guided practice models.

Chapter 1

Nursing Theory and the Discipline of Nursing

MARLAINE C. SMITH AND
MARILYN E. PARKER

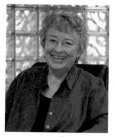

Marilyn E. Parker

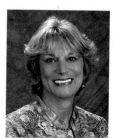

Marlaine C. Smith

What is nursing? At first glance, the question may appear to be one with an obvious answer, but when it is posed to nurses, many define nursing by providing a litany of functions and activities. Some answer with the elements of the nursing process: nurses assess, plan, implement, and evaluate the patient. Others might answer that nurses coordinate a patient's care.

Defining nursing in terms of the nursing process, or by functions or activities performed is problematic. The phases of the nursing process are the same as those that delineate the solution of any problem we encounter, from a broken computer to a failing vegetable garden. We assess the situation to determine what is going on and then identify the problem; we plan what to do about it, implement our plan, and then evaluate if it works. The nursing process does nothing to define nursing.

Defining ourselves by tasks presents other problems. What nurses do, that is, the functions associated with practice, differs based on the setting. For example, nurses might start IVs, administer medications, and perform treatments in an acute care setting. In a community-based clinic, nurses might teach a young mother the principles of infant feeding or place phone calls to connect a child with special needs to community resources. Multiple professionals and non-professionals perform the same tasks as nurses, and persons with the ability and authority to perform certain tasks change based on time and setting. For example, both physicians and nurses may listen to breath sounds and recognize the presence of rales. Both nurses and social workers might do discharge planning. Both nurses and family members might change dressings, monitor vital signs, and administer medications, so defining nursing based solely on functions or activities performed is not useful.

To answer the question "What is nursing?" we must formulate nursing's unique perspective as a field of study or discipline. Florence Nightingale is credited as the founder of modern Nursing, the one who articulated its distinctive focus. In her book *Notes on Nursing: What It Is and What It Is Not* (Nightingale, 1859/1992), she differentiated nursing from medicine, stating that they were two distinct practices. She defined nursing as putting the person in the best condition for nature to act, insisting that the focus of nursing was on health and the natural healing process, and not on disease and reparation. For her, creating an environment that provided the conditions for natural healing to occur was the focus of nursing. Her beginning conceptualizations were the seeds for the theoretical development of nursing as a professional discipline.

In this chapter, we situate the understanding of nursing theory within the context of the discipline of nursing. We define the discipline of nursing and theory, describe the purpose of theory for the discipline of nursing, identify the structure of the discipline of nursing, and speculate on the future place of nursing theory in the discipline.

The Discipline of Nursing

Every discipline has a unique focus that directs the inquiry within it and distinguishes it from other fields of study (Smith, 2008, p. 1). Nursing knowledge guides its professional practice; therefore, it is classified as a professional discipline. Donaldson and Crowley (1978) stated that a discipline "offers a unique perspective, a distinct way of viewing...phenomena, which ultimately defines the limits and nature of its inquiry" (p. 113). Any discipline includes networks of philosophies, theories, concepts, approaches to inquiry, research findings, and practices

that both reflect and illuminate its distinct perspective. **The discipline of nursing is formed by a community of scholars, including nurses in all nursing venues, who share a commitment to values, knowledge, and processes to guide the thought and work of the discipline.**

The classic work of King and Brownell (1976) is consistent with the thinking of nursing scholars (Donaldson & Crowley, 1978; Meleis, 1977) about the discipline of nursing. These authors have elaborated attributes that characterize all disciplines. The attributes of King and Brownell provide a framework that contextualizes nursing theory within the discipline of nursing. Each of the attributes of disciplines is described in the text that follows.

Expression of Human Imagination

Members of any discipline imagine and create structures that offer descriptions and explanations of the phenomena that are of concern to that discipline. These structures are the theories of that discipline. Nursing theory is dependent on the imagination of nurses in practice, administration, research, and teaching, as they create and apply theories to improve nursing practice and ultimately the lives of those we serve. To remain dynamic and useful, our discipline requires openness to new ideas and innovative approaches that grow out of members' reflections and insights.

Domain

A professional discipline must be clearly defined by a statement of its domain—the boundaries or focus of that discipline. The domain of nursing includes the phenomena of interest, problems to be addressed, main content and methods used, and roles required of the discipline's members (Kim, 1997; Meleis, 1997). The processes and practices claimed by members of the disciplinary community grow out of these domain statements. Nightingale provided some direction for the domain of the discipline of nursing. While the disciplinary focus has been debated, there is some degree of consensus. Donaldson and Crowley (1978, p. 113) identified the following as the domain of the discipline of nursing:

1. Concern with principles and laws that govern the life processes, well-being, and optimum functioning of human beings, sick or well
2. Concern with the patterning of human behavior in interactions with the environment in critical life situations
3. Concern with the processes by which positive changes in health status are affected

Fawcett (1984) described the metaparadigm as a way to distinguish nursing from other disciplines. The metaparadigm is very general and is intended to reflect agreement among members of the discipline about the field of nursing. This is the most abstract level of nursing knowledge and closely mirrors beliefs held about nursing. By virtue of being nurses, all nurses have some awareness of nursing's metaparadigm. However, because the term may not be familiar, it offers no direct guidance for research and practice (Kim, 1997; Walker & Avant, 1995). The metaparadigm consists of four concepts: persons, environment, health, and nursing. According to Fawcett, nursing is the study of the interrelationship among these four concepts.

Modifications and alternative concepts for this framework have been explored throughout the discipline (Fawcett, 2000). For example, nursing scholars have suggested that "caring" replace "nursing" in the metaparadigm (Stevenson & Tripp-Reimer, 1989). Kim (1987, 1997) set forth four domains: client, client–nurse encounters, practice, and environment. In recent years, increasing attention has been directed to the nature of nursing's relationship with the environment (Kleffel, 1996; Schuster & Brown, 1994).

Others have defined nursing as the study of: "the health or wholeness of human beings as they interact with their environment" (Donaldson & Crowley, 1978, p. 113); the life process of unitary human beings (Rogers, 1970); care or caring (Leininger,

1978; Watson, 1985); and human–universe–health interrelationships (Parse, 1998). A widely accepted focus statement for the discipline was published by Newman, Sime, and Corcoran-Perry (1991) as "Nursing is the study of caring in the human health experience" (p. 3). A consensus statement of philosophical unity in the discipline was published by Roy and Jones (2007). Statements include:

- The human being is characterized by wholeness, complexity, and consciousness.
- The essence of nursing involves the nurse's true presence in the process of human-to-human engagement.
- Nursing theory expresses the values and beliefs of the discipline, creating a structure to organize knowledge and illuminate nursing practice.
- The essence of nursing practice is the nurse–patient relationship.

In 2008, Newman, Smith, Dexheimer-Pharris, and Jones revisited the disciplinary focus asserting that relationship was central to the discipline, and the convergence of seven concepts—health, consciousness, caring, mutual process, presence, patterning, and meaning—specified relationship in the professional discipline of nursing. Willis, Grace, and Roy (2008) posited that the central unifying focus for the discipline is facilitating humanization, meaning, choice, quality of life, and healing in living and dying (p. E28). Finally, Litchfield and Jondorsdottir (2008) defined the discipline as the study of humanness in the health circumstance. Smith (1994) defined the domain of the discipline of nursing as "the study of human health and healing through caring" (p. 50). For Smith, "nursing knowledge focuses on wholeness of human life and experience and the processes that support relationship, integration, and transformation" (p. 3). Nursing conceptual models, grand theories, middle-range theories, and practice theories explicate the phenomena within the domain of nursing. In addition, the focus of the nursing discipline is a clear statement of social mandate and service used to direct the study and practice of nursing (Newman, Sime, & Corcoran-Perry, 1991).

Syntactical and Conceptual Structures

Syntactical and conceptual structures are essential to any discipline and are inherent in nursing theories. The conceptual structure delineates the proper concerns of nursing, guides what is to be studied, and clarifies accepted ways of knowing and using content of the discipline. This structure is grounded in the focus of the discipline. The conceptual structure relates concepts within nursing theories. The syntactical structures help nurses and other professionals to understand the talents, skills, and abilities that must be developed within the community. This structure directs descriptions of data needed from research, as well as evidence required to demonstrate the impact on nursing practice. In addition, these structures guide nursing's use of knowledge in research and practice approaches developed by related disciplines. It is only by being thoroughly grounded in the discipline's concepts, substance, and modes of inquiry that the boundaries of the discipline can be understood and possibilities for creativity across disciplinary borders can be created and explored.

Specialized Language and Symbols

As nursing theory has evolved, so has the need for concepts, language, and forms of data that reflect new ways of thinking and knowing specific to nursing. The complex concepts used in nursing scholarship and practice require language that can be specific and understood. The language of nursing theory facilitates communication among members of the discipline. Expert knowledge of the discipline is often required for full understanding of the meaning of these theoretical terms.

Heritage of Literature and Networks of Communication

This attribute calls attention to the array of books, periodicals, artifacts, and aesthetic expressions, as well as audio, visual, and electronic media that have developed over centuries to communicate the nature of nursing knowledge and practice. Conferences and forums on every aspect of nursing held throughout the world are part of this network. Nursing organizations and societies also provide critical communication links. Nursing theories are part of this heritage of literature, and those working with these theories present their work at conferences, societies, and other communication networks of the nursing discipline.

Tradition

The tradition and history of the discipline is evident in the study of nursing over time. There is recognition that theories most useful today often have threads of connection with ideas originating in the past. For example, many theorists have acknowledged the influence of Florence Nightingale, and have acclaimed her leadership in influencing nursing theories of today. In addition, nursing has a rich heritage of practice. Nursing's practical experience and knowledge have been shared and transformed as the content of the discipline and are evident in many nursing theories (Gray & Pratt, 1991).

Values and Beliefs

Nursing has distinctive views of persons and strong commitments to compassionate and knowledgeable care of persons through nursing. Fundamental nursing values and beliefs include a holistic view of person, the dignity and uniqueness of persons and the call to care. There are both shared and differing values and beliefs within the discipline. The metaparadigm reflects the shared beliefs while the paradigms reflect the differences.

Systems of Education

A distinguishing mark of any discipline is the education of future and current members of the community. Nursing is recognized as a professional discipline within institutions of higher education because it has an identifiable body of knowledge that is studied, advanced, and used to underpin its practice. Students of any professional discipline study its theories and learn its methods of inquiry and practice.

Nursing theories, by setting directions for the substance and methods of inquiry for the discipline, should provide the basis for nursing education and the framework for organizing nursing curricula.

Definitions of Nursing Theory

A *theory*, as a general term, is a notion or an idea that explains experience, interprets observation, describes relationships, and projects outcomes. Parsons (1949), often quoted by nursing theorists, wrote that theories help us know what we know and decide what we need to know. Theories are mental patterns or frameworks created to help understand and create meaning from our experience, organize and articulate our knowing, and ask questions leading to new insights. As such, theories are not discovered in nature, but are human inventions.

Theories are organizing structures of our reflections, observations, projections, and inferences. Many describe theories as lenses because they color and shape what is seen. The same phenomena will be seen differently depending on the theoretical perspective assumed. For these reasons, theory and related terms have been defined and described in a number of ways according to individual experience and what is useful at the time. Theories, as reflections of understanding, guide our actions, help us set forth desired outcomes, and give evidence of what has been achieved. A theory, by traditional definition, is an organized, coherent set of concepts and their relationships to each other that offers descriptions, explanations, and predictions about phenomena.

Early writers on nursing theory brought definitions of theory from other disciplines to direct future work within nursing. Dickoff and James (1968, p. 198) define theory as a "conceptual system or framework invented for some purpose." Ellis (1968, p. 217) defined theory as "a coherent set of hypothetical, conceptual, and pragmatic principles forming a general frame of reference for a field of inquiry." McKay (1969, p. 394) asserted that theories are the capstone of scientific work, and that the term refers to "logically interconnected sets of confirmed hypotheses." Barnum (1998, p. 1) later offers a more open definition of theory as a "construct that accounts for or organizes some phenomenon," and simply states that a nursing theory describes or explains nursing.

Definitions of theory emphasize its various aspects. Those developed in recent years are more open and conform to a broader conception of science. The following definitions of theory are consistent with general ideas of theory in nursing practice, education, administration, or research:

• Theory is a set of concepts, definitions, and propositions that project a systematic view of phenomena by designating specific interrelationships among concepts for purposes of describing, explaining, predicting, and/or controlling phenomena (Chinn & Jacobs, 1987, p. 71).

• Theory is a creative and rigorous structuring of ideas that projects a tentative, purposeful, and systematic view of phenomena (Chinn & Kramer, 2004, p. 268).

• Nursing theory is a conceptualization of some aspect of reality (invented or discovered) that pertains to nursing. The conceptualization is articulated for the purpose of describing, explaining, predicting, or prescribing nursing care (Meleis, 1997, p. 12).

• Nursing theory is an inductively and/or deductively derived collage of coherent, creative, and focused nursing phenomena that frame, give meaning to, and help explain specific and selective aspects of nursing research and practice (Silva, 1997, p. 55).

• A theory is an imaginative grouping of knowledge, ideas, and experience that are represented symbolically and seek to illuminate a given phenomenon." (Watson, 1985, p. 1).

The Purpose of Theory in a Professional Discipline

All professional disciplines have a body of knowledge consisting of theories, research, and methods of inquiry and practice. They organize knowledge, guide practice, enhance the care of patients, and guide inquiry to advance science. Nursing theories address the phenomena of interest to nursing, including the focus of nursing; the person, group, or population nursed; the nurse; the relationship of nurse and nursed; and the hoped-for goal or purposes of nursing. **Based on strongly held values and beliefs about nursing, and within contexts of various worldviews, theories are patterns that guide the thinking about, being, and doing of nursing.**

They provide structures for making sense of the complexities of reality for both practice and research. Theory-based research is needed in order to explain and predict nursing outcomes essential to the delivery of nursing care that is both humane and cost-effective (Gioiella, 1996). Some conceptual structure either implicitly or explicitly directs all avenues of nursing, including nursing education and administration. Nursing theories provide concepts and designs that define the place of nursing in health care. Through theories, nurses are offered perspectives for relating with professionals from other disciplines who join with nurses to provide human services. Nursing has great expectations of its theories. At the same time, theories must provide structure and substance to ground the practice and scholarship of nursing and must also be flexible and dynamic to keep pace with the growth and changes in the discipline and practice of nursing.

The major reason for structuring and advancing nursing knowledge is for the sake of nursing practice. The primary purpose of nursing theories is to further the development and understanding of nursing practice. Because nursing theory exists to improve practice, the test of nursing theory is a test of its usefulness in professional practice (Colley, 2003; Fitzpatrick, 1997). The work of nursing theory is moving from academia into the realm of nursing practice. Chapters in the remaining sections of this book highlight the use of nursing theories in nursing practice.

Nursing practice is both the source and goal of nursing theory. From the viewpoint of practice, Gray and Forsstrom (1991) suggest

that theory provides nurses with different ways of looking at and assessing phenomena, rationale for their practice, and criteria for evaluating outcomes. Many of the theories in this book have been used to guide nursing practice, stimulate creative thinking, facilitate communication, and clarify purposes and processes in practice. The practicing nurse has an ethical responsibility to use the discipline's theoretical knowledge base, just as it is the nurse scholar's ethical responsibility to develop the knowledge base specific to nursing practice (Cody, 1997, 2003).

At the empirical level of theory, abstract concepts are operationalized, or made concrete, for practice and research (Fawcett, 2000; Smith & Liehr, 2008). Empirical indicators provide specific examples of how the theory is experienced in reality; they are important for bringing theoretical knowledge to the practice level. These indicators include procedures, tools, and instruments to determine the impact of nursing practice and are essential to research and management of outcomes of practice (Jennings & Staggers, 1998). The resulting data form the basis for improving the quality of nursing care and influencing healthcare policy. Empirical indicators, grounded carefully in nursing concepts, provide clear demonstration of the utility of nursing theory in practice, research, administration, and other nursing endeavors (Allison & McLaughlin-Renpenning, 1999; Hart & Foster, 1998).

Meeting the challenges of systems of care delivery and interdisciplinary work demands practice from a theoretical perspective. Nursing's disciplinary focus is essential within an interdisciplinary environment (Allison & McLaughlin-Renpenning, 1999); otherwise its unique contribution to the interdisciplinary team is unclear. Nursing actions reflect nursing concepts and thought. Careful, reflective, and critical thinking are the hallmarks of expert nursing, and nursing theories should undergird these processes. Appreciation and use of nursing theory offer opportunity for successful collaboration with colleagues from other disciplines, and provide definition for nursing's overall contribution to health care.

Nurses must know what they are doing, why they are doing it, what the range of outcomes of nursing may be, and indicators for documenting nursing's impact. These nursing theoretical frameworks serve as powerful guides for articulating, reporting, and recording nursing thought and action.

One of the assertions referred to most often in the nursing theory literature is that theory is given birth in nursing practice and, after examination and refinement through research, must be returned to practice (Dickoff, James, & Wiedenbach, 1968). Nursing theory is stimulated by questions and curiosities arising from nursing practice. Development of nursing knowledge is a result of theory-based nursing inquiry. The circle continues as data, conclusions, and recommendations of nursing research are evaluated and developed for use in practice. Nursing theory must be seen as practical and useful to practice, and the insights of practice must in turn continue to enrich nursing theory.

The Structure of Knowledge in the Discipline of Nursing

Theories are part of the knowledge structure of any discipline. The domain of inquiry, metaparadigm, or focus of the discipline is the foundation of the structure. The knowledge of the discipline is related to its general domain or focus. For example, knowledge of biology relates to the study of living things; psychology is the study of the mind; sociology is the study of social structures and behaviors. Nursing's domain was discussed earlier and relates to the focus statement or metaparadigm. Other levels of the knowledge structure include paradigms, conceptual models or grand theories, middle-range theories, practice theories, and research and practice traditions. These levels of nursing knowledge are interrelated; each level of development is influenced by work at other levels. Theoretical work in nursing must be dynamic; that is, it must be continually in process and useful for the purposes and work of the discipline. It must be open to adapting

and extending in order to guide nursing endeavors and to reflect development within nursing. Although there is diversity of opinion among nurses about terms used to describe the levels of theory, the following discussion of theoretical development in nursing is offered as a context for further understanding nursing theory.

Paradigm

Paradigm is the next level of the disciplinary structure of nursing. The notion of paradigm can be useful as a basis for understanding nursing knowledge. *Paradigm* is a global, general framework made up of assumptions about aspects of the discipline held by members to be essential in development of the discipline. The concept of paradigm comes from the work of Kuhn (1970, 1977), who used the term to describe models that guide scientific activity and knowledge development in disciplines. Because paradigms are broad, shared perspectives held by members of the discipline, they are often called "worldviews." Kuhn set forth the view that science does not always evolve as a smooth, regular, continuing path of knowledge development over time, but that periodically there are times of revolution when traditional thought is challenged by new ideas, and "paradigm shifts" occur.

Kuhn's ideas provide a way for us to think about the development of science. Before any discipline engages in the development of theory and research to advance its knowledge, it is in a pre-paradigmatic period of development. Typically, this is followed by a period of time when a single paradigm emerges to guide knowledge development. Research activities initiated around this paradigm advance its theories. This is a time during which knowledge advances at a regular pace. At times, a new paradigm can emerge to challenge the worldview of the existing paradigm. It can be revolutionary, overthrowing the previous paradigm, or multiple paradigms can coexist in a discipline, providing different worldviews that guide the scientific development of the discipline.

Kuhn's work has meaning for nursing and other scientific disciplines because of his recognition that science is the work of a community of scholars in the context of society. Paradigms and worldviews of nursing are subtle and powerful, reflecting different values and beliefs about the nature of human beings, human–environment relationships, health, and caring. Kuhn's (1970, 1977) description of scientific development is particularly relevant to nursing today as new perspectives are being articulated, some traditional views are being strengthened, and some views are taking their places as part of our history. As we continue to move away from the historical conception of nursing as a part of biomedical science, developments in the nursing discipline are directed by at least two paradigms or worldviews outside of the medical model. These are described below.

Several nursing scholars have named the existing paradigms in the discipline of nursing (Fawcett, 1995; Newman et al. 1991; Parse, 1987); each is slightly different. Parse (1987) described two paradigms: the totality and the simultaneity. The totality paradigm reflects a worldview that humans are integrated beings with biological, psychological, sociocultural, and spiritual dimensions. Humans adapt to their environments, and health and illness are states on a continuum. In the simultaneity paradigm, humans are unitary, irreducible, and in continuous mutual process with the environment (Rogers, 1970, 1992). Health is subjectively defined and reflects a process of becoming or evolving. Three paradigms in nursing were identified by Newman and her colleagues (Newman et al., 1991): particulate–deterministic, interactive–integrative, and unitary–transformative. From the perspective of the particulate–deterministic paradigm, humans are known through parts; health is the absence of disease; and predictability and control are essential for its management. In the interactive–integrative paradigm, humans are viewed as systems with interrelated dimensions interacting with the environment, and change is probabilistic. The worldview of the unitary–transformative paradigm describes humans as patterned, self-organizing fields within larger patterned, self-organizing fields.

Change is characterized by fluctuating rhythms of organization–disorganization toward more complex organization. Health is a reflection of this continuous change. Fawcett (1995, 2000) provides another model for the nursing paradigms: reaction, reciprocal interaction, and simultaneous action. In the reaction paradigm, humans are the sum of their parts, reaction is causal, and stability is valued. In the reciprocal interaction worldview, the parts are seen within the context of a larger whole, there is a reciprocal nature to the relationship with the environment, and change is based on multiple factors. Finally, the simultaneous action worldview includes a belief that humans are known by pattern and are in an open ever-changing process with the environment. Change is unpredictable and evolving toward greater complexity (Smith, 2008, pp. 4–5).

Theories are clustered within these paradigms. There will be many theories that share the worldview established by a particular paradigm. Nursing is in a phase whereby multiple paradigms coexist.

Grand Theories and Conceptual Models

Grand theories and conceptual models are at the next level in the structure of the discipline. They are less abstract than the focus of the discipline and paradigms, but more abstract than middle-range theories. Conceptual models and grand theories focus on the phenomena of concern to the discipline such as persons as adaptive systems, self-care deficits, unitary human beings, human becoming, or health as expanding consciousness. The grand theories, or conceptual models, are composed of concepts and relational statements. Relational statements upon which the theories are built are called assumptions and often reflect the foundational philosophies of the conceptual model/grand theory. These philosophies are statements of enduring values and beliefs; they may be practical guides for the conduct of nurses applying the theory and can be used to determine the compatibility of the model/theory with personal, professional, organizational, and societal beliefs and values. Fawcett (2000) differentiates conceptual models and grand theories. For her, conceptual models, also called conceptual frameworks or conceptual systems, are sets of general concepts and propositions that provide perspectives on the major concepts of the metaparadigm: person, environment, health, and nursing. Fawcett (1993, 2000) points out that direction for research must be described as part of the conceptual model in order to guide development and testing of nursing theories. We do not differentiate between conceptual models and grand theories and use the terms interchangeably.

Middle-Range Theories

Middle-range theories comprise the next level in the structure of the discipline. Robert Merton (1968) described this level of theory in the field of sociology stating that they are theories broad enough to be useful in complex situations and appropriate for empirical testing. Nursing scholars proposed using this level of theory because of the difficulty in testing grand theory (Jacox, 1974). Middle-range theories are more narrow in scope than grand theories and offer an effective bridge between grand theories and the description and explanation of specific nursing phenomena. They present concepts and propositions at a lower level of abstraction and hold great promise for increasing theory-based research and nursing practice strategies (Smith and Liehr, 2008). Several middle-range theories are included in this book. Middle-range theories may have their foundations in a particular paradigmatic perspective or may be derived from a grand theory or conceptual model. The literature presents a growing number of middle-range theories. This level of theory is expanding most rapidly in the discipline, and represents some of the most exciting work published in nursing today. Some of these new theories are synthesized from knowledge from related disciplines and transformed through a nursing lens (Eakes, Burke, & Hainsworth, 1998; Lenz, Suppe, Gift, Pugh, & Milligan, 1995; Polk, 1997). The literature also offers middle-range nursing

theories that are directly related to grand theories of nursing (Ducharme, Ricard, Duquette, Levesque, & Lachance, 1998; Dunn, 2004; Olson & Hanchett, 1997). Reports of nursing theory developed at this level include implications for instrument development, theory testing through research, and nursing practice strategies.

Practice Level Theories

Practice level theories have the most limited scope and level of abstraction and are developed for use within a specific range of nursing situations. Theories developed at this level have a more direct impact on nursing practice than do more abstract theories. Nursing practice theories provide frameworks for nursing interventions/activities and suggest outcomes and/or the impact of nursing practice. Nursing actions may be described or developed as nursing practice theories. Ideally, nursing practice theories are interrelated with concepts from middle-range theories or developed under the framework of grand theories. Theory developed at this level has been called prescriptive theory (Crowley, 1968; Dickoff, James, & Wiedenbach, 1968), situation-specific theory (Meleis, 1997), and micro theory (Chinn & Kramer, 2004). The day-to-day experience of nurses is a major source of nursing practice theory.

The depth and complexity of nursing practice may be fully appreciated as nursing phenomena and relations among aspects of particular nursing situations are described and explained. Dialogue with expert nurses in practice can be fruitful for discovery and development of practice theory. Research findings on various nursing problems offer data to develop nursing practice theories. Nursing practice theory has been articulated using multiple ways of knowing through reflective practice (Johns & Freshwater, 1998). The process includes quiet reflection on practice, remembering and noting features of nursing situations, attending to one's own feelings, reevaluating the experience, and integrating new knowing with other experience (Gray & Forstrom, 1991). The LIGHT model (Andersen & Smereck, 1989) and the attendant nurse caring model (Watson & Foster, 2003) are examples of the development of practice level theories.

Associated Research and Practice Traditions

Research traditions are the associated methods, procedures, and empirical indicators that guide inquiry related to the theory. For example, the theories of health as expanding consciousness, human becoming, and cultural care diversity and universality have specific associated research methods. Other theories have specific tools that have been developed to measure constructs related to the theories. The practice tradition of the theory consists of the activities, protocols, processes, tools, and practice wisdom emerging from the theory. Several conceptual models/grand theories have specific associated practice methods.

Nursing Theory and the Future

Nursing theory is essential to the continuing evolution of the discipline of nursing. Several trends are evident in the development and use of nursing theory. First, there seems to be more agreement on the focus of the discipline of nursing that provides a meaningful direction for our study and inquiry. This disciplinary dialogue has extended beyond the confines of Fawcett's metaparadigm and explicates the importance of caring and relationship as central to the discipline of nursing (Newman, Smith, Dexheimer-Pharris, & Jones, 2008; Roy & Jones, 2007; Willis, Grace, & Roy, 2008). The development of new grand theories and conceptual models has decreased. Dossey's (2008) theory of integral nursing, included in this book, is the only new theory at this level that has been developed in nearly 20 years. Instead, the growth in theory development is at the middle range and practice levels. There has been a significant increase in middle-range theories, and many practice scholars are

working on developing and implementing practice models based on grand theories/conceptual models.

There have been changes in the teaching and learning of nursing theory that are troubling. Many baccalaureate programs have very little nursing theory included in their curricula. Similarly, some graduate programs are eliminating or decreasing their emphasis on nursing theory. This alarming trend deserves our attention. If nursing is to continue to thrive, and to make a difference in the lives of people, our practitioners and researchers need to practice and expand knowledge within the structure of the discipline. As practice becomes more interdisciplinary, the focus of nursing becomes even more important. If nurses do not learn and practice based on the knowledge of their discipline, they may be co-opted into the practice of another discipline. Even worse, another discipline could emerge that will assume practices associated with the discipline of nursing. For example, health coaching is emerging as an area of practice focused on providing people with help as they make health-related changes in their lives. However, this is the practice of nursing, as articulated by many nursing theories.

On a positive note, nursing theories are being embraced by health care organizations to structure nursing practice. For example, organizations embarking on the journey toward magnet status (www.nursecredentialing.org/magnet) are required to identify a theoretical perspective that guides nursing practice and many are choosing existing nursing models. This work has great potential to refine and extend nursing theories.

The use of nursing theory in research is inconsistent at best. Often, outcomes research is not contextualized within any theoretical perspective; however, reviewers of proposals for most funding agencies request theoretical frameworks, and scoring criteria give points for having one. This encourages theoretical thinking and organizing findings within a broader perspective. Nurses often use theories from other disciplines instead of their own and this expands the knowledge of another discipline.

We are hopeful about the growth, continuing development, and expanded use of nursing theory. We hope that there will be continued growth in the development of all levels of nursing theory. The students of all professional disciplines study the theories of their disciplines in their courses of study. We must continue to include the study of nursing theories within our baccalaureate, master's, and doctoral programs. Baccalaureate students need to understand the foundations for the discipline, our historical development, and the place of nursing theory in its history and future. They should learn about conceptual models and grand theories. Didactic and practice courses should reflect theoretical values and concepts so that students learn to practice nursing from a theoretical perspective. Middle-range theories should be included in the study of particular phenomena such as self-transcendence, sorrow, and uncertainty. As they prepare to become practice leaders of the discipline, Doctor of Nursing Practice students should learn to develop and test nursing theory-guided models. PhD students will learn to develop and extend nursing theories in their research. New and expanded nursing specialties, such as nursing informatics, call for development and use of nursing theory (Effken, 2003). New, more open, and inclusive ways to theorize about nursing will be developed. These new ways will acknowledge the history and traditions of nursing, but will move nursing forward into new realms of thinking and being. Reed (1995) notes the "ground shifting" with the reforming of philosophies of nursing science and calls for a more open philosophy, grounded in nursing's values, which connects science, philosophy, and practice. Gray and Pratt (1991, p. 454) project that nursing scholars will continue to develop theories at all levels of abstraction and that theories will be increasingly interdependent with other disciplines such as politics, economics, and

aesthetics. These authors expect a continuing emphasis on unifying theory and practice that will contribute to the validation of the nursing discipline. Theorists will work in groups to develop knowledge in an area of concern to nursing, and these phenomena of interest, rather than the name of the author, will define the theory (Meleis, 1992). Newman (2003) calls for a future in which we transcend competition and boundaries that have been constructed between nursing theories and instead appreciate the links among theories, thus moving toward a fuller, more inclusive, and richer understanding of nursing knowledge.

Nursing's philosophies and theories must increasingly reflect nursing's values for understanding, respect, and commitment to health beliefs and practices of cultures throughout the world. **It is important to question to what extent theories developed and used in one major culture are appropriate for use in other cultures.** To what extent must nursing theory be relevant in multicultural contexts? Despite efforts of many international scholarly societies, how relevant are American nursing theories for the global community? Can nursing theories inform us about how to stand with and learn from peoples of the world? Can we learn from nursing theory how to come to know those we nurse, how to be with them, to truly listen and hear? Can these questions be recognized as appropriate for scholarly work and practice for graduate students in nursing? Will these issues offer direction for studies of doctoral students? If so, nursing theory will offer new ways to inform nurses for humane leadership in national and global health policy. Perspectives of various time and worlds in relation to present nursing concerns were described by Schoenhofer (1994). Abdellah (McAuliffe, 1998) proposed an international electronic "think tank" for nurses around the globe to dialogue about nursing theory. Such opportunities could lead nurses to truly listen, learn, and adapt theoretical perspectives to accommodate cultural variations.

■ Summary

This chapter focused on the place of nursing theory within the discipline of nursing. The relationship and importance of nursing theory to the characteristics of a professional discipline were reviewed. A variety of definitions of theory was offered, and the structure of knowledge in the discipline was outlined. Finally, we reviewed trends and speculated about the future of nursing theory development and application. One challenge of nursing theory is the perspective that theory is always in the process of developing, and that, at the same time, it is useful for the purposes and work of the discipline.

This may be seen as ambiguous or as full of possibilities. Continuing students of the discipline are required to study and know the basis for their contributions to nursing and to those we serve, while at the same time, be open to new ways of thinking, knowing, and being in nursing. Exploring structures of nursing knowledge and understanding the nature of nursing as a professional discipline, provide a frame of reference to clarify nursing theory. The wise study and use of nursing theory is an essential companion through the unfolding of this new millennium.

References

Allison, S. E., & McLaughlin-Renpenning, K. E. (1999). *Nursing administration in the 21st century: A self-care theory approach.* Thousand Oaks, CA: Sage.

Andersen, M. D., & Smereck, G. A. D. (1989). Personalized nursing LIGHT model. *Nursing Science Quarterly, 2,* 120–130.

Barnum, B. S. (1998). *Nursing theory: Analysis, application, evaluation* (5th ed.). Philadelphia: Lippincott.

Chinn, P., & Jacobs, M. (1987). *Theory and nursing: A systematic approach.* St. Louis, MO: C. V. Mosby.

Chinn, P., & Kramer, M. (2004). *Integrated knowledge development in nursing.* St. Louis, MO: C. V. Mosby.

Cody, W. K. (1997). Of tombstones, milestones, and gemstones: A retrospective and prospective on nursing theory. *Nursing Science Quarterly, 10*(1), 3–5.

Cody, W. K. (2003). Nursing theory as a guide to practice. *Nursing Science Quarterly, 16*(3), 225–231.

Colley, S. (2003). Nursing theory: Its importance to practice. *Nursing Standard, 17*(56), 33–37.

Crowley, D. (1968). Perspectives of pure science. *Nursing Research, 17*(6), 497–501.

Dickoff, J., & James, P. (1968). A theory of theories: A position paper. *Nursing Research, 17*(3), 197–203.

Dickoff, J., James, P., & Wiedenbach, E. (1968). Theory in a practice discipline. *Nursing Research, 17*(5), 415–435.

Donaldson, S. K., & Crowley, D. M. (1978). The discipline of nursing. *Nursing Outlook, 26*(2), 113–120.

Dossey, B. (2008). Theory of integral nursing. *Advances in Nursing Science, 31*(1), E52–E73.

Ducharme, F., Ricard, N., Duquette, A., Levesque, L., & Lachance, L. (1998). Empirical testing of a longitudinal model derived from the Roy Adaptation Model. *Nursing Science Quarterly, 11*(4), 149–159.

Dunn, K. S. (2004). Toward a middle-range theory of adaptation to chronic pain. *Nursing Science Quarterly, 17*(1), 78–84.

Eakes, G., Burke, M., & Hainsworth, M. (1998). Middle-range theory of chronic sorrow. *Image: Journal of Nursing Scholarship, 30*(2), 179–184.

Effken, J. A. (2003). An organizing framework for nursing informatics research. *Computers Informatics Nursing, 21*(6), 316–325.

Ellis, R. (1968). Characteristics of significant theories. *Nursing Research, 17*(3), 217–222.

Fawcett, J. (1993). *Analysis and evaluation of nursing theory.* Philadelphia: F. A. Davis.

Fawcett, J. (1984). The metaparadigm of nursing: Current status and future refinements. *Image: Journal of Nursing Scholarship, 16,* 84–87.

Fawcett, J. (1995). *Analysis and evaluation of conceptual models of nursing* (3rd ed.). Philadelphia: F. A. Davis.

Fawcett, J. (2000). *Analysis and evaluation of contemporary nursing knowledge: Nursing models and nursing theories.* Philadelphia: F. A. Davis.

Fitzpatrick, J. (1997). Nursing theory and metatheory. In: I. King & J. Fawcett (Eds.), *The language of nursing theory and metatheory.* Indianapolis, IN: Center Nursing Press.

Gioiella, E. C. (1996). The importance of theory-guided research and practice in the changing health care scene. *Nursing Science Quarterly, 9*(2), 47.

Gray, J., & Forsstrom, S. (1991). Generating theory for practice: The reflective technique. In: J. Gray & R. Pratt (Eds.), *Towards a discipline of nursing.* Melbourne: Churchill Livingstone.

Gray, J., & Pratt, R. (Eds.). (1991). *Towards a discipline of nursing.* Melbourne: Churchill Livingstone.

Hart, M., & Foster, S. (1998). Self-care agency in two groups of pregnant women. *Nursing Science Quarterly, 11*(4), 167–171.

Jacox, A. (1974). Theory construction in nursing: An overview. *Nursing Research, 23*(1), 4–13.

Jennings, B. M., & Staggers, N. (1998). The language of outcomes. *Advances in Nursing Science, 20*(4), 72–80.

Johns, C., & Freshwater, D. (1998). *Transforming nursing through reflective practice.* London: Oxford.

Kim, H. (1987). Structuring the nursing knowledge system: A typology of four domains. *Scholarly Inquiry for Nursing Practice: An International Journal, 1*(1), 99–110.

Kim, H. (1997). Terminology in structuring and developing nursing knowledge. In: I. King & J. Fawcett (Eds.), *The language of nursing theory and metatheory.* Indianapolis, IN: Center Nursing Press.

King, A. R., & Brownell, J. A. (1976). *The curriculum and the disciplines of knowledge.* Huntington, NY: Robert E. Krieger.

Kleffel, D. (1996). Environmental paradigms: Moving toward an ecocentric perspective. *Advances in Nursing Science, 18*(4), 1–10.

Kuhn, T. (1970). *The structure of scientific revolutions* (2nd ed.). Chicago: The University of Chicago Press.

Kuhn, T. (1977). *The essential tension: Selected studies in scientific tradition and change.* Chicago: The University of Chicago Press.

Leininger, M. (1987). *Transcultural nursing.* New York: John Wiley & Sons.

Lenz, E., Suppe, F., Gift, A., Pugh, L., & Milligan, R. (1995). Collaborative development of middle-range theories: Toward a theory of unpleasant symptoms. *Advances in Nursing Science, 17*(3), 1–13.

Litchfield, M., & Jondorsdottir, H. (2008). The practice discipline that's here and now. *Advances in Nursing Science, 31*(1), E79–91.

McAuliffe, M. (1998). Interview with Faye G. Abdellah on nursing research and health policy. *Image: Journal of Nursing Scholarship, 30*(3), 215–219.

McKay, R. (1969). Theories, models and systems for nursing. *Nursing Research, 18*(5), 393–399.

Meleis, A. (1992). Directions for nursing theory development in the 21st century. *Nursing Science Quarterly, 5,* 112–117.

Meleis, A. (1997). *Theoretical nursing: Development and progress.* Philadelphia: Lippincott.

Merton, R. (1968). *Social theory and social structure.* New York: The Free Press.

Newman, M. (2003). A world of no boundaries. *Advances in Nursing Science, 26*(4), 240–245.

Newman, M., Sime, A., & Corcoran-Perry, S. (1991). The focus of the discipline of nursing. *Advances in Nursing Science, 14*(1), 1–6.

Newman, M., Smith, M. C., Dexheimer-Pharris, M., & Jones, D. (2008). The focus of the discipline of nursing revisited. *Advances in Nursing Science, 31*(1), E16–E27.

Nightingale, F. (1859/1992). *Notes on nursing: What it is and what it is not.* Philadelphia: Lippincott.

Olson, J., & Hanchett, E. (1997). Nurse-expressed empathy, patient outcomes, and development of a middle-range theory. *Image: Journal of Nursing Scholarship, 29*(1), 71–76.

Parse, R. (1987). *Nursing science: Major paradigms, theories and critiques.* Philadelphia: W. B. Saunders.

Parse, R. (1997). Nursing and medicine: Two different disciplines. *Nursing Science Quarterly, 6*(3), 109.

Parse, R. (1998). *The human becoming school of thought: A perspective for nurses and other health professionals.* Thousand Oaks, CA: Sage.

Parsons, T. (1949). *Structure of social action.* Glencoe, IL: The Free Press.

Polk, L. (1997). Toward a middle-range theory of resilience. *Advances in Nursing Science, 19*(3), 1–13.

Reed, P. (1995). A treatise on nursing knowledge development for the 21st century: Beyond postmodernism. *Advances in Nursing Science, 17*(3), 70–84.

Rogers, M. E. (1970). *An introduction to the theoretical basis of nursing.* Philadelphia: F. A. Davis.

Rogers, M. E. (1992). Nursing science and the space age. *Nursing Science Quarterly, 5,* 27–34.

Roy, C., & Jones, D. (Eds). (2007). *Nursing knowledge development and clinical practice.* New York: Springer.

Schoenhofer, S. (1994). Transforming visions for nursing in the timeworld of *Einstein's Dreams. Advances in Nursing Science, 16*(4), 1–8.

Schuster, E., & Brown, C. (1994). *Exploring our environmental connections.* New York: National League for Nursing.

Silva, M. (1997). Philosophy, theory, and research in nursing: A linguistic journey to nursing practice. In: I. King & J. Fawcett (Eds.), *The language of nursing theory and metatheory.* Indianapolis, IN: Center Nursing Press.

Smith, M. C. (1994). Arriving at a philosophy of nursing: In: J. F. Kikuchi & H. Simmons (Eds.), *Developing a philosophy of nursing* (pp. 43–60). Thousand Oaks, CA: Sage.

Smith, M. C. (2008). Disciplinary perspectives linked to middle range theory. In: M. J. Smith & P. R. Liehr (Eds.), *Middle range theory for nursing* (2nd ed., pp. 1–12). New York: Springer.

Smith, M. J., & Liehr, P. R. (2008). *Middle range theory for nursing* (2nd ed.). New York: Springer.

Stevenson, J. S., & Tripp-Reimer, T. (Eds.). *Knowledge about care and caring. Proceedings of a Wingspread Conference.* February 1–3, 1989. Kansas City, MO: American Academy of Nursing, 1990.

Walker, L., & Avant, K. (1995). *Strategies for theory construction in nursing.* Norwalk, CT: Appleton-Century-Crofts.

Watson, J. (1985). *Nursing: Human science and human care.* Norwalk, CT: Appleton-Century-Crofts.

Watson, J., & Foster, R. (2003). The attending nurse caring model: Integrating theory, evidence and advanced caring-healing therapeutics for transforming professional practice. *Journal of Clinical Nursing, 12,* 360–365.

Willis, D., Grace, P., & Roy, C. (2008). A central unifying focus for the discipline: Facilitating humanization, meaning, quality of life and healing in living and dying. *Advances in Nursing Science, 31*(1), E28–E40.

Chapter 2

A Guide for the Study of Theories for Practice

MARILYN E. PARKER AND
MARLAINE C. SMITH

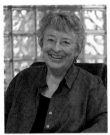

Marilyn E. Parker

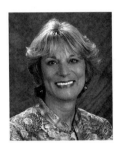

Marlaine C. Smith

Nursing is a professional discipline, a field of study, focused on human health and healing through caring (Smith, 1994). The knowledge base of the discipline consists of diverse components such as nursing science, art, philosophy, and ethics. Nursing science comprises the conceptual models, theories, and research findings specific to the discipline. As in other sciences such as biology, psychology, or sociology, the study of nursing science requires a disciplined approach. This chapter offers a guide to this disciplined approach in the form of a set of questions that facilitate reflection, exploration, and a deeper study of the selected nursing theories.

As you read the chapters in this book, the questions in the guide can facilitate your study. These chapters offer a marvelous beginning on the journey of studying nursing theories, which we hope will ignite interest in deeper exploration of some of the theories through reading the books written by the theorists and other published articles related to the use of the theories in practice and research. This book's online resources can provide additional materials as you continue your exploration. The questions in this guide can lead you toward this deeper study of the selected nursing theories.

Rapid and dramatic changes are affecting nurses everywhere. Health care delivery systems are in crisis and in need of real change. Hospitals continue to be the largest employers of nurses, and some hospitals are recognizing the need to develop nursing theory-guided practice models. A criterion for hospitals seeking magnet hospital designation by the American Nurses Credentialing Center (www.nursecredentialing.org/magnet) includes the selection of a theoretical model for practice. The list of questions in this chapter can be useful to nurses as they select theories to guide practice.

Increasingly, nurses are practicing in diverse settings and often develop organized nursing practices through which accessible health care to communities can be provided. Community members may be active participants in selecting, designing, and evaluating the nursing they receive. In these situations, it is important for nurses to identify with communities the approach to nursing that is most consistent with the community's values. The questions in this chapter can be helpful in the mutual exploration of theoretical approaches to practice.

In the current health care environment, interdisciplinary practice is frequently the norm. This does not mean that practicing from a nursing theoretical base is any less important. Interdisciplinary practice means that each discipline brings its own lens or perspective to the patient's situation. Nursing's lens is essential for a complete picture of the person's health and the goals of caring and healing. The nursing theory selected will provide this lens, and the questions in this chapter can assist nurses in selecting the theory/theories that will guide their unique contribution to the interdisciplinary team.

Theories and practices from a variety of disciplines inform the practice of nursing. The scope of nursing practice is continually being expanded to include additional knowledge and skills from related disciplines, such as medicine and psychology. Again, this does not diminish the need for practice based on a nursing theory, and these guiding questions help to differentiate the knowledge and practice of nursing from those of other disciplines.

Groups of nurses working together as colleagues to provide care often realize that they share the same values and beliefs about nursing. The study of nursing theories can clarify the purposes of nursing and facilitate building a cohesive practice to meet them. Regardless of the setting of nursing practice, nurses may choose to study nursing theories together in order to design and articulate theory-guided practice.

The study of nursing theory precedes the activities of analysis and evaluation. The evaluation of a theory involves preparation, judgment, and justification (Smith, 2008). In the preparation phase, the student of the theory spends time coming to know it by reading and reflecting on it. The best approach involves intellectual empathy, curiosity, honesty, and responsibility (Smith, 2008). Through reading and dwelling with the theory, the student tries to understand it from the point of view of the theorist. Curiosity leads to raising questions in the quest for greater understanding. It involves imagining ways the theory might work in practice, as well as the challenges it might present. Honesty involves knowing oneself and being true to one's own values and beliefs in the process of understanding. Some theories may resonate with deeply held values; others may conflict with them. It is important to listen to these inner messages of comfort/discomfort, for they will be important in the selection of theories for practice. Each member of a professional discipline has a responsibility to take the time and effort to understand the theories of that discipline. In nursing, there is an even greater responsibility to understand and be true to those that are selected to guide nursing practice.

Responses to questions offered and points summarized in the guides may be found in nursing literature, as well as in audiovisual and electronic resources. Primary source material, including the writing of nurses who are recognized authorities in specific nursing theories and the use of nursing theory, should be used.

Study of Theory for Nursing Practice

Four main questions have been developed and refined to facilitate study of nursing theories for use in nursing practice (Parker, 1993). They focus on concepts within the theories, as well as on points of interest and general information about each theory. This guide was developed for use by practicing nurses and students in undergraduate and graduate nursing education programs. Many nurses and students have used these questions and have contributed to their continuing development. The guide may be used to study most of the nursing theories developed at all levels.

A Guide for Study of Nursing Theory for Use in Practice

1. **How is nursing conceptualized in the theory?**
   Is the focus of nursing stated?
   - What does the nurse attend to when practicing nursing?
   - What guides nursing observations, reflections, decisions, and actions?
   - What does the nurse think about when considering nursing?
   - What are illustrations of use of the theory to guide practice?

   What is the purpose of nursing?
   - What do nurses do when they are practicing nursing based on the theory?
   - What are exemplars of nursing assessments, designs, plans, and evaluations?
   - What indicators give evidence of quality and quantity of nursing practice?
   - Is the richness and complexity of nursing practice evident?

   What are the boundaries or limits for nursing?
   - How is nursing distinguished from other health-related services?
   - How is nursing related to other disciplines and services?
   - What is the place of nursing in interdisciplinary practice?
   - What is the range of nursing situations in which the theory is useful?

   How can nursing situations be described?
   - What are attributes of the one nursed?
   - What are characteristics of the nurse?
   - How can interactions of the nurse and the recipient of nursing be described?
   - Are there environmental requirements for the practice of nursing?

2. **What is the context of the theory development?**
   Who is the nursing theorist as person and as nurse?
   - Why did the theorist develop the theory?
   - What is the background of the theorist as a nursing scholar?
   - What are central values and beliefs set forth by the theorist?

   What are major theoretical influences on this theory?
   - What nursing models and theories influenced this theory?
   - What are the relationships between this theory and other theories?
   - What nursing-related theories and philosophies influenced this theory?

   What were major external influences on development of the theory?
   - What were the social, economic, and political influences that shaped the theory?
   - What images of nurses and nursing influenced the theory development?
   - What was the status of nursing as a discipline and profession at the time of its development?

3. **Who are authoritative sources for information about development, evaluation, and use of this theory?**
   Who are nursing authorities who speak about, write about, and use the theory?
   - What are the professional attributes of these persons?

- What are the attributes of authorities, and how does one become one?
- Which other nurses should be considered authorities?

What major resources are authoritative sources on the theory?

- What books, articles, audiovisual and electronic media exist to elucidate the theory?
- What nursing societies share and support work of the theory?
- What service and academic programs are authoritative sources for practicing and teaching the theory?

4. **How can the overall significance of the nursing theory be described?**

What is the importance of the nursing theory over time?

- What are exemplars of the theory's use that structure and guide individual practice?
- How has the theory been used to guide programs of nursing education?
- How has the theory been used to guide nursing administration and organizations?

- How does published nursing scholarship reflect the significance of the theory?

What is the experience of nurses who report consistent use of the theory?

- What is the range of reports from practice?
- Has nursing research led to further theoretical formulations?
- Has the theory been used to develop new nursing practices?
- Has the theory influenced the design of methods of nursing inquiry?
- What has been the influence of the theory on nursing and health policy?

What are projected influences of the theory on nursing's future?

- How has the theory influenced the community of scholars?
- In what ways has nursing as a professional practice been strengthened by the theory?
- What future possibilities for nursing are open because of this theory?
- What will be the continuing social value of the theory?

■ Summary

This chapter contains a guide designed for the study of nursing theory for use in practice. As members of the professional discipline of nursing, the serious study of the theories of nursing is essential. The implementation of theory-guided practice models is important for nursing practice in all settings. The guide presented in this chapter can lead students on a journey from a beginning to a deeper understanding of nursing theory. The study of nursing theory precedes its analysis and evaluation. Students should approach the study of nursing theory with intellectual empathy, curiosity, honesty, and responsibility. This guide is composed of four main questions to foster reflection and facilitate the study of nursing theory for practice.

References

Parker, M. (1993). *Patterns of nursing theories in practice.* New York: National League for Nursing.

Smith, M. C. (1994). Arriving at a philosophy of nursing: Discovering? Constructing? Evolving? In: J. Kikuchi & H. Simmons (Eds.), *Developing a philosophy of nursing* (pp. 43–60). Thousand Oaks, CA: Sage.

Smith, M. C. (2008). Evaluation of middle range theories for the discipline of nursing. In: M. J. Smith & P. Liehr (Eds.), *Middle range theory for nursing* (2nd ed., pp. 293–306). New York: Springer.

Chapter 3

Choosing, Evaluating and Implementing Nursing Theories for Practice

MARILYN E. PARKER AND
MARLAINE C. SMITH

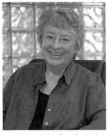
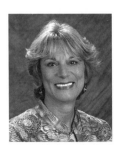

Marilyn E. Parker   *Marlaine C. Smith*

The primary purpose of nursing theory is to improve nursing practice, and therefore, the health and quality of life of persons, families, and communities served. Nursing theories provide coherent ways of viewing and approaching the care of persons in their environment. When a theoretical model is used to organize care in any setting, it strengthens the nursing focus of care and provides consistency to the communication and activities related to nursing care. The development of nursing theories and theory-guided practice models advances the discipline and professional practice of nursing.

One of the most urgent issues facing the discipline of nursing is the artificial separation of nursing theory and practice. Nursing can no longer afford to see these dimensions as disconnected territories, belonging to either scholars or practitioners. The examination and use of nursing theories are essential for closing the gap between nursing theory and nursing practice. Nurses in practice have a responsibility to study and value nursing theories, just as nursing theory scholars must understand and appreciate the day-to-day practice of nurses. Nursing theory informs and guides the practice of nursing, and nursing practice informs and guides the process of developing theory.

The theories of any professional discipline are useless if they have no impact on practice. Just as psychotherapists, educators, and economists base their approaches and decisions on particular theories, so should the practice of nursing be guided by selected nursing theories.

When practicing nurses and nurse scholars work together, both the discipline and practice of nursing benefit, and nursing service to our clients is enhanced. There are many examples throughout the book of how nursing theories have been, or can be, used to guide nursing practice. Many of the nursing theorists in this book developed or refined their theories based on dialogue with nurses who shared descriptions of their practice. This kind of work must continue for nursing theories to be relevant and meaningful to the discipline.

The need to bridge the gap between nursing theory and practice is highlighted by considering the following brief encounter during a question-and-answer period at a conference. A nurse in practice, reflecting her experience, asked a nurse theorist, "What is the meaning of this theory to my practice? I'm in the real world! I want to connect—but how can connections be made between your ideas and my reality?" The nurse theorist responded by describing the essential values and assumptions of her theory. The nurse said, "Yes, I know what you are talking about. I just didn't know I knew it, and I need help to use it in my practice" (Parker, 1993, p. 4). To remain current in the discipline, all nurses must join in community to advance nursing knowledge in practice and must accept their obligations to engage in the continuing study of nursing theories. Today, agencies that employ nurses are increasingly receiving recognition when they adopt a nursing theory as a guiding framework for nursing practice. This decision provides an excellent opportunity for nurses in practice and in administration to study, implement, and evaluate nursing theories for use in practice. Communicating the outcomes of this process with the community of scholars advancing the theories is a useful way to initiate dialogue among nurses and to form new bridges between the theory and practice of nursing.

The purpose of this chapter is to describe the processes leading to implementation of nursing theory-guided practice models. These processes include choosing possible theories for use in practice, analyzing and evaluating these theories, and implementing theory in practice. The chapter begins with responses to the questions: Why study nursing theory? What do the practicing nurses gain from nursing theory? Methods of analysis and evaluation of nursing theory set forth in the literature are presented. Finally, steps in implementing nursing theory in practice are described.

Significance of Nursing Theory for Practice

Nursing practice is essential for developing, testing, and refining nursing theory. The development of many nursing theories has been enhanced by reflection and dialogue about actual nursing situations. The everyday practice of nursing enriches nursing theories. When nurses think about nursing, they consider the content and structure of the discipline of nursing. Even if nurses do not conceptualize them theoretically, their values and perspectives are often consistent with particular nursing theories. Making these values and perspectives explicit through the use of a nursing theory results in a more scholarly, professional practice.

Creative nursing practice is the direct result of ongoing theory-based thinking, decision-making, and action. Nursing practice must continue to contribute to thinking and theorizing in nursing, just as nursing theory must be used to advance practice.

Nursing practice and nursing theory often reflect the same abiding values and beliefs. Nurses in practice are guided by their values and beliefs, as well as by knowledge. These values, beliefs, and knowledge often are reflected in the literature about nursing's metaparadigm, philosophies, and theories. In addition, nursing theorists and nurses in practice think about and work with the same phenomena, including the person nursed, the actions and relationships in the nursing situation, and the context of nursing. It is no wonder that nurses often sense a connection and familiarity with many of the concepts in nursing theories.

They often say, "I knew this, but didn't have the words for it." This is another value of nursing theory. It provides a vehicle for us to share and communicate the important concepts within nursing practice.

It is not possible to practice without some theoretical frame of reference. The question is what frame of reference is being used in practice. As stated in Chapter 1, theories are ways to organize our thinking about the complexities of any situation. Theories are lenses that we select that will color the way that we view reality. In the case of nursing, the theories we choose to use will frame the way we think about a particular person and his/her health situation. It will inform the ways that we approach the person, how we relate, and what we do. Many nurses practice according to ideas and directions from other disciplines, such as medicine, psychology, and public health. If your approach to a person is framed by his or her medical diagnosis, you are influenced by the medical model that focuses your attention on diagnosis, treatment, and cure. If you are thinking about disease prevention as you work with a community group, you are influenced by public health theory and approaches. While we use this knowledge in practice, nursing theory focuses us on the distinctive perspective of the discipline which is more than and different from these approaches.

Historically, nursing practice has been deeply rooted in the medical model and this model continues today. The depth and scope of the practice of nurses who follow notions about nursing held by other disciplines are limited to practices understood and accepted by those disciplines. Nurses who learn to practice from nursing perspectives are awakened to the challenges and opportunities of practicing nursing more fully and with a greater sense of autonomy, respect, and satisfaction for themselves. Hopefully, they also provide different and more expansive opportunities for health and healing for those they serve. Nurses who practice from a nursing perspective approach clients and families in ways unique to nursing. They ask questions, receive and process information about needs for nursing differently, and they create nursing responses that are more holistic and client-focused. These nurses learn to reframe their thinking about nursing knowledge and practice and are then able to bring knowledge from other disciplines within the context of their practice—not to direct their practice.

Nurses who practice from a nursing theoretical base see beyond immediate facts and delivery systems; they can integrate other health sciences and technologies as the background or context and not the essence of their practice. Nurses who study nursing theory realize that although no group actually owns ideas, professional disciplines do claim a unique perspective that defines their practice. In the same way, no group actually owns the technologies of practice, though disciplines do claim them for their practice. For example, before World War II, nurses rarely took blood pressure readings and did not give intramuscular injections. This was not because nurses lacked the skill, but because they did not claim the use of these techniques to facilitate their nursing. Such a realization can also lead to understanding that the things nurses do that are often called nursing are not nursing at all. The skills and technologies used by nurses, such as taking blood pressure readings, giving injections, and auscultating heart sounds, are actually activities that are part of the context, but not the essence, of nursing practice. Nursing theories provide an organizing framework that directs nurses to the essence of their purpose and places the use of knowledge from other disciplines in their proper perspective.

If nursing theory is to be useful—or practical—it must be brought into practice. At the same time, nurses can be guided by nursing theory in a full range of nursing situations. Nursing theory can change nursing practice: It provides direction for new ways of being present with clients, helps nurses realize ways of expressing caring, and provides approaches to understanding needs for nursing and designing care to address these needs. The chapters of this book affirm the use of nursing theory in practice and the study and assessment of theory to ultimately use in practice.

Responses to Questions from Practicing Nurses About Using Nursing Theory

Study of nursing theory may either precede or follow selection of a nursing theory for use in nursing practice. Analysis and evaluation of nursing theory follow the study of a nursing theory. These activities are demanding and deserve the full commitment of nurses who undertake the work. Because it is understood that the study of nursing theory is not a simple, short-term endeavor, nurses often question doing such work. The following questions about studying and using nursing theory have been collected from many conversations with nurses about nursing theory. These queries also identify specific issues that are important to nurses who consider the study of nursing theory.

My Nursing Practice
- Does this theory reflect nursing practice as I know it? Can it be understood in relation to my nursing practice? Will it support what I believe to be excellent nursing practice?
- Conceptual models and grand theories can guide practice in any setting and situation. Middle-range theories address circumscribed phenomena in nursing that are directly related to practice. These levels of theory can enrich perspectives on practice and should foster an excellent professional level of practice.
- Is the theory specific to my area of nursing? Can the language of the theory help me explain, plan, and evaluate my nursing? Will I be able to use the terms to communicate with others?
- Can this theory be considered in relation to a wide range of nursing situations? How does it relate to more general views of nursing people in other settings?
- Will my study and use of this theory support nursing in my interdisciplinary setting?

- Will those from other disciplines be able to understand, facilitating cooperation?
- Will my work meet the expectations of those I serve? Will other nurses find my work helpful and challenging?

Conceptual models and grand theories are not specific to any nursing specialty. Theories in any discipline introduce new terminology that are not part of general language. For example, the id, ego, and superego are familiar terms in a particular psychological theory, but were unknown at the time of the theory's introduction. The language of the theory facilitates thinking differently through naming new concepts or ideas. Members of disciplines do share specific language that may be less familiar to members outside the discipline. In interprofessional communication, new terms can be defined and explained to facilitate communication as needed. Nursing's unique perspective needs to be represented clearly within the interprofessional team. The diversity of each discipline's perspective is important to provide the best care possible for patients. People deserve and expect high-quality care. Nursing theory has the potential to bring to bear the importance of relationship and caring in the process of health and healing; the interrelationship of the environment and health; an understanding of the wholeness of persons in their life situations; and an appreciation of the person's experiences, values, and choices in care. These are essential contributions to a multidisciplinary perspective.

My Personal Interests, Abilities, and Experiences
- Is the study of nursing theories consistent with my talents, interests, and goals? Is this something I want to do?
- Will I be stimulated by thinking about and trying to use this theory? Will my study of nursing be enhanced by use of this theory?
- What will it be like to think about nursing theory in nursing practice?
- Will my work with nursing theory be worth the effort?

The study of nursing theory does take an investment in time and attention. It is a responsibility of a professional nurse who engages in a scholarly level of practice. Learning about nursing theory is a conceptual activity that can be challenging and intellectually stimulating. We need nurses who will invest in these activities so that knowledgeable theory-guided practice is the norm in all health care settings.

Resources and Support
• Will this be useful to me outside the classroom?
• What resources will I need to understand fully the terms of the theory?
• Will I be able to find the support I need to study and use the theory in my practice?

The purpose of nursing theory goes beyond its study within courses. Nursing theory becomes alive when the ideas are brought to practice. The usefulness of theory in practice is one way that we judge its value and worth. It is helpful to read about the theory from primary sources or the most notable scholars and practitioners who have studied the theory. Nurses interested in particular theories can join listservs where issues related to the theory are discussed. Many of the theory groups have formed professional societies and hold conferences that support lifelong learning and growing with those applying the theory in practice, administration, research, and education.

The Theorist, Evidence, and Opinion
• Who is the author of this theory? What background of nursing education and experience does the theorist bring to this work? Is the author an authoritative nursing scholar?
• How is the theorist's background of nursing education and experience brought to this work?
• What is the evidence that use of the theory may lead to improved nursing care? Has the theory been useful to guide nursing organizations and administrations? What about influencing nursing and health care policy?
• What is the evidence that this nursing theory has led to nursing research, including questions and methods of inquiry? Did the

theory grow out of research findings or out of practice issues and concerns?
• Does the theory reflect the latest thinking in nursing? Has the theory kept pace with the times in nursing? Is this a nursing theory for the future?

Approaching the study of nursing theory with openness, curiosity, imagination, and skepticism is important. The search for the support that the theory makes a difference is part of the evaluation of any theory. Theories must have pragmatic value, that is, they need to generate research questions and provide models that can be applied in practice. Theory-guided practice models should be evaluated to support that the theory makes a difference in the lives of persons. You will find examples of how the theory has been used in research and practice in the nursing literature. In some cases, especially with newly formed theories, this evidence may be unavailable. In these situations, imagine the potential related to application of the theory. Theories have heuristic value in that they can lead to new ways of thinking about situations. Consider the heuristic value of the theory as you read it. The theory should ignite your passion about nursing.

Choosing a Nursing Theory to Study

It is important to give adequate attention to selection of theories. Results of this decision will have lasting influences on nursing practice. It is not unusual for nurses who begin to work with nursing theory to realize their practice is changing and that their future efforts in the discipline and practice of nursing are markedly altered.

There is always some measure of hope mixed with anxiety as nurses seriously explore nursing theory for the first time. Individual nurses who practice with a group of colleagues often wonder how to select and study nursing theories. Nurses and nursing students in courses considering nursing theory have similar questions. Nurses in new practice settings designed and developed by nurses have the same concerns about getting started as do nurses in hospital organizations who want more from their practice.

The following exercise is grounded in the belief that the study and use of nursing theory in nursing practice must have roots in the practice of the nurses involved. Moreover, the nursing theory used by particular nurses must reflect elements of practice that are essential to those nurses, while at the same time bringing focus and freshness to that practice. This exercise calls on the nurse to think about the major components of nursing and bring forth the values and beliefs most important to nurses. In these ways, the exercise begins to parallel knowledge development reflected in the nursing metaparadigm (focus of the discipline) and nursing philosophies described in Chapter 1. From this point on, the nurse is guided to connect nursing theory and nursing practice in the context of nursing situations.

A Reflective Exercise for Choosing a Nursing Theory for Practice

Select a comfortable, private, and quiet place to reflect and write. Relax by taking some deep, slow breaths. Think about the reasons you went into nursing in the first place. Bring your nursing practice into focus. Consider your practice today. Continue to reflect and, while avoiding distractions, make notes to record your thoughts and feelings. When you have been thinking for a time and have taken the opportunity to reflect on your practice, proceed with the following questions. Continue to reflect and to make notes as you consider each one.

Enduring Values
• What are the enduring values and beliefs that brought me to nursing?
• What beliefs and values keep me in nursing today?
• What are those values that I hold most dear?
• What are the ties of these values to my personal values?

• How do my personal and nursing values connect with what is important to society?

Reflect on an instance of nursing in which you interacted with a person, family, or community for nursing purposes. This can be a situation from your current practice or may be from your nursing in years past. Consider the purpose or hoped-for outcome.

Nursing Situations
• Who was this person, family or community? How did I come to know him or them as unique?
• What were the needs for nursing the person, family or community?
• Who was I as a person in the nursing situation?
• Who was I as a nurse in the situation?
• What was the relationship between the person, family or community and myself?
• What nursing actions emerged in the context of the relationship?
• What other nursing responses might have been possible?
• What was the environment of the nursing situation?
• What about the environment was important to the needs for nursing and to my nursing responses?

Nursing can change when we consciously connect values and beliefs to nursing situations. Consider that values and beliefs are the basis for our nursing. Briefly describe the connections of your values and beliefs with your chosen nursing situation.

Connecting Values and the Nursing Situation
• How are my values and beliefs reflected in any nursing situation?
• Are my values and beliefs in conflict or frustrated in this situation?
• Do my values come to life in the nursing situation?

Verifying Awareness and Appreciation

In reflecting and writing about values and situations of nursing that are important to us, we often come to a fuller awareness and appreciation of nursing. Make notes about your insights. You might consider these initial notes the beginning of a journal in which you record your study of nursing theories and their use in nursing practice. This is a valuable way to follow your progress and is a source of nursing questions for future study. You may want to share this process and experience with your colleagues. These are ways to clarify and verify views about nursing and to seek and offer support for nursing values and situations that are critical to your practice. If you are doing this exercise in a group, share your essential values and beliefs with your colleagues.

Multiple Ways of Knowing and Reflecting on Nursing Theory

Multiple ways of knowing are used in theory-guided nursing practice. Carper (1978) studied the nursing literature and described four essential patterns of knowing in nursing. Using the Phenix (1964) model of realms of meaning, Carper described personal, empirical, ethical, and esthetic ways of knowing in nursing. Chinn and Kramer (2007) use Carper's patterns of knowing and a fifth pattern, called emancipatory knowing, to develop an integrated framework for nursing knowledge development. Additional patterns of knowing in nursing have been explored and described, and the initial four patterns have been the focus of much consideration in nursing (Boykin, Parker, & Schoenhofer, 1994; Leight, 2002; Munhall, 1993; Parker, 2002; Pierson, 1999; Ruth-Sahd, 2003; Thompson, 1999; White, 1995).

Each of Carper's patterns of knowing and its relationship to theory-guided practice is articulated below.

Empirical knowing is the most familiar of the ways of knowing in nursing. Empirical knowing is how we come to know the science of nursing and other disciplines that are used in nursing practice. This includes knowing the actual theories, concepts, principles, and research findings from nursing, pathophysiology, pharmacology, psychology, sociology, epidemiology, etc. Nursing theory is within the pattern of empirical knowing. The theoretical framework for practice integrates the concepts, principles, laws, and facts essential for practice.

Personal knowing is about striving to know the self and to actualize authentic relationships between the nurse and the one nursed. Using this pattern of knowing in nursing, the client is not seen as an object, but as a person moving toward fulfillment of potential (Carper, 1978). The nurse is recognized as continuously learning and growing as a person and practitioner. Reflecting on a person as a client and a person as a nurse in the nursing situation can enhance understanding of nursing practice and the centrality of relationships in nursing. These insights are useful for choosing and studying nursing theory. Knowing the self is essential in selecting nursing theory to guide practice. Ultimately, the choice of theoretical perspective reflects personal values and beliefs.

Ethical knowing is increasingly important to the study and practice of nursing today. According to Carper (1978), ethics in nursing is the moral component guiding choices within the complexity of health care. Ethical knowing informs us of what is right, what is our obligation, and what the nurse ought to do in any situation. Ethical knowing is essential in every action of the nurse in day-to-day nursing.

Esthetic knowing is described by Carper (1978) as the art of nursing; it is the creative and imaginative use of nursing knowledge in practice (Rogers, 1988). Although nursing is often referred to as art, this aspect of nursing may not be as highly valued as the science and ethics of nursing. Each nurse is an artist, expressing and interpreting the guiding theory uniquely in his or her practice. Reflecting on the *experience* of nursing is primary in understanding esthetic knowing. Through such reflection, the nurse understands that nursing practice has in fact been *created*, that each instance of nursing is unique, and that outcomes of nursing cannot be precisely predicted. Besides the art of nursing, knowing through artistic forms is part of esthetic knowing. Often human experiences and relationships can best be appreciated and understood through art forms such as stories, paintings, music, or poetry. Some assert that esthetic knowing allows for understanding the wholeness of experience. Examples of this most complete knowing are frequent in nursing situations in which even momentary connection and genuine presence between the nurse and the person, family or community is realized.

The notes describing your experience will help in selecting a nursing theory to study and consider for guiding practice. You will want to answer these questions:

Using Insights to Choose Theory
• What nursing theory seems consistent with the values and beliefs that guide my practice?
• What theories are consistent with my personal values and beliefs?
• What do I hope to achieve from the use of nursing theory?
• Given my reflection on a nursing situation, how can I use theory to support this description of my practice?
• How can I use nursing theory to improve my practice for myself and for my patients?

Evaluation of Nursing Theory

Evaluation of nursing theory follows its study and analysis, and is the process of making a determination about its value, worth, and significance (Smith, 2008). There are many sets of criteria for evaluating conceptual models and grand theories (Chinn & Kramer, 2007; Fawcett, 2004; Fitzpatrick & Whall, 2004; Parse, 1987; Stevens, 1998). Smith (2008) has published criteria for evaluating middle-range theories. After reading and studying the primary sources of the theory, the research and practice applications of the theory, and other critiques and evaluations of the theory; it is important for the evaluator to come to his or her own judgments supported by logical analysis and examples from the theory.

The whole theory must be studied. Parts of the theory without the whole will not be fully meaningful and may lead to misunderstanding.

Before selecting a guide for theory evaluation, consider the level and scope of the theory. Is the theory a conceptual model or grand nursing theory? A middle-range nursing theory? A practice theory? Not all aspects of theory described in an evaluation guide will be evident in all levels of theory. Whall (2004) recognizes this in offering particular guides for analysis and evaluation that vary according to three types of nursing theory: models, middle-range theories, and practice theories. Fawcett's (2004) criteria for analysis and evaluation pertain to conceptual models and grand theories. Smith's (2008) criteria specifically address the evaluation of middle-range theories.

Theory analysis and evaluation may be thought of as one process or as a two-step sequence. It may be helpful to think of analysis of theory as necessary for in-depth study of a nursing theory and evaluation of theory as the assessment of a theory's significance, structure, and utility. Guides for theory evaluation are intended as tools to inform us about theories and to encourage further development, refinement, and use of theory. There are no guides for theory analysis and evaluation that are adequate and appropriate for every nursing theory.

Johnson (1974) wrote about three basic criteria to guide evaluation of nursing theory. These have continued in use over time and offer direction for guides in use today. These criteria state that the theory should:

• Define the congruence of nursing practice with societal expectations of nursing decisions and actions
• Clarify the social significance of nursing, or the impact of nursing on persons receiving nursing
• Describe social utility, or usefulness of the theory in practice, research, and education.

The following are summaries of the most frequently used guides for theory evaluation. These guides are components of the entire work about nursing theory of the individual nursing scholar and offer various interesting approaches to theory evaluation. Each guide should be studied in more detail than is offered in this introduction and should be examined in context of the whole work of the individual nurse scholar.

The approach to theory evaluation set forth by Chinn and Kramer (2007) is to use guidelines for describing nursing theory that are based on their definition of theory as "a creative and rigorous structuring of ideas that projects a tentative, purposeful, and systematic view of phenomena" (p. 58). The guidelines set forth questions that clarify the facts about aspects of theory: purpose, concepts, definitions, relationships and structure, and assumptions. These authors suggest that the next step in the evaluation process is critical reflection about whether and how the nursing theory works. Questions are posed to guide this reflection:

• How clear is this theory?
• How simple is this theory?
• How general is this theory?
• How accessible is this theory?
• How important is this theory?

Fawcett (2000) developed two different frameworks for the analysis and evaluation of conceptual models and theories. The questions for *analysis* of conceptual models (Fawcett, 2000, p. 63) address:

• Origins of the nursing model
• Unique focus of the nursing model
• Content of the nursing model

The questions for *evaluation* of conceptual models (Fawcett, 2000, p. 63) address:

• Explication of origins
• Comprehensiveness of content
• Logical congruence
• Generation of theory
• Credibility of nursing model

The framework for *analysis* of grand and middle-range theories (Fawcett, 2000, p. 501) includes:

• Theory scope
• Theory context
• Theory content

The questions for *evaluation* of grand and middle-range theories (Fawcett, 2000, p. 501) address:

• Significance
• Internal consistency
• Parsimony
• Testability
• Empirical adequacy
• Pragmatic adequacy

Meleis (2004) states that the structural and functional components of a theory should be studied before evaluation. The structural components are assumptions, concepts, and propositions of the theory. Functional components include descriptions of the following: focus, client, nursing, health, nurse–client interactions, environment, nursing problems, and interventions. After studying these dimensions of the theory, critical examination of these elements may take place, as summarized here:

• Relations between structure and function of the theory, including clarity, consistency, and simplicity
• Diagram of theory to elucidate the theory by creating a visual representation
• Contagiousness, or adoption of the theory by a wide variety of students, researchers, and practitioners, as reflected in the literature
• Usefulness in practice, education, research, and administration
• External components of personal, professional, social values, and significance

Smith (2008) developed a framework for the evaluation of middle-range theories and includes the following criteria:

Substantive foundation relates to meaning or how the theory corresponds to existing knowledge in the discipline. The questions for evaluation ask about its fit with the disciplinary focus of nursing; its specification of assumptions; its substantive meaning of a phenomenon; and its origins in practice and/or research.

Structural integrity relates to the structure or internal organization of the theory. Questions for evaluation ask about the clarity of definitions of concepts, the consistency of level of abstraction, the simplicity of the theory, and the logical represention of relationships among concepts.

Functional adequacy refers to the ability of the theory to be used in practice and research. Questions are related to its applicability to practice and client groups, the identification of empirical indicators, the presence of published examples of practice and research using the theory and the evolution of the theory through inquiry (p. 299).

Implementing Theory-Guided Practice

Every nurse should develop a practice that is guided by nursing theory. Most conceptual models or grand theories have actual practice methods or processes that can be adopted. The scope and generality of middle-range theories makes them less appropriate to guide nursing practice within a unit or hospital. Instead, they can be used to understand and respond to phenomena that are encountered in nursing situations. For example, Boykin and Schoenhofer's Nursing as Caring theory has been adopted as a practice model by several hospitals. Reed's middle-range theory of self-transcendence can be used to guide a nurse who is leading a support group for women with breast cancer. Hospital units or entire nursing departments may adopt a model that guides nursing practice within their unit or organization. The following are suggestions that can facilitate this process of adoption and implementation of theory-guided practice within units or organizations:

Gaining administrative support. Organizational leaders need to support the initiative to begin the process of implementing nursing theory-guided practice. While the impetus to begin this initiative might not originate in formal leadership, the organizational leaders and managers need to be on board. If it is to succeed, the implementation of a model for practice requires the support of administration at the highest levels.

Selecting the theory or model to be used in practice. The entire nursing staff should be fully involved and invested in the process of deciding on the theoretical model that will guide practice. This can be done is several ways. An organization's governance structure can be used to develop the most appropriate selection process. As stated previously, the selection of a nursing theory or model is based on values. Some nursing organizations have used their mission, values, and vision statements as a blueprint that helps them select nursing theories that are most consistent with these values. Another approach is to survey all nurses about the practice models they would like to see implemented. The top three or four can then be studied by the nursing staff in greater detail so that the staff can make an informed decision. Staff development can be involved in planning educational offerings related to the models. A process of voting or gaining consensus can be used for the final selection.

Launching the initiative. Once the model has been selected, the leaders (formal and informal) begin to plan for its implementation. This involves creating a timeline, planning the phases and stages of implementation including activities, and using all methods of communication to be sure that all are informed of these plans. Unit champions, informal leaders who are enthusiastic and positive about the initiative, can be key to the building excitement for the intiative. A structure to lead and manage the implementation is essential. Consultants who are experts in the theory itself or who have experience in implementing the theory-guided practice model can be very helpful. For example, Watson's Caring Science Consortium consists of hospitals who have experience implementing the theory in practice. New hospitals can join the consortiuim for consultation and support as they launch initiatives. Watson herself often serves as a consultant to hospitals adopting her caring theory. A kick-off event, such as an inspirational presentation, can build excitement and visibility for the initiative.

Creating a plan for evaluation. It is important to build in a systematic plan for evaluation of the new model from the beginning. An evaluation study should be designed to track process and outcome indicators. Consultation from an evaluation researcher is essential. For example, outcomes of nurse satisfaction, patient satisfaction, nurse retention, and core measures might be considered as outcomes to be measured before and after the implementation of the model. Focus groups might be held at intervals to identify nurses' experiences and attitudes related to implementation of the model.

Consistent and constant support and education. As the model is implemented, a process to support continuing learning and growth with the theory needs to be in place. The nurses implementing the model will have questions and suggestions, so resident experts should be available for this education and support. Those working with the model will grow in their expertise, and their experiences need to be recorded and shared with the community of scholars advancing the theory in practice. Ways to foster staying on track must be developed. Some hospitals have created unit bulletin boards, newsletters, or signage to prevent slippage and cement new behaviors. Staff need opportunities to dialogue about their experiences: what is working and what is not. They need the freedom to develop new ways of implementing the model so that their scholarship and creativity flourishes.

Periodic feedback on outcomes and opportunities for re-energizing is essential. Planned change involves anticipating the ebb and flow of enthusiasm. In the stressful health care environment it is important to find opportunities to provide feedback on how the project is going, to reward and celebrate the successes, and to fan any dying embers of enthusiasm for the project. This can be accomplished through inviting study champions to attend regional or national conferences, bringing in speakers, or holding recognition events.

Re-visioning of the theory-guided practice model based on feedback. Any theory-guided practice model will become richer through its testing in practice. The nurses working with the model will help to modify and revise the model based on evaluation data. This re-visioning should be done in partnership with theorists and other practice scholars working with the model.

■ Summary

This chapter focused on the important connection between nursing theory and nursing practice and the processes of choosing, evaluating, and implementing theory for practice. The selection of a nursing theory for practice is based on values and beliefs, and a reflective process can help to identify the most important qualities of practice that need to be present in a chosen theory. Evaluation of nursing theory is a judgment of its value or worth. Several models of theory evaluation are available for use. Implementing a theory-based practice model in a health care setting can be challenging and rewarding. Suggestions for successful implementation were offered.

References

Boykin, A., Parker, M., & Schoenhofer, S. (1994). Aesthetic knowing grounded in an explicit conception of nursing. *Nursing Science Quarterly, 7*(4), 158–161.

Carper, B. A. (1978). Fundamental patterns of knowing in nursing. *Advances in Nursing Science, 1*(1), 13–23.

Chinn, P., & Jacobs, M. (1987). *Theory and nursing: A systematic approach.* St. Louis, MO: C. V. Mosby.

Chinn, P., & Kramer, M. (2004). *Integrated knowledge development in nursing* (6th ed.). St. Louis, MO: C. V. Mosby.

Chinn, P., & Kramer, M. (2007). *Integrated knowledge development in nursing* (7th ed.). St. Louis, MO: C. V. Mosby.

Fawcett, J. (2000). *Analysis and evaluation of contemporary nursing knowledge.* Philadelphia: F. A. Davis.

Fawcett, J. (2004). *Analysis and evaluation of contemporary nursing knowledge*. Philadelphia: F. A. Davis.

Fitzpatrick, J., & Whall, A. (2004). *Conceptual models of nursing*. Stamford, CT: Appleton & Lange.

Johnson, D. (1974). Development of theory: A requisite for nursing as a primary health profession. *Nursing Research, 23*(5), 372–377.

Leight, S. B. (2002). Starry night: Using story to inform aesthetic knowing in women's health nursing. *Journal of Advanced Nursing, 37*(1), 108–114.

Meleis, A. (1997). *Theoretical nursing: Development and progress*. Philadelphia: Lippincott.

Meleis, A. (2004). *Theoretical nursing: Development and progress*. Philadelphia: Lippincott.

Munhall, P. (1993). Unknowing: Toward another pattern of knowing in nursing. *Nursing Outlook, 41*, 125–128.

Parker, M. (1993). *Patterns of nursing theories in practice*. New York: National League for Nursing.

Parker, M. E. (2002). Aesthetic ways in day-to-day nursing. In: D. Freshwater (Ed.), *Therapeutic nursing: Improving patient care through self-awareness and reflection* (pp. 100–120). Thousand Oaks, CA: Sage.

Parse, R. R. (1987). *Nursing science: Major paradigms, theories and critiques*. Philadelphia: W. B. Saunders.

Phenix, P. H. (1964). *Realms of meaning*. New York: McGraw-Hill.

Pierson, W. (1999). Considering the nature of intersubjectivity within professional nursing. *Journal of Advanced Nursing, 30*(2), 294–302.

Rogers, M. E. (1988). Nursing science and art: A prospective. *Nursing Science Quarterly, 1*(3), 99–102.

Ruth-Sahd, L. A. (2003). Intuition: A critical way of knowing in a multicultural nursing curriculum. *Nursing Education Perspectives, 24*(3), 129–134.

Silva, M. (1997). Philosophy, theory, and research in nursing: A linguistic journey to nursing practice. In: I. King & J. Fawcett (Eds.), *The language of nursing theory and metatheory*. Indianapolis, IN: Center Nursing Press.

Smith, M. C. (2008). Evaluation of middle range theories for the discipline of nursing. In: M. J. Smith & P. R. Liehr (Eds.), *Middle range theory for nursing* (pp. 293–306). New York: Springer.

Stevens, B. (1998). *Nursing theory: Analysis, application, evaluation*. Boston: Little, Brown.

Thompson, C. (1999). A conceptual treadmill: The need for 'middle ground' in clinical decision making theory in nursing. *Journal of Advanced Nursing, 30*(5), 1222–1229.

Whall, A. (2004). The structure of nursing knowledge: Analysis and evaluation of practice, middle-range, and grand theory. In: J. Fitzpatrick & A. Whall (Eds.), *Conceptual models of nursing: Analysis and application* (4th ed., pp. 5–20). Stamford, CT: Appleton & Lange.

White, J. (1995). Patterns of knowing: Review, critique and update. *Advances in Nursing Science, 17*(4), 73–86.

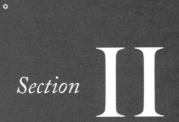

Section **II**

Evolution of Nursing Theory

Conceptual Influences on the Evolution of Nursing Theory

The second section of the book has three chapters that describe conceptual influences on the development of nursing theory. Thomas Kuhn calls the stage of scientific development before formal theories are structured as the "pre-paradigm" stage. These scholars were working in this stage of our development, planting the seeds that grew into nursing theories. Nursing theorists today have stood on the shoulders of these "giants," building on their brilliant conceptualizations of the nature of nursing and the nurse–patient relationship. In Chapter 4 Dr. Lynne Dunphy, a noted historian and Nightingale scholar, illuminates the core ideas from Nightingale's work that have been essential foundations for the development of nursing theories. Although Nightingale did not develop a theory of nursing, she did provide a direction for the development of the profession and discipline. She believed in the natural or inherent healing ability of human beings, and that the goal of nursing was to facilitate the emergence of health and healing through attending to the person–environment relationship. She said that the goal of nursing was to put the patient in the best condition for nature to act, and she identified five environmental components essential to health. Nightingale saw nursing and medicine as separate fields, and emphasized the importance of systematic inquiry. Her spiritual nature and vision of nursing as an art continue to influence practice today. In Chapter 5, Dr. Shirley Gordon and her contributors summarized the work of Ernestine Wiedenbach, Virginia Henderson, and Lydia Hall. Wiedenbach emphasized the importance of reverence for life, respect for dignity, autonomy, worth, and uniqueness of each person, and a commitment to act on these values as the essence of a personal philosophy of nursing. Henderson described nursing as "getting into the skin" of the patient so that nurses would be able to provide the strength, will, or knowledge that was needed by the patient to heal or maintain health. Lydia Hall is an inspiration to all who envision nursing as an autonomous discipline and practice. She created a model of nursing consisting of The Core, The Cure, and The Care, and implemented that model in the Loeb Center for Nursing and Rehabilitation. Physicians referred their patients to the Center, and nurses admitted the patients for nursing care. Nurses worked independently with patients to foster learning, growth, and healing. Chapter 6, written by a group of authors, focused on three nursing leaders who described the nurse–patient relationship: Hildegard Peplau, Ida Jean Orlando, and Joyce Travelbee. A psychiatric nurse, Peplau viewed the purpose of nursing as helping the patient gain the intellectual and interpersonal competencies necessary to heal. She articulated stages of the nurse–patient relationship, a framework for anxiety and nursing interventions to decrease anxiety. Travelbee emphasized the human-to-human relationship between nurse and person nursed, and spoke of the purpose of nursing as assisting the person(s) to prevent or cope with the experience of illness and suffering. Orlando described attributes of the nurse–patient relationship. She valued that relationship as central to the practice of nursing, and was the first to describe nursing process as identifying needs and responding to those needs.

Chapter *4*

Florence Nightingale's Legacy of Caring and Its Applications

LYNNE M. DUNPHY

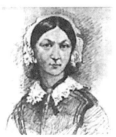

Florence Nightingale

Introducing the Theorist

Florence Nightingale, the acknowledged founder of modern nursing, remains a compelling and transformative figure. Not a year goes by in which new scholarship on Nightingale does not emerge. *Florence Nightingale and the Health of the Raj* was published in 2003 documenting Nightingale's 40-year long interest and involvement in Indian affairs, a previously not well explored area of scholarship (Gourley, 2003). In 2004 a new biography of Nightingale, *Nightingales: The Extraordinary Upbringing and Curious Life of Miss Florence Nightingale* by Gillian Gill, was published. In 2008, yet another new biography, entitled *Florence Nightingale: The Making of an Icon*, by Mark Bostridge, was published. Lynn McDonald's prodigious, ambitious, and long overdue *Collected Works of Florence Nightingale* has seen the publication of 10 out of a projected 16 volumes as of this writing. In 2005 the American Nurses Association published *Florence Nightingale Today: Healing, Leadership, Global Action,* an ambitious casting of Nightingale as 21st century nursing's inspiration and savior. At the time you are perusing this chapter, it will be a century since the death of Florence Nightingale in 1910, and almost 200 hundred years since her birth on May 12 in 1820.

Nightingale transformed a "calling from God" and an intense spirituality into a new social role for women: that of nurse. Her caring was a public one. "Work your true work," she wrote, "and you will find God within you" (Woodham-Smith, 1983, p. 74). A reflection on this statement appears in a well-known quote from *Notes on Nursing* (1859/1992): "Nature [i.e., the manifestation of God] alone cures . . . what nursing has to do . . . is put the patient in the best condition for nature to act upon him" (Macrae, 1995, p. 10). Although Nightingale never defined human care or caring in *Notes on Nursing,* there is no doubt that her life in nursing exemplified and personified an ethos of caring. Jean Watson (1992, p. 83), in the 1992 commemorative edition of *Notes on Nursing,* observed, "Although Nightingale's feminine-based caring-healing model has transcended time and is prophetic for this century's health reform, the model is yet to truly come of age in nursing or the health care system." In a reflective essay, Boykin and Dunphy (2002) extended this thinking and related Nightingale's life, rooted in compassion and caring, as an exemplar of justice-making (p. 14). *Justice-making* is understood as a manifestation of compassion and caring, "for it is our actions that bring about justice" (p. 16).

This chapter reiterates Nightingale's life from the years 1820 to 1860, delineating the formative influences on her thinking and providing historical context for her ideas about nursing as we recall them today. Part of what follows is a well-known tale; yet it remains a tale that is irresistible, casting an age-old spell on the reader, like the flickering shadow of Nightingale and her famous lamp in the dark and dreary halls of the Barrack Hospital, Scutari, on the outskirts of Constantinople, circa 1854 to 1856. It is a tale that carries even *more* relevance for nursing practice today.

Early Life and Education

A profession, a trade, a necessary occupation, something to fill and employ all my faculties, I have always felt essential to me, I have always longed for, consciously or not. . . . The first thought I can remember, and the last, was nursing work. . . .

—FLORENCE NIGHTINGALE, CITED IN COOK (1913, P. 106)

Nightingale was born in 1820 in Florence, Italy—the city she was named for. The Nightingales were on an extended European tour, begun in 1818 shortly after their marriage. This was a common journey for those of their class and wealth. Their first daughter, Parthenope, had been born in the city of that name in the previous year.

A legacy of humanism, liberal thinking, and love of speculative thought was bequeathed to Nightingale by her father. His views on the education of women were far ahead of his time. W. E. N., as her father, William, was called, undertook the education of both his daughters. Florence and her sister studied music; grammar; composition; modern languages; classical Greek and Latin; constitutional history and Roman, Italian, German, and Turkish history; and mathematics (Barritt, 1973).

From an early age, Florence exhibited independence of thought and action. The sketch (Fig. 4-1) of W. E. N. and his daughters was done by Nightingale's beloved aunt,

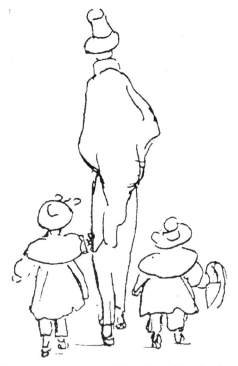

Figure 4 • 1 A sketch of W. E. N. and his daughters by one of his wife Fanny's sisters, Julia Smith. *(From Woodham-Smith, p. 9, with permission of Sir Henry Verney, Bart.)*

Julia Smith. It is Parthenope, the older sister, who clutches her father's hand and Florence who, as described by her aunt, "independently stumps along by herself" (Woodham-Smith, 1983, p. 7).

Travel also played a part in Nightingale's education. Eighteen years after Florence's birth, the Nightingales and both daughters made an extended tour of France, Italy, and Switzerland between the years of 1837 and 1838 and later Egypt and Greece (Sattin, 1987). From there, Nightingale visited Germany, making her first acquaintance with Kaiserswerth, a Protestant religious community that contained the Institution for the Training of Deaconesses, with a hospital school, penitentiary, and orphanage. A Protestant pastor, Theodore Fleidner, and his young wife had established this community in 1836, in part to provide training for women deaconesses (Protestant "nuns") who wished to nurse. Nightingale was to return there in 1851 against much family opposition to stay from July through October, participating in a period of "nurse's training" (Cook, Vol. I, 1913; Woodham-Smith, 1983).

Life at Kaiserswerth was spartan. The trainees were up at 5 A.M., ate bread and gruel, and then worked on the hospital wards until noon. Then they had a 10-minute break for broth with vegetables. Three P.M. saw another 10-minute break for tea and bread. They worked until 7 P.M., had some broth, and then Bible lessons until bed. What the Kaiserswerth training lacked in expertise it made up for in a spirit of reverence and dedication. Florence wrote, "The world here fills my life with interest and strengthens me in body and mind" (Huxley, 1975, p. 24).

In 1852, Nightingale visited Ireland, touring hospitals and keeping notes on various institutions along the way. Nightingale took two trips to Paris in 1853, hospital training again was the goal, this time with the sisters of St. Vincent de Paul, an order of nursing nuns. In August 1853, she accepted her first "official" nursing post as superintendent of an "Establishment for Gentlewomen in Distressed Circumstances during Illness," located at 1 Harley Street, London.

After 6 months at Harley Street, Nightingale wrote in a letter to her father: "I am in the hey-day of my power" (Nightingale, cited in Woodham-Smith, 1983, p. 77).

By October 1854, larger horizons beckoned.

Spirituality

Today I am 30—the age Christ began his Mission. Now no more childish things, no more vain things, no more love, no more marriage. Now, Lord let me think only of Thy will, what Thou willest me to do. O, Lord, Thy will, Thy will. . . .

—FLORENCE NIGHTINGALE, PRIVATE NOTE, 1850, CITED IN WOODHAM-SMITH (1983, P. 130)

By all accounts, Nightingale was an intense and serious child, always concerned with the poor and the ill, mature far beyond her years. A few months before her 17th birthday, Nightingale recorded in a personal note dated February 7, 1837, that she had been called to God's service. What that service was to be was unknown at that point in time. This was to be the first of four such experiences that Nightingale documented.

The fundamental nature of her religious convictions made her service to God, through service to humankind, a driving force in her life. She wrote: "The kingdom of Heaven is within; but we must make it without" (Nightingale, private note, cited in Woodham-Smith, 1983).

It would take 16 long and torturous years, from 1837 to 1853, for Nightingale to actualize her calling to the role of nurse. This was a revolutionary choice for a woman of her social standing and position, and her desire to nurse met with vigorous family opposition for many years. Along the way, she turned down proposals of marriage, potentially, in her mother's view, "brilliant matches," such as that of Richard Monckton Milnes. However, her need to serve God and to demonstrate her caring through meaningful activity proved stronger. She did not think that she could be married and also do God's will.

Calabria and Macrae (1994) note that for Nightingale there was no conflict between science and spirituality; actually, in her view, science is necessary for the development of a mature concept of God. The development of science allows for the concept of one perfect God Who regulates the universe through universal laws as opposed to random happenings. Nightingale referred to these laws, or the organizing principles of the universe, as "Thoughts of God" (Macrae, 1995, p. 9). As part of God's plan of evolution, it was the responsibility of human beings to discover the laws inherent in the universe and apply them to achieve well-being. In *Notes on Nursing* (1860/1969, p. 25), she wrote:

God lays down certain physical laws. Upon his carrying out such laws depends our responsibility (that much abused word). . . . Yet we seem to be continually expecting that He will work a miracle— i.e. break his own laws expressly to relieve us of responsibility.

Influenced by the Unitarian ideas of her father and her extended family, as well as by the more traditional Anglican Church she attended, Nightingale remained for her entire life a searcher of religious truth, studying a variety of religions and reading widely. She was a devout believer in God. Nightingale wrote: "I believe that there is a Perfect Being, of whose thought the universe in eternity is the incarnation" (Calabria & Macrae, 1994, p. 20). Dossey (1998) recasts Nightingale in the mode of "religious mystic." However, to Nightingale, mystical union with God was not an end in itself but was the source of strength and guidance for doing one's work in life. For Nightingale, service to God was service to humanity (Calabria & Macrae, 1994, p. xviii).

In Nightingale's view, nursing should be a search for the truth; it should be a discovery of God's laws of healing and their proper application. This is what she was referring to in *Notes on Nursing* when she wrote about the Laws of Health, as yet unidentified. It was the Crimean War that provided the stage for her to actualize these foundational beliefs, rooting

forever in her mind certain "truths." In the Crimea, she was drawn closer to those suffering injustice. It was in the Barracks Hospital of Scutari that Nightingale acted justly and responded to a call for nursing from the prolonged cries of the British soldiers (Boykin & Dunphy, 2002, p. 17).

War

I stand at the altar of those murdered men and while I live I fight their cause.

—Nightingale, cited in Woodham-Smith (1983)

Nightingale had powerful friends and had gained prominence through her study of hospitals and health matters during her travels. When Great Britain became involved in the Crimean War in 1854, Nightingale was ensconced in her first official nursing post at 1 Harley Street. Britain had joined France and Turkey to ward off an aggressive Russian advance in the Crimea (Fig. 4-2). A successful advance of Russia through Turkey could threaten the peace and stability of the European continent.

The first actual battle of the war, the Battle of Alma, was fought in September 1854. It was written of that battle that it was a "glorious and bloody victory." The best communication technology of the times, the telegraph, was to have an effect on what was to follow. In prior wars, news from the battlefields trickled home slowly. However, the telegraph enabled war correspondents to transmit reports home with rapid speed. The horror of the battlefields was relayed to a concerned citizenry. Descriptions of wounded men, disease, and illness abounded. Who was to care for these men? The French had the Sisters of Charity to care for their sick and wounded. What were the British to do? (Goldie, 1987; Woodham-Smith, 1983).

The minister of war was Sidney Herbert, Lord Herbert of Lea, who was the husband of Liz Herbert; both were close friends of Nightingale. Herbert had an innovative

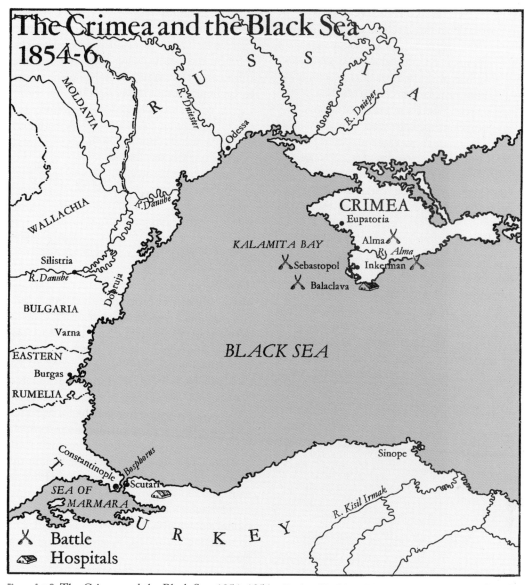

Figure 4 • 2 The Crimea and the Black Sea, 1854–1856. *(Designed by Manuel Lopez Parras in Huxley, E. [1975]. Florence Nightingale, p. 998. G. P. Putnam's Sons, New York.)*

solution: appoint Miss Nightingale and charge her to head a contingent of nurses to the Crimea to provide help and organization to the deteriorating battlefield situation. It was a brave move on the part of Herbert. Medicine and war were exclusively male domains. To send a woman into these hitherto uncharted waters was risky at best. But, as is well known, Nightingale was no ordinary woman, and she more than rose to the occasion. In a passionate letter to Nightingale, requesting her to accept this post, Herbert wrote:

Your own personal qualities, your knowledge and your power of administration, and among greater things, your rank and position in society, give you advantages in such a work that no other person possesses. (Dolan, 1971, p. 2)

At the same time, such that their letters actually crossed, Nightingale wrote to Herbert, offering her services. Accompanied by 38 handpicked "nurses" who had no formal training, she arrived on November 4, 1854 to "take charge" and did not return to England until August 1856.

Biographer Woodham-Smith and Nightingale's own correspondence, as cited in a number of sources (Cook, 1913; Goldie, 1987; Huxley, 1975; Summers, 1988; Vicinus & Nergaard, 1990), paint the most vivid picture of the experiences that Nightingale sustained there, experiences that cemented her views on disease and contagion, as well as her commitment to an environmental approach to health and illness:

The filth became indescribable. The men in the corridors lay on unwashed floors crawling with vermin. As the Rev. Sidney Osborne knelt to take down dying messages, his paper became thickly covered with lice. There were no pillows, no blankets; the men lay, with their heads on their boots, wrapped in the blanket or greatcoat stiff with blood and filth which had been their sole covering for more than a week . . . [S]he [Miss Nightingale] estimated . . . . there were more than 1000 men suffering from acute diarrhea and only 20 chamber pots. . . . [T]here was liquid filth which floated over the floor an inch deep. Huge wooden tubs stood in the halls and corridors for the men to use. In this filth lay the men's food—Miss Nightingale saw the skinned carcass of a sheep lie in a ward all night . . . the stench from the hospital could be smelled outside the walls (Woodham-Smith, 1983).

On her arrival in the Crimea, the immediate priority of Nightingale and her small band of nurses was not in the sphere of medical or surgical nursing as currently known; rather, their order of business was *domestic management*. This is evidenced in the following exchange between Nightingale and one of her party as they approached Constantinople: "Oh, Miss Nightingale, when we land don't let there be any red-tape delays, let us get straight to nursing the poor fellows!" Nightingale's reply: "The strongest will be wanted at the wash tub" (Cook, 1913; Dolan, 1971).

Although the bulk of this work continued to be done by orderlies after Nightingale's arrival (with the laundry farmed out to the soldiers' wives), it was accomplished under Nightingale's eagle eye: "She insisted on the huge wooden tubs in the wards being emptied, standing [obstinately] by the side of each one, sometimes for an hour at a time, never scolding, never raising her voice, until the orderlies gave way and the tub was emptied" (Cook, 1913; Summers, 1988; Woodham-Smith, 1983).

Nightingale set up her own extra "diet kitchen." Small portions, helpings of such things as arrowroot, port wine, lemonade, rice pudding, jelly, and beef tea, whose purpose was to tempt and revive the appetite, were provided to the men. It was therefore a logical sequence from cooking to feeding, from administering food to administering medicines. Because no antidote to infection existed at this time, the provision—by Nightingale and her nurses—of cleanliness, order, encouragement to eat, feeding, clean bed linen, clean bodies, and clean wards, was essential to recovery (Summers, 1988).

Mortality rates at the Barrack Hospital in Scutari fell. In February, at Nightingale's insistence, the prime minister had sent to the Crimea a sanitary commission to investigate the high mortality rates. Beginning their work in March, they described the conditions at the Barrack Hospital as "murderous." Setting to work immediately, they opened the channel through which the water supplying the hospital flowed, where a dead horse was found. The commission cleared "556 handcarts and large baskets full of rubbish ... 24 dead animals and 2 dead horses buried." In addition, they flushed and cleansed sewers, limewashed walls, tore out shelves that harbored rats, and got rid of vermin. The commission, Nightingale said, "saved the British Army." Miss Nightingale's anticontagionism was sealed as the mortality rates began showing dramatic declines (Rosenberg, 1979).

Figure 4-3 illustrates Nightingale's own hand-drawn "coxcombs" (as they were referred to), as Nightingale, always aware of the necessity of documenting outcomes of care, kept copious records of all sorts (Cook, 1913; Rosenberg, 1979; Woodham-Smith, 1983).

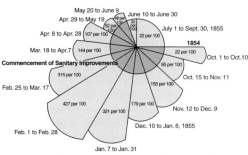

Diagram Representing the Mortality in the Hospitals
at Scutari and Kulali from Oct. 1st 1854 to Sept. 30th 1855

Figure 4 • 3 Diagram by Florence Nightingale showing declining mortality rates. *(From Cohen, I. B. [1981]. Florence Nightingale: The passionate statistician. Scientific American, 250(3), 128–137.)*

Florence Nightingale possessed *moral authority*, so firm because it was grounded in caring and was in a larger mission that came from her spirituality. For Miss Nightingale, spirituality was a much broader, more unifying concept than that of religion. Her spirituality involved the sense of a presence higher than humanity, the divine intelligence that creates, sustains, and organizes the universe, and an awareness of our inner connection to this higher reality. Through this inner connection flows creative endeavors and insight, a sense of purpose and direction. For Miss Nightingale, spirituality was intrinsic to human nature and was the deepest, most potent resource for healing. In *Suggestions for Thought* (Calabria & Macrae, 1994, p. 58), Nightingale wrote that "human consciousness is tending to become what God's consciousness is—to become One with the consciousness of God." This progression of consciousness to unity with the divine was an evolutionary view and not typical of either the Anglican or Unitarian views of the time (Calabria & Macrae, 1994; Macrae, 1995; Rosenberg, 1979; Slater, 1994; Welch, 1986; Widerquist, 1992).

There were 4 miles of beds in the Barrack Hospital at Scutari, a suburb of Constantinople. A letter to the *London Times* dated February 24, 1855, reported the following: "When all the medical officers have retired for the night and silence and darkness have settled upon those miles of prostrate sick, she may be observed, alone with a little lamp in her hand, making her solitary rounds" (Kalisch & Kalisch, 1987, p. 46).

In April 1855, after having been in Scutari for 6 months, Florence wrote to her mother, "[A]m in sympathy with God, fulfilling the purpose I came into the world for" (Woodham-Smith, 1983, p. 97). Henry Wadsworth Longfellow authored "Santa Filomena" to commemorate Miss Nightingale.

Lo! In That House of Misery
A lady with a lamp I see
Pass through the glimmering gloom
And flit from room to room
And slow as if in a dream of bliss
The speechless sufferer turns to kiss
Her shadow as it falls
Upon the darkening walls
As if a door in heaven should be
Opened and then closed suddenly
The vision came and went
The light shone and was spent.
A lady with a lamp shall stand
In the great history of the land
A noble type of good
Heroic womanhood
(Longfellow, cited in Dolan, 1971, p. 5).

Miss Nightingale slipped home quietly, arriving at Lea Hurst in Derbyshire on August 7, 1856, after 22 months in the Crimea and after sustained illness from which she was never to recover, after ceaseless work and after witnessing suffering, death, and despair that would haunt her for the remainder of her life. Her hair was shorn; she was pale and drawn (Fig. 4-4). She took her family by surprise. The next morning, a peal of the village church bells and a prayer of Thanksgiving were, her sister wrote, "'all the innocent greeting' except for those provided by the spoils of war that had proceeded her—a one-legged sailor boy, a small Russian orphan, and a large puppy found in some rocks near Balaclava. All England was ringing with her name, but she had left her heart on the battlefields of the Crimea and in the graveyards of Scutari" (Huxley, 1975, p. 147).

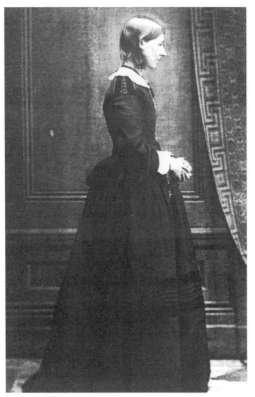

Figure 4 • 4 A rare photograph of Florence taken on her return from the Crimea. Although greatly weakened by her illness, she refused to accept her friends' advice to rest, and pressed on relentlessly with her plans to reform the army medical services. *(From Huxley, E. [1975]. Florence Nightingale, p. 139, G. P. Putnam's Sons, New York.)*

Introducing the Theory

In watching disease, both in private homes and public hospitals, the thing which strikes the experienced observer most forcefully is this, that the symptoms or the sufferings generally considered to be inevitable and incident to the disease are very often not symptoms of the disease at all, but of something quite different— of the want of fresh air, or light, or of warmth, or of quiet, or of cleanliness, or of punctuality and care in the administration of diet, of each or of all of these.

—FLORENCE NIGHTINGALE, *NOTES ON NURSING* (1860/1969, P. 8)

The Medical Milieu

To gain a better understanding of Nightingale's ideas on nursing, one must enter the particular world of 19th-century medicine and its views on health and disease. Considerable new medical knowledge had been gained by 1800. Gross anatomy was well known; chemistry promised to shed light on various body processes. Vaccination against smallpox existed. There were some established drugs in the pharmacopoeia: cinchona bark, digitalis, and mercury. Certain major diseases, such as leprosy and the bubonic plague, had almost disappeared. The crude death rate in western Europe was falling, largely related to decreasing infant mortality as a result of improvement in hygiene and standard of living (Ackernecht, 1982; Shyrock, 1959).

Yet, in 1800, physicians still had only the vaguest notion of diagnosis. Speculative philosophies continued to dominate medical thought, although inroads continued to be made that eventually gave way to a new outlook on the nature of disease: from belief in general states common to all illnesses to an understanding of disease-specificity symptoms. It was this shift in thought—a paradigm shift of the first order— that gave us the triumph of 20th-century medicine, with all its attendant glories and concurrent sterility.

The 18th century was host to two major traditions or paradigms in the healing arts: one based on "empirics" or "experience," trial and error, with an emphasis on curative remedies; the other based on Hippocratic notions and learning. Evidence of both these trends persisted into the 19th century and can be found in Nightingale's philosophy.

Consistent with the philosophical nature of her superior education (Barritt, 1973), Nightingale, like many of the physicians of her time, continued to emphatically disavow the reality of specific states of disease. She insisted on a view of sickness as an "adjective," not a substantive noun. Sickness was not an "entity" somehow separable from the body. Consistent with her more holistic view, sickness was an aspect or quality of the body as a whole. Some physicians, as she phrased it, taught that diseases were like cats and dogs, distinct species necessarily descended from other cats and dogs. She found such views misleading (Nightingale, 1860/1969).

At this point in time, in the mid-19th century, there were two competing theories regarding the nature and origin of disease. One view was known as "contagionism," postulating that some diseases were communicable, spread via commerce and population migration. A strategic consequence of this explanatory model was *quarantine,* and its attendant bureaucracy aimed at shutting down commerce and trade to keep disease away from noninfected areas. To the new and rapidly emerging merchant classes, quarantine represented government interference and control (Ackernecht, 1982; Arnstein, 1988).

The second school of thought on the nature and origin of disease, of which Nightingale was an ardent champion, was known as "anti-contagionism." It postulated that disease resulted from local environmental sources and arose out of "miasmas"—clouds of rotting filth and matter, activated by a variety of things such as meteorologic conditions (note the similarity to elements of water, fire, air, and earth on humors); the filth must be eliminated from *local* areas to prevent the spread of disease. Commerce and "infected" individuals were left alone (Rosenberg, 1979).

William Farr, another Nightingale associate and avid anti-contagionist, was Britain's statistical superintendent of the General Register Office. Farr categorized epidemic and infectious diseases as *zygomatic,* meaning pertaining to or caused by the process of fermentation. The debate as to whether fermentation was a chemical process or a "vitalistic" one had been raging for some time (Swazey & Reed, 1978). The familiarity of the process of fermentation helps to explain its appeal. Anyone who had seen bread rise could immediately grasp how a minute amount of some contaminating substance could in turn "pollute" the entire atmosphere, the very air that was breathed.

What was at issue was the *specificity* of the contaminating substance. Nightingale, and the anti-contagionists, endorsed the position that a "sufficiently intense level of atmospheric contamination could induce both endemic and epidemic ills in the crowded hospital wards [with particular configurations of environmental circumstances determining which]" (Rosenberg, 1979).

Anti-contagionism reached its peak before the political revolutions of 1848; the resulting wave of conservatism and reaction brought contagionism back into dominance, where it remained until its reformulation into the germ theory in the 1870s. Leaders of the contagionists were primarily high-ranking military physicians, politically united. These divergent worldviews accounted in some part for Nightingale's clashes with the military physicians she encountered during the Crimean War.

Given the intellectual and social milieu in which Nightingale was raised and educated, her stance on contagionism seems preordained and logically consistent (Rosenberg, 1979). Likewise, the eclectic religious philosophy she evolved contained attributes of the philosophy of Unitarianism with the fervor of Evangelicalism, all based on an organic view of humans as part of nature. The treatment of disease and dysfunction was inseparable from the nature of man as a whole, and likewise, the environment. And all were linked to God.

The emphasis on "atmosphere" (or "environment") in the Nightingale model is consistent with the views of the "anti-contagionists" of her time. This worldview was reinforced by Nightingale's Crimean experiences, as well as her liberal and progressive political thought. In addition, she viewed all ideas as being distilled through a distinctly *moral* lens (Rosenberg, 1979). As such, Nightingale was typical of a number of her generation's intellectuals. These thinkers struggled to come to grips with an increasingly complex and changing world order and frequently combined a language of two disparate realms of authority: the moral realm and the emerging scientific paradigm that has assumed dominance in the 20th century. Traditional religious and moral assumptions were garbed in a mantle of "scientific objectivity," often spurious at best, but more in keeping with the increasingly rationalized and bureaucratic society accompanying the growth of science.

The Feminist Context of Nightingale's Caring

I have an intellectual nature which requires satisfaction and that would find it in him. I have a passionate nature which requires satisfaction and that would find it in him. I have a moral, an active nature which requires satisfaction and that would not find it in his life.

—FLORENCE NIGHTINGALE, PRIVATE NOTE, 1849, CITED IN WOODHAM-SMITH (1983, P. 51)

Florence Nightingale wrote the following tortured note upon her final refusal of Richard Monckton Milnes's proposal of marriage: "I know I could not bear his life," she wrote, "that to be nailed to a continuation, an exaggeration of my present life without hope of another would be intolerable to me—that voluntarily to put it out of my power ever to be able to seize the chance of forming for myself a true and rich life would seem to be like suicide" (Nightingale, personal note cited in Woodham-Smith, 1983, p. 52). For Miss Nightingale there was no compromise. Marriage and pursuit of her "mission" were not compatible. She chose the mission, a clear repudiation of the mores of her time, which were rooted in the time-honored role of family and "female duty."

The census of 1851 revealed that there were 365,159 "excess women" in England, meaning women who were not married. These women were viewed as redundant, as described in an essay about the census entitled, "Why Are Women Redundant?" (Widerquist, 1992, p. 52). Many of these women had no acceptable means of support,

and Nightingale's development of a suitable occupation for women, that of nursing, was a significant historical development and a major contribution by Nightingale to women's plight in the 19th century. However, in other ways, her views on women and the question of women's rights were quite mixed.

Notes on Nursing: What It Is and What It Is Not (1859/1969) was written not as a manual to teach nurses to nurse, but rather to help all women to learn how to nurse.

Nightingale believed all women required this knowledge in order to take proper care of their families during times of sickness and to promote health—specifically what Nightingale referred to as "the health of houses," that is, the "health" of the environment, which she espoused. Nursing, to her, was clearly situated within the context of female duty.

In *Ordered to Care: The Dilemma of American Nursing* (1987, p. 43), historian Susan Reverby traces contemporary conflicts within the nursing profession back to Nightingale herself. She asserts that Nightingale's ideas about female duty and authority, along with her views on disease causality, brought about an independent field—that of nursing—that was separate, and in the view of Nightingale, equal, if not superior, to that of medicine. But this field was dominated by a female hierarchy and insisted on both deference and loyalty to the physician's authority. Reverby sums it up as follows: "Although Nightingale sought to free women from the bonds of familial demand, in her nursing model she rebound them in a new context."

Does the record support this evidence? Was Nightingale a champion for women's rights or a regressive force? As noted earlier, the answer is far from clear.

The shelter for all moral and spiritual values, threatened by the crass commercialism that was flourishing in the land, as well as the spirit of critical inquiry that accompanied this age of expanding scientific progress, was agreed upon: the home. All considered this to be a "sacred place, a Temple" (Houghton, 1957, p. 343). And who was the head of this home? Woman. Although the Victorian family was patriarchal in nature, in that women had virtually no economic and/or legal rights, they nonetheless yielded a major *moral* authority (Arnstein, 1988; Houghton, 1957; Perkins, 1987).

There was hostility on the part of men as well as some women toward women's emancipation. Many intelligent women—for example, Beatrice Webb, George Eliot, and, at times, Nightingale herself—viewed their gender's emancipation with apprehension. In Nightingale's case, the best word might be "ambivalence." There was a fear of weakening women's moral influence, coarsening the feminine nature itself.

This stance is best equated with *cultural feminism,* defined as a belief in inherent gender differences. Women, in contrast to men, are viewed as morally superior, the holders of family values and continuity; they are refined, delicate, and in need of protection. This school of thought, important in the 19th century, used arguments for women's suffrage such as the following: "[W]omen must make themselves felt in the public sphere because their *moral* perspective would improve corrupt masculine politics." In the case of Nightingale, these cultural feminist attitudes "made her impatient with the idea of women seeking rights and activities just because men valued these entities" (Bunting & Campbell, 1990, p. 21).

Nightingale had chafed at the limitations and restrictions placed on women, especially "wealthy" women with nothing to do: "What these [women] suffer—even physically—from the want of such work no one can tell. The accumulation of nervous energy, which has had nothing to do during the day, makes them feel every night, when they go to bed, as if they were going mad. . . ." Despite these vivid words, authored by Nightingale (1852/1979) in the fiery polemic "Cassandra," which was used as a rallying cry in many feminist circles, her view of the solution was measured. Her own resolution, painfully arrived at, was to break from her family and actualize her caring mission, that of nurse. One of the many results of this was that a useful occupation for other women to pursue was founded. Although Nightingale approved of this occupation outside of the home for other women, certain other occupations—that of doctor, for example—she viewed with hostility and as inappropriate for women. Why should these women not be nurses or nurse midwives, a far superior calling in Nightingale's view than that of a medicine "man" (Monteiro, 1984)?

Welch (1990) termed Nightingale a "Christian feminist" on the eve of her departure to the Crimea. She returned even more skeptical of women. Writing to her close friend Mary Clarke Mohl, she described women whom she worked with in the Crimea as being incompetent and incapable of independent thought (Welch, 1990; Woodham-Smith, 1983). According to Palmer (1977), by this time in her life, the concerns of the British people and the demands of service to God took precedence over any concern she had ever had about women's rights.

In other words, Nightingale, despite the clear freedom in which she lived her own life, nonetheless genderized the nursing role, leaving it rooted in 19th-century morality. Nightingale is seen constantly trying to improve the existing order and to work within that order; she was above all a reformer, seeking to improve the existing order, not to change the terrain radically.

In Nightingale's mind, the specific "scientific" activity of nursing—hygiene—was the central element in health care, without which medicine and surgery would be ineffective:

> The Life and Death, recovery or invaliding of patients generally depends not on any great and isolated act, but on the unremitting and thorough performance of every minute's practical duty. (Nightingale, 1860/1969)

This "practical duty" was the work of women, and the conception of the proper division of labor resting upon work demands internal to each respective "science," nursing and medicine, obscured the professional inequality. The later successes of medical science heightened this inequity. The scientific grounding espoused by Nightingale for nursing was ephemeral at best, as later 19th-century discoveries proved much of her analysis wrong, although nonetheless powerful. Much of her strength was in her rhetoric; if not always logically consistent, it certainly was morally resonant (Rosenberg, 1979).

Despite exceptional anomalies, such as women physicians, what Nightingale effectively accomplished was a genderization of the division of labor in health care: male physicians and female nurses. This appears to be a division that Nightingale supported. Because this "natural" division of labor was rooted in the family, women's work outside the home ought to resemble domestic tasks and complement the "male principle" with the "female." Thus, nursing was left on the shifting sands of a soon-outmoded "science"; the main focus of its authority grounded in an equally shaky moral sphere, also subject to change and devaluation in an increasingly secularized, rationalized, and technological 20th century.

Nightingale failed to provide institutionalized nursing with an autonomous future, on an equal parity with medicine. She did, however, succeed in providing women's work in the public sphere, establishing for numerous women an identity and source of employment. Although that public identity grew out of women's domestic and nurturing roles in the family, the conditions of a modern society required public as well as private forms of care. It is questionable whether more could have been achieved at that point in time (King, 1988).

A woman, Queen Victoria, presided over the age: "Ironically, Queen Victoria, that panoply of family happiness and stubborn adversary of female independence, could not help but shed her aura upon single women." The queen's early and lengthy widowhood, her "relentlessly spreading figure and commensurately increasing empire, her obstinate longevity which engorged generations of men and the collective shocks of history, lent an epic quality to the lives of solitary women" (Auerbach, 1982, pp. 120–121). Both Nightingale and the queen saw themselves as working through men, yet their lives added new, unexpected, and powerful dimensions to the myth of Victorian womanhood, particularly that of a woman alone and in command (Auerbach, 1982, pp. 120–121).

Nightingale's clearly chosen spinsterhood repudiated the Victorian family. Her unmarried life provides a vision of a powerful life lived on her own terms. This is not the spinsterhood of convention—one to be pitied, one of broken hearts—but a *radically* new image. She is freed from the trivia of family complaints and scorns the feminist collectivity; yet in this seemingly solitary life, she finds union not with one man but with all men, personified by the British soldier.

Lytton Strachey's well-known evocation of Nightingale, iconoclastic and bold, is perhaps closest to the decidedly masculine imagery she selected to describe herself, as evidenced in this imaginary speech to her mother written in 1852:

Well, my dear, you don't imagine with my "talents," and my "European reputation" and my "beautiful letters" and all that, I'm going to stay dangling around my mother's drawing room all my life! . . . [Y]ou must look upon me as your vagabond son . . . . I shan't cost you nearly as much as a son would have done, or had I married. You must consider me married or a son. (Woodham-Smith, 1983, p. 66)

Ideas About Nursing

Every day sanitary knowledge, or the knowledge of nursing, or in other words, of how to put the constitution in such a state as that it will have no disease, or that it can recover from disease, takes a higher place.

—FLORENCE NIGHTINGALE, NOTES ON NURSING (1860/1969), PREFACE

Evelyn R. Barritt, professor of nursing and Nightingale scholar, suggested that nursing became a science when Nightingale identified the laws of nursing, also referred to as the laws of health, or nature (Barritt, 1973; Nightingale, 1860/1969). The remainder of all nursing theory may be viewed as mere branches and "acorns," all fruit of the roots of Nightingale's ideas. Early writings of Nightingale, compiled in *Notes on Nursing: What It Is and What It Is Not* (1860/1969), provided the earliest systematic perspective for defining nursing. According to Nightingale, analysis and application of universal "laws" would promote well-being and relieve the suffering of humanity. This was the goal of nursing.

As noted by the caring theorist Madeline Leininger, Nightingale never defined human care or caring in Nightingale's *Notes on Nursing* (1859/1992, p. 31), and she goes on to wonder if Nightingale considered "components of care such as comfort, support, nurturance, and many other care constructs and characteristics and how they would influence the reparative process." Although Nightingale's conceptualizations of nursing, hygiene, the laws of health, and the environment never explicitly identify the construct of caring, an underlying ethos of care and commitment to others echoes in her words and, most importantly, resides in her actions and the drama of her life.

Nightingale did not theorize in the way to which we are accustomed today. Patricia Winstead-Fry (1993), in a review of the 1992 commemorative edition of Nightingale's *Notes on Nursing* (1859/1992, p. 161), states: "Given that theory is the interrelationship of concepts which form a system of propositions that can be tested and used for predicting practice, Nightingale was not a theorist. None of her major biographers present her as a theorist. She was a consummate politician and health care reformer." And our emerging 21st century has never been more in need of nurses who *are* consummate politicians and health care reformers. Her words and ideas, contextualized in the earlier portion of this chapter, ring differently than those of the other nursing theorists you will study in this book. However, her underlying ideas continue to be relevant and, some would argue, prescient.

Lynn McDonald, Canadian professor of sociology and editor of the *Collected Works of Florence Nightingale*, a 16-volume work still in progress, places Nightingale among the most prominent "Women Methodologists" identified in *The Women Founders of the Social Sciences* (McDonald, 1994). McDonald notes that Nightingale was firmly committed to ". . . a determined, probabilistic social science" and goes on to state that: "Indeed, she [Nightingale] described the laws of social science as God's laws for the right operation of the world" (p. 186). Nightingale was convinced of the necessity for evaluative statistics to underpin rational approaches to public administrations. Consistently she used the presentation of statistical data to prove her case that the costs of disease, crime, and excess mortality was greater than the cost of sanitary improvements. In later life, Nightingale endeavored to establish a chair or readership at Oxford University to teach Quetelet's statistical approaches and probability theory. In today's world, this would translate to a commitment to evidence-based practice as justification for nursing's value.

Karen Dennis and Patricia Prescott (1985) note that including Nightingale among the nurse theorists has been a recent development. They make the case that nurses today continue to incorporate in their practice the insight, foresight, and, most important, the clinical acumen of Nightingale's more than century and a half vision of nursing. As part of a larger study, they collected a large base of descriptions from both nurses and physicians describing "good" nursing practice. More than 300 individual interviews were subjected to content analysis; categories were named inductively and validated by four members of the project staff, separately.

Noting no marked differences in the descriptions obtained from either the nurses or physicians, the authors report that despite their independent derivation, the categories that emerged during the study bore a striking resemblance to nursing practice as described by Nightingale: prevention of illness and promotion of health, observation of the sick, and attention to the physical environment. Also referred to by Nightingale as the "health of houses," this physical environment included ventilation of both the patient's rooms and the larger environment of the "house": light, cleanliness, and the taking of food; attention to the interpersonal milieu, which included variety; and not indulging in superficialities with the sick or giving them false encouragement.

The authors note that "the words change but the concepts do not" (Dennis & Prescott, 1985, p. 80). In keeping with the tradition established by Nightingale, they note that nurses continue to foster an interpersonal milieu that focuses on the person, while manipulating and mediating the environment to "put the patient in the best condition for nature to act upon him" (Nightingale, 1860/1969, p. 133).

Afaf I. Meleis (1997), nurse scholar, does not compare Nightingale to contemporary nurse theorists; nonetheless, she refers to her frequently. Meleis states that it was Nightingale's conceptualization of environment as the focus of nursing activity and her de-emphasis of pathology, emphasizing instead the "laws of health" (which she said were yet to be identified), that were the earliest differentiation of nursing and medicine. Meleis (1997, pp. 114–116) describes Nightingale's concept of nursing as including "the proper use of fresh air, light, warmth, cleanliness, quiet, and the proper selection and administration of diet, all with the least expense of vital power to the patient." These ideas clearly had evolved from Nightingale's observations and experiences. The art of observation was identified as an important nursing function in the Nightingale model. And this observation was what should form the basis for nursing ideas. Meleis speculates on how differently the theoretical base of nursing might have evolved if we had continued to consider extant nursing practice as a source of ideas.

Pamela Reed and Tamara Zurakowski (1983/1989, p. 33) call the Nightingale model "visionary." They state: "At the core of all theory development activities in nursing today is the tradition of Florence Nightingale." They also suggest four major factors that influenced

her model of nursing: religion, science, war, and feminism, all of which are discussed in this chapter.

The assumptions in the following section were identified by Victoria Fondriest and Joan Osborne (1994).

Nightingale's Assumptions

1. Nursing is separate from medicine.
2. Nurses should be trained.
3. The environment is important to the health of the patient.
4. The disease process is not important to nursing.
5. Nursing should support the environment to assist the patient in healing.
6. Research should be utilized through observation and empirics to define the nursing discipline.
7. Nursing is both an empirical science and an art.
8. Nursing's concern is with the person in the environment.
9. The person is interacting with the environment.
10. Sickness and wellness are governed by the same laws of health.
11. The nurse should be observant and confidential.

The goal of *nursing* as described by Nightingale is assisting the patient in his or her retention of "vital powers" by meeting his or her needs, and thus, putting the patient in the best condition for nature to act upon (Nightingale, 1860/1969). This must not be interpreted as a "passive state," but rather one that reflects the patient's capacity for self-healing facilitated by nurses' ability to create an environment conducive to health. The focus of this nursing activity was the proper use of fresh air, light, warmth, cleanliness, quiet, proper selection and administration of diet, monitoring the patient's expenditure of energy, and observing. This activity was directed toward the environment and the patient (see Nightingale's Assumptions).

Health was viewed as an additive process, the result of environmental, physical, and psychological factors, not just the absence of disease. Disease was the reparative process of the body to correct a problem and could provide an opportunity for spiritual growth. The laws of health, as defined by Nightingale, were those to do with keeping the person, and the population, healthy. They were dependent on proper environmental control, for example, sanitation. The environment was what the nurse manipulated; it included the physical elements external to the patient.

Nightingale isolated five environmental components essential to an individual's health: clean air, pure water, efficient drainage, cleanliness, and light.

The patient is at the center of the Nightingale model, which incorporates a holistic view of the person as someone with psychological, intellectual, and spiritual components. This is evidenced in her acknowledgment of the importance of "variety." For example, she wrote of "the degree . . . to which the nerves of the sick suffer from seeing the same walls, the same ceiling, the same surroundings" (Nightingale, 1860/1969). Likewise, her chapter on "chattering hopes and advice" illustrates an astute grasp of human nature and of interpersonal relationships. She remarked upon the spiritual component of disease and illness, and she felt they could present an opportunity for spiritual growth. In this, all persons were viewed as equal.

A *nurse* was defined as any woman who had "charge of the personal health of somebody," whether well, as in caring for babies and children, or sick, as an "invalid" (Nightingale, 1860/1969). It was assumed that all women, at one time or another in their lives, would nurse. Thus, all women needed to know the laws of health. Nursing proper, or "sick" nursing, was both an art and a science and required organized, formal education to care for those suffering from disease. Above all, nursing was "service to God in relief of man"; it was a "calling" and "God's work" (Barritt, 1973). Nursing activities served as an "art form" through which spiritual development might occur (Reed & Zurakowski, 1983/1989). All nursing actions were guided by the nurses' *caring*, which was guided by underlying ideas about God.

Consistent with this caring base is Nightingale's views on *nursing as an art and a science.* Again, this was a reflection of the marriage, essential to Nightingale's underlying worldview, of science and spirituality. On the surface, these might appear to be odd bedfellows; however, this marriage flows directly from Nightingale's underlying religious and philosophic views, which were operationalized in her nursing practice. Nightingale was an empiricist, valuing the "science" of observation with the intent of using that knowledge to better the life of humankind. The application of that knowledge required an artist's skill, far greater than that of the painter or sculptor:

> Nursing is an art; and if it is to be made an art, it requires as exclusive a devotion, as hard a preparation, as any painter's or sculptor's work; for what is the having to do with dead canvas or cold marble, compared with having to do with the living body—the Temple of God's spirit? It is one of the Fine Arts; I had almost said, the finest of the Fine Arts. (Florence Nightingale, cited in Donahue, 1985, p. 469)

Nightingale's ideas about nursing health, the environment, and the person were grounded in experience; she regarded one's sense observations as the only reliable means of obtaining and verifying knowledge. Theory must be reformulated if inconsistent with empirical evidence. This experiential knowledge was then to be transformed into empirically based generalizations, an inductive process, to arrive at, for example, the laws of health. Regardless of Nightingale's commitment to empiricism and experiential knowledge, her early education and religious experience also shaped this emerging knowledge (Hektor, 1992).

According to Nightingale's model, nursing contributes to the ability of persons to maintain and restore health directly or indirectly through managing the environment. The person has a key role in his or her own health, and this health is a function of the interaction between person, nurse, and environment. However, neither the person nor the environment is discussed as influencing the nurse (Fig. 4-5).

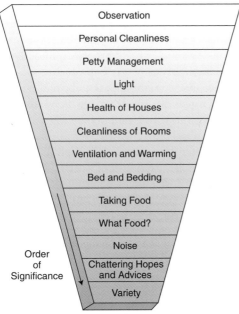

Order of Significance

Observation
Personal Cleanliness
Petty Management
Light
Health of Houses
Cleanliness of Rooms
Ventilation and Warming
Bed and Bedding
Taking Food
What Food?
Noise
Chattering Hopes and Advices
Variety

Figure 4 • 5 Perspective on Nightingale's 13 canons. *(Illustration developed by V. Fondriest, RN, BSN, and J. Osborne, RN, C BSN in October 1994.)*

Although it is difficult to describe the interrelationship of the concepts in the Nightingale model, Figure 4-6 is a schema that attempts to delineate this. Note the prominence of "observation" on the outer circle (important to all nursing functions) and the interrelationship of the specifics of the interventions, such as "bed and bedding" and "cleanliness of rooms and walls," that go into making up the "health of houses" (Fondriest & Osborne, 1994).

Nightingale's Legacy for 21st Century Nursing Practice

Philip and Beatrice Kalisch (1987, p. 26) described the popular and glorified images that arose out of the portrayals of Florence Nightingale during and after the Crimean War—that of nurse as self-sacrificing, refined, virginal, and an "angel of mercy," a far less threatening image than one of educated and

"Nursing"

Observation

Management

Ventilation & Warming

"Environment"

Health of Houses (Pure Air, Water & Light)

Bed & Bedding

Light, Noise & Variety

Cleanliness of Rooms & Walls

Taking Food

Chattering Hopes & Advices

Personal Cleanliness

What Food ?

Figure 4 • 6 Nightingale's model of nursing and the environment. *(Illustration developed by V. Fondriest, RN, BSN, and J. Osborne, RN, C BSN.)*

skilled professional nurses. They attribute nurses' low pay to the perception of nursing as a "calling," a way of life for devoted women with private means, such as Florence Nightingale (Kalisch & Kalisch, 1987, p. 20). Well over 100 years later, the amount of scholarship on Nightingale provides a more realistic portrait of a complex and brilliant woman. To quote Auerbach (1982) and Strachey (1918), she was "a demon, a rebel . . ."

Florence Nightingale's legacy of caring and the activism it implies is carried on in nursing today. There is a resurgence and inclusion of concepts of spirituality in current nursing practice and a delineation of nursing's caring base that in essence began with the nursing life of Florence Nightingale. Nightingale's caring, as demonstrated in this chapter, extended beyond the individual patient, beyond the individual person. She herself said that the specific business of nursing was the least important of the functions into which she had been forced in the Crimea. Her caring encompassed a broadened sphere—that of the British Army and, indeed, the entire British Commonwealth.

Themes in contemporary nursing practice focusing on evidence-based practice and curricula championing cultures of safety and quality are all found in the life and works of Florence Nightingale. I would venture to say that almost all contemporary nursing practice settings echo some aspect of the ideas—and ideals—of Nightingale. Themes of Nightingale, the environmentalist, are critical to nursing practice for the individual, the community, and global health. An exemplar of practice personifying Nightingale's approach and practice would be a larger-than-life nurse hero/heroine championing current health care reform by designing health care systems that are truly responsive to the needs of the populace and that extend cross-culturally and globally.

■ Summary

The unique aspects of Florence Nightingale's personality and social position, combined with historical circumstances, laid the groundwork for the evolution of the modern discipline of nursing. Are the challenges and obstacles that we face today any more daunting than what confronted Nightingale when she arrived in the Crimea in 1854? Nursing for Florence Nightingale was what we might call today her "centering force." It allowed her to express her spiritual values as well as enabled her to fulfill her needs for leadership and authority. As historian Susan Reverby noted, today we are challenged with the dilemma of how to practice our integral values of caring in an unjust health care system that does not value caring. Let us look again to Florence Nightingale for inspiration, for she remains a role model par excellence on the transformation of values of caring into an *activism* that could potentially transform our current health care system into a more humanistic and *just* one. Her activism situates her in the context of justice-making. *Justice-making* is understood as a manifestation of compassion and caring, for it is actions that bring about justice (Boykin & Dunphy, 2002, p. 16). Florence Nightingale's legacy of connecting caring with activism can then truly be said to continue.

References

Ackernecht, E. (1982). *A short history of medicine.* Baltimore: Johns Hopkins University Press.

Arnstein, W. (1988). *Britain: Yesterday and today.* Lexington, MA: D. C. Heath.

Auerbach, N. (1982). *Women and the demon: The life of a Victorian myth.* Cambridge, MA: Harvard University Press.

Barritt, E. R. (1973). Florence Nightingale's values and modern nursing education. *Nursing Forum, 12,* 7–47.

Boykin, A., & Dunphy, L. M. (2002). Justice-making: Nursing's call. *Policy, Politics, & Nursing Practice, 3,* 14–19.

Bunting, S., & Campbell, J. (1990). Feminism and nursing: An historical perspective. *Advances in Nursing Science, 12,* 11–24.

Calabria, M., & Macrae, J. (Eds.). (1994). *Suggestions for thought by Florence Nightingale: Selections and commentaries.* Philadelphia: University of Pennsylvania Press.

Cohen, I. B. (1981). Florence Nightingale: The passionate statistician. *Scientific American, 250*(3), 128–137.

Cook, E. T. (1913). *The life of Florence Nightingale* (vols. 1–2). London: Macmillan.

Dennis, K. E., & Prescott, P. A. (1985). Florence Nightingale: Yesterday, today and tomorrow. *Advances in Nursing Science, 7*(2), 66–81.

Dolan, J. (1971). *The grace of the great lady.* Chicago: Medical Heritage Society.

Donahue, P. (1985). *Nursing: The finest art.* St. Louis, MO: C. V. Mosby.

Dossey, B. (1998). Florence Nightingale: A 19th century mystic. *Journal of Holistic Nursing, 16*(2), 111–164.

Fondriest, V., & Osborne, J. (1994). A theorist before her time? Presentation, NGR 5110, Nursing Theory and Advanced Practice Nursing, School of Nursing, Florida International University, N. Miami, FL.

Goldie, S. (1987). *I have done my duty: Florence Nightingale in the Crimean War, 1854–1856.* Iowa City: University of Iowa Press.

Gourley, J. (2003). *Florence Nightingale and the health of the Raj.* Cornwall, UK: MPG Books.

Hektor, L. M. (1992). *Nursing, science, and gender: Florence Nightingale and Martha E. Rogers.* Unpublished doctoral dissertation, University of Miami.

Houghton, W. (1957). *The Victorian frame of mind.* New Haven, CT: Yale University Press.

Huxley, E. (1975). *Florence Nightingale.* New York: G. P. Putnam's Sons.

Kalisch, P. A., & Kalisch, B. J. (1987). *The changing image of the nurse.* Menlo Park, CA: Addison-Wesley.

King, M. G. (1988). Gender: A hidden issue in nursing's professionalizing reform movement. Boston: Boston University School of Nursing. In *Strategies for Theory Development V,* March 10–12.

Macrae, J. (1995). Nightingale's spiritual philosophy and its significance for modern nursing. *Image: Journal of Nursing Scholarship, 27,* 8–10.

Meleis, A. I. (1997). *Theoretical nursing: Development and progress* (3rd ed.). Philadelphia: J. B. Lippincott.

Monteiro, L. (1984). On separate roads: Florence Nightingale and Elizabeth Blackwell. *Signs: Journal of Women in Culture & Society, 9,* 520–533.

Newman, M. A. (1972). Nursing's theoretical evolution. *Nursing Outlook, 20,* 449–453.

Nightingale, F. (1852/1979). *Cassandra,* with an introduction by Myra Stark. Westbury, NY: Feminist Press.

Nightingale, F. (1859). *Notes on nursing: What it is and what it is not.* London: Harrison & Sons.

Nightingale, F. (1859/1992). *Notes on nursing: Commemorative edition with commentaries by contemporary nursing leaders.* Philadelphia: J. B. Lippincott.

Nightingale, F. (1860). *Suggestions for thought to searchers after religious truths* (vols. 2–3). London: George E. Eyre & William Spottiswoode.

Nightingale, F. (1860/1969). *Notes on nursing: What it is and what it is not.* New York: Dover.

Palmer, I. S. (1977). Florence Nightingale: Reformer, reactionary, research. *Nursing Research, 26,* 84–89.

Perkins, J. (1987). *Women and marriage in nineteenth century England.* Chicago: Lyceum Books.

Quinn, V., & Prest, J. (Eds.). (1981). *Dear Miss Nightingale: A selection of Benjamin Jowett's letters to Florence Nightingale, 1860–1893.* Oxford: Clarendon Press.

Reed, P. G., & Zurakowski, T. L. (1983/1989). Nightingale: A visionary model for nursing. In: J. Fitzpatrick & A. Whall (Eds.), *Conceptual models of nursing: Analysis and application.* Bowie, MD: Robert J. Brady.

Reverby, S. M. (1987). *Ordered to care: The dilemma of American nursing (1865–1945).* New York: Cambridge University Press.

Rosenberg, C. (1979). *Healing and history.* New York: Science History Publications.

Sattin, A. (Ed.). (1987). *Florence Nightingale's letters from Egypt: A journey on the Nile, 1849–1850.* New York: Weidenfeld & Nicolson.

Shyrock, R. (1959). *The history of nursing.* Philadelphia: W. B. Saunders.

Slater, V. E. (1994). The educational and philosophical influences on Florence Nightingale, an enlightened conductor. *Nursing History Review, 2,* 137–152.

Strachey, L. (1918). *Eminent Victorians: Cardinal Manning, Florence Nightingale, Dr. Arnold, General Gordon.* London: Chatto & Windus.

Summers, A. (1988). *Angels and citizens: British women as military nurses, 1854–1914.* London: Routledge & Kegan Paul.

Swazey, J., & Reed, K. (1978). Louis Pasteur: Science and the application of science. In J. Swazey & K. Reed (Eds.), *Today's medicine, tomorrow's science.* U.S. Government Printing Office: DHEW Pub. No. NIH 78–244. Washington, DC: U.S. Government Printing Office.

Vicinus, M., & Nergaard, B. (Eds.). (1990). *Ever yours, Florence Nightingale: Selected letters.* Cambridge, MA: Harvard University Press.

Watson, J. (1992). Commentary. In *Notes on nursing: What it is and what it is not* (pp. 80–85). Commemorative edition. Philadelphia: J. B. Lippincott.

Welch, M. (1986). Nineteenth-century philosophic influences on Nightingale's concept of the person. *Journal of Nursing History, 1*(2), 3–11.

Welch, M. (1990). Florence Nightingale: The social construction of a Victorian feminist. *Western Journal of Nursing Research, 12,* 404–407.

Widerquist, J. G. (1992). The spirituality of Florence Nightingale. *Nursing Research, 41,* 49–55.

Winstead-Fry, P. (1993). Book review: *Notes on nursing: What it is and what it is not.* Commemorative edition. *Nursing Science Quarterly, 6*(3), 161–162.

Woodham-Smith, C. (1983). *Florence Nightingale.* New York: Atheneum 97.

Chapter 5

Twentieth-Century Nursing: Ernestine Wiedenbach, Virginia Henderson, and Lydia Hall's Contributions to Nursing Theory and Their Use in Practice

SHIRLEY C. GORDON,
THERIS A. TOUHY, THERESA GESSE,
MARCIA DOMBRO, AND NETTIE BIRNBACH

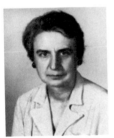

Ernestine Wiedenbach

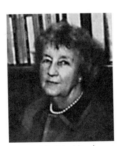

Virginia Henderson

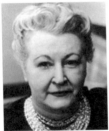

Lydia Hall

Introducing the Theorists

Ernestine Wiedenbach, Virginia Henderson, and Lydia Hall are three of the most important influences on nursing theory development of the 20th century. Indeed, their work continues to ground nursing thought in the new century. The work of each of these nurse scholars was based on nursing practice, and today some of this work might be referred to as practice theories. Concepts and terms they first used are heard today around the globe.

This chapter provides a brief overview of three important 20th-century nursing theorists. The content of this chapter is partially based on work from scholars who have studied or worked with these theorists and who wrote chapters for the first and/or second editions of *Nursing Theories and Nursing Practice* (Gesse, Dombro, Gordon, & Rittman, 2006; Gordon, 2001; Touhy & Birnbach, 2006). For a wealth of additional information on these nurses, scholars, researchers, thinkers, writers, practitioners, and educators, please consult the reference and bibliography sections at the end of this chapter.

Ernestine Wiedenbach

Wiedenbach was born in 1900 in Germany to an American mother and a German father who emigrated to the United States when

Ernestine was a child. She received a bachelor of arts degree from Wellesley College in 1922 and graduated from Johns Hopkins School of Nursing in 1925 (Nickel, Gesse, & MacLaren, 1992). After completing a master of arts at Columbia Univeristy in 1934, she became a professional writer for the *American Journal of Nursing* and played a critical role in the recruitment of nursing students and military nurses during World War II. At age 45, she began her studies in nurse-midwifery. Wiedenbach's roles as practitioner, teacher, author, and theorist were consolidated as a member of the Yale University School of Nursing, where Yale colleagues William Dickoff and Patricia James encouraged her development of prescriptive theory (Dickoff, James, & Wiedenbach, 1968). Even after her retirement in 1966, she and her lifelong friend Caroline Falls offered informal seminars in Miami, always reminding students and faculty of the need for clarity of purpose, based on reality. She even continued to use her gift for writing to transcribe books for the blind, including a Lamaze childbirth manual, which she prepared on her Braille typewriter. Ernestine Wiedenbach died in April 1998 at the age of 98.

Virginia Henderson

Born in Kansas City, Missouri, in 1897, Virginia Avenel Henderson was the fifth of eight children. With two of her brothers serving in the armed forces during World War I, and in anticipation of a critical shortage of nurses, Virginia Henderson entered the Army School of Nursing at Walter Reed Army Hospital. It was there that she began to question the regimentalization of patient care and the concept of nursing as ancillary to medicine (Henderson, 1991). She described her introduction to nursing as a "series of almost unrelated procedures, beginning with an unoccupied bed and progressing to aspiration of body cavities" (Henderson, 1991, p. 9). It was also at Walter Reed Army Hospital that she met Annie W. Goodrich, the dean of the School of Nursing. Henderson admired Goodrich's intellectual abilities and stated: "Whenever she visited our unit, she lifted our sights above techniques and routine" (Henderson, 1991, p. 11). Henderson credited Goodrich with inspiring her with the "ethical significance of nursing" (Henderson, 1991, p. 10).

As a member of society during a war, Henderson considered it a privilege to care for sick and wounded soldiers (Henderson, 1960). This wartime experience forever influenced her ethical understanding of nursing and her appreciation of the importance and complexity of the nurse–patient relationship.

She continued to explore the nature of nursing as her student experiences exposed her to different ways of being in relationships with patients and their families. For instance, a pediatric experience as a student at Boston Floating Hospital introduced Henderson to patient-centered care in which nurses were assigned to patients instead of tasks, and warm, nurse–patient relationships were encouraged (Henderson, 1991). After a summer spent with the Henry Street Visiting Nurse Agency in New York City, Henderson began to appreciate the importance of getting to know the patients and their environments. She enjoyed the less formal visiting nurse approach to patient care and became skeptical of the ability of hospital regimes to alter patients' unhealthy ways of living upon returning home (Henderson, 1991). She entered Teachers College at Columbia University, earning her baccalaureate degree in 1932 and her master's degree in 1934. She continued at Teachers College as an instructor and associate professor of nursing for the next 20 years.

Virginia Henderson presented her definition of the nature of nursing in an era when few nurses had ventured into describing the complex phenomena of modern nursing. Henderson wrote about nursing the way she lived it: focusing on what nurses do, how nurses function, and on nursing's unique role in health care. Her works are beautifully written in jargon-free, everyday language. Her search for a definition of nursing ultimately influenced the practice and education of nursing around the world. Her pioneer work in the area of identifying and structuring nursing knowledge has provided the foundation for nursing scholarship for generations to come.

Henderson has been heralded as the greatest advocate for nursing libraries worldwide. Of all her contributions to nursing, Virginia Henderson's work on the identification and control of nursing literature is perhaps her greatest. In the 1950s, there was an increasing interest on the part of the profession to establish a research basis for the nursing practice. It was also recognized that the body of nursing knowledge was unstructured and therefore inaccessible to practicing nurses and educators. After the completion of her revised text in 1955, Henderson moved to Yale University and began what would become a distinguished career in library science research. Henderson encouraged nurses to become active in the work of classifying nursing literature. In 1990, the Sigma Theta Tau International Library was named in her honor. Henderson insisted that if the library was to bear her name, the electronic networking system would have to advance the work of staff nurses by providing them with current, jargon-free information wherever they were based (McBride, 1997).

Lydia Hall

Visionary, risk taker, and consummate professional, Lydia Hall touched all who knew her in a special way. Born in 1906, she inspired commitment and dedication through her unique conceptual framework for nursing practice that viewed professional nursing as the key to the care and rehabilitation of patients.

A 1927 graduate of the York Hospital School of Nursing in Pennsylvania, Hall held various nursing positions during the early years of her career. In the mid-1930s, she enrolled at Teachers College, Columbia University, where she earned a Bachelor of Science degree in 1937, and a Master of Arts degree in 1942. She worked with the Visiting Nurse Service of New York from 1941 to 1947 and was a member of the nursing faculty at Fordham Hospital School of Nursing from 1947 to 1950. Hall was subsequently appointed to a faculty position at Teachers College, where she developed and implemented a program in nursing consultation and joined a community of nurse leaders. At the same time, she was involved in research activities for the U.S. Health Service. Active in nursing's professional organizations, Hall also provided volunteer service to the New York City Board of Education, Youth Aid, and other community associations (Birnbach, 1988).

Hall's model, which she designed and put into place in the Loeb Center for Nursing and Rehabilitation at Montefiore Medical Center in Bronx, New York, was her most significant contribution to nursing practice. Opened in 1963, the Loeb Center was the culmination of five years of planning and construction under Hall's direction. The circumstances that brought Hall and the Loeb Center together date back to 1947, when Dr. Martin Cherkasky was named director of the new hospital-based home care division of Montefiore Medical Center in Bronx, New York. At that time, Hall was employed by the Visiting Nurse Service at its Bronx office and had frequent contact with the Montefiore home care program. Hall and Cherkasky shared congruent philosophies regarding health care and the delivery of quality service, which served as the foundation for a long-standing professional relationship (Birnbach, 1988).

In 1950, Cherkasky was appointed director of the Montefiore Medical Center. During the early years of his tenure, existing traditional convalescent homes fell into disfavor. Convalescent treatment was undergoing rapid change owing largely to medical advances, new pharmaceuticals, and technological developments. One of the homes that closed as a result of the emerging trends was the Solomon and Betty Loeb Memorial Home in Westchester County, New York. Cherkasky and Hall collaborated in convincing the board of the Loeb Home to join with Montefiore in founding the Loeb Center for Nursing and Rehabilitation. Using the proceeds from the sale of the Loeb Home, plans for the Loeb Center construction proceeded over a 5-year period, from 1957 to 1962. The Loeb Center was separately administered, with its own board of trustees that interrelated with the Montefiore board, giving Hall considerable autonomy in developing the centers policies and procedures.

For example, under Hall's direction, nurses selected patients for the Loeb Center based on a nursing assessment of an individual patient's potential for rehabilitation. Qualified professional nurses provided direct care to patients and coordinated needed services. Hall frequently described the center as "a halfway house on the road home" (Hall, 1963, p. 2), where the nurse worked with the patients as active participants in achieving desired outcomes. Over time, the effectiveness of Hall's practice model was validated by the significant decline in the number of readmissions among former Loeb patients as compared with those who received other types of posthospital care ("Montefiore cuts," 1966).

In 1967, Hall received the Teachers College Nursing Alumni Award for distinguished achievement in nursing practice. She shared her innovative ideas about the nursing practice with numerous audiences around the country and contributed articles to nursing journals. In those articles, she referred to nurses using feminine pronouns. Because gender-neutral language was not yet an accepted style, and women comprised 96 percent of the nursing workforce, the feminine pronoun was used almost exclusively.

Hall died of heart disease on February 27, 1969, at Queens Hospital in New York. In 1984, she was inducted into the American Nurses' Association Hall of Fame. Following Hall's death, her legacy was kept alive at the Loeb Center until 1984, under the capable leadership of her friend and colleague Genrose Alfano.

Remembered by her colleagues for her passion for nursing, her flamboyant personality, and the excitement she generated, Hall was indeed a force for change. At a time when task-oriented team nursing was the preferred practice model in most institutions, she implemented a professional patient-centered framework whereby patients received a standard of care unequaled anywhere else. At the Loeb Center, Lydia Hall created an environment in which nurses were empowered, in which patients' needs were met through a continuum of care, and in which, according to Genrose Alfano, "nursing was raised to a high therapeutic level" (personal communication, January 27, 1999).

Overview of 20th-Century Nursing: Wiedenbach, Henderson, and Hall's Conceptualizations of Nursing

Virginia Henderson, sometimes known as the modern day Florence Nightingale, developed the definition of nursing that is most well known internationally. Ernestine Wiedenbach gave us new ways to think about nursing practice and nursing scholarship, introducing us to the ideas of (1) nursing as a professional practice discipline and (2) nursing practice theory. Lydia Hall challenged us to think in new ways about the key role of professional nursing in the care and rehabilitation of patients. Each of these nurses helped us focus on the patient, instead of on the tasks to be done, and to plan care to meet needs of the person. Each of these women emphasized caring based on the perspective of the individual being cared for— through observing, communicating, designing, and reporting. Each was concerned with the unique aspects of nursing practice and scholarship and with the essential question of "What is nursing?"

Wiedenbach's Conceptualizations of Nursing

Initial work on Wiedenbach's prescriptive theory is presented in her article in the

American Journal of Nursing (1963) and her book, *Meeting the Realities in Clinical Teaching* (1969).

Her explanation of prescriptive theory is that "Account must be taken of the motivating factors that influence the nurse not only in doing what she does, but also in doing it the way she does it with the realities that exist in the situation in which she is functioning" (Wiedenbach, 1970, p. 2). Three ingredients essential to the prescriptive theory are:

1. *The nurse's central purpose in nursing is the nurse's professional commitment.* For Wiedenbach, the central purpose in nursing is to motivate the individual and/or facilitate his efforts to overcome the obstacles that may interfere with his ability to respond capably to the demands made of him by the realities in his situation (Wiedenbach, 1970, p. 4). She emphasized that the nurse's goals are grounded in the nurse's philosophy, "those beliefs and values that shape her attitude toward life, toward fellow human beings and toward herself." The three concepts that epitomize the essence of such a philosophy are: (1) reverence for the gift of life; (2) respect for the dignity, autonomy, worth, and individuality of each human being; and (3) resolution to act dynamically in relation to one's beliefs (Wiedenbach, 1970, p. 4). She recognized that nurses have different values and various commitments to nursing and that to formulate one's purpose in nursing is a "soul-searching experience." She encouraged each nurse to undergo this experience and be "willing and ready to present your central purpose in nursing for examination and discussion when appropriate" (Wiedenbach, 1970, p. 5).

2. *The prescription indicates the broad general action that the nurse deems appropriate to fulfillment of her central purpose.* The nurse will have thought through the kind of results to be sought and will take action to obtain these results, accepting accountability for what she does and for the outcomes of her action. Nursing action, then, is deliberate action that is mutually understood and agreed upon and that is both patient-directed and nurse-directed (Wiedenbach, 1970, p. 5).

3. The realities are the aspects of the immediate nursing situation that influence the results the nurse achieves through what she does (Wiedenbach, 1970, p. 3). These include the physical, psychological, emotional, and spiritual factors in which nursing action occurs. Within the situation are these components:

   • The agent, who is the nurse supplying the nursing action
   • The recipient, or the patient receiving this action or on whose behalf the action is taken
   • The framework, comprised of situational factors that affect the nurse's ability to achieve nursing results
   • The goal, or the end to be attained through nursing activity on behalf of the patient
   • The means, the actions and devices through which the nurse is enabled to reach the goal

Henderson's Definition of Nursing and Components of Basic Nursing Care

While working on the 1955 revision of the *Textbook of the Principles and Practice of Nursing,* Henderson focused on the need to be clear about the function of nurses. She opened the first chapter with the following question: What is nursing and what is the function of the nurse? (Harmer & Henderson, 1955, p. 1). Henderson believed this question was fundamental to anyone choosing to pursue the study and practice of nursing.

Definition of Nursing

Her often-quoted definition of nursing first appeared in the fifth edition of Textbook of the Principles and Practice of Nursing (Harmer & Henderson, 1955, p. 4):

Nursing is primarily assisting the individual (sick or well) in the performance of those activities contributing to health or its recovery (or to a peaceful death), that he would perform unaided if he had the necessary strength, will, or knowledge. It is likewise the unique contribution of nursing to help people be independent of such assistance as soon as possible.

In presenting her definition of nursing, Henderson hoped to encourage others to develop their own working concept of nursing and nursing's unique function in society. She believed the definitions of the day were too general and failed to differentiate nurses from other members of the health team, which led to the following questions: "What is nursing that is not also medicine, physical therapy, social work, etc.?" and "What is the unique function of the nurse?" (Harmer & Henderson, 1955, p. 4).

Based on Henderson's definition, and after coining the term "basic nursing care," Henderson identified 14 components of basic nursing care that reflect needs pertaining to personal hygiene and healthful living, including helping the patient carry out the physician's therapeutic plan (Henderson, 1960; 1966, pp. 16–17):

1. Breathe normally.
2. Eat and drink adequately.
3. Eliminate bodily wastes.
4. Move and maintain desirable postures.
5. Sleep and rest.
6. Select suitable clothes—dress and undress.
7. Maintain body temperature within normal range by adjusting clothing and modifying the environment.
8. Keep the body clean and well groomed and protect the integument.
9. Avoid dangers in the environment and avoid injuring others.
10. Communicate with others in expressing emotions, needs, fears, or opinions.
11. Worship according to one's faith.
12. Work in such a way that there is a sense of accomplishment.
13. Play or participate in various forms of recreation.
14. Learn, discover, or satisfy the curiosity that leads to normal development and health and use the available health facilities.

Hall's Care, Cure, and Core Model

Hall enumerated three aspects of the person as patient: the person, the body, and the disease. She envisioned these aspects as overlapping circles of care, core, and cure that influence each other.

"Everyone in the health professions either neglects or takes into consideration any or all of these, but each profession, to be a profession, must have an exclusive area of expertness with which it practices, creates new practices, new theories, and introduces newcomers to its practice" (Hall, 1965, p. 4).

Hall believed that medicine's responsibility was the areas of pathology and treatment. The area of person, which, according to Hall, had been sadly neglected, belongs to a number of professions, including psychiatry, social work, and the ministry, among others. She saw nursing's expertise as the area of body as body, and also as influenced by the other two areas. Hall clearly stated that the focus of nursing is the provision of intimate bodily care. She reflected that the public has long recognized this as belonging exclusively to nursing (Hall, 1958, 1964, 1965). To be expert, the nurse must know how to modify the care depending on the pathology and treatment while considering the patient's unique needs and personality.

Based on her view of the person as patient, Hall conceptualized nursing as having three aspects, and she delineated the area that is the specific domain of nursing and those areas that are shared with other professions (Hall, 1955, 1958, 1964, 1965) (Fig. 5-1). Hall believed that this model reflected the nature of nursing as a professional interpersonal process. She visualized each of the three overlapping circles as an "aspect of the nursing process related to the patient, to the supporting sciences and to the underlying philosophical dynamics" (Hall, 1958, p. 1). The circles overlap and change in size as the patient progresses through a medical crisis to the rehabilitative phase of the illness. In the acute care

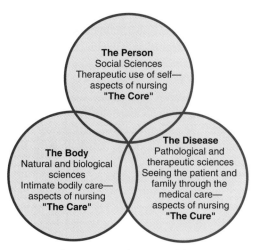

Figure 5 • 1 Care, core, and cure model. *(From Hall, L. [1964, February]. Nursing: What is it? The Canadian Nurse, 60[2], 151. Reproduced with permission from The Canadian Nurse.)*

phase, the cure circle is the largest. During the evaluation and follow-up phase, the care circle is predominant. Hall's framework for nursing has been described as the Care, Core, and Cure Model (Chinn & Jacobs, 1987; Marriner-Tomey, Peskoe, K & Gumm, S. 1989; Stevens-Barnum, 1990).

Care

Hall suggested that the part of nursing that is concerned with intimate bodily care (e.g., bathing, feeding, toileting, positioning, moving, dressing, undressing, and maintaining a healthful environment) belongs exclusively to nursing. Nursing is required when people are not able to undertake these activities for themselves. This aspect provided the opportunity for closeness and required seeing the process as an interpersonal relationship (Hall, 1958). Hall labeled this aspect "care" and identified knowledge in the natural and biological sciences as foundational to practice. The intent of bodily care is to comfort the patient. Through this comforting, the patient as a person, as well as his or her body, responds to the physical care. Hall cautioned against viewing intimate bodily care as a task that can be performed by anyone:

To make the distinction between a trade and a profession, let me say that the laying on of hands to wash around a body is an activity, it is a trade; but if you look behind the activity for the rationale and intent, look beyond it for the opportunities that the activity opens up for something more enriching in growth, learning and healing production on the part of the patient—you have got a profession. Our intent when we lay hands on the patient in bodily care is to comfort. While the patient is being comforted, he feels close to the comforting one. At this time, his person talks out and acts out those things that concern him—good, bad, and indifferent. If nothing more is done with these, what the patient gets is ventilation or catharsis, if you will. This may bring relief of anxiety and tension but not necessarily learning. If the individual who is in the comforting role has in her preparation all of the sciences whose principles she can offer a teaching-learning experience around his concerns, the ones that are most effective in teaching and learning, then the comforter proceeds to something beyond—to what I call "nurturer"—someone who fosters learning, someone who fosters growing up emotionally, someone who even fosters healing (Hall, 1969, p. 86).

Cure

The second area of the nursing process is shared with medicine and is labeled the "cure." Hall (1958) asserted that this medical aspect of nursing may be viewed as the nurse assisting the doctor by assuming medical tasks/functions or viewed as the nurse helping the patient through his or her medical, surgical, and rehabilitative care in the role of comforter and nurturer. Hall felt that the nursing profession was assuming more and more of the medical aspects of care while at the same time relinquishing the nurturing process of nursing to less well-prepared persons.

Interestingly enough, physicians do not have practical doctors. They don't need them . . . they have nurses. Interesting, too, is the fact that most nurses show by their delegation of nurturing to others, that they prefer being second class doctors to being first class nurses. This is the prerogative of any nurse. If she feels better in this role, why not? One good reason why not for more and more nurses is that with this increasing trend, patients receive from professional nurses second class doctoring; and from practical nurses, second class nursing. Some nurses would like the public to get first class nursing. Seeing the patient through [his or her] medical care without giving up the nurturing will keep the unique opportunity that personal closeness provides to further [the] patient's growth and rehabilitation. (Hall, 1958, p. 3)

Core

The third area that nursing shares with all of the helping professions is that of using relationships for therapeutic effect—the core. This area emphasizes the social, emotional, spiritual, and intellectual needs of the patient in relation to family, institution, community, and the world (Hall, 1955, 1958, 1965). Knowledge that is foundational to the core is based on the social sciences and on therapeutic use of self. Through the closeness offered by the provision of intimate bodily care, the patient will feel comfortable enough to explore with the nurse "who he is, where he is, where he wants to go, and will take or refuse help in getting there—the patient will make amazingly more rapid progress toward recovery and rehabilitation" (Hall, 1958, p. 3). Hall believed that through this process, the patient would emerge as a whole person.

Knowledge and skills the nurse needs to use self therapeutically include knowing self and learning interpersonal skills. The goals of the interpersonal process are to help patients to understand themselves as they participate in problem focusing and problem solving. Hall discussed the importance of nursing with the patient as opposed to nursing at, to, or for the patient. Hall reflected on the value of the therapeutic use of self by the professional nurse when she stated:

The nurse who knows self by the same token can love and trust the patient enough to work *with* him professionally, rather than for him technically, or at him vocationally.

Her goals cease being tied up with "where can I throw my nursing stuff around," or "how can I explain my nursing stuff to get the patient to do what we want him to do," or "how can I understand my patient so that I can handle him better." Instead her goals are linked up with "what is the problem?" and "how can I help the patient understand himself?" as he participates in problem facing and solving. In this way, the nurse recognizes that the power to heal lies in the patient and not in the nurse, unless she is healing herself. She takes satisfaction and pride in her ability to help the patient tap this source of power in his continuous growth and development. She becomes comfortable working cooperatively and consistently with members of other professions, as she meshes her contributions with theirs in a concerted program of care and rehabilitation. (Hall, 1958, p. 5)

Hall believed that the role of professional nursing was enacted through the provision of *care* that facilitates the interpersonal process and invites the patient to learn to reach the *core* of his difficulties while seeing him through the *cure* that is possible. Through the professional nursing process, the patient has the opportunity to see the illness as a learning experience from which he may emerge even healthier than before his illness (Hall, 1965).

Practice Applications

The practice of clinical nursing is goal directed, deliberately carried out, and patient centered.

—WIEDENBACH (1964, P. 23)

Wiedenbach

Figure 5-2 represents a spherical model that depicts the "experiencing individual" as the central focus (Wiedenbach, 1964). This model and detailed charts were later edited and published in *Clinical Nursing: A Helping Art* (Wiedenbach, 1964).

In a paper entitled "A Concept of Dynamic Nursing" Wiedenbach (1962, p. 7), described the model as follows:

In its broadest sense, Practice of Dynamic Nursing may be envisioned as a set of concentric circles, with the experiencing individual in the circle at its

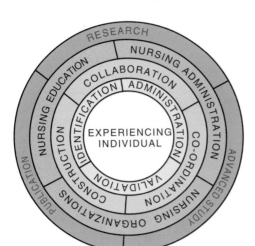

Figure 5 • 2 Professional nursing practice focus and components. *(Reprinted with permission from the Wiedenbach Reading Room [1962], Yale University School of Nursing.)*

core. Direct service, with its three components, identification of the individual's experienced need for help, ministration of help needed, and validation that the help provided fulfilled its purpose, fills the circle adjacent to the core. The next circle holds the essential concomitants of direct service: coordination, i.e., charting, recording, reporting, and conferring; consultation, i.e., conferencing, and seeking help or advice; and collaboration, i.e., giving assistance or cooperation with members of other professional or nonprofessional groups concerned with the individual's welfare. The content of the fourth circle represents activities which are essential to the ultimate well-being of the experiencing individual, but only indirectly related to him: nursing education, nursing administration, and nursing organizations. The outermost circle comprises research in nursing, publication, and advanced study, the key ways to progress in every area of practice.

Wiedenbach's nursing practice application of her prescriptive theory was evident in her practice examples. These often related to general basic nursing procedures and to maternity nursing practice.

Henderson

Based on the assumption that nursing has a unique function, Henderson believed that nursing independently initiates and controls

activities related to basic nursing care. Relating the conceptualization of basic care components with the unique functions of nursing provided the initial groundwork for introducing the concept of independent nursing practice. In her 1966 publication, *The Nature of Nursing,* Henderson stated: "It is my contention that the nurse is, and should be legally, an independent practitioner and able to make independent judgments as long as he, or she, is not diagnosing, prescribing treatment for disease, or making a prognosis, for these are the physician's functions" (Henderson, 1966, p. 22).

Furthermore, Henderson believed that functions pertaining to patient care could be categorized as nursing and non-nursing. She believed that limiting nursing activities to "nursing care" was a useful method of conserving professional nurse power (Harmer & Henderson, 1955). She defined non-nursing functions as those that are not a service to the person (mind and body) (Harmer & Henderson, 1955). For Henderson, examples of non-nursing functions included ordering supplies, cleaning and sterilizing equipment, and serving food (Harmer & Henderson, 1955).

At the same time, Henderson was not in favor of the practice of assigning patients to lesser trained workers on the basis of complexity level. For Henderson, "all 'nursing care' is essentially complex because it involves constant adaptation of procedures to the needs of the individual" (Harmer & Henderson, 1955, p. 9).

As the authority on basic nursing care, Henderson believed that the nurse has the responsibility to assess the needs of the individual patient, help individuals meet their health needs, and/or provide an environment in which the individual can perform activities unaided. It is the nurse's role, according to Henderson, "to 'get inside the patient's skin' and supplement his strength, will or knowledge according to his needs" (Harmer & Henderson, 1955, p. 5). Conceptualizing the nurse as a substitute for the patient's lack of necessary will, strength, or knowledge to attain good health and to complete or make the patient whole, highlights the complexity and uniqueness of nursing.

Based on the success of *Textbook of the Principles and Practice of Nursing* (fifth edition), Henderson was asked by the International Council of Nurses (ICN) to prepare a short essay that could be used as a guide for nursing in any part of the world. Despite Henderson's belief that it was difficult to promote a universal definition of nursing, *Basic Principles of Nursing Care* (Henderson, 1960) became an international sensation. To date, it has been published in 29 languages and is referred to as the 20th-century equivalent of Florence Nightingale's *Notes on Nursing*. After visiting countries worldwide, Henderson concluded that nursing varied from country to country and that rigorous attempts to define it have been unsuccessful, leaving the "nature of nursing" largely an unanswered question (Henderson, 1991).

Henderson's definition of nursing has had a lasting influence on the way nursing is practiced around the globe. She was one of the first nurses to articulate that nursing had a unique function yielding a valuable contribution to the health care of individuals. In writing reflections on the nature of nursing, Henderson (1966) states that her concept of nursing anticipates universally available health care and a partnership among doctors, nurses, and other health-care workers.

Hall

In 1963, Lydia Hall was able to actualize her vision of nursing through the creation of the Loeb Center for Nursing and Rehabilitation at Montefiore Medical Center. The center's major orientation was rehabilitation and subsequent discharge to home or to a long-term care institution, if further care was needed. Doctors referred patients to the center, and a professional nurse made admission decisions. Criteria for admission were based on the patient's need for rehabilitation nursing. What made the Loeb Center unique was the model of professional nursing that was implemented under Lydia Hall's guidance. The center's guiding philosophy was Hall's belief that during the rehabilitation phase of an illness experience, professional nurses were the best prepared to foster the rehabilitation process, decrease complications and recurrences, and promote health and prevent new illnesses.

Hall saw these outcomes being accomplished by the special and unique way nurses work with patients in a close interpersonal process with the goal of fostering learning, growth, and healing.

Practice Exemplars

Wiedenbach

The focus of practice is the experiencing individual, i.e., the individual for whom the nurse is caring, and the way he and only he perceived his condition or situation. For example, a mother had a red vaginal discharge on her first postpartum day. The doctor had recognized it as lochi, a normal concomitant of the phenomenon of involution, and had left an order for her to be up and move about. Instead of trying to get up, the mother remained, immobile in her bed. The nurse who wanted to help her out of bed expressed surprise at the mother's unwillingness to get up when she seemed to be progressing so well. The mother explained that she had a red discharge, and this to her was evidence of onset of hemorrhage. This terrified her and made her afraid to move. Her sister, she added, had hemorrhaged and almost lost her life the day after she had her baby two years ago. The nurse expressed her understanding of the mother's fear, but then encouraged her to compare her current experience with that of her sister. When the mother tried to do this, she recognized gross differences, and accepted the nurse's explanation of the origin of the discharge. The mother then voiced her relief, and validated it by getting out of bed without further encouragement (Wiedenbach, 1962, pp. 6–7).

Continued

Wiedenbach considered nursing a "practical phenomenon" that involved action. She believed that this was necessary to understand the theory that underlies the "nurse's way of nursing." This involved "knowing what the nurse wanted to accomplish, how she went about accomplishing it, and in what context she did what she did" (Wiedenbach, 1970, p. 1058).

Henderson

Henderson's definition of nursing and 14 components of basic nursing care can be useful in guiding the assessment and care of patients preparing for surgical procedures. For example, in assessing Mr. G.'s preoperative vital signs, the nurse noticed he seemed anxious. The nurse encouraged Mr. G. to express his concerns about the surgery. Mr. G. told the nurse that he had a fear of not being able to control his body and that he felt general anesthesia represented the extreme limit of loss of bodily control. The nurse recognized this concern as being directly related to Henderson's fourth component of basic nursing care: *Move and maintain desirable postures.* The nurse explained to Mr. G. that her role was to "perform those acts he would do for himself if he was not under the influence of anesthesia" (Gillette, 1996, p. 267) and that she would be responsible for maintaining his body in a comfortable and dignified position. She explained how he would need to be positioned during the surgical procedure, what part of his body would be exposed, and how long the procedure was expected to take. Mr. G. also told the nurse about an experience he had following an earlier surgical procedure in which he experienced pain in his right shoulder. Mr. G. expressed concern that being in one position too long during the surgery would damage his shoulder and result in waking up with shoulder pain again. Together they discussed positions that would be most comfortable for his shoulder during the upcoming proce-

dure, and she assured Mr. G. that she would be assessing his position throughout the procedure.

Hall

Hall envisioned that outcomes were accomplished by the special and unique way nurses work with patients in a close interpersonal process with the goal of fostering learning, growth, and healing. Her work at the Loeb Center serves as an administative exemplar of the application of her theory. At the Loeb Center, nursing was the chief therapy, with medicine and the other disciplines ancillary to nursing. In this new model of organization of nursing services, nursing was in charge of the total health program for the patient and was responsible for integrating all aspects of care. Only registered professional nurses were hired. The 80-bed unit was staffed with 44 professional nurses employed around the clock. Professional nurses gave direct patient care and teaching and were responsible for eight patients and their families. Senior staff nurses were available on each ward as resources and mentors for staff nurses. For every two professional nurses there was one nonprofessional worker called a "messenger-attendant." The messenger-attendants did not provide hands-on care to the patients. Instead, they performed such tasks as getting linen and supplies, thus freeing the nurse to nurse the patient (Hall, 1969). In addition, there were four ward secretaries. Morning and evening shifts were staffed at the same ratio. Night-shift staffing was less; however, Hall (1965) noted that there were "enough nurses at night to make rounds every hour and to nurse those patients who are awake around the concerns that may be keeping them awake" (p. 2). In most institutions of that time, the number of nurses was decreased during the evening and night shifts because it was felt that larger numbers of nurses were needed during the day to get the work done. Hall took exception to the idea that nursing service was organized around work to be done rather than the needs of the patients.

The patient was the center of care at Loeb and actively participated in all care decisions. Families were free to visit at any hour of the day or night. Rather than strict adherence to institutional routines and schedules, patients at the Loeb Center were encouraged to maintain their own usual patterns of daily activities, thus promoting independence and an easier transition to home. There was no chart section labeled "Doctor's Orders." Hall believed that to order a patient to do something violated the right of the patient to participate in his or her treatment plan. Instead, nurses shared the treatment plan with the patient and helped him or her to discuss his or her concerns and become an active learner in the rehabilitation process. In addition, there were no doctor's progress notes or nursing notes. Instead, all charting was done on a form entitled "Patient's Progress Notes." These notes included the patient's reaction to care, his concerns and feelings, his understanding of the problems, the goals he has identified, and how he sees his progress toward those goals. Patients were also encouraged to keep their own notes to share with their caregivers.

Staff conferences were held at least twice weekly as forums to discuss concerns, problems, or questions. A collaborative practice model between physicians and nurses evolved, and the shared knowledge of the two professions led to more effective team planning (Isler, 1964). The nursing stories published by nurses who worked at Loeb describe nursing situations that demonstrate the effect of professional nursing on patient outcomes. In addition, they reflect the satisfaction derived from practicing in a truly professional role (Alfano, 1971; Bowar, 1971; Bowar-Ferres, 1975; Englert, 1971).

◾ Summary

Among other theorists featured in Section II of this book, Wiedenbach, Henderson, and Hall introduced nursing theory to us in the mid-20th century. Each of these nurses reflected on her nursing practice and explored nurse–patient interactions using nursing practice as the basis for their thought and for their published scholarship. These nurse scholars defined the ways nursing is thought about, practiced, and researched, both in the United States and other countries around the world. Perhaps most importantly, each of these scholars stated and responded to the question "What is nursing?" Their responses helped all who followed to understand that the one nursed is a person, not an object, and that the relationship of nurse and patient is valuable to all.

References

Alfano, G. (1971). Healing or caretaking—which will it be? *Nursing Clinics of North America, 6,* 273–280.

Barron, M. A. (1966). The effects varied nursing approaches have on patients' complaints of pain. *Nursing Research, 15*(1), 90–91.

Birnbach, N. (1988). Lydia Eloise Hall, 1906–1969. In: V. L. Bullough, O. M. Church, & A. P. Stein (Eds.), *American nursing: A biographical dictionary* (pp. 161–163). New York: Garland Publishing.

Bochnak, M. A. (1963). The effect of an automatic and deliberative process of nursing activity on the relief of patients' pain: A clinical experiment. *Nursing Research, 12*(3), 191–193.

Bowar, S. (1971). Enabling professional practice through leadership skills. *Nursing Clinics of North America, 6,* 293–301.

Bowar-Ferres, S. (1975). Loeb Center and its philosophy of nursing. *American Journal of Nursing, 75,* 810–815.

Chinn, P. L., & Jacobs, M. K. (1987). *Theory and nursing.* St. Louis, MO: C. V. Mosby.

Dickoff, J., James, P., & Wiedenbach, E. (1968). Theory in a practice discipline. *Nursing Research, 14*(5), 415–437.

Dumas, R. G., & Leonard, R. C. (1963). The effect of nursing on the incidence of post-operative vomiting. *Nursing Research, 12*(1), 12–15.

Elms, R. R., & Leonard, R. C. (1966). The effects of nursing approaches during admission. *Nursing Research, 15*(1), 39–48.

Englert, B. (1971). How a staff nurse perceives her role at Loeb Center. *Nursing Clinics of North America, 6*(2), 281–292.

Gesse, T., & Dombro, M. (2001). Ernestine Wiedenbach clinical nursing: A helping art. In: M. Parker (Ed.), *Nursing theories and nursing practice* (pp. 69–84). Philadelphia: F. A. Davis.

Gesse, T., Dombro, M., Gordon, S. C. & Rittman, M. R. (2006). Twentieth-Century nursing: Wiedenbach, Henderson, and Orlando's theories and their applications. In: M. Parker (Ed.), *Nursing theories and nursing practice* (2nd ed., pp. 70–78). Philadelphia: F. A. Davis.

Gillette, V. A. (1996). Applying nursing theory to perioperative nursing practice. *AORN, 64*(2), 261–270.

Gordon, S. C. (2001). Virginia Avenel Henderson definition of nursing. In: M. Parker (Ed.), *Nursing theories and nursing practice* (pp. 143–149). Philadelphia: F. A. Davis.

Gowan, N. I., & Morris, M. (1964). Nurses' responses to expressed patient needs. *Nursing Research, 13*(1), 68–71.

Hall, L. E. (1955). *Quality of nursing care.* Manuscript of an address before a meeting of the Department of Baccalaureate and Higher Degree Programs of the New Jersey League for Nursing, February 7, 1955, at Seton Hall University, Newark, New Jersey. Montefiore Medical Center Archives, Bronx, New York.

Hall, L. E. (1958). *Nursing: What is it?* Manuscript. Montefiore Medical Center Archives, Bronx, New York.

Hall, L. E. (1963, March). *Summary of project report: Loeb Center for Nursing and Rehabilitation.* Unpublished report. Montefiore Medical Center Archives, Bronx, New York.

Hall, L. E. (1964). Nursing—what is it? *Canadian Nurse, 60,* 150–154.

Hall, L. E. (1965). *Another view of nursing care and quality.* Address delivered at Catholic University, Washington, DC. Unpublished report. Montefiore Medical Center Archives, Bronx, New York.

Harmer, B., & Henderson, V. A. (1955). *Textbook of the principles and practice of nursing.* New York: Macmillan.

Henderson, V. A. (1960). *Basic principles of nursing care.* Geneva: International Council of Nurses.

Henderson, V. A. (1966). *The nature of nursing.* New York: The National League for Nursing Press.

Henderson, V. A. (1991). *The nature of nursing: Reflections after 25 years.* New York: The National League for Nursing Press.

Isler, C. (June, 1964). New concept in nursing therapy: Care as the patient improves. *RN,* 58–70.

Marriner-Tomey, A., Peskoe, K., & Gumm, S. (1989). Lydia E. Hall core, care, and cure model. In A. M. Marriner-Tomey (Ed.), *Nursing theorists and their work* (pp. 109–117). St. Louis, MO: C. V. Mosby.

McBride, A. B. (Narrator). (1997). Celebrating Virginia Henderson (video). Available from Center for Nursing Press, 550 West North Street, Indianapolis, IN 46202.

Montefiore cuts readmissions 80%. (1966, February 23). *The New York Times.*

Nickel, S., Gesse, T., & MacLaren, A. (1992). Her professional legacy. *Journal of Nurse Midwifery, 3,* 161.

Stevens-Barnum, B. J. (1990). *Nursing theory analysis, application, evaluation* (3rd ed.). Glenview, IL: Scott, Foresman/Little Brown.

Touhy, T., & Birnbach, N. (2006). Lydia Hall: The Care, Core, and Cure Model and its applications. In: M. Parker (Ed.), *Nursing theories and nursing practice* (2nd ed., pp. 113–124). Philadelphia: F. A. Davis.

Tryson, P. A. (1963). An experiment of the effect of patients' participation in planning the administration of a nursing procedure. *Nursing Research, 12*(4), 262–265.

Wiedenbach, E. (1962). *A concept of dynamic nursing: Philosophy, purpose, practice and process.* Paper presented at the Conference on Maternal and Child Nursing, Pittsburgh, PA. Archives, Yale University School of Nursing, New Haven, CT.

Wiedenbach, E. (1963). The helping art of nursing. *American Journal of Nursing, 63*(11), 54–57.

Wiedenbach, E. (1964). *Clinical nursing: A helping art.* New York: Springer.

Wiedenbach, E. (1969). *Meeting the realities in clinical teaching.* New York: Springer.

Wiedenbach, E. (1970). *A systematic inquiry: Application of theory to nursing practice.* Paper presented at Duke University, Durham, NC (author's personal files).

Chapter **6**

Nurse–Patient Relationship Theories: Hildegard Peplau, Joyce Travelbee, and Ida Jean Orlando

ANN R. PEDEN, KAITLIN A. LAUBHAM,
AUTUMN WELLS, JACQUELINE STAAL,
AND MAUDE RITTMAN

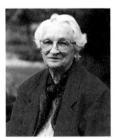

Hiledegard Peplau

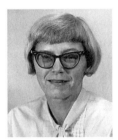

Joyce Travelbee

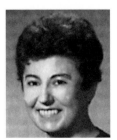

Ida Jean Orlando

The nurse–patient relationship was a significant focus of early conceptualizations of nursing. Hildegard Peplau, Joyce Travelbee, and Ida Jean Orlando were three early nursing scholars who explicated the nature of this relationship. Their work situated the focus of nursing from performance of tasks to engagement in a therapeutic relationship designed to facilitate health and healing. Each of these conceptualizations will be described in Parts One, Two, and Three of the chapter.

Introducing the Theorist

Hildegard Peplau was an outstanding leader and pioneer in psychiatric nursing whose career spanned seven decades. A review of the events in her life also serves as an introduction to the history of modern psychiatric nursing. With the publication of *Interpersonal Relations in Nursing* in 1952, Peplau provided a framework for the practice of psychiatric nursing that would result in a paradigm shift in this field of nursing. Before this, patients were viewed as objects to be observed. Peplau taught that patients were not objects, but were subjects, and that psychiatric nurses must participate with the patients, engaging in the nurse–patient relationship. This was a revolutionary idea. Although *Interpersonal Relations in Nursing* was not well received when it was first published in 1952, later the book's influence was widespread, and it was reprinted in 1988 and has been translated into at least six languages.

Hildegard Peplau entered nursing for practical reasons, seeing it as a way to leave home and have an occupation. As she adapted to nursing school, she made the conscious decision that if she was going to be a nurse, then she would be a good one (Peplau, 1998).

Peplau served as the college head nurse and later as executive officer of the Health Service at Bennington College, Vermont. While working there, she began taking courses that would lead to a Bachelor of Arts degree in interpersonal psychology. Dr. Eric Fromm

was one of her teachers at Bennington. An experience while working in the Health Service piqued Peplau's interest in psychiatric nursing. A young student with symptoms of schizophrenia came to the clinic seeking help. Peplau did not know what to do for her. The student left Bennington to receive treatment and returned to complete her education. Observing the successful recovery of this young woman was a positive experience for Peplau.

On graduation from Bennington, Peplau joined the Army Nurse Corps. She was assigned to the School of Military Neuropsychiatry in England. This experience introduced her to the psychiatric problems of soldiers at war and allowed her to work with many great psychiatrists. After the war, Peplau attended Columbia University on the GI Bill and earned her master's degree in psychiatric–mental health nursing.

After her graduation in 1948, Peplau was invited to remain at Columbia and teach in their master's program. She immediately searched the library for books to use with students, but found very few. At that time, the psychiatric nurse was viewed as a companion to patients, someone who would play games and take walks, but talk about nothing substantial. In fact, nurses were instructed not to talk to patients about their problems, thoughts, or feelings. Peplau began teaching at Columbia, knowing that she wanted to change the education and practice of psychiatric nursing. There was no direction for what to include in graduate nursing programs. She took educational experiences from psychiatry and psychology and adapted them to her conceptualization of nursing. Peplau described this as a time of "innovation or nothing."

Her goal was to prepare nurse psychotherapists, referring to this training as "talking to patients" (Peplau, 1960, 1962). She arranged clinical experiences for her students at Brooklyn State Hospital, the only hospital in the New York City area that would take them. At the hospital, students were assigned to back wards, working with the most chronic and severely ill patients. Each student met twice weekly with the same patient, for a session lasting 1 hour. According to Peplau, the nurses resisted this practice tremendously and thought it was an awful thing to do (Peplau, 1998). Using carbon paper, verbatim notes were taken during the session. Students then met individually with Peplau to go over the interaction in detail. Through this process, both Peplau and her students began to learn what was helpful and what was harmful in the interaction.

In 1955, Peplau left Columbia to teach at Rutgers, where she began the Clinical Nurse Specialist program in psychiatric–mental health nursing. The students were prepared as nurse psychotherapists, developing expertise in individual, group, and family therapies. Peplau required of her students "unflinching self-scrutiny," examining their own verbal and nonverbal communication and its effects on the nurse–patient relationship. Students were encouraged to ask, "What message am I sending?"

In 1956, Peplau began spending her summers touring the country, offering week-long clinical workshops in state hospitals. This activity was instrumental in teaching interpersonal theory and the importance of the nurse–patient relationship to psychiatric nurses. The workshops also provided a forum from which Peplau could promote advanced education for psychiatric nurses. Her belief that psychiatric nurses must have advanced degrees encouraged large numbers of psychiatric nurses to seek master's degrees and eventual certification as psychiatric–mental health clinical specialists.

During her career as a nursing educator, a total of 100 students had the opportunity to study with Peplau. These students have become leaders in psychiatric nursing. Many went on to earn doctoral degrees, becoming psychoanalysts, writing prolifically in the field of psychiatric nursing, and entering and influencing the academic world. Their influence has resulted in the integration of the nurse–patient relationship and the concept of anxiety into the culture of nursing. In 1974, Peplau retired from Rutgers, which allowed her more time to devote to the larger profession of nursing. Throughout her career,

Peplau actively contributed to the American Nurses' Association (ANA) by serving on various committees and task forces. She was the only person who had been both the executive director and president of ANA. Peplau served on the ANA committee that wrote the Social Policy Statement. For the first time in nursing's history, nursing had a phenomenological focus—human responses.

Peplau held 11 honorary degrees. In 1994, she was inducted into the American Academy of Nursing's Living Legends Hall of Fame. She was named one of the 50 great Americans by *Marquis Who's Who* in 1995. In 1997, Peplau received the Christiane Reiman Prize. In 1998, she was inducted into the ANA Hall of Fame.

Internationally, Peplau was an advisor to the World Health Organization (WHO); she was a member of their First Nursing Advisory Committee and contributed to WHO's first paper on psychiatric nursing. She served as a consultant to the Pan-American Health Association and she served two terms on the International Council of Nurses' Board of Directors. Even after her retirement, she continued to mentor nurses in many countries.

Hildegard Peplau died in March 1999 at her home in Sherman Oaks, California.

Overview of Peplau's Nurse–Patient Relationship Theory

Peplau (1952) defined nursing as a "significant, therapeutic, interpersonal process" that is an "educative instrument, a maturing force, that aims to promote foreward movement of personality in the direction of creative, constructive, productive, personal, and community living" (p. 16). Peplau was the first nursing theorist to identify the nurse–patient relationship as being central to all nursing care. In fact, nursing cannot occur if there is no relationship, or connection, between the patient and the nurse. Her work, while written for all nursing specialties, provides specific guidelines for the psychiatric nurse.

The nurse brings to the relationship professional expertise which includes clinical knowledge. Peplau valued knowledge, believing that the psychiatric nurse must possess extensive knowledge about the potential problems that emerge during a nurse–patient interaction. The nurse must understand psychiatric illnesses and their treatments (Peplau, 1987). The nurse interacts with the patients as both a resource person and a teacher (Peplau, 1952). Through education and supervision, the nurse develops the knowledge base required to select the most appropriate nursing intervention. In order to fully engage in the nurse–patient relationship, the nurse must possess intellectual, interpersonal, and social skills. These are the same skills often diminished or lacking in psychiatric patients. For nurses to promote growth in patients, they must themselves use these skills competently (Peplau, 1987).

There are four components of the nurse–patient relationship: two individuals (nurse and patient), professional expertise, and patient need (Peplau, 1992). The goal of the nurse–patient relationship is to further the personal development of the patient (Peplau, 1960). Nurse and patient meet as "strangers" who interact differently than friends would. The role of stranger implies respect and positive interest in the patient as an individual. The nurse "accepts the patients as they are and interacts with them as emotionally able strangers and relating on this basis until evidence shows otherwise" (Peplau, 1952, p. 44). Peplau valued therapeutic communication as a key component of nurse–patient interactions. She advised strongly against the use of "social chit-chat." In fact, she would view this as wasting valuable time with your patient. Every interaction must focus on being therapeutic. Even something as simple as sharing a meal with psychiatric patients can be a therapeutic encounter.

The nurse–patient relationship, viewed as growth-promoting with forward movement, is enhanced when nurses are aware of how their own behavior affects the patient. The "behavior of the nurse-as-a-person interacting with the patient-as-a person has significant impact on the patient's well-being and the quality and outcome of nursing care" (Peplau, 1992, p. 14). An essential component of this relationship is the continuing process of the nurse becoming more self-aware. This occurs via supervision.

Peplau (1989a) recommended that nurses participate in weekly supervision meetings with an expert nurse clinician. The focus of the supervisory meetings is on the nurses' interactions with patients. The primary purpose is to review observations and interpersonal patterns that the nurse has made or used. The goal is always to develop the nurse's skills as an expert in interpersonal relations. Peplau (1989a) emphasized "the slow but sure growth of nurses" (p. 166) as they developed their competencies in working with patients. Not only are patient problems reviewed but treatment options and the nurses' own pattern of responding to the patient are explored. If an interaction between a nurse and a patient has not gone well, the nurse's response is to examine his/her own behaviors first. Asking questions such as, "Did my own anxiety interfere with this interaction?" or "Is there something in my experiences that influenced how I interacted with this patient?" leads to continual growth and development as a skilled clinician. This process also assures the delivery of quality care in psychiatric settings. Supervision continues to be an important aspect in advanced practice psychiatric nursing and is a requirement for certification as a psychiatric clinical specialist or nurse practitioner. Supervision is essential as the nurse assumes the role of counselor. In this role, the nurse assists the patient to integrate the thoughts and feelings associated with the illness into the patient's own life experiences (Lakeman, 1999).

The nurse–patient relationship is objective and its focus is on the needs of the patient. To focus on the patient's needs, the nurse must be a skilled listener and able to respond in ways that foster the patient's growth and return to health. Active listening facilitates the nurse–patient relationship. As Peplau wrote in 1960, nursing is an "opportunity to further the patient's learning about himself (sic), the focus in the nurse-patient relationship will be upon the patient – his (sic) needs, difficulties, lack in interpersonal competence, interest in living" (Peplau, 1960, p. 966). Within the nurse–patient relationship, the nurse works "to create a mood that encourages clients to reflect, to restructure perceptions and views of situations as needed, to get in touch with their feelings, and to connect interpersonally with other people" (Peplau, 1988, p. 10). While the nurse-patient relationship is "time-limited in both duration and frequency, the aim is to create an interpersonally intimate encounter, however brief, as if two whole persons are involved in a purposive, enduring relationship; this requires discipline and skill on the part of the nurse" (p. 11). Peplau continued to emphasize that nurses must possess "well-developed intellectual competencies, and disciplined attention to the work at hand" (p. 13).

Communication, both verbal and nonverbal, is an essential component of the nurse–patient relationship. However, in Peplau's view, verbal communication is required in order for the nurse-patient relationship to develop. She writes, "anything clients act out with nurses will most probably not be talked about, and that which is not discussed cannot be understood" (Peplau, 1989a, p. 197). One objective of the nurse–patient relationship is to talk about the problem or need that has resulted in the patient interacting with the nurse. Peplau provided descriptions of phrases commonly used by patients that require clarification on the part of the nurse. These included referring to "they," using the phrase, "you know," and overgeneralizing responses to situations. The nurse clarifies who "they" are, responds that she/he does not know and needs further information, and assists patients to be more specific as they describe their experiences (Forchuk, 1993).

Phases of the Nurse–Patient Relationship

Peplau introduced the phases of the nurse–patient relationship in her Interpersonal Relations Theory (1952). This time-limited relationship is interpersonal in nature and has a starting point, proceeds through identifiable phases, and ends. Initially, Peplau included four phases in the relationship: orientation, identification, exploitation, and resolution (Peplau, 1952). In 1991, Forchuk, a Canadian researcher who has tested and refined some of Peplau's work, proposed three phases: orientation, working, and resolution (Peplau, 1992). Forchuk's recommendation of a three-phase nurse–patient relationship resolves the lack of easy differentiation between the identification and exploitation stages. These two phases were collapsed into the working phase. By renaming theses two phases the working phase, a more accurate reflection of what actually occurs in this important aspect of the nurse–patient relationship is provided. Although the nurse–patient relationship is time limited in nature, much of this relationship is spent "working."

Orientation Phase

The relationship begins with the orientation phase (Peplau, 1952). This phase is particularly important because it sets the stage for the development of the relationship. During the orientation period, the nurse and patient's relationship is still new and unfamiliar. Nurse and patient get to know each other as people; their expectations and roles are understood. During this first phase, the patient expresses a "felt need" and seeks professional assistance from the nurse. In reaction to this need, the nurse helps the individual by recognizing and assessing his or her situation. It is during the assessment that the patient's needs are evaluated by the patient and nurse working together as a team. Through this process, trust develops between the patient and the nurse. Also, the parameters for the relationship are clarified. Based on the assessment information, nursing diagnoses; goals; and outcomes for the patient are created. Nursing interventions are implemented and the evaluations of the patient's goals are also incorporated (Peplau, 1992).

Working Phase

The working phase incorporates identification and exploitation. The focus of the working phase is twofold: first is the patient, who "exploits" resources to improve health; second is the nurse, who enacts the roles of "resource person, counselor, surrogate, and teacher in facilitating...development toward well-being" (Fitzpatrick & Wallace, 2005, p. 460). This phase of the relationship is meant to be flexible, so that the patient is able to function "dependently, independently, or interdependently with the nurse, based on...developmental capacity, level of anxiety, self-awareness, and needs" (Fitzpatrick, 2005, p. 460). A balance between independence and dependence must exist here, and it is the nurse who must aid the patient in its development (Lakeman, 1999).

During the exploitation phase of the working phase, the client assumes an active role in the health team by taking advantage of available services and determining the degree to which they are used (Erci, 2008). Within this phase, the client begins to develop responsibility and independence, becoming better able to face new challenges in the future (Erci, 2008). Peplau writes that "Exploiting what a situation offers gives rise to new differentiations of the problem and the development and improvement of skill in interpersonal relations" (Peplau, 1992, pp. 41–42).

Resolution Phase

The resolution phase is the last phase and involves the patient's continual movement from dependence to independence, based on both a distancing from the nurse and a strengthening of individual's ability to manage care (Peplau, 1952). According to Peplau, resolution can take place only when the patient has gained the ability to be free from nursing assistance and act independently (Lloyd, Hancock, & Campbell, 2007). At this point, old needs are abandoned and new goals are adopted (Lakeman, 1999). The completion of the resolution phase results in the mutual termination of the nurse–patient relationship and involves planning for future sources of support (Peplau, 1952). Completion of this final phase

"is one measure of the success of...all the other phases" (Lloyd et al., 2007, p. 50).

Practice Applications

Almost all of the research that has tested Peplau's nurse–patient relationship has been conducted by Forchuk (1994, 1995) and colleagues (Forchuk & Brown, 1989; Forchuk, Westwell, Martin, Azzapardi, Kosterewa-Tolman, & Hus, 2000; Forchuk, Jewell, Schofield, Sircelj, & Vallendor, 1998). Much of Forchuk's work has focused on the orientation phase. Forchuk and Brown emphasized the importance of being able to identify the orientation phase and not rush movement into the working phase. To assist in this, Forchuk and Brown (1989) developed a one-page instrument, the Relationship Form, which they have used to determine the current phase of the relationship and overall progression from phase to phase. For additional information, please visit DavisPlus at http://davisplus.fadavis.com.

Peplau first wrote about the nurse–patient relationship in 1952. She hoped that through this work nurses would change how they interacted with their patients. She wanted nurses to "do with" clients rather than "do to" (Forchuk, 1993). The majority of the work that has tested Peplau's nurse–patient relationship has been conducted with individuals with severe mental illness, many of them in psychiatric hospitals. In these studies, patients did move through the phases of the nurse–patient relationship. As psychiatric nurses have changed the location of their practice from hospital to community, they have carried Peplau's work to this new arena. Unfortunately, there has been limited testing of the nurse–patient relationship in community settings. Parrish, Peden, and Staten (2008) explored strategies used by advanced practice psychiatric nurses treating individuals with depression. All the participants in this study practiced in community settings. When describing the strategies used, the nurse–patient relationship was the primary vehicle by which strategies were delivered. These strategies included active listening, partnering with the client, and a holistic view of the client. This work supports the integration of Peplau's nurse–patient relationship into the work of the psychiatric nurse.

However, more studies are needed that focus on the use of the nurse–patient relationship in community settings. The delivery of psychiatric care has radically changed in the last 10 years; however, the nurse–patient relationship continues to be the vehicle by which psychiatric nursing care is delivered. Further studies must examine the progression of the phases of the nurse–patient relationship in the managed care environment in psychiatry.

Practice Exemplar

Karen Thomas is a 49-year-old married woman who has a scheduled appointment with an advanced practice psychiatric nurse (APPN). She appears anxious and uncomfortable in the encounter with the APPN. In an effort to help Ms. Thomas feel more comfortable, the APPN offers her a glass of water or cup of coffee. Ms. Thomas announces that she has not eaten all day and would like something to drink. The APPN provides a cup of water and several crackers for Ms. Thomas to eat. Once they are both seated, the APPN asks Ms. Thomas about the reason for the appointment (what brought her here today). Ms. Thomas replies that she does not know; her husband made the appointment for her. In order to more fully understand the reason for her husband making the appointment, the APPN asks Ms. Thomas to tell her what aspects of her behavior were viewed by her husband as calling for attention. Once again, Ms. Thomas shares that she does not know. Continuing to focus on getting acquainted and enhancing Ms. Thomas's comfort in this beginning relationship, the APPN asks Ms. Thomas to tell her about herself. Ms. Thomas shares that she has been depressed in the past and was treated by a psychiatric nurse practitioner who prescribed an antidepressant medication. Becoming tearful, she also shares that she has left her husband several days ago and has moved in with her oldest son, stating that she just needs some time to think. For the next 15 minutes, Ms. Thomas talks about her marriage, her love for her husband, and her lack of trust in him. She also shares symptoms of depression that are present. Ms. Thomas speaks tangentially and is a poor historian when recalling events in the marriage that have caused her pain. Her responses are guarded as she alludes to marital infidelity on the part of her husband. Interspersed throughout the conversation are statements about her dislike of medications. The APPN then begins to ask more pointed assessment questions related to depressive symptoms. Ms. Thomas shares that she has very poor sleep, cannot concentrate, is isolating herself, has difficulties making decisions, and feels hopeless about her future. At this point, Ms. Thomas also shares that she had never taken the antidepressant prescribed for her. By sharing this, Ms. Thomas indicates the beginning of a trusting relationship with the APPN. Once the initial assessment is complete, a preliminary diagnosis is determined, and client and nurse are ready to move into the working phase.

The working phase is initiated with problem identification. For Ms. Thomas, the primary problem is major depression with a secondary problem, partner-relational issues. The APPN, acting as a resource person, provides education about the illness, major depression. Included is information about the biological causes of the illness, genetic predisposition, and explanations about the symptoms. A partnership is formed as the APPN and Ms. Thomas discuss treatment options. While Ms. Thomas shares that she does not like to take medications, she agrees to an appointment with a psychiatric nurse practitioner who will conduct a medication evaluation. That appointment is scheduled later in the week. Ms. Thomas also shares that she really wants to talk about her relationship with her husband and come to some decision about the future of their marriage. Marital counseling is mentioned as a possible treatment option, but the APPN suggests that this be delayed until

Continued

Ms. Thomas's depressive symptoms have decreased. The first session ends with both client and nurse committed to working to decrease Ms. Thomas's depressive symptoms. Ms. Thomas is reminded about her appointment for a medication evaluation and a second therapy appointment is made with the APPN.

At the second visit, Ms. Thomas reports that she has started taking an antidepressant but as of yet has not seen any relief of her symptoms. The APPN provides information about the usual length of time required for results to occur. While Ms. Thomas does not see noticeable results from the medication, the APPN shares that Ms. Thomas looks more relaxed and seems less anxious. Ms. Thomas states that she would like to spend this session talking about her relationship with her husband. She describes what was once a very happy marriage. The APPN listens, asks for clarification when needed, and encourages Ms. Thomas to share her perceptions of her marriage. The APPN asks Ms. Thomas again to talk about what might have caused her husband to call and make the therapy appointment for her. Ms. Thomas shares that her husband does not want their marriage to end; however, she is not sure yet about their future. Her perception is that her husband thinks she is the one with the problem and once she is "fixed" that their marriage will return to its former state of happiness. The session ends with the APPN asking Ms. Thomas to focus on her own physical and mental health. Possible interventions include beginning an exercise program, practicing stress reduction strategies, and reconnecting with individuals who have been supportive in the past.

At the next session, Ms. Thomas is noticeably improved. She states that she is sleeping, she is not crying as much, she is concentrating better, and she is feeling more hopeful about her marriage. She also shares that she and her husband have met for dinner several times and that he is willing to come with her for marital counseling. However, she shares that she is not yet ready for this, preferring to spend time focusing on her own mental health. Over the course of several months, Ms. Thomas and the APPN meet. In these sessions, Ms. Thomas explores her childhood, talks about the recent death of her mother, decides to begin a new exercise program, and reconnects with childhood friends. Through this work, Ms. Thomas grows more secure in who she is and in how she wants to live. During this same time period, she continues to meet her husband regularly for dinner, and sometimes, a movie.

At their final session, Ms. Thomas shares that she is ready to go with her husband to marital counseling. As a result of antidepressant medication and therapy, the problem of major depression has been resolved. However, the focus of this last session returns to depression. This is done in order to help Ms. Thomas recognize the early symptoms of depression in order to prevent a relapse. Ms. Thomas shares that her first symptoms were not sleeping well and withdrawing from friends and family. The APPN emphasizes the importance of monitoring this and calling for an appointment if these early symptoms occur. The focus now is on the secondary problem of partner-relationship issues. With this, the APPN makes a referral to a marital and family therapist.

References

Beck, A. T., Ward, C. H., Mendelson, M., Mock, L., & Erbaugh, J. (1961). An inventory for measuring depression. *Archives of General Psychiatry, 4,* 561–571.

Coatsworth-Puspoky, Forchuk, C., & Ward-Griffin, C. (2006). Nurse-client processes in mental health:

Recipient's perspectives. *Journal of Psychiatric and Mental Health Nursing, 13,* 347–355.

Erci, B. (2008). Nursing theories applied to vulnerable populations: Examples from Turkey. In: M. de Chesney & B. A. Anderson, (Eds.), *Caring for the vulnerable: Perspectives in nursing theory, practice and research* (2nd ed., pp. 45-60). Sudbury, MA: Jones and Bartlett.

Fitzpatrick, J. J., & Wallace, M. (2005). *Encyclopedia of nursing research.* New York: Springer.

Forchuk, C. (1993). *Hildegard E. Peplau: Interpersonal nursing.* Newbury Park, CA: Sage.

Forchuk, C. (1994). The orientation phase of the nurse-client relationship: Testing Peplau's theory. *Journal of Advanced Nursing, 20*(3), 532–537.

Forchuk, C. (1995). Development of nurse-client relationship: What helps? *Journal of the American Psychiatric Nurses Association, 1*, 146–151.

Forchuk, C., & Brown, B. (1989). Establishing a nurse-client relationship. *Journal of Psychosocial Nursing, 27*(2), 30–34.

Forchuk, C., Jewell, J., Schofield, R., Sircelj, M., & Valledor, T. (1998). From hospital to community: Bridging therapeutic relationships. *Journal of Psychiatric and Mental Health Nursing, 5*, 197–202.

Forchuk, C., Westwell, J., Martin, A., Azzapardi, W. B., Kosterewa-Tolman, D., & Hux, M. (1998). Factors influencing movement of chronic psychiatric patients from the orientation to the working phase of the nurse-client relationship on an inpatient unit. *Perspectives in Psychiatric Care, 34*, 36–44.

Forchuk, C., Westwell, J., Martin, M., Bamber-Azzaparadi, W., Kosterewa-Tolman, D., & Hux, M. (2000). The developing nurse-client relationship: Nurses' perspectives. *Journal of the American Psychiatric Nurses Association, 6*, 3–10.

Lakeman, R. (1999). *Remembering Hildegard Peplau. Vision, 5*(8), 29–31.

Lloyd, H., Hancock, H., & Campbell, S. (2007). *Principles of care.* London: Blackwell.

Morrison, E. G. (1992). Inpatient practice: An integrated framework. *Journal of Psychosocial Nursing and Mental Health Services, 30*(1), 26–29.

O'Toole, A., & Welt, S. R. (1989). *Interpersonal theory in nursing practice: Selected works of Hildegard Peplau.* New York: Springer.

Parrish, E., Peden, A. R., & Staten, R. R. (2008). Strategies used by advanced practice psychiatric nurses in treating adults with depression. *Perspectives in Psychiatric Care, 44*, 232–240.

Peplau, H. E. (1952). *Interpersonal relations in nursing.* New York: G. P. Putnam's Sons. (English edition reissued as a paperback in 1988 by Macmillan Education, London.)

Peplau, H. E. (1960). Talking with patients. *American Journal of Nursing, 60*, 964–967.

Peplau, H. E. (1962). The crux of psychiatric nursing. *American Journal of Nursing, 62*, 50–54.

Peplau, H. E. (1987). Tomorrow's world. *Nursing Times, 83*, 29–33.

Peplau, H. E. (1988). The art and science of nursing: Similarities, differences and relations. *Nursing Science Quarterly, 1*, 8–15.

Peplau, H. E. (1989a). Clinical supervision of staff nurses. In: A. O'Toole, & S. R. Welt (Eds.), *Interpersonal theory in nursing practice: Selected works of Hildegard Peplau* (pp. 164–167). New York: Springer.

Peplau, H. E. (1989b). Therapeutic nurse–patient interactions. In: A. O'Toole & S. R. Welt (Eds.), *Interpersonal theory in nursing practice: Selected works of Hildegard Peplau* (pp. 192–204). New York: Springer.

Peplau, H. E. (1992). Interpersonal relations: A theoretical framework for application in nursing practice. *Nursing Science Quarterly, 5*(1), 13–18.

Peplau, H. E. (1998). *Life of an angel: Interview with Hildegard Peplau (1998).* Hatherleigh Co. Audiotape available from the American Psychiatric Nurses Association. www.apna.org/items.htm

Part Two   Travelbee's Human-to-Human Relationship Model

Introducing the Theorist

Joyce Travelbee (1926–1973) was a nurse educator and psychiatric nurse practitioner and was enrolled in doctoral study at the time of her death at age 47 (O'Brien, 2008). She is best known for her human-to-human relationship model, a mid-range theory based on the nursing process. Travelbee graduated from the diploma nursing program at Charity Hospital in New Orleans, received her Bachelor of Science degree from Louisiana State University, and obtained her Master of Science in Nursing degree from Yale University (Meleis, 1997). She taught psychiatric and mental health nursing and was a professor of nursing at Louisiana State University, New Orleans, an instructor in the Department of Nursing Education at New York University, a professor in the University of Mississippi School of Nursing in Jackson, and a professor at the Hotel Dieu School of Nursing in New Orleans, Louisiana (Meleis, 1997; Travelbee, 1971). Her human-to-human relationship model was based on the work of nurse theorists Hildegard Peplau and Ida Jean Orlando (Tomey & Alligood, 2006).

Overview of Travelbee's Human-to-Human Relationship Model Theory

Caring, in the human-to-human relationship model, involves the dynamic, reciprocal, interpersonal connection between the nurse and patient, developed through communication and the mutual commitment to perceive self and other as unique and valued. Through the therapeutic use of self and the integration of evidence-based knowledge, the nurse provides quality patient care that can foster the patient's trust and confidence in the nurse (Travelbee, 1971). The meaning of the illness experience becomes self-actualizing for the patient as the nurse helps the patient find meaning in the experience. The human-to-human relationship "refers to an experience or series of experiences between the human being who is nurse and an ill person," culminating in the nurse meeting the ill person's unique needs (Travelbee, 1971, pp. 16–17). The term "patient" is not used in Travelbee's model, as "patient" refers to a label or category of people, rather than a unique individual in need of nursing care. The purpose of nursing, according to Travelbee (1971), is "to assist an individual, family or community to prevent or cope with the experience of illness and suffering and, if necessary, to find meaning in these experiences" (p. 16). Simply caring about an individual is not sufficient for providing quality care, but rather the integration of a broad knowledge base with the therapeutic use of self is needed.

Transcendence of the traditional titles of "nurse" and "patient" is necessary to prevent dehumanization of the ill person. With the rapid expansion of health technology, combined with financial constraints leading to restructuring of nurse–patient ratios, competing demands are placed on the nurse's time and attention. An emotional detachment between the nurse and ill person is created when the nurse views the ill person as the category of "patient," rather than as a unique individual with his own understanding of the illness experience. By performing nursing tasks without an emotional investment in the nurse–patient relationship, the ill person's physical needs are met. However, the ill person recognizes the lack of caring in the transaction and is left alone to suffer with the symptoms of illness. Dehumanization occurs when the ill person is left alone to find meaning in his illness experience.

Questions such as "why me?" or "why my loved one?" may be asked by many ill persons and their family members. By inquiring into the individual's perception of his illness and how he has derived meaning from his illness experience, the nurse can assess his coping ability and provide nursing interventions to prevent suffering and despair. Hope and motivation are important nursing tasks in caring for an ill person in despair. However, the nurse "cannot 'give' hope to another person; she can, however, strive to provide some ways and means for an ill person to experience hope" (Travelbee, 1971, p. 83).

All human beings endure suffering, though the experience of suffering differs from one individual to another (Travelbee, 1971). According to Meleis (1997), "a person's attitude toward suffering ultimately determines how effectively he copes with illness" (p. 361). If the patient's needs are not met in his suffering, he may develop "despairful not-caring," in which he does not care if he dies or recovers, or "apathetic indifference," in which he has "lost the will to live" (Travelbee, 1971, pp. 180–181). Hope helps the suffering person to cope, and it is an assumption of Travelbee's (1971) that "the role of the nurse...(is) to assist the ill person (to) experience hope in order to cope with the stress of illness and suffering" (p. 77).

To relieve the patient's suffering and to foster hope, the nurse provides care based on the individual's unique needs. Nursing care, according to Travelbee (1971), is delivered through five stages: observation, interpretation, decision-making, action (or nursing intervention), and appraisal (or evaluation). The nursing intervention is designed to achieve the purpose of nursing and is communicated to the patient. The goals of communication in the nursing process are "to know (the) person, (to) ascertain and meet the nursing needs of ill persons, and (to) fulfill the purpose of nursing" (Travelbee, 1971, p. 96).

In the observation stage of nursing care, the nurse "does not observe signs of illness," but rather collects sensory data in order to identify a problem or need (Travelbee, 1971, p. 99). The nurse validates her interpretation of the problem or need with the ill person and decides whether or not to act upon her interpretation. A nursing intervention is developed in alignment with the purpose of nursing, and requires the nurse to "assist ill persons to find meaning in the experience of illness, suffering, and pain" (Travelbee, 1971, p. 158). However, the nurse may not assume she understands the meaning of the illness experience to the ill person without first inquiring into this meaning. To do so would communicate to the ill person that his or her experience is not of value to the nurse, resulting in dehumanization. The nurse evaluates the outcomes of her nursing intervention based on objectives developed before the phase of appraisal.

In meeting the ill person's needs through the human-to-human relationship, the nurse employs a disciplined intellectual approach or a logical approach consistent with nursing standards and clinical practice guidelines in order to identify, manage, and evaluate the ill person's problem (Travelbee, 1971). Each stage in the nursing process may be employed without the establishment of a human-to-human relationship. An acute medical need may be met, but the patient's deeper spiritual and emotional needs are neglected. These spiritual and emotional needs are addressed in the human-to-human relationship in the progression through five phases: the original encounter, emerging identities, empathy, sympathy, and rapport.

In the phase of the original encounter, the nurse and ill person form judgments about each other that will guide and shape future nurse–person interactions. Past experiences, the media, and stereotypes may influence one's perception of another, blocking the development of a human-to-human relationship. In the phase of emerging identities, a bond begins to form between nurse and person as each individual begins to "appreciate the uniqueness of the other" (Travelbee, 1971, p. 132). The bond is created and shaped through each nurse–person interaction and is facilitated by the therapeutic use of self, combined with nursing knowledge. The nurse must recognize how she perceives the person, in order to create a foundation of empathy.

In the phase of empathy, the nurse begins to see the individual "beyond outward behavior and sense accurately another's inner experience at a given point in time" (Travelbee, 1971, p. 136). Empathy enables the nurse to predict what the person is experiencing and requires acceptance, as empathy involves the "intellectual and…emotional comprehension of another person" (Travelbee, 1964). Empathy is the precursor to sympathy, or the "desire, almost an urge, to help or aid an individual in order to relieve his distress" (Travelbee, 1964). Sympathy is not pity, but rather a demonstration to the person that he is not carrying the burden of illness alone. Trust develops between the nurse and person in the phase of sympathy, and the person's distress is diminished.

Rapport, according to Meleis (1997) is "both the goal and the process" of the human-to-human relationship (p. 367). Travelbee (1971) defines rapport as "a process, a happening, and experience, or series of experiences, undergone simultaneously by nurse and the recipient of her care" (p. 150). Rapport "is composed of a cluster of interrelated thoughts and feelings: interest in and concern for, others; empathy, compassion, and sympathy; a non-judgmental attitude, and respect for each individual as a unique human being" (Travelbee, 1963). Through the establishment of rapport, the nurse is able to foster a meaningful relationship with the ill person during multiple points of contact in the care setting. Rapport is not established in every nurse–person encounter; however, emotional involvement is required from the nurse. To establish this emotional bond with one's patient, the nurse must first ensure her own emotional needs are met.

Practice Applications

Cook (1989) used Travelbee's nursing concepts to design a support group for nurses facing organizational restructuring at a New York hospital. The purpose of the support group was to help nurses develop more meaningful perceptions of their roles during a nursing shortage created during a financial crisis that resulted in a restructuring of patient care delivery and nurse/patient ratios. Group morale was low in the beginning, and nurses were frustrated with higher nurse/patient ratios. The support group met over 2 weeks, and the group intervention was designed by incorporating Hoff's theory on crisis intervention with Travelbee's phases of observation and communication. Travelbee's human-to-human relationship was used to guide supportive discussions and problem-solving as nurses struggled to regain a sense of meaning and purpose related to their professional identity.

Participants shared their perceptions of their work environment during the initial encounter. Support group members discussed the similarities and differences in their work perceptions during the phase of emerging identities. Empathy and trust developed as nurses became more accepting and nonjudgmental of each other's perceptions, culminating in the establishment of rapport as group members were able to "recapture" the meaning of nursing (Cook, 1989).

Cook (1989) found that nurses who had threatened to quit earlier had remained in the system by the end of the support group. Nurse productivity had increased over time, and the number of sick days taken by the nurses had diminished over the 6-month period after program cessation. Nurses regained a sense of meaning of their work and reported increased job satisfaction after completion of the program. Travelbee's ideas hold potential as an effective nursing intervention for improving nurse retention rates. However, further research is necessary, as the exact number of nurses recruited into the support group and the actual number of nurses who completed the program are unknown.

References

Cook, L. (1989). Nurses in crisis: A support group based on Travelbee's nursing theory. *Nursing and Health Care, 10*(4), 203–205.

Meleis, A. I. (1997). *Theoretical nursing: Development & progress* (3rd ed.). New York: Lippincott.

O'Brien, M. E. (2008). *Spirituality in nursing: Standing on holy ground* (3rd ed.). Boston: Jones and Bartlett.

Tomey, A. M., & Alligood, M. R. (2006). *Nursing theorists and their work* (6th ed.). St. Louis, MO: Mosby Elsevier.

Travelbee, J. (1963). What do we mean by rapport? *American Journal of Nursing, 63*(2), 70–72.

Travelbee, J. (1964). What's wrong with sympathy? *American Journal of Nursing, 64*(1), 68–71.

Travelbee, J. (1971). *Interpersonal aspects of nursing* (2nd ed.). Philadelphia: F. A. Davis.

Part Three	Orlando's Theory of the Dynamic Nurse–Patient Relationship

Introducing the Theorist

Ida Jean Orlando was born in 1926 in New York. Her nursing education began at New York Medical College School of Nursing where she received a diploma in nursing. In 1951, she received a bachelor of science degree in public health nursing from St. John's University in Brooklyn, New York, and in 1954 she completed a master's degree in nursing from Columbia University. Orlando's early nursing practice experience included obstetrics, medicine, and emergency room nursing. Her first book, *The Dynamic Nurse–Patient Relationship: Function, Process and Principles* (1961), was based on her research and blended nursing practice, psychiatric–mental health nursing, and nursing education. It was published when she was director of the graduate program in mental health and psychiatric nursing at Yale University School of Nursing.

Orlando's theoretical work is both practice and research based and was funded by the National Institute of Mental Health to improve education of nurses about concepts and interpersonal relationships. The method of her study was qualitative and inductive, using naturalistic inquiry methods. As a consultant at McLean Hospital in Belmont, Massachusetts, Orlando continued to study nursing practice and developed a training program and nursing service department based on her theory. From evaluation of this program, she published her second book, *The Discipline and Teaching of Nursing Process* (Orlando, 1972; Rittman, 1991).

Overview of Orlando's Theory of the Dynamic Nurse–Patient Relationship

Nursing is responsive to individuals who suffer or anticipate a sense of helplessness; it is focused on the process of care in an immediate experience; it is concerned with providing direct assistance to individuals in whatever setting they are found for the purpose of avoiding, relieving, diminishing or curing the individual's sense of helplessness. (Orlando, 1972)

The essence of Orlando's theory, the Dynamic Nurse–Patient Relationship, reflects her beliefs that practice should be based on needs of the patient and that communication with the patient is essential to understanding needs and providing effective nursing care. Following is an overview of the major components of Orlando's work.

1. *The nursing process* includes identifying the needs of patients, responses of the nurse, and nursing action. The nursing process, as envisioned and practiced by Orlando, is not the linear model often taught today, but is more reflexive and circular, and occurs during encounters with patients.
2. *Understanding the meaning* of patient behavior is influenced by the nurse's perceptions, thoughts, and feelings. It may be validated through communication between the nurse and the patient. Patients experience distress when they cannot cope with unmet needs. Nurses use direct and indirect observations of patient behavior to discover distress and meaning.
3. *Nurse–patient interactions* are unique, complex, and dynamic processes. Nurses help patients express and understand the meaning of behavior. The basis for nursing action is the distress experienced and expressed by the patient.
4. *Professional nurses* function in an independent role from physicians and other health-care providers.

Practice Applications

Orlando's theoretical work was based on analysis of thousands of nurse–patient interactions to describe major attributes of the relationship. Based on this work, her later book provided direction for understanding and using the nursing process (Orlando, 1972). This has been known as the first theory of nursing process and has been widely used in nursing education and practice in the United States and across the globe. Orlando considered her overall work to be a theoretical framework for the practice of professional nursing, emphasizing the essentiality of the nurse–patient relationship. Orlando's theoretical work reveals and bears witness to the essence of nursing as a practice discipline.

Although there is little evidence in the literature that Orlando's theory has been directly used in nursing practice, it is highly probable that nurses familiar with her writing used her work to guide or more fully understand their practice. During the 1960s, several studies were published that explored nursing practice issues. These works focused on patients' complaints of pain (Barron, 1966; Bochnak, 1963), incidence of postoperative vomiting (Dumas & Leonard, 1963), patient admission processes (Elms & Leonard, 1966), nurses' responses to expressed patient needs (Gowan & Morris, 1964), and the effects of patient assistance with planning nursing procedure administration (Tryson, 1963).

The most important contribution of Orlando's theoretical work is what it says about the values underpinning nursing practice. Inherent in this theory is a strong statement: What transpires between the patient and the nurse is of the highest value. The true worth of her nursing theory is that it clearly states what nursing is or should be today. Regardless of the changes in the health care system, the human transaction between the nurse and the patient in any setting holds the greatest value, not only for nursing, but also for society at large. Orlando's theory can serve as a philosophy as well as a theory, because it is the foundation upon which our profession has been built. With all of the benefits that modern technology and modern health care bring—and there are many—we need to pause and ask the question "What is at risk in health care today"? The answer to that question may lead to reconsideration of the value of Orlando's theory as perhaps the critical link for enhancing relationships between nursing and patient today (Rittman, 1991).

References

Barron, M. A. (1966). The effects varied nursing approaches have on patients' complaints of pain. *Nursing Research, 15*(1), 90–91.

Bochnak, M. A. (1963). The effect of an automatic and deliberative process of nursing activity on the relief of patients' pain: A clinical experiment. *Nursing Research, 12*(3), 191–193.

Dumas, R. G., & Leonard, R. C. (1963). The effect of nursing on the incidence of post-operative vomiting. *Nursing Research, 12*(1), 12–15.

Elms, R. R., & Leonard, R. C. (1966). The effects of nursing approaches during admission. *Nursing Research, 15*(1), 39–48.

Gowan, N. I., & Morris, M. (1964). Nurses' responses to expressed patient needs. *Nursing Research, 13*(1), 68–71.

Orlando, I. J. (1961/1990). *The dynamic nurse-patient relationship: Function, process and principles.* New York: National League for Nursing (reprinted from 1961 edition). New York: G. P. Putnam's Sons.

Orlando, I. J. (1972). *The discipline and teaching of nursing process: An evaluative study.* New York: G. P. Putnam's Sons.

Rittman, M. R. (1991). Ida Jean Orlando (Pelletier)—the dynamic nurse–patient relationship. In: M. Parker (Ed.), *Nursing theories and nursing practice* (pp. 125–130). Philadelphia: F. A. Davis.

Tryson, P. A. (1963). An experiment of the effect of patients' participation in planning the administration of a nursing procedure. *Nursing Research, 12*(4), 262–265.

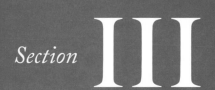

Conceptual Models/Grand Theories in the Interactive/Integrative Paradigm

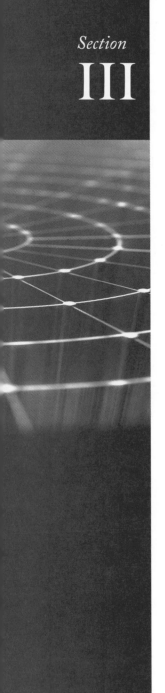

III

Conceptual Models/Grand Theories in the Interactive/Integrative Paradigm

Section III includes eight chapters on the conceptual models or grand theories situated in the inter-active–integrative nursing paradigm. These chapters are written by either the theorist or an author designated as an authority on the theory by the theorist or the community of scholars advancing that theory. Theories in the interactive–integrative paradigm view persons (families, groups, com-munities) as integrated wholes or integrated systems interacting with the larger environmental sys-tem. The integrated dimensions of the person (family, group, community) are influenced by envi-ronmental factors leading to some change that impacts health or well-being. The subjectivity of the person and the multidimensional nature of any outcome are considered. Most of the theories are based explicitly on a systems perspective. Levine's Conservation Model, described in Chapter 7, focuses on promotion of adaptation and maintaining integrity of the system in interaction with the environment. The goal of nursing is to promote health or integrity as the person is confronted with challenges or life situations. According to Levine, energy conservation in the midst of organismic response to stress is essential for integrity. In Chapter 8, Johnson's Behavioral Systems Model is described. It includes principles of wholeness and order, stabilization, reorganization, hierarchic interaction, and dialectic contradiction. The person is viewed as a compilation of subsystems. According to Johnson, the goal of nursing is to restore, maintain, or attain behavioral system bal-ance and stability at the highest possible level. Chapter 9 features Orem's Self-Care Deficit Nursing Theory, a conceptual model with three interrelated theories associated with it: Theory of Nursing Systems, Theory of Self-Care Deficit, and the Theory of Self-Care. According to Orem, when requirements for self-care exceed capacity for self-care, self-care deficits occur. Nursing systems are designed to address these self-care deficits. King's Theory of Goal Attainment presented in Chap-ter 10 offers a view that the goal of nursing is to help persons maintain health or regain health. This is accomplished through a transaction or setting a goal with the patient. In Chapter 11, Sr. Callista Roy and her colleague, Dr. Lin Zhan, describe the Roy Adaptation Model and its appli-cations. In this model, the person is viewed as a holistic adaptive system with coping processes to maintain adaptation and promote person–environment transformations. The adaptive system can be integrated, compensatory, or compromised depending on the level of adaptation. Nurses pro-mote coping and adaptation within health and illness. Patricia Deal Aylward authored Chapter 12 on Neuman's Systems Model. The model includes the client–client system with a basic structure protected from stressors by lines of defense and resistance. The concern of nursing is to keep the client stable by assessing the actual or potential effects of stressors and assisting client adjustments for optimal wellness. In Chapter 13, Erickson, Tomlin, and Swain's Modeling and Role Modeling Theory is presented by Helen Erickson. Modeling and Role Modeling Theory provides a guide for the practice or process of nursing. The theory integrates a holistic philosophy with concepts from a variety of theoretical perspectives such as adaptation, need status, and developmental task res-olution. The final chapter in this section is Dossey's Theory of Integral Nursing, a relatively new grand theory that posits an integral worldview and body–mind–spirit connectedness. The theory is informed by a variety of ideas including Nightingale's tenets, holism, multidimensionality, spiral dynamics, chaos theory, and complexity. It includes the major concepts of healing, the metapara-digm of nursing, patterns of knowing, and Wilber's integral theory and Wilber's all quadrants, all levels, all lines.

Chapter 7

Myra Levine's Conservation Model

KAREN MOORE SCHAEFER

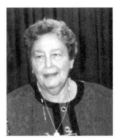

Myra Levine

Introducing the Theorist

Myra Levine has been called a Renaissance woman—highly principled, remarkable, and committed to what happens to the patient's quality of life (Loyola University, 1992). She was a daughter, sister, wife, mother, friend, educator, administrator, student of humanities, scholar, facilitator, and confidante. She was amazingly intelligent, opinionated, quick to respond, loving, caring, trustworthy, and global in her vision of nursing.

Levine was born in Chicago and was raised with a sister and a brother with whom she shared a close, loving relationship (Levine, 1988b). She was also very fond of her father, who was a hardware man. He was often ill and frequently hospitalized with gastrointestinal problems. She thinks that this might have been why she had such a great interest in nursing. Levine's mother was a strong woman who kept the home filled with love and warmth. She was very supportive of Levine's choice to be a nurse. "[My mother] probably knew as much about nursing as I did" (Levine, 1988b) because she was devoted to caring for her father when he was ill.

Levine began attending the University of Chicago but chose to attend Cook County School of Nursing when she could no longer afford the university. Being in nursing school was a new experience for her; she called it a "great adventure" (Levine, 1988b). She received her diploma from Cook County in 1944. She later received her Bachelor of Science degree from the University of Chicago in 1949 and her Master of Science in nursing from Wayne State University in 1962.

Aside from her husband and children, education was Levine's primary interest, although she had clinical experience in the operating room and in oncology nursing. She was a civilian nurse at the Gardiner General Hospital; Director of Nursing at Drexel Home in Chicago; Clinical Instructor at Bryan Memorial Hospital in Lincoln, Nebraska; and Administrative Supervisor at University of Chicago Clinics and Henry Ford Hospital in Michigan. She was Chairperson of Clinical Nursing at Cook County School of Nursing and a faculty member at Loyola University, Rush University, and University of Illinois. She was a visiting professor at Tel Aviv University in Israel and Recanti School of Nursing at Ben Gurion University of the Negev in Beer Sheeva, Israel. She was Professor Emeritus in Medical Surgical Nursing, University of Chicago; a Charter Fellow of the American Academy of Nursing, and a member of Sigma Theta Tau International, from which she received the Elizabeth Russell Belford Award as distinguished educator. She received an honorary doctorate from Loyola University in 1992.

Overview of the Model

The F. A. Davis Company published the first edition of Myra Levine's textbook, *Introduction to Clinical Nursing,* in 1969 and the second and last editions in 1973. In discussing the first edition of her book, Levine (1969a, p. 39) said: "I decided against using 'holistic' in favor of 'organismic,' largely because the term 'holistic' had been appropriated by pseudoscientists endowing it with the mythology of transcendentalism. I used 'holism' in the second edition in 1973 because I realized it was too important to be abandoned to the mystics. I believed that it was the proper description of the way the internal environment and the external environment were joined in the real world." In the introduction to the second edition, she wrote:

There is something very final about a printed page, and yet books do have a life all their own. They gather life from the use to which they are put, and when they succeed in communicating among many individuals in many places, then their intent is most truly served. The most remarkable fact about the first edition of this book has been the exchange of interests that has resulted from the willingness with which its readers and users have communicated with its author. (Levine, 1973, p. vii)

Levine's original book (1969b) provided a model for teaching medical surgical nursing and created a dialogue among colleagues about the plan itself. The text has continued to create dialogue about the art and science of nursing with ongoing research serving as a testament to its value (Delmore, 2003; Mefford, 1999, 2004).

Foundations of Clinical Nursing

Levine's original reason for writing the book was to find a way to teach the foundations of nursing that would focus on nursing itself and was organized in such a way that students would learn the skill as well as the rationale for it. She felt that too often the focus was on skill alone. Her intent was to bring practice and research together to establish nursing as an applied science. The book was used as a beginning nursing text by Levine and many of her colleagues.

The first chapter of her text was entitled, "Introduction to Patient-Centered Nursing Care," a model of care delivery that is now acclaimed as the answer to cost-effective delivery of health care services today. She believed that patient-centered care was "individualized nursing care" (Levine, 1973, p. 23). She discussed the theory of causation, a unified theory of health and disease, the meaning of the conservation principles, the hospital as environment, and patient-centered intervention. The nursing care chapters in her text focus on care of the patient with:

1. Failure of the nervous system
2. Failure of integration resulting from hormonal imbalance
3. Disturbance of homeostasis: fluid and electrolyte imbalance
4. Disturbance of homeostasis: nutritional needs
5. Disturbance of homeostasis: systemic oxygen needs
6. Disturbance of homeostasis: cellular oxygen needs

7. Disease arising from aberrant cellular growth
8. Inflammatory problems
9. Holistic response

Her way of organizing the material was a shift from teaching nursing based on the disease model. Her final chapter on the holistic response represented a major change from disease to systems thinking. Informed by other disciplines, she discussed the integrated system, the interaction of systems creating the sense of well-being, energy exchange at the organismic level and at the cellular level, perception of self, the effect of space on self-perception, and the circadian rhythm.

As Levine wrote her book, major changes occurred in the curriculum at Cook County Hospital (Levine, 1988b). She and her colleagues began to focus on the importance of nursing research and taught perception, sleep, distance (space), and periodicity as factors in health and disease (see Box 7-1).

Box 7-1   Influences on the Conservation Model

Levine used the inductive method to develop her model. She borrowed information from other disciplines while retaining the basic structure of nursing in the model (Levine, 1988a). As she continued to write about her model, she integrated information from other sciences and increasingly cited personal experiences as evidence of her work's validity. The following is a list of the influences in the development of her philosophy of nursing and the Conservation Model.

1. Levine indicated that Florence Nightingale, through her focus on observation (Nightingale, 1859), provided great attention to energy conservation and recognized the need for structural integrity. Levine relates Nightingale's discussion of social integrity to Nightingale's concern for sanitation, which she says implies an interaction between the person and the environment.
2. Irene Beland influenced Levine's thinking about nursing as a compassionate art and rigid intellectual pursuit (Levine, 1988b). Levine also credited Beland (1971) for the theory of specific causation and multiple factors.
3. Feynman (1965) provided support for Levine's position that conservation was a natural law, arguing that the development of theory cannot deny the importance of natural law (Levine, 1973).
4. Bernard (1957) is recognized for his contribution in the identification of the interdependence of bodily functions (Levine, 1973).
5. Levine (1973) emphasized the dynamic nature of the internal milieu, using Waddington's (1968) term "homeophoresis."
6. Use of Bates's (1967) formulation of the external environment as having three levels of factors (perceptual, operational, and conceptual) challenging the integrity of the individual helped to emphasize the complexity of the environment.
7. The description of illness is based on Wolf's (1961) description of disease as adaptation to noxious environmental forces.
8. Selye's (1956) definition of "stress" is included in Levine's (1989c) description of her organismic stress response as "being recorded over time and . . . influenced by the accumulated experience of the individual" (p. 30).
9. The perceptual organismic response incorporates Gibson's (1966) work on perception as a mediator of behavior. His identification of the five perceptual systems, including hearing, sight, touch, taste, and smell, contributed to the development of the perceptual response.
10. The notion that individuals seek to defend their personhood is grounded in Goldstein's (1963) explanation of soldiers who, despite brain injury, sought to cling to some semblance of self-awareness.
11. Dubos' (1965) discussion of the adaptability of the organism helped support Levine's explanation that adaptation occurs within a range of responses.
12. Levine's personal experiences influenced her thinking. When hospitalized, she said, "the experience of wholeness is universally acknowledged" (Levine, 1996, p. 39).

Assumptions and Values of the Conservation Model

Assumptions

The person is viewed as a holistic being: "The experience of wholeness is the foundation of all human enterprises" (Levine, 1991, p. 3).

Human beings respond in a singular yet integrated fashion.

Each individual responds wholly and completely to every alteration in his or her life pattern.

Individuals cannot be understood out of the context of their environment.

"Ultimately, decisions for nursing care are based on the unique behavior of the individual patient. . . . A theory of nursing must recognize the importance of unique detail of care for a single patient within an empiric framework which successfully describes the requirements of all patients" (Levine, 1973, p. 6).

"Patient-centered care means individualized nursing care. It is predicated on the reality of common experience: every man (sic) is a unique individual, and as such requires a unique constellation of skills, techniques, and ideas designed specially for him (sic)" (Levine, 1973, p. 23).

"Every self-sustaining system monitors its own behavior by conserving the use of resources required to define its unique identity" (Levine, 1991, p. 4).

The nurse is responsible for recognizing the state of altered health and the patient's organismic response to altered health.

Nursing is a unique contributor to patient care (Levine, 1988a).

The patient is in an altered state of health (Levine, 1973). A patient is someone who seeks health care because of a desire to remain healthy or someone who identifies a known risk behavior or a desire to reduce a possible one.

A guardian-angel activity assumes that the nurse accepts responsibility and shows concern based on knowledge that makes it possible to decide on the patient's behalf and in his [or her] best interest (Levine, 1973).

Values

All nursing actions are moral actions.

The sanctity of life and the relief of suffering are moral imperatives.

Ethical behavior "is the day-to-day expression of one's commitment to other persons and the ways in which human beings relate to one another in their daily interactions" (Levine, 1977, p. 846).

A fully informed individual should make decisions regarding life and death in advance of crises. These decisions are not the role of the health care provider or the family (Levine, 1989b).

Judgments by nurses or doctors about quality of life are inappropriate and should not be used as a basis for the allocation of care (Levine, 1989b).

"Persons who require the intensive interventions of critical care units enter with a contract of trust. To respect trust ... is a moral responsibility" (Levine, 1988b, p. 88).

The Composition of the Conservation Model

As an organizing framework for nursing practice, the goal of the Conservation Model is to promote adaptation and maintain wholeness using the principles of conservation.

The model guides the nurse to focus on the influences and responses at the organismic level. The nurse accomplishes the goals of the model through the conservation of energy, structure, and personal and social integrity (Levine, 1967). Interventions are provided to improve the patient's condition (therapeutic) or to promote comfort (supportive) when change in the patient's condition is not possible. The outcomes of the interventions are assessed through the organismic response.

Although Levine identified two concepts critical to the use of her model—adaptation and wholeness—conservation is fundamental to the outcomes expected when the model is used. Conservation is addressed as the third major concept of the model. Using the model in practice requires that the nurse understand the commonplaces (Barnum, 1994) of health, person, environment, and nursing.

Before delving into the inner workings of Levine's model, it is necessary to understand its components.

Adaptation

Adaptation is the process of change, and conservation is the outcome of adaptation. Adaptation is the process whereby the patient maintains integrity within the realities of the environment (Levine, 1966, 1989a). Adaptation is achieved through the "frugal, economic, contained, and controlled use of environmental resources by the individual in his or her best interest" (Levine, 1991, p. 5). In her view:

> The environmental "fit" that underscores successful adaptation suggests that every species has fixed patterns of response uniquely designed to ensure success in essential life activities, demonstrating that adaptation is both historical and specific. However, tremendous opportunities for individual accommodations are locked into the gene structure of each species; every individual is one of a kind. (p. 5)

Every individual has a unique range of adaptive responses. These responses will vary based on heredity, age, gender, or challenges of an illness experience. For example, the response to weakness of the cardiac muscle is increased heart rate, dilation of the ventricle, and thickening of the myocardial muscle. Although the responses are the same, the timing and the manifestation of the organismic response (e.g., pulse rate) will be unique for each individual.

Redundancy, history, and specificity characterize adaptation. These characteristics are "rooted in history and awaiting the specific circumstances to which they respond" (Levine, 1991, p. 6). The genetic structure develops over time and provides the foundation for these responses. Specificity refers to the fact that while sharing traits with a species, individual potential creates a variety of adaptation outcomes. For example, diabetes has a genetic component, which explains the fundamental decrease in sugar metabolism. However, the

organismic responses vary (renal perfusion, blood vessel integrity) based on genetic alterations, age, gender, and therapeutic management techniques.

Redundancy represents the fail-safe options available to the individual to ensure continued adaptation. Levine (1991) believed that health is dependent on the ability to select from redundant options. She hypothesized that aging may be the result of the failure of redundant systems. If this is the case, then survival is dependent on redundant options, which are often challenged and limited by illness, disease, and the normal aging process. When the compensatory response to cardiac disease is no longer able to maintain an adequate blood flow to vital organs during activity, survival becomes increasingly difficult. Adaptation represents the accommodation between the internal and external environments.

Conservation

> Conservation is the product of adaptation and is a common principle underlying many of the basic sciences. It is critical to understanding an essential element of human life: Implicit in the knowledge of conservation is the fact of wholeness, integrity, unity—all of the structures that are being conserved … conservation of the integrity of the person is essential to ensuring health and providing the strength to confront disability … the importance of conservation in the treatment of illness is precisely focused on the reclamation of wholeness, of health. … Every nursing act is dedicated to the conservation, or "keeping together," of the wholeness of the individual. (Levine, 1991, p. 3)

Individuals are continuously defending their wholeness to keep together the life system. Individuals defend themselves in constant interaction with their environment, choosing the most economic, frugal, and energy-sparing options that safeguard their integrity. Conservation seeks to achieve a balance of energy supply and demand that is within the unique biological capabilities of the individual (Schaefer, 1991a).

Maintaining the proper balance requires that the nursing intervention be coupled with the patient's participation to ensure that activities are within the safe limits of the patient's ability to participate. Although energy cannot be directly observed, the consequences of energy exchanges are predictable, recognizable, and manageable (Levine, 1973, 1991).

Wholeness

Wholeness is based on Erikson's (1964) description of wholeness as an open system: "Wholeness emphasizes a sound, organic, progressive mutuality between diversified functions and parts within an entirety, the boundaries of which are open and fluid" (p. 63). Levine (1973) stated that "the unceasing interaction of the individual organism with its environment does represent an 'open and fluid' system, and a condition of health, wholeness, exists when the interaction or constant adaptations to the environment, permit ease—the assurance of integrity ... in all the dimensions of life" (p. 11). This continuously dynamic, open interaction between the internal and external environment provides the basis for holistic thought: the view of the individual as whole.

Health, Person, Environment, and Nursing

Health and disease are patterns of adaptive change. From a social perspective, health is the ability to function in social roles. Health is culturally determined: "[I]t is not an entity, but rather a definition imparted by the ethos and beliefs of the groups to which the individual belongs" (M. Levine, personal communication, February 21, 1995).

Health is an individual response that may change over time in response to new situations; new life challenges; aging; or social, political, economic, or spiritual factors. Health implies unity and integrity. The goal of nursing is to promote health.

Levine (1991) clarified what she meant by health as "...the avenue of return to the daily activities compromised by illness. It is not only the insult or the injury that is repaired but the person himself or herself. ... It is not merely the healing of an afflicted part. It is rather a return to selfhood, where the encroachment of the disability can be set aside entirely, and the individual is free to pursue once more his or her own interests without constraint" (p. 4). In all of life's challenges, individuals will constantly attempt to attain, retain, maintain, or protect their integrity (health, wholeness, and unity).

To Levine, the holistic individual is a thinking being who is aware of the past and oriented to the future. The wholeness (integrity) of the person demands that the "individual life has meaning only in the context of social life" (Levine, 1973, p. 17). The person responds to change in an integrated, sequential, yet singular fashion while in constant interaction with the environment. Levine (1996) defined "the person" as a spiritual being, quoting Genesis 1:27: "And God created man in his own image, in the image of God created He him. Male and female created He them. ... Sanctity of life is manifested in everyone. The holiness of life itself [testifies] to its spiritual reality" (p. 40). "Person" can be an individual, a family, or a community.

Levine (1968a, 1968b, 1973) recognizes that the *person* is defined to a certain degree based on the boundaries defined by Hall (1966) as "personal space." Levine rejected the notion that energy can be manipulated and transferred from one human to another as in therapeutic touch. Yet someone is affected by the presence of another relative to his or her personal space boundaries. Admittedly, some of this is based on cultural ethos, yet what is it about the "bubble" that results in a specific organismic response? It may be that the energy involved in the interaction is not clearly defined, fueling the skeptic's criticism and challenging scientists to examine the question. Levine encouraged creativity to explore this question, but rejected activities that were not scientifically supported.

The *environment* completes the wholeness of the individual. The individual has both an internal and external environment. The internal environment combines the physiological and pathophysiological aspects of the individual and is constantly challenged by the external environment.

The external environment includes factors that impinge on and challenge the individual. The environment as described by Levine (1973) was adapted from the following three levels of environment identified by Bates (1967).

The *perceptual* environment includes aspects of the world that individuals are able to seize or interpret through the senses. The individual "seeks, selects, and tests information from the environment in the context of his [her] definition of himself [herself], and so defends his [her] safety, his [her] identity, and in a larger sense, his [her] purpose" (Levine, 1971, p. 262).

The *operational* environment includes factors that may physically affect individuals but are not directly perceived by them, such as radiation, microorganisms, and pollution.

The *conceptual* environment includes the cultural patterns characterized by spiritual existence and mediated by language, thought, and history. Factors that affect behavior, such as norms, values, and beliefs, are also part of the conceptual environment.

Nursing is "human interaction" (Levine, 1973, p. 1). "The nurse enters into a partnership of human experience where sharing moments in time—some trivial, some dramatic—leaves its mark forever on each patient" (Levine, 1977, p. 845). The goal of nursing is to promote adaptation and maintain wholeness (health). The goal is accomplished through the use of the conservation principles: energy and structural, personal, and social integrity.

The Model

Energy conservation is dependent on the free exchange of energy with the internal and external environment to maintain the balance of energy supply and demand. Conservation of structural integrity is dependent on an intact defense system (immune system) that supports healing and repair to preserve the structure and function of the whole being.

The conservation of personal integrity acknowledges the individual as one who strives

for recognition, respect, self-awareness, humanness, selfhood, and self-determination. The conservation of social integrity recognizes the individual as a social being who functions in a society that helps to establish boundaries of the self. The value of the individual is recognized, together with an appreciation that the individual resides within a family, a community, a religious group, an ethnic group, a political system, a nation and a global world (Levine, 1973).

The outcome of nursing involves the assessment of organismic responses. The nurse is responsible for responding to a request for health care and for recognizing altered health and the patient's organismic response to altered health. An organismic response is a change in behavior or change in the level of functioning during an attempt to adapt to the environment. Organismic responses are intended to maintain the patient's integrity. According to Levine (1973), the levels of organismic response include:

1. *Response to fear (flight/fight response).* The most primitive response is the physiological and behavioral readiness to respond to a sudden and unexpected environmental change. It is an instantaneous response to a real or imagined threat.
2. *Inflammatory response.* The second level of response is intended to provide for structural integrity (as a defense against noxious stimuli) and the promotion of healing.
3. *Response to stress.* The third level of response is developed over time and influenced by each stressful experience encountered by the patient. If the experience is prolonged, the stress can lead to damage to the systems.
4. *Perceptual response.* The fourth level of response involves gathering information from the environment and converting it to a meaningful experience.

The organismic responses are redundant in the sense that they coexist. The four responses help individuals protect and maintain their integrity. They are integrated by cognitive abilities, the wealth of previous experiences, the ability to define relationships, and the strength of adaptive abilities.

The nurse uses the scientific process and creative abilities to provide nursing care to the patient (Schaefer, 1991a). The nursing process incorporates these abilities, thereby improving the patient's care (see Table 7-1).

Applications to Practice

The model's universality is supported by its use in a variety of situations and patient conditions across the life span. A growing body of research provides evidence to support its application to nursing practice. The focus of

Table 7 • 1 Use of the Nursing Process According to Levine

Process	Application of the Process
Assessment	Collection (through observation and interview) of challenges to the internal and external environments. The nurse observes the patient for organismic responses to illness, reads medical reports, evaluates results of diagnostic studies, and talks with patients and their families (support persons) about their needs for assistance. The nurse assesses for physiological and pathophysiological challenges to the internal environment and the factors in the perceptual, operational, and conceptual levels of the external environment that challenge the individual.
Trophicognosis*	Nursing diagnosis that gives the provocative facts meaning. The nurse arranges the provocative facts in a way that provides meaning to the patient's predicament. A judgment is the trophicognosis.**
Hypotheses	Direct the nursing interventions with the goal of maintaining wholeness and promoting adaptation. Nurses seek validation of the patients' problems with the patients or support persons. The nurses then propose hypotheses about the problems and the solutions, such as "Eight glasses of water a day will improve bowel evacuation." These become the plan of care.
Interventions	Test the hypotheses. Nurses use hypotheses to direct care. The nurse tests proposed hypotheses and designs interventions based on the conservation principles: conservation of energy, structural integrity, person integrity, and social integrity. Interventions are not imposed but are determined to be mutually acceptable. The expectation is that this approach will maintain wholeness and promote adaptation.
Evaluation	Observation of organismic response to interventions. The outcome of hypothesis-testing is evaluated by assessing for organismic response that means the hypotheses are supported or not supported. Consequences of care are either therapeutic or supportive: therapeutic measures improve the sense of well-being; supportive measures provide comfort when the downward course of illness cannot be influenced. If the hypotheses are not supported, the plan is revised and new hypotheses are proposed.

*The novice nurse may use the conservation principles at this point to assist with the organization of the provocative facts. The expert nurse integrates this into the environmental assessments.

**Trophicognosis is a nursing care judgment arrived at through the use of the scientific process (Levine, 1965). The scientific process is used to make observations and select relevant data to form hypothetical statements about the patients' predicaments (Schaefer, 1991a).

Source: Levine's Nursing Process Using Critical Thinking. In: M. R. Alligood & A. Marriner-Tomey (Eds.). (1997). *Nursing theory: Utilization and application*. St. Louis, MO: C. V. Mosby. Revised and used with permission of C. V. Mosby.

this section is on how practitioners have used the model to provide care with evidence appropriately integrated with use.

Roberts, Fleming, and Yeates-Giese (1991) designed interventions to maintain perineal integrity for women in labor based on the Conservation Model. The findings support that the normal adaptations of the birthing process "provide the most physically, emotionally and socially beneficial means for this physiological function" (p. 69). Episiotomy should be reserved for specific situations where it is warranted, rather than being used prophylactically, because it does not appear to be protective.

Langer (1990) used the Conservation Model to develop a protocol for minimal handling of premature infants. Based on the goal of maintaining the integrity of the infant and family, the integrities were used to identify activities that would help reduce the handling of each infant while maintaining the wholeness of the infant–family unit. For example, swaddling was used to maintain the personal integrity of the infant to limit agitation from suctioning, and to make sure parents were part of the health care team in order to maintain their social integrity.

Savage and Culbert (1989) adopted the Conservation Model as a framework to establish a care plan for a family with a developmentally disabled child. The integrities were used to conduct an assessment, identify short-term goals, plan nursing actions, and evaluate outcomes. A case study identified nutritional intake as a threat to energy conservation. One nursing action was to help the mother position her child for optimal alignment and demonstrate manual jaw closure and placement of food in the mouth using a spoon. The outcome was achieved when the mother demonstrated proper positioning and noted that feeding was easier using the new techniques. The child's limited cognition was a challenge to the family's personal integrity. A standardized assessment revealed that the child had the cognitive function of a 2-month-old with some skills up to those of a 6-month-old. The short-term goal was to

determine the child's tolerance of activities and to respond to his cues. The nurse encouraged the mother to communicate through touch and language. The mother successfully recognized the child's cues and discontinued activities when he became tired.

Mefford (1999, 2004) tested a theory of health promotion for preterm infants derived from Levine's Conservation Model. She found a significant inverse relationship between the consistency of caregiver and the age at which the infant achieved health. An inverse relationship also existed between the use of resources by preterm infants during the initial hospital stay and the consistency of caregivers. This suggests that with increasing age (and perhaps experience) of the care provider, the infants may receive a higher quality of care. These findings can be helpful in making assignments to patient care units. Mefford has indicated that she plans to continue her work with the model to develop the theory of health promotion across the life span (L. C. Mefford, personal communication, 2008).

Using a case study approach, Dever (1991) demonstrated how the use of the Conservation Model can assist nurses in the care of children. She based care on the assumption that children have an amazing capacity to adapt and recover if the right mix of interventions is provided. The conservation principles served as a guide to ensure comprehensive care.

Cooper (1990) developed a framework for wound care focusing on structural integrity while noting that conservation must be understood as part of the integrated role of the nurse. She noted that energy conservation was essential to protecting the patient and that nursing processes should be dedicated to the promotion of healing. Dibble, Bostrom-Ezerati, and Ruzzuto (1991) used the model to identify nursing actions that would promote structural integrity and limit the development of phlebitis and infiltration at an intravenous site.

O'Laughlin (1986) approached nursing care of a patient after a radical hysterectomy using the Conservation Model. She outlined the role of the nurse according to the integrities and indicated that the nurse (1) conserves energy when energy is needed for healing by maintaining good catheter care to reduce the chance of infection, (2) ensures that the bladder is emptied regularly to prevent overdistension and structural damage, (3) assesses the patient for how changes in micturition will affect her lifestyle and encourages the patient to participate in decisions about how to manage her bladder and adapt to lifestyle changes, and (4) integrates aspects of the patient's social life into her plan of care.

Neswick (1997) used a case study of a patient with an ostomy to demonstrate how the model helps provide holistic care. Energy focused on the nutrition needed to heal; structural focused on maintaining skin integrity; personal addressed issues associated with going public with an ostomy; and social integrity stressed the importance of rehabilitation. After the completion of a prevalence and incidence study of skin care, Burd et al. (1994) used the model to evaluate strategies in the prevention of skin breakdown.

Leach (2006) published a white paper on the use of the Conservation Model to guide wound care practices, specifically venous leg ulcers (VLUs). In the context of VLUs, nurses focus on the maintenance of energy conservation and structural integrity by providing external dressings and compression devices to improve venous flow. In contrast to Mefford (2004), Leach uses Levine for short-term goal achievement only. He does not support the use of the Levine Conservation Model as a basis for health promotion or maintenance. This conflicts with Levine's (1973) view of individuals as past-aware and future-oriented.

Webb (1993) used the Conservation Model to provide care for patients undergoing Hartman's procedure. Using a case study approach, the author demonstrated how the use of trophicognoses (see Table 9-1) can be successful in developing a plan of care for a surgical patient.

Roberts, Brittin, and deClifford (1995) and Roberts, Brittin, Cook, and deClifford (1994) used the Conservation Model to study the effect of the boomerang pillow technique on respiratory capacity. The findings supported that boomerang pillows provide comfort without compromising respiratory capacity. Dow and Mest (1997) used the Conservation Model to design interventions to meet the psychosocial needs of the client with chronic obstructive pulmonary disease (COPD) living in the community. They focused on the personal and social integrities. The client's personal integrity can be challenged by forced early retirement, feelings of guilt from not being able to provide for the family, and managing personal issues such as being overweight. Consideration was given to the need for the spouse to take on new roles, which can add stress to the family structure. Recommended interventions included counseling, exercise, and relaxation as well as teaching about medications.

Several practitioners have used the Conservation Model to assist patients with fatigue and develop interventions to reduce this disabling symptom (Schaefer & Shober-Rotylycki, 1993; Schaefer, Swavely, Rothenberger, Hess, & Willistin, 1996). Schaefer (1991b) used the model to conceptualize the experience of fatigue in patients with congestive heart failure. In talking with clients, she learned that the feeling of fatigue affects one's way of being by overcoming the entire body. Interventions for fatigue must take into consideration all of the integrities in order to have a positive organismic response. Mock et al. (2007) used the model to design and test interventions for the fatigue experienced by patients with cancer. The four conservation principles guided the development of an exercise intervention that is currently being tested. For example, energy conservation addresses fatigue and sleep; structural integrity focuses on physical function; personal integrity includes emotional desires and quality of life; and social integrity focuses on social function.

In the critical care environment, the Conservation Model has been used by several practitioners to provide care for a variety of clients. Brunner (1985) used the model to develop a conceptual plan of care for patients in critical care. She used the integrities to develop an assessment and showed how the data could be used to determine the nursing diagnosis, short-term goals, nursing actions, and outcomes. Ballard, Robley, Barrett, Fraser, and Mendoza (2006) approached the complex experience of therapeutic paralysis from a systems perspective, and asked how the system adapts and functions to maintain the internal and external environment. Guided by the Conservation Model, she learned that patients reconstructed their lives; living through a life-threatening ordeal resulted in a modification of the stress response.

The nurse's role is to maintain integrity while helping patients live with themselves in new ways. Use of the Conservation Model facilitates this process. Using the principle of conservation of energy, Littrell and Schumann (1989) explained the importance of promoting sleep for the patient with a myocardial infarction. They linked their discussion to the requirement to balance energy resources and needs in order to promote healing related to the infarction. The nurse's goals are to ensure undisturbed restful sleep by clustering activities, creating a familiar sleep environment, using monitors, minimizing noise and pain, avoiding care activities during REM sleep, and limiting visitors. McCall (1991) used the model to develop an assessment tool and provide care for patients with epilepsy in a neurological intensive care unit. Schaefer (1991b) used the model to design care for patients with congestive heart failure, and Bayley (1991) showed how the model can be used to develop a plan of care for clients with burns.

Using the model, Pond and Taney (1991) provided care for emergency room clients while developing a collaborative practice, a project sustained by the emergency room practitioners' (physicians and nurses) interest in collaborating. The model worked because it was precise and useful; physicians were able to communicate the clients' needs with clarity and common understanding between all practitioners. Crawford-Gamble (1986) used

the Conservation Principles to explain the perioperative experience and the role of the nurse in maintaining wholeness. She briefly explained the model to provide a context for care and stressed the importance of the unique approach to each patient. Conservation of energy focused on maintaining physiological function during the operative experience; maintenance of structural integrity focused on the prevention of injury and the promotion of healing; personal integrity addressed the possibility that patients admitted to the operating room might be unfamiliar with the environment and were, at times, away from their support system such that the nurse had to focus on helping the patient manage feelings of loneliness and loss; and finally the nurse determined the patient's needs relative to family and friends to maintain social integrity. Lynn-McHale and Smith (1991) developed a family assessment tool based on the Conservation Model with the goal of providing comprehensive care. Examples of assessment criteria included: energy—perception of the event; structural—family function; personal—life events; and social—work patterns.

Taylor (1974) used the model to explain how to develop outcomes of nursing care. She argued that by using a framework, nurses would be able to identify critical points along the continuum of care to assure the achievement of outcomes. Using the neurological patient as the paradigm case, Taylor clustered potential problems encountered by the patient and listed examples of outcomes. For example, in the early phase of illness, energy is compromised by respiratory paralysis and immobility. Early outcomes include the successful maintenance of respiratory function and adequate control of pain and discomfort. As the patient approaches recovery, possible issues associated with energy conservation include poor appetite and becoming easily fatigued. Outcomes might include normal weight and activity consistent with pathology.

Pond (1991) used the model in her nurse practitioner practice to care for the homeless population. She recognized that individuals who were homeless had severe health and social service needs. Her goal was to promote health for this aggregate. Levine's (1973) concept of the environment was particularly relevant to the person living on the street. The integrities were used to assess and meet the needs of the homeless. For example, energy conservation focused on food and nutrition programs; structural integrity addressed injury prevention and safety in shelters; personal integrity focused on privacy for interpersonal interactions and community education about the homeless; and social integrity included self-awareness, parenting and interaction group interventions.

Schaefer (2006a, 2006b) has used the model to organize the care of individuals with chronic illness. The model provides an inclusive framework for assessing the needs of the individuals, identifying trophicognoses, developing a plan of care based on hypothetical statements, and evaluating for organismic patient responses. Use of this process also forms potential research questions, because of the use of hypothetical statements that are tested based on the organismic outcomes.

Hirschfeld (1976) has used the principles of conservation in the care of older adults. Cox (1991) used the model to provide long-term care to older clients. She describes how she instructed staff to provide care according to the conservation principles and identify goals for each principle. She extended care beyond the walls of the agency by encouraging staff to help residents maintain ties to the local community, preserving their social integrity. Happ, Williams, Strumpf, and Burger (1996) applied the Conservation Model to the case of the frail elderly. She used the concept of wholeness to encourage staff to build and maintain relationships with elderly clients. Foreman (1989, 1991) claims that the model works well in caring for clients with dementia when all the conservation principles are used to assess, organize, and evaluate care.

The Conservation Model has also been used to develop programs in administration and education. Jost (2000) used the Conservation Model to assess and develop interventions for staff during the process of change. The following are examples of how the integrities were operationalized in the assessment: energy conservation included sleep patterns and nutrition; structural integrity addressed skin and body movement; personal integrity included self-esteem, independence, and control; and social integrity addressed stable support and family.

Levine's Conservation Model was used successfully as a basis for the undergraduate and graduate programs at Allentown College (now DeSales University). The model was operationalized through the nursing process for students in the undergraduate program (Grindley & Paradowski, 1991). Levine's approach to care and philosophical discussions about nursing provided a context for the graduate program (Schaefer, 1991c). The faculty believed that graduate students should learn about more than one nursing model or theory. They agreed that the match between individual practice and the nature of the model must be a good fit, making it imperative that the student select or work with a model appropriate for the setting and the type of client in their practice.

The Model Modified for Use in Community-Based Care

The principles of community health nursing that are fundamental to community-based care can be practiced in any setting. The discussion that follows focuses on community-based care using Levine's Conservation Model to provide a foundation for the future of nursing practice, demonstrating the model's utility for community nursing practice.

The focus of health in the community is based on the assumption that community-based care is often informed by the one-on-one care provided to individuals. Using Levine's Conservation Model, community was initially defined as "a group of people living together within a larger society, sharing common characteristics, interests, and location" (*National League for Nursing Self Study Report*, 1978). Clark (1992) provided examples of the use of the conservation principles with the individual, family, and community as a testament to the model's flexibility/universality.

The approach begins with the collection of facts and a thorough community assessment (provocative facts). The internal environment assessment directs the nurse to examine the patterns of health and disease among the people and their use of programs available to promote a healthy community. The assessment of the external environment directs the nurse to examine the perceptual, operational, and conceptual levels of the environment in which the people live.

The perceptual environment incorporates the factors that are processed by the senses. On a community basis, these factors might include an assessment of how the media affects the health of the people; the influence of air quality on health patterns and housing development; the availability of nutritious and affordable foods throughout the community; noise pollution; and relationships among the community's subcultures.

Understanding the operational environment requires a more detailed assessment of the factors in the environment that affect the individual's health but are not perceived by the people. These might include surveillance of communicable diseases; assessment for the use of toxins in industry; disposal of waste products; consideration for exposure to electromagnetic fields from power lines; and examination of buildings for asbestos, lead, and radon.

The conceptual environment focuses the assessment on the ethnic and cultural patterns in the community. An assessment of types of houses of worship and health care settings might be included. In this area, the effect of communities external to the one being assessed would be addressed to determine factors that may influence the function of the target community.

The novice nurse will benefit from using the conservation principles to guide continued assessment to assure a thorough understanding of the community. When considering energy conservation, areas to assess might include:

1. Hours of employment
2. Water supply
3. Community budget
4. Food sources

An assessment of structural integrity might include:

1. City planning
2. Availability of resources
3. Transportation
4. Traffic patterns
5. Public services

An assessment of personal integrity might include:

1. Community identity
2. Mission of the government
3. Political environment

An assessment of the social integrity might include:

1. Recreation
2. Social services
3. Opportunities for employment

See Table 7-2, Levine's Conservation Model—Nursing Process in the Community.

Table 7 • 2 **Levine's Conservation Model – Nursing Process in the Community**	
Process	**Application of the Process**
Assessment	Collection of provocative facts through observation and interview. The nurse uses observation, review of census data, statistics, data from community member interviews, and so on to collect provocative facts about the community. Use of windshield assessments or other formally developed community assessments are helpful in the collection of data.

Continued

Table 7 · 2 **Levine's Conservation Model – Nursing Process in the Community—cont'd**

Process	Application of the Process
Trophicognosis	Community diagnosis. The nurse organizes the data in such a way as to provide meaning. A judgment or trophicognosis is made.
Hypotheses	Direct the nurse to provide interventions that will promote adaptation and maintain wholeness of the community. In discussion with the community members, the nurse validates her judgments about the community's predicament. The nurse then proposes hypotheses about the problems and solutions, such as "Providing shelter to abused women will reduce the morbidity associated with continuous uninterrupted abuse."
Interventions	Test the hypotheses. The nurse uses the hypotheses to direct the plan of care for the community. The nurse tests the proposed hypotheses to try to remedy the predicament. The nurse selects the most appropriate solutions with the help of the community members. Interventions are based on the conservation principles of energy, structural integrity, personal integrity, and social integrity. The shelter for abused women provides for structural integrity of the community while preserving the energy, personal, and social integrity of the women who choose shelter.
Evaluation	Observation of organismic response to interventions. The outcome of hypothesis-testing is evaluated by assessing for organismic response. For example, an expected outcome of shelters for abused women might be a reduction in emergency room visits for injury resulting from suspected abuse or an increase in the number of women who are able to remove themselves from an abusive relationship.

Practice Exemplar

Missy is a 32-year-old woman who is currently in her third trimester of pregnancy. She and her husband have been married for 5 years; she works as a consultant for a retail business. Although her job is demanding, she can choose to work at home 2 days a week. She considers herself healthy, except that she was diagnosed with fibromyalgia (FM) at age 26. She has been able to manage her FM with amitriptyline (Elavil) 25 mg nightly and exercise. Deciding to become pregnant was difficult because little is known about how FM might affect pregnancy and whether the child would be in any way affected by the illness. Her physician assured her that she would be fine and that there was no evidence that FM affects or is passed on to the fetus.

It took several years before Missy and her husband were able to become pregnant. Needless to say they were very pleased with the news. Because there was limited information on how medication used to treat FM might affect the fetus, Missy stopped the Elavil while trying to become pregnant. She used relaxation, warm baths, and stretching to help her sleep and to control the muscular discomfort associated with FM with limited success.

The first trimester of pregnancy was "normal." She was tired and experienced some "morning sickness" in the evening. She did not feel the need for medicinal intervention, primarily because she wanted to be sure she did not put her child at risk. She noted that she felt a bit "down and out" when she thought she would be "on cloud nine" because she was pregnant. She was comfortable during her second trimester, although she still felt tired. Compared to her friends who were also pregnant, she rated her tiredness as being worse. Working 2 days a week from home did give her the chance to rest more when needed, while still meeting the deadlines and needs of her employer.

When Missy arrived at the office for her 32-week check-up, the nurse noted that she did not seem to be herself, was more reserved than normal, and seemed to be moving very slowly. In casual conversation, Missy said that she had been feeling "down in the dumps" and was having trouble sleeping.

On careful assessment the nurse found that Missy was sleeping about 6 interrupted hours a night and was anxious about her delivery because her FM symptoms had come back with a vengeance. She did not know how she would ever be able to go through labor, and she could not sleep because she was having so much lower back pain and indigestion. Because she was tired, she was not walking every day as she was accustomed to doing. Her husband was supportive and tried to do as much as he could for her. He worked full-time and commuted to New York by train 2 days a week. The following objective data were obtained:

Blood pressure	136/86 mm Hg
Temperature	98.2°F (36.8°C)
Respirations	18 breaths/min
Pulse	88 beats/min
Weight	166 lbs (75.5 kg; normal weight 120 lbs [54.5 kg]; last visit 150 lbs [68 kg])
Urine	No ketones, blood, or glucose

Baby	Vertex position
	Heart rate assessed at 140 beats/min
	Movement is vigorous

Using the Levine Conservation Model, the nurse's goal is to promote wholeness in the context of Missy's pregnancy.

Assessment

Challenges to Missy's Internal Environment

Missy is experiencing a normal pregnancy with the exception of weight gain of 16 pounds in one month. Her vital signs are normal; her diastolic pressure is 86 mm Hg. She rates her pain level as 7 on a scale of 0 to 10. The nurse questions Missy and learns that because of her fatigue, she is not eating as well as she had before. She is more likely to eat fast food to cut down on preparation time. Her husband is gone 2 days a week and she does not feel like cooking for herself.

Challenges to Missy's External Environment

Missy's perceptual environment is affected by her high level of pain and fatigue (feeling more tired than normal). Her operational environmental assessment reveals that she is bothered by the summer heat. She thinks heat might be the source of her fatigue and feeling down in the dumps. Her conceptual environment is challenged by her concerns about being able to manage labor, given her generalized discomfort and more severe pain in her lower back. She is disappointed about the return of her FM symptoms because she fears that this will interfere with her ability to go through natural childbirth. She is also concerned about her ability to be a good mother because of the aches and pain associated with the FM.

Energy Conservation

Missy's fatigue serves as a clue to an alteration in function. Missy may not be getting an adequate supply of nutrients to support

Continued

bodily functions. In addition she reports dyspepsia. She is taking her daily prenatal vitamins, yet her nutrition may be inadequate because of eating fast foods. She is more fatigued than usual, and the fatigue is affecting her ability to engage in activities of daily living.

Structural Integrity

Missy's pregnancy is progressing normally. Indicators suggest that the baby is growing and behaving normally. Fetal movement is as expected. Missy reports lower back pain which is making it difficult for her to sleep.

Personal Integrity

Missy is frustrated by the return of her FM symptoms and is afraid they may make labor and delivery difficult. These symptoms are challenging her ability to go through a natural delivery, something both she and her husband have planned for.

Social Integrity

The possibility of not being able to go through natural childbirth with her husband as coach challenges their social integrity, changing how they had expected to experience the birth of their child. Because she has felt down in the dumps, she is beginning to question her ability to be a good mother. She wants to breastfeed her child and is concerned about the demands that this may place on her ability to function.

Trophigcognoses

Inadequate nutrition based on frequent fast food meals

Lower back pain related to normal pregnancy changes and fibromyalgia

Lack of restful sleep related to lower back pain and indigestion

Inadequate self-esteem related to fear of not being able to fulfill her role as a mother

Anxiety related to anticipated discomfort during delivery

Hypotheses

Alteration in sleep position will improve the quality of Missy's sleep.

Exploring comfort options for her lower back pain will result in improved comfort and more restful sleep.

Identifying challenges related to delivery will help to reduce her anxiety.

Reviewing the expected changes post delivery will help Missy anticipate when she might need assistance because of her FM.

Discussing ways to parent in the context of FM will improve her self-esteem as a new mother.

Referring Missy for a nutritional consult will help her meet her nutritional needs and control her indigestion during her last trimester.

Nursing Interventions

Energy Conservation

The nutritional consultation will help Missy identify simple ways to meet her nutritional needs. The nutritionist will conduct a brief assessment of food normally eaten during a 24-hour period. Potentially helpful interventions that can be reinforced by nurses include: selecting healthier fast foods; eating smaller meals several times a day (fruit, vegetables, protein); preparing foods in larger quantities to reduce the anxiety and fatigue associated with always cooking; and avoiding gas-forming food such as carbonated beverages, beans and some green vegetables, like cucumber and broccoli.

Restful sleep is important for both physiological and emotional renewal. The goal is to help Missy sleep comfortably so that she actually feels rested. For Missy, pregnancy and the fibromyalgia are partners in the challenges associated with sleeping and the subsequent back pain. Discuss the use of pillows to support the body in a comfortable position. She currently uses several pillows at night to make it easier for her to breathe. Suggestions to support this modified sleeping position include using soft pillows to support her lower back and arms. This will help reduce pressure on tender points, relieving some discomfort. Advise her to take a brief nap in the morning and the afternoon to help her reenergize her emotions and prevent physiological disruptions.

Encourage her to discuss the possibility of using very low dose amitriptyline for sleep and pain management. Discussing this with the physician or nurse practitioner will help alleviate any fears about the effect of the medication on the baby, and the medication may help relieve the patient's discomfort. Additional interventions for sleep and pain include a warm bath before bed, the use of aromatherapy such as lavender, mild exercise (walking several times a day for 10 minutes each time), use of music or environmental sounds to induce relaxation, keeping the room temperature comfortable and constant, and establishing a routine bedtime and time to arise in the morning.

Structural Conservation

Improving Missy's nutrition will support the healing process needed after delivery of her child. The nurse will want to stress the importance of blood work to assess physiological nutrition and follow-up in response to changes in her eating habits. Acknowledge Missy's commitment to taking her prenatal vitamins and how important this is for the health and well-being of her baby.

Personal Integrity

Missy is anxious about delivery. Additional information is needed to determine what it is about delivery that concerns her. Once the challenges are identified, the nurse can reassure Missy that every effort will be made to support a normal delivery with the least amount of discomfort. Interventions will need to be adjusted to accommodate her FM. For example, the intensity of sustained contractions may require greater distraction (preferred music) and careful coaching.

It is important to reassure Missy that she can be a good mother even with the FM. She may need some assistance in adjusting activities to reduce discomfort when caring for her child across the spectrum of growth and development. Because she wants to breast feed, it is important that she be referred to a lactation consultant who will work with her to assure adequate latching and positions of comfort for the feedings. Women with FM have more difficulty with endurance than with ability to physically function. This means that Missy may need to reposition during breastfeeding to avoid stiffness and aching associated with FM. It is also important to begin a discussion about how she will care for her child. It is appropriate to recommend that she have some help for the first 2 to 4 weeks after the baby comes home, so that she can get the rest she needs and still bond with her child. It is also helpful to talk about things that she hopes to do with her child, so that she can begin to develop a healthy positive approach to motherhood. For example, throwing a ball for a long time challenges the endurance. However, she will be able to throw the ball for short periods of time without the fatigue associated with low endurance. She will learn through trial and error how long she can tolerate an activity. Usually at the first sign of muscle fatigue or aching, the activity should be stopped. Reading is wonderful for children and can be a source of great interaction and mothering, yet it requires limited use of muscles and energy.

Social Integrity

It is recommended that Missy's husband join her for the last several health visits before birth so that he is included in the discussions and planning for the baby. This will give him a chance to have questions answered and can be a great way to foster the parenting relationship. Missy acknowledges his support and willingness to help. If they have difficulty communicating concerns and

Continued

desires related to the pregnancy and recovery, they might benefit from a referral to a counselor familiar with FM. To maintain her social integrity, she will want to maintain a balance in her life so that her sense of being is not stressed.

Organismic Responses

In response to the above interventions, the nurse will observe for the following organismic responses.

Reduced lower back pain and restful sleep
Controlled dyspepsia
Normal hemoglobin and hematocrit

No protein in her urine
Average weight gain of 1 pound per week until delivery
Meeting with her husband and a lactation consultant
Reports that she has made arrangements for her mother (or other support person) to spend 2 weeks with her after the baby is born. Her sister will then spend a week so that she will have help for 3 weeks.
Discomfort controlled during delivery
Successful delivery of a healthy child
Expresses excitement about becoming a new mother

▓ Summary

Levine's notion of the environment as complex provides an excellent basis for continuing to develop an improved understanding of the environment. Studying the interactions between the external and the internal environment will provide for a better understanding of adaptation. This focus will provide for additional information about the challenges in the external environment and how they change over time. It is important that we understand the changes that occur and how the person who adapted before now changes the adaptive response in order to maintain balance or integrity. This adaptive response will inform the organismic response. With an improved repertoire of organismic responses, we can test how to predict these responses, and thus assure that adaptive responses occur. This acknowledges that the nurse may recognize that the most appropriate goal is to maintain comfort only (e.g., supportive interventions).

Moving to a more global perspective, the environment as defined according to Levine (1973) provides nurses with the opportunity to enhance their understanding of it and to provide interventions for communities that suffer from environmental disasters. An assessment of the internal environment's response to the challenge of the external environment (e.g., destruction from hurricanes) will immediately identify the altered health status of the community and the community needs. An assessment of the external environment will provide an understanding of the changes occurring due to the assault on the internal environment and a more detailed assessment of the perceptual, organismic, and conceptual levels of the environmental challenges. There is no question that this approach to describing, defining, and planning for environmental challenges will identify (1) the perceptual challenges; (2) the organismic challenges that may not be immediately known to the residents (e.g., pollution of air and water); and (3) the conceptual issues that increase nurses' awareness of the social, political, economic, and global impact on the predicament. This provides nurses with the opportunity to develop a political agenda and perhaps design public policy that might improve interventions in the context of a disaster. The Conservation Model has the components needed to provide nurses with a global perspective of the environment.

The methods of nurses and advanced practice nurses are changing rapidly to keep up with the current speed of health care system changes. Levine's Conservation Model provides an approach that educates good nurses and provides a foundation for their practice, whatever the role or the setting. Nurse practitioners, case managers, program planners, nurse midwives, nurse anesthetists, and nurse entrepreneurs are encouraged to test the model as a basis for improving and guiding their practice.

There is a renewed interest in the use of the model as a basis of nursing research. Zalon (2004) noted that the use of the integrities as guiding principles for research and identification of variables continues to result in wholeness. Delmore (2006) found that the model was an appropriate frame work for examining the effect of ventilator weaning on the patient's energy and structural integrity. Researchers must replicate these studies and publish their findings to ensure the continued development of the art and science of nursing. Levine will applaud their efforts.

> Theory is the poetry of science. The poet's words are familiar, each standing alone, but brought together they sing, they astonish, they teach. The theorist offers a fresh vision, familiar concepts brought together in bold, new designs. . . . The theorist and poet seek excitement in the sudden insights that make ordinary experience extraordinary, but theory caught in the intellectual exercises of the academy becomes alive only when it is made a true instrument of persuasion. (Levine, 1995, p. 14)

References

Alligood, M. R., & Marriner-Tomey, A. (Eds.) (1997). *Nursing theory: Utilization and application* (pp. 31–45). St. Louis, MO: C. V. Mosby.

Ballard, N., Robley, L., Barrett, D., Fraser, D., & Mendoza, I. (2006). Patients' recollections of therapeutic paralysis in the intensive care unit. *American Journal of Critical Care, 15*, 86–94.

Barnum, B. J. S. (1994). *Nursing theory: Analysis, application, evaluation* (4th ed.). Philadelphia: J. B. Lippincott.

Bates, M. (1967). A naturalist at large. *Natural History, 76*, 8–16.

Bayley, E. (1991). Care of the burn patients. In: K. M. Schaefer & J. B. Pond (Eds.), *The conservation model: A framework for nursing practice* (pp. 91–100). Philadelphia: F. A. Davis.

Beland, I. (1971). *Clinical nursing: Pathophysiological and psychological implications* (2nd ed.). New York: Dover.

Bernard, C. (1957). *An introduction to the study of experimental medicine.* New York: Dover.

Brunner, M. (1985). A conceptual approach to critical care nursing using Levine's model. *Focus on Critical Care, 12*(2), 39–44.

Burd, C., Olson, B., Langemo, D., Hunter, S., Hanson, D., Osowski, K. F., & Sauvage, T. (1994). Skin care strategies in a skilled nursing home. *Journal of Gerontological Nursing, 20*(11), 28–34.

Clark, M. J. (1992). *Nursing in the community.* Norwalk, CT: Appleton & Lange.

Cooper, D. H. (1990). Optimizing wound healing: A practice within nursing's domain. *Nursing Clinics of North America, 25*(1), 165–180.

Cox, R. A. Sr. (1991). A tradition of caring: Use of Levine's model in long-term care. In K. M. Schaefer & J. B. Pond (Eds.), *The conservation model: A framework for nursing practice* (pp. 179–197). Philadelphia: F. A. Davis.

Crawford-Gamble, P. E. (1986). An application of Levine's conceptual model. *Perioperative Nursing Quarterly, 2*(1), 64–70.

Delmore, B. A. (2003). Fatigue and prealbumin levels during the weaning process in long-term ventilated patients (Doctoral dissertation, New York University, 2003). *Dissertation Abstracts International, 64-05B,* 2127.

Delmore, B. A. (2006). Levine's framework in long-term ventilated patients during the weaning course. *Nursing Science Quarterly, 19*(3), 247–258.

Dever, M. (1991). Care of children. In: K. M. Schaefer & J. B. Pond (Eds.), *The conservation model: A framework for nursing practice* (pp. 71–83). Philadelphia: F. A. Davis.

Dibble, S. L., Bostrom-Ezerati, J., & Ruzzuto, C. (1991). Clinical predictors of intravenous site symptoms. *Research in Nursing & Health, 14,* 413–420.

Dow, J. S., & Mest, C. G. (1997). Psychosocial interventions for patients with chronic obstructive pulmonary disease. *Home-Healthcare-Nurse, 15*(6), 414–420.

Dubos, R. (1965). *Man adapting.* New Haven: Yale University Press.

Erickson, E. H. (1964). *Insight and responsibility.* New York: W. W. Norton.

Feynman, R. (1965). *The character of physical law.* Cambridge, MA: MIT Press.

Foreman, M. D. (1989). Confusion in the hospitalized elderly: Incidence, onset, and associated factors. *Research in Nursing & Health, 12*(1), 21–29.

Foreman, M. D. (1991). Conserving cognitive integrity of the hospitalized elderly. In: K. M. Schaefer & J. B. Pond (Eds.), *The conservation model: A framework for nursing practice* (pp. 133–150). Philadelphia: F. A. Davis.

Gibson, J. E. (1966). *The senses considered as perceptual systems.* Boston: Houghton Mifflin.

Goldstein, K. (1963). *The organism.* Boston: Beacon Press.

Grindley, J., & Paradowski, M. B. (1991). Developing an undergraduate program using Levine's model. In: K. M. Schaefer & J. B. Pond (Eds.), *The conservation model: A framework for nursing practice* (pp. 199–208). Philadelphia: F. A. Davis.

Hall, E. (1966). *The hidden dimension.* Garden City, NY: Doubleday.

Happ, M. B., Williams, C. C., Strumpf, N. E., & Burger, S. G. (1996). Individualized care for frail elderly: Theory and practice. *Journal of Gerontological Nursing, 22*(3), 7–14.

Hirschfeld, M. H. (1976). The cognitively impaired older adult. *American Journal of Nursing, 76,* 1981–1984.

Jost, S. G. (2000). An assessment and intervention strategy for managing staff needs during change. *Journal of Nursing Administration, 30*(1), 34–40.

Langer, V. S. (1990). Minimal handling protocol for the intensive care nursery. *Neonatal Network, 9*(3), 23–27.

Leach, M. J. (2006). Wound management: Using Levine's Conservation Model to guide practice. *Ostomy Wound Management.* Retrieved from http://www.o-wm.com/article/6024 (Accessed September 9, 2007).

Levine, M. E. (1965). Trophicognosis: An alternative to nursing diagnosis. *ANA Regional Clinical Conferences, 2,* 55–70.

Levine, M. E. (1966). Adaptation and assessment: A rationale for nursing intervention. *American Journal of Nursing, 66,* 2450–2453.

Levine, M. E. (1967). The four conservation principles of nursing. *Nursing Forum, 6,* 45–59.

Levine, M. E. (1968a). Knock before entering personal space bubbles (Part I). *Chart, 65*(1), 58–62.

Levine, M. E. (1968b). Knock before entering personal space bubbles (Part II). *Chart, 65*(2), 82–84.

Levine, M. E. (1969a). *Introduction to clinical nursing.* Philadelphia: F. A. Davis.

Levine, M. E. (1969b). The pursuit of wholeness. *American Journal of Nursing, 69,* 93–98.

Levine, M. E. (1971). Holistic nursing. *Nursing Clinics of North America, 6*(2), 253–263.

Levine, M. E. (1973). *Introduction to clinical nursing* (2nd ed.). Philadelphia: F. A. Davis.

Levine, M. E. (1977). Nursing ethics and the ethical nurse. *American Journal of Nursing, 77*(5), 845–849.

Levine, M. E. (1988a). Antecedents from adjunctive disciplines: Creation of nursing theory. *Nursing Science Quarterly, 1*(1), 16–21.

Levine, M. E. (1988b). Myra Levine. In: T. M. Schoor & A. Zimmerman (Eds.), *Making choices, taking chances: Nurse leaders tell their stories* (pp. 215–228). St. Louis, MO: C. V. Mosby.

Levine, M. E. (1989a). The conservation model: Twenty years later. In: J. P. Riehl-Sisca (Ed.), *Conceptual models for nursing practice* (pp. 325–337). Norwalk, CT: Appleton & Lange.

Levine, M. E. (1989b). Ration or rescue: The elderly in critical care. *Critical Care Nursing, 12*(1), 82–89.

Levine, M. E. (1989c). The ethics of nursing rhetoric. *Image: Journal of Nursing Scholarship, 21*(1), 4–5.

Levine, M. E. (1991). The conservation model: A model for health. In: K. M. Schaefer & J. B. Pond (Eds.), *The conservation model: A framework for nursing practice* (pp. 1–11). Philadelphia: F. A. Davis.

Levine, M. E. (1995). The rhetoric of nursing theory. *Image: Journal of Nursing Scholarship, 27*(2), 11–14.

Levine, M. E. (1996). The conservation principles: A retrospective. *Nursing Science Quarterly, 9*(1), 38–41.

Littrell, K., & Schumann, L. (1989). Promoting sleep for the patient with a myocardial infarction. *Critical Care Nurse, 9*(3), 44–49.

Loyola University, Chicago. Mid-Year Convocation: The Conferring of Honorary Degrees by R. C. Baumhart. Candidate for the degree of Doctor of Humane Letters, 1992, p. 6.

Lynn-McHale, D. J., & Smith, A. (1991). Comprehensive assessment of families of the critically ill. In J. S. Leske (Ed.), *AACN clinical issues in critical care nursing* (pp. 195–209). Philadelphia: J. B. Lippincott.

McCall, B. H. (1991). Neurological intensive monitoring. In: K. M. Schaefer & J. B. Pond (Eds.), *The conservation model: A framework for nursing practice* (pp. 83–90). Philadelphia: F. A. Davis.

Mefford, L. C. (1999). The relationship of nursing care to health outcomes of preterm infants: Testing a theory of health promotion for preterm infants based on Levine's Conservation Model of Nursing. Doctoral dissertation, the University of Tennessee, 1999. *Dissertation Abstracts International,* 60–098, 4522.

Mefford, L. C. (2004). A theory of health promotion for preterm infants based on Levine's conservation model of nursing. *Nursing Science Quarterly, 17*(3), 260–266.

Mock, V., St. Ours, C., Hall. H., Bositis, A., Tilley, M., Belcher, A., et al. (2007). Using a conceptual model in nursing research – mitigating fatigue in cancer patients. *Journal of Advanced Nursing, 59*(5), 503–512.

Molchany, C. A. (1992). Ventricular septal and free wall rupture complicating acute MI. *Journal of Cardiovascular Nursing, 6*(4), 38–45.

National League for Nursing Self Study Report (1978). Allentown College of St. Francis de Sales, Department of Nursing.

Neswick, R. S. (1997). Myra E. Levine: A theoretical basis for ET nursing. *Professional Practice, 24*(1), 6–9.

Nightingale, F. (1859). *Notes on nursing: What it is, and what it is not.* London: Harrison & Sons.

O'Laughlin, K. M. (1986). Change in bladder function in the woman undergoing radical hysterectomy for cervical cancer. *Journal of Obstetric, Gynecologic and Neonatal Nursing, 15*(5), 380–385.

Pond, J. B. (1991). Ambulatory care of the homeless. In: K. M. Schaefer & J. B. Pond (Eds.), *The conservation model: A framework for nursing practice* (pp. 167–178). Philadelphia: F. A. Davis.

Pond, J. B., & Taney, S. G. (1991). Emergency care in a large university emergency department. In: K. M. Schaefer & J. B. Pond (Eds.), *The conservation model: A framework for nursing practice* (pp. 151–166). Philadelphia: F. A. Davis.

Roberts, J. E., Fleming, N., & Yeates-Giese, D. (1991). Perineal integrity. In: K. M. Schaefer & J. B. Pond (Eds.), *The conservation model: A framework for nursing practice* (pp. 61–70). Philadelphia: F. A. Davis.

Roberts, K. L., Brittin, M., Cook, M., & deClifford, J. (1994). Boomerang pillows and respiratory capacity. *Clinical Nursing Research, 3*(2), 157–165.

Roberts, K. L., Brittin, M., & deClifford, J. (1995). Boomerang pillows and respiratory capacity in frail elderly women. *Clinical Nursing Research, 4*(4), 465–471.

Savage, T. A., & Culbert, C. (1989). Early interventions: The unique role of nursing. *Journal of Pediatric Nursing, 4*(5), 339–345.

Schaefer, K. M. (1991a). Levine's conservation principles and research. In K. M. Schaefer & J. B. Pond (Eds.), *The conservation model: A framework for nursing practice* (pp. 45–59). Philadelphia: F. A. Davis.

Schaefer, K. M. (1991b). Care of the patient with congestive heart failure. In K. M. Schaefer & J. B. Pond (Eds.), *The conservation model: A framework for nursing practice* (pp. 119–132). Philadelphia: F. A. Davis.

Schaefer, K. M. (1991c). Developing a graduate program in nursing: integrating Levine's philosophy. In: K. M. Schaefer & J. B. Pond (Eds.), *The conservation model: A framework for nursing practice* (pp. 209–218). Philadelphia: F. A. Davis.

Schaefer, K. M. (2006a). Levine's conservation model in practice. In: M. R. Alligood & A. Marriner-Tomey (Eds.), *Nursing theory: Utilization and application* (pp. 207–226). St. Louis, MO: C. V. Mosby.

Schaefer, K. M. (2006b). Myra Estrin Levine: The conservation model. In: A. M. Tomey & M. R. Alligood (Eds.), *Nursing theorists and their work* (pp. 227–243). St. Louis, MO: C. V. Mosby.

Schaefer, K. M., & Shober-Potylycki, M. J. (1993). Fatigue associated with congestive heart failure: Use of Levine's Conservation Model. *Journal of Advanced Nursing, 18*, 260–268.

Schaefer, K. M., Swavely, D., Rothenberger, C., Hess, S., & Willistin, D. (1996). Sleep disturbances post coronary artery bypass surgery. *Progress in Cardiovascular Nursing, 11*(1), 5–14.

Selye, H. (1956). *The stress of life.* New York: McGraw-Hill.

Taylor, J. W. (1974). Measuring the outcomes of nursing care. *Nursing Clinics of North America, 9*, 337–348.

Taylor, J. W. (1989). Levine's conservation principles: Using the model for nursing diagnosis in a neurological setting. In: J. P. Riehl-Sisca (Ed.), *Conceptual models for nursing practice* (3rd ed., pp. 349–358). Norwalk, CT: Appleton & Lange.

Tribotti, S. (1990). Admission to the neonatal intensive care unit: Reducing the risks. *Neonatal Network, 8*(4), 17–22.

Waddington, C. H. (Ed.). (1968). *Towards a theoretical biology: I. Prolegomena.* Chicago: Aldine.

Webb, H. (1993). Holistic care following palliative Hartmann's procedure. *British Journal of Nursing, 2*(2), 128–132.

Wolf, S. (1961). Disease as a way of life: Neural integration in systemic pathology. *Perspectives on Biological Medicine, 5*, 288–303.

Zalon, M. L. (2004). Correlates of recovery among older adults after major abdominal surgery. *Nursing Research, 53*(2), 99–106.

Chapter 8

Dorothy Johnson's Behavioral System Model and Its Applications

BONNIE HOLADAY

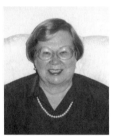

Dorothy Johnson

Introducing the Theorist

Dorothy Johnson's earliest publications pertained to the knowledge base nurses needed for nursing care (Johnson, 1959, 1961). Throughout her career, Johnson stressed that nursing had a unique, independent contribution to health care that was distinct from "delegated medical care." Johnson was one of the first "grand theorists" to present her views as a conceptual model. Her model was the first to provide both a guide to understanding and a guide to action. These two ideas—understanding seen first as a holistic, behavioral system process mediated by a complex framework and second as an active process of encounter and response—are central to the work of other theorists who followed her lead and developed conceptual models for nursing practice.

Dorothy Johnson was born on August 21, 1919, in Savannah, Georgia. She received her associate of arts degree from Armstrong Junior College in Savannah, Georgia, in 1938 and her bachelor of science in nursing degree from Vanderbilt University in 1942. She practiced briefly as a staff nurse at the Chatham-Savannah Health Council before attending Harvard University, where she received her master of public health (MPH) in 1948. She began her academic career at Vanderbilt University School of Nursing. A call from Lulu Hassenplug, Dean of the School of Nursing, enticed her to go to the University of California at Los Angeles (UCLA) in 1949. She served there as an assistant, associate, and professor of pediatric nursing until her retirement in 1978. She passed away in 1999.

During her academic career, Dorothy Johnson addressed issues related to nursing practice, nursing education, and nursing science. While she was a pediatric nursing advisor at the Christian Medical College School of Nursing in Vellare, South India, she wrote a series of clinical articles for the *Nursing Journal of India* (Johnson, 1956, 1957). She worked with the California Nurses' Association, the National League for Nursing, and the American Nurses' Association to examine the role of the clinical nurse specialist, the scope of nursing practice, and the need for nursing research. She also completed a Public Health Service–funded research project ("Crying as a Physiologic State in the Newborn Infant") in 1963 (Johnson & Smith, 1963). The foundations of her model and her beliefs about nursing are clearly evident in these early publications.

Overview of Johnson's Behavioral System Model

Johnson has noted that her theory, the Johnson Behavioral System Model (JBSM), evolved from philosophical ideas, theory, and research; her clinical background; and many years of thought, discussions, and writing (Johnson, 1968). She cited a number of sources for her theory. From Florence Nightingale came the belief that nursing's concern is a focus on the person rather than the disease. Systems theorists (Buckley, 1968; Chin, 1961; Parsons & Shils, 1951; Rapoport, 1968; Von Bertalanffy, 1968) were all sources for her model. Johnson's background as a pediatric nurse is also evident in the development of her model. In her papers, Johnson cited developmental literature to support the validity of a behavioral system model (Ainsworth, 1964; Crandal, 1963; Gerwitz, 1972; Kagan, 1964; Sears, Maccoby, & Levin, 1954). Johnson also noted that a number of her subsystems had biological underpinnings.

Johnson's theory and her related writings reflect her knowledge about both development and general systems theories. The combination of nursing, development, and general systems introduces into the rhetoric about nursing theory development some of the specifics that make it possible to test hypotheses and conduct critical experiments.

Five Core Principles

Johnson's model incorporates five core principles of system thinking: wholeness and order, stabilization, reorganization, hierarchic interaction, and dialectical contradiction. Each of these general systems principles has analogs in developmental theories that Johnson used to verify the validity of her model (Johnson, 1980, 1990). Wholeness and order provide the basis for continuity and identity, stabilization for development, reorganization for growth and/or change, hierarchic interaction for discontinuity, and dialectical contradiction for motivation. Johnson conceptualized a person as an open system with organized, interrelated, and interdependent subsystems. By virtue of subsystem interaction and independence, the whole of the human organism (system) is greater than the sum of its parts (subsystems). Wholes and their parts create a system with dual constraints: Neither has continuity and identity without the other.

The overall representation of the model can also be viewed as a behavioral system within an environment. The behavioral system and the environment are linked by interactions and transactions. We define the person (behavioral system) as comprising subsystems and the environment as comprising physical, interpersonal (e.g., father, friend, mother, sibling), and sociocultural (e.g., rules and mores of home, school, country, and other cultural contexts) components that supply the sustenal imperatives (Grubbs, 1980; Holaday, 1997; Johnson, 1990; Meleis, 1991).

Wholeness and Order

The developmental analogy of wholeness and order is continuity and identity. Given the behavioral system's potential for plasticity, a basic feature of the system is that both continuity and change can exist across the life span. The presence of or potentiality for at least some plasticity means that the key way of casting the issue of continuity is not a matter of deciding what exists for a given process or function of a subsystem. Instead, the issue should be cast in terms of determining patterns of interactions among levels of the behavioral system that may promote continuity for a particular subsystem at a given point in time. Johnson's work infers that continuity is in the relationship of the parts rather than in their individuality. Johnson (1990) noted that at the psychological level, attachment (affiliative) and dependency are examples of important specific behaviors that change over time while the representation (meaning) may remain the same. Johnson stated: "[D]evelopmentally, dependence behavior in the socially optimum case evolves from almost total dependence on others to a greater degree of dependence on self, with a certain amount of interdependence essential to the survival of social groups" (1990, p. 28). In terms of behavioral system balance, this pattern of dependence to independence may be repeated as the behavioral system engages in new situations during the course of a lifetime.

Stabilization

Stabilization or behavioral system balance is another core principle of the JBSM. Dynamic systems respond to contextual changes by either a homeostatic or homeorhetic process. Systems have a set point (like a thermostat) that they try to maintain by altering internal conditions to compensate for changes in external conditions. Human thermoregulation is an example of a homeostatic process that is primarily biological but is also behavioral (turning on the heater). Narcissism or the use of attribution of ability or effort are behavioral homeostatic processes we use to interpret activities so they are consistent with our mental organization.

From a behavioral system perspective, homeorrhesis is a more important stabilizing process than is homeostasis. In homeorrhesis, the system stabilizes around a trajectory rather than a set point. A toddler placed in a body cast may show motor lags when the cast is removed but soon shows age-appropriate motor skills. An adult newly diagnosed with asthma who does not receive proper education until a year after diagnosis can successfully incorporate the material into her daily activities. These are examples of homeorhetic processes or self-righting tendencies that can occur over time.

What we as nurses observe as development or adaptation of the behavioral system is a product of stabilization. When a person is ill or threatened with illness, he or she is subject to biopsychosocial perturbations. The nurse, according to Johnson (1980, 1990), acts as the external regulator and monitors patient response, looking for successful adaptation to occur. If behavioral system balance returns, there is no need for intervention. If not, the nurse intervenes to help the patient restore behavioral system balance. It is hoped that the patient matures and with additional hospitalizations the previous patterns of response have been assimilated and there are few disturbances.

Reorganization

Adaptive reorganization occurs when the behavioral system encounters new experiences in the environment that cannot be balanced by existing system mechanisms. Adaptation is defined as change that permits the behavioral system to maintain its set points best in new situations. To the extent that the behavioral system cannot assimilate the new conditions with existing regulatory mechanisms, accommodation must occur either as a new relationship between subsystems or by the establishment of a higher order or different cognitive schema (set, choice). The nurse acts to provide conditions or resources essential to help the accommodation process, may impose regulatory or control mechanisms to stimulate or reinforce certain behaviors, or may attempt to repair structural components (Johnson, 1980).

The difference between stabilization and reorganization is that the latter involves change or evolution. A behavioral system is embedded in an environment, but it is capable of operating independently of environmental constraints through the process of adaptation. The diagnosis of a chronic illness, the birth of a child, or the development of a healthy lifestyle regimen to prevent problems in later years are all examples wherein accommodation not only promotes behavioral system balance, but also involves a developmental process that results in the establishment of a higher order or more complex behavioral system.

Hierarchic Interaction

Each behavioral system exists in a context of hierarchical relationships and environmental relationships. From the perspective of general systems theory, a behavioral system that has the properties of wholeness and order, stabilization, and reorganization will also demonstrate a hierarchic structure (Buckley, 1968). Hierarchies, or a pattern of relying on particular subsystems, lead to a degree of stability. A disruption or failure will not destroy the whole system but instead lead to decomposition to the next level of stability.

The judgment that a discontinuity has occurred is typically based on a lack of correlation between assessments at two points of time. For example, one's lifestyle before surgery is not a good fit postoperatively. These discontinuities can provide opportunities for reorganization and development.

Dialectical Contradiction

The last core principle is the motivational force for behavioral change. Johnson (1980) described these as drives and noted that these responses are developed and modified over time through maturation, experience, and learning. A person's activities in the environment lead to knowledge and development. However, by acting on the world, each person is constantly changing it and his or her goals, and therefore changing what he or she needs to know. The number of environmental domains that the person is responding to include the biological, psychological, cultural, familial, social, and physical setting. The person needs to resolve (maintain behavioral system balance of) a cascade of contradictions between goals related to physical status, social

roles, and cognitive status when faced with illness or the threat of illness. Nurses' interventions during these periods can make a significant difference in the lives of the persons involved. Behavioral system balance is restored and a new level of development is attained.

Johnson's model is unique, in part, because it takes from both general systems and developmental theories. One may analyze the patient's response in terms of behavioral system balance, and, from a developmental perspective ask, "Where did this come from and where is it going?" The developmental component necessitates that we identify and understand the processes of stabilization and sources of disturbances that lead to reorganization. These need to be evaluated by age, gender, and culture. The combination of systems theory and development identifies "nursing's unique social mission and our special realm of original responsibility in patient care" (Johnson, 1990, p. 32).

Major Concepts of the Model

Next, we review the model as a behavioral system within an environment.

Person

Johnson conceptualized a nursing client as a behavioral system. The behavioral system is orderly, repetitive, and organized with interrelated and interdependent biological and behavioral subsystems. The client is seen as a collection of behavioral subsystems that interrelate to form the behavioral system. The system may be defined as "those complex, overt actions or responses to a variety of stimuli present in the surrounding environment that are purposeful and functional" (Auger, 1976, p. 22). These ways of behaving form an organized and integrated functional unit that determines and limits the interaction between the person and environment and establishes the relationship of the person to the objects, events, and situations in the environment. Johnson (1980, p. 209) considered such "behavior to be orderly, purposeful and predictable; that is, it is functionally efficient and effective most of the time, and is sufficiently stable and recurrent to be amenable to description and exploration."

Subsystems

The parts of the behavioral system are called subsystems. They carry out specialized tasks or functions needed to maintain the integrity of the whole behavioral system and manage its relationship to the environment. Each of these subsystems has a set of behavioral responses that is developed and modified through motivation, experience, and learning.

Johnson identified seven subsystems. However, in this author's operationalization of the model, as in Grubbs (1980), I have included eight subsystems. These eight subsystems and their goals and functions are described in Table 8-1. Johnson noted that these subsystems are found cross-culturally and across a broad range of the phylogenetic scale. She also noted the significance of social and cultural factors involved in the development of the subsystems. She did not consider the seven subsystems as complete, because "the ultimate group of response systems to be identified in the behavioral system will undoubtedly change as research reveals new subsystems or indicated changes in the structure, functions, or behavioral groupings in the original set" (Johnson, 1980, p. 214).

Each subsystem has functions that serve to meet the conceptual goal. Functional behaviors are the activities carried out to meet these goals. These behaviors may vary with each individual, depending on the person's age, sex,

Table 8 • 1   The Subsystems of Behavior

Achievement Subsystem

Goal	Mastery or control of self or the environment
Function	To set appropriate goals To direct behaviors toward achieving a desired goal To perceive recognition from others To differentiate between immediate goals and long-term goals To interpret feedback (input received) to evaluate the achievement of goals

Affiliative Subsystem

Goal	To relate or belong to someone or something other than oneself; to achieve intimacy and inclusion
Function	To form cooperative and interdependent role relationships within human social systems To develop and use interpersonal skills to achieve intimacy and inclusion To share To be related to another in a definite way To use narcissistic feelings in an appropriate way

Aggressive/Protective Subsystem

Goal	To protect self or others from real or imagined threatening objects, persons, or ideas; to achieve self-protection and self-assertion
Function	To recognize biological, environmental, or health systems that are potential threats to self or others To mobilize resources to respond to challenges identified as threats To use resources or feedback mechanisms to alter biological, environmental, or health input or human responses in order to diminish threats to self or others To protect one's achievement goals To protect one's beliefs To protect one's identity or self-concept

Table 8 • 1   The Subsystems of Behavior—cont'd

Dependency Subsystem

Goal	To obtain focused attention, approval, nurturance, and physical assistance; to maintain the environmental resources needed for assistance; to gain trust and reliance
Function	To obtain approval, reassurance about self To make others aware of self To induce others to care for physical needs To evolve from a state of total dependence on others to a state of increased dependence on the self To recognize and accept situations requiring reversal of self-dependence (dependence upon others) To focus on another or oneself in relation to social, psychological, and cultural needs and desires

Eliminative Subsystem

Goal	To expel biological wastes; to externalize the internal biological environment
Function	To recognize and interpret input from the biological system that signals readiness for waste excretion To maintain physiological homeostasis through excretion To adjust to alterations in biological capabilities related to waste excretion while maintaining a sense of control over waste excretion To relieve feelings of tension in the self To express one's feelings, emotions, and ideas verbally or nonverbally

Ingestive Subsystem

Goal	To take in needed resources from the environment to maintain the integrity of the organism or to achieve a state of pleasure; to internalize the external environment
Function	To sustain life through nutritive intake To alter ineffective patterns of nutritive intake To relieve pain or other psychophysiological subsystems To obtain knowledge or information useful to the self To obtain physical and/or emotional pleasure from intake of nutritive or nonnutritive substances

Restorative Subsystem

Goal	To relieve fatigue and/or achieve a state of equilibrium by reestablishing or replenishing the energy distribution among the other subsystems; to redistribute energy
Function	To maintain and/or return to physiological homeostasis To produce relaxation of the self system

Sexual Subsystem

Goal	To procreate, to gratify or attract; to fulfill expectations associated with one's gender; to care for others and to be cared about by them
Function	To develop a self-concept or self-identity based on gender To project an image of oneself as a sexual being To recognize and interpret biological system input related to sexual gratification and/or procreation To establish meaningful relationships in which sexual gratification and/or procreation may be obtained

Sources: Based on J. Grubbs (1980). An interpretation of the Johnson behavioral system model. In: J. P. Riehl & C. Roy (Eds.), *Conceptual models for nursing practice* (2nd ed., pp. 217–254). New York: Appleton-Century-Crofts; D. E. Johnson (1980). The behavioral system model for nursing. In: J. P. Riehl & C. Roy (Eds.), *Conceptual models for nursing practice* (2nd ed., pp. 207–216). New York: Appleton-Century-Crofts; D. Wilkie (1987). *Operationalization of the JBSM.* Unpublished paper. University of California, San Francisco; and B. Holaday (1972). *Operationalization of the JBSM.* Unpublished paper. University of California, Los Angeles.

motives, cultural values, social norms, and self-concepts. For the subsystem goals to be accomplished, behavioral system structural components must meet functional requirements of the behavioral system.

Each subsystem is composed of at least four structural components that interact in a specific pattern: goal, set, choice, and action. The goal of a subsystem is defined as the desired result or consequence of the behavior. The basis for the goal is a universal drive whose existence can be supported by scientific research. In general, the drive of each subsystem is the same for all people, but there are variations among individuals (and within individuals over time) in the specific objects or events that are drive-fulfilling, in the value placed on goal attainment, and in drive strength. With drives as the impetus for the behavior, goals can be identified and are considered universal.

The behavioral set is a predisposition to act in a certain way in a given situation. The behavioral set represents a relatively stable and habitual behavioral pattern of responses to particular drives or stimuli. It is learned behavior and is influenced by knowledge, attitudes, and beliefs. The set contains two components: perseveration and preparation. The perseveratory set refers to a consistent tendency to react to certain stimuli with the same pattern of behavior. The preparatory set is contingent upon the function of the perseveratory set. The preparatory set functions to establish priorities for attending or not attending to various stimuli.

The conceptual set is an additional component to the model (Holaday, 1982). It is a process of ordering that serves as the mediating link between stimuli from the preparatory and perseveratory sets. Here attitudes, beliefs, information, and knowledge are examined before a choice is made. There are three levels of processing—an inadequate conceptual set, a developing conceptual set, and a sophisticated conceptual set.

The third and fourth components of each subsystem are choice and action. Choice refers to the individual's repertoire of alternative behaviors in a situation that will best meet the goal and attain the desired outcome. The larger the behavioral repertoire of alternative behaviors in a situation, the more adaptable is the individual. The fourth structural component of each subsystem is the observable action of the individual. The concern is with the efficiency and effectiveness of the behavior in goal attainment. Actions are any observable responses to stimuli.

For the eight subsystems to develop and maintain stability, each must have a constant supply of functional requirements (sustenal imperatives). The concept of functional requirements tends to be confined to conditions of the system's survival, and it includes biological as well as psychosocial needs. The problems are related to establishing the types of functional requirements (universal versus highly specific) and finding procedures for validating the assumptions of these requirements. It also suggests a classification of the various states or processes on the basis of some principle and perhaps the establishment of a hierarchy among them. The Johnson model proposes that, for the behavior to be maintained, it must be protected, nurtured, and stimulated: It requires protection from noxious stimuli that threaten the survival of the behavioral system; nurturance, which provides adequate input to sustain behavior; and stimulation, which contributes to continued growth of the behavior and counteracts stagnation. A deficiency in any or all of these functional requirements threatens the behavioral system as a whole, or the effective functioning of the particular subsystem with which it is directly involved.

Environment

Johnson referred to the internal and external environment of the system. She also referred to the interaction between the person and the environment and to the objects, events, and situations in the environment. She also noted that there are forces in the environment that impinge on the person and to which the person adjusts. Thus, the environment consists of all elements that are not a part of the individual's behavioral system but influence the system and can serve as a source of sustenal imperatives.

Some of these elements can be manipulated by the nurse to achieve health (behavioral system balance or stability) for the patient. Johnson provided no other specific definition of the environment, nor did she identify what she considered internal versus external environment. But much can be inferred from her writings, and system theory also provides additional insights into the environment component of the model.

The external environment may include people, objects, and phenomena that can potentially permeate the boundary of the behavioral system. This external stimulus forms an organized or meaningful pattern that elicits a response from the individual. The behavioral system attempts to maintain equilibrium in response to environmental factors by assimilating and accommodating to the forces that impinge upon it. Areas of external environment of interest to nurses include the physical settings, people, objects, phenomena, and psychosocial–cultural attributes of an environment.

Johnson provided detailed information about the internal structure and how it functions. She also noted that "[i]llness or other sudden internal or external environmental change is most frequently responsible for system malfunction" (Johnson, 1980, p. 212). Such factors as physiology; temperament; ego; age; and related developmental capacities, attitudes, and self-concept are general regulators that may be viewed as a class of internalized intervening variables that influence set, choice, and action. They are key areas for nursing assessment. For example, a nurse attempting to respond to the needs of an acutely ill hospitalized 6-year-old would need to know something about the developmental capacities of a 6-year-old, and about self-concept and ego development, to understand the child's behavior.

Health

Johnson viewed health as efficient and effective functioning of the system and as behavioral system balance and stability. Behavioral system balance and stability are demonstrated by observed behavior that is purposeful, orderly, and predictable. Such behavior is maintained when it is efficient and effective in managing the person's relationship to the environment.

Behavior changes when efficiency and effectiveness are no longer evident or when a more optimal level of functioning is perceived. Individuals are said to achieve efficient and effective behavioral functioning when their behavior is commensurate with social demands, when they are able to modify their behavior in ways that support biologic imperatives, when they are able to benefit to the fullest extent during illness from the physician's knowledge and skill, and when their behavior does not reveal unnecessary trauma as a consequence of illness (Johnson, 1980, p. 207).

Behavior system imbalance and instability are not described explicitly but can be inferred from the following statement to be a malfunction of the behavioral system:

> The subsystems and the system as a whole tend to be self-maintaining and self-perpetuating so long as conditions in the internal and external environment of the system remain orderly and predictable, the conditions and resources necessary to their functional requirements are met, and the interrelationships among the subsystems are harmonious. If these conditions are not met, malfunction becomes apparent in behavior that is in part disorganized, erratic, and dysfunctional. Illness or other sudden internal or external environmental change is most frequently responsible for such malfunctions. (Johnson, 1980, p. 212)

Thus, Johnson equates behavioral system imbalance and instability with illness. However, as Meleis (1991) has pointed out, we must consider that illness may be separate from behavioral system functioning. Johnson also referred to physical and social health, but did not specifically define wellness. Just as the inference about illness may be made, it may be inferred that wellness is behavioral system balance and stability, as well as efficient and effective behavioral functioning.

Nursing and Nursing Therapeutics

Nursing is viewed as "a service that is complementary to that of medicine and other health professions, but which makes its own distinctive contribution to the health and well-being of people." (Johnson, 1980, p. 207) She distinguished nursing from medicine by noting that nursing views the patient as a behavioral system, and medicine views the patient as a biological system. In her view, the specific goal of nursing action is "to restore, maintain, or attain behavioral system balance and stability at the highest possible level for the individual" (Johnson, 1980, p. 214). This goal may be expanded to include helping the person achieve an optimal level of balance and functioning when this is possible and desired.

The goal of the system's action is behavioral system balance. For the nurse, the area of concern is a behavioral system threatened by the loss of order and predictability through illness or the threat of illness. The goal of a nurse's action is to maintain or restore the individual's behavioral system balance and stability or to help the individual achieve a more optimal level of balance and functioning.

Johnson did not specify the steps of the nursing process but clearly identified the role of the nurse as an external regulatory force. She also identified questions to be asked when analyzing system functioning, and she provided diagnostic classifications to delineate disturbances and guidelines for interventions.

Johnson (1980) expected the nurse to base judgments about behavioral system balance and stability on knowledge and an explicit value system. One important point she made about the value system is that "given that the person has been provided with an adequate understanding of the potential for and means to obtain a more optimal level of behavioral functioning than is evident at the present time, the final judgment of the desired level of functioning is the right of the individual" (Johnson, 1980, p. 215).

The source of difficulty arises from structural and functional stresses. Structural and functional problems develop when the system is unable to meet its own functional requirements.

As a result of the inability to meet functional requirements, structural impairments may take place. In addition, functional stress may be found as a result of structural damage or from the dysfunctional consequences of the behavior. Other problems develop when the system's control and regulatory mechanisms fail to develop or become defective.

Four diagnostic classifications to delineate these disturbances are differentiated in the model. A disorder originating within any one subsystem is classified as either an insufficiency, which exists when a subsystem is not functioning or developed to its fullest capacity due to inadequacy of functional requirements, or as a discrepancy, which exists when a behavior does not meet the intended conceptual goal. Disorders found between more than one subsystem are classified either as an incompatibility, which exists when the behaviors of two or more subsystems in the same situation conflict with each other to the detriment of the individual, or as dominance, which exists when the behavior of one subsystem is used more than any other, regardless of the situation or to the detriment of the other subsystems. This is also an area where Johnson believed additional diagnostic classifications would be developed. Nursing therapeutics deal with these three areas.

The next critical element is the nature of the interventions the nurse would use to respond to the behavioral system imbalance. The first step is a thorough assessment to find the source of the difficulty or the origin of the problem. There are at least three types of interventions that the nurse can use to bring about change. The nurse may attempt to repair damaged structural units by altering the individual's set and choice. The second would be for the nurse to impose regulatory and control measures. The nurse acts outside the patient environment to provide the conditions, resources, and controls necessary to restore behavioral system balance. The nurse also acts within and upon the external environment and the internal interactions of the subsystem to create change and restore stability. The third, and most common, treatment modality is to supply or to help the client find his or her own supplies of essential functional requirements. The nurse may provide nurturance (resources and conditions necessary for survival and growth; the nurse may train the client to cope with new stimuli and encourage effective behaviors), stimulation (provision of stimuli that brings forth new behaviors or increases behaviors, that provides motivation for a particular behavior, and that provides opportunities for appropriate behaviors), and protection (safeguarding from noxious stimuli, defending from unnecessary threats, and coping with a threat on the individual's behalf). The nurse and the client negotiate the treatment plan.

Applications of the Model

Fundamental to any professional discipline is the development of a scientific body of knowledge that can be used to guide its practice. JBSM has served as a means for identifying, labeling, and classifying phenomena important to the nursing discipline. Nurses have used the JBSM model since the early 1970s, and the model has demonstrated its ability to provide a medium for theoretical growth; organization for nurses' thinking, observations, and interpretations of what was observed; a systematic structure and rationale for activities; direction to the search for relevant research questions; solutions for patient care problems; and, finally, criteria to determine if a problem has been solved.

Practice-Focused Research

Stevenson and Woods (1986) state: "Nursing science is the domain of knowledge concerned with the adaptation of individuals and groups to actual or potential health problems, the environments that influence health in humans and the therapeutic interventions that promote health and affect the consequences of illness" (1986, p. 6). This position focuses efforts in nursing science on the expansion of knowledge about clients' health problems and nursing therapeutics. Nurse

researchers have demonstrated the usefulness of Johnson's model in a clinical practice in a variety of ways. The majority of the research focuses on clients' functioning in terms of maintaining or restoring behavioral system balance, understanding the system and/or subsystems by focusing on the basic sciences, or focusing on the nurse as an agent of action who uses the JBSM to gather diagnostic data or to provide care that influences behavioral system balance.

Derdiarian (1990, 1991) examined the nurse as an action agent within the practice domain. She focused on the nurses' assessment of the patient using the DBSM and the effect of using this instrument on the quality of care (Derdiarian, 1990, 1991). This approach expanded the view of nursing knowledge from exclusively client-based to knowledge about the context and practice of nursing that is model-based. The results of these studies found a significant increase in patient and nurse satisfaction when the DBSM was used. Derdiarian (1983, 1983b, 1988) also found that a model-based, valid, and reliable instrument could improve the comprehensiveness and the quality of assessment data; the method of assessment; and the quality of nursing diagnosis, interventions, and outcome. Derdiarian's body of work reflects the complexity of nursing's knowledge as well as the strategic problem-solving capabilities of the JBSM. Her article (Derdiarian, 1991) demonstrated the clear relationship between Johnson's theory and nursing practice.

Others have demonstrated the utility of Johnson's model for clinical practice. Coward and Wilke (2000) used the JBSM to examine cancer pain control behaviors. D'Huyvetter (2000) found that defining trauma as a disease, and approaching it within the context of the JBSM, helps the practitioner develop effective interventions. Box 8-1 highlights the research on this theory.

Lewis and Randell (1990) used the JBSM to identify the most common nursing diagnoses of hospitalized geopsychiatric patients. They found that 30 percent of the diagnoses were related to the achievement subsystem.

Box 8-1	Bonnie Holaday's Research Highlighted

My program of research has examined normal and atypical patterns of behavior of children with a chronic illness and the behavior of their parents and the interrelationship between the children and the environment. My goal was to determine the causes of instability within and between subsystems (e.g., breakdown in internal regulatory or control mechanisms) and to identify the source of problems in behavioral system balance.

My first study (Holaday, 1974) compared the achievement behavior of chronically ill and healthy children. The study showed that chronically ill children differed in attributional tendencies when compared with healthy children and showed that the response patterns differed within the chronically ill group when compared on certain dimensions (e.g., gender, age at diagnosis). Males and children diagnosed at birth attributed both success and failure to the presence or absence of ability and little to effort. This is a pattern found in children with low achievement needs. The results indicated behavioral system imbalance and focused my attention on interventions directed toward set, choice, and action.

The next series of studies used the concept of "behavioral set" and examined how mothers and their chronically ill infants interacted (Holaday, 1981, 1982, 1987). Patterns of maternal response provided information related to the setting of the "set goal" or behavioral set; that is, the degree of proximity and speed of maternal response. Mothers with chronically ill infants rarely did not respond to a cry indicating a narrow behavioral set. Further analysis of the data led to the identification of a new structural component of the model-conceptual set. A person's conceptual set was defined as an organized cluster of cognitive units that were used to interpret the content information from the preparatory and perseveratory sets. A conceptual set may differ both in the number of cognitive units involved and in the degree of organization exhibited. The various cognitive units that make up a conceptual set may vary in complexity depending on the situation. Three levels of conceptual set have been identified, ranging from a very simple to a complex "set" with a high degree of connectedness between multiple perspectives (Holaday, 1982). Thus, the conceptual set functions as an information collection and processing unit. Examining a person's set, choice, and conceptual set offered a way to examine issues of individual cognitive patterns and its impact on behavioral system balance.

The most recent study (Holaday, Turner-Henson, & Swan, 1997) drew from the knowledge gained from previous studies. This study viewed the JBSM as holistic, in that it assumed that all part processes—biological, physical, psychological, and sociocultural—are interrelated; developmental, in that it assumed that development proceeds from a relative lack of differentiation toward a goal of differentiation and hierarchic integration of organismic functioning; and system-oriented, in that a unit of analysis was the person in the environment where the person's physical and/or biological (e.g., health), psychological, interpersonal, and sociocultural levels of organization are operative and interrelated with the physical, interpersonal, and sociocultural levels of organization in the environment. Our results indicate that it was possible to determine the impact of a lack of functional requirements on a child's actions and to identify behavioral system imbalance and the need for specific types of nursing intervention.

The goal of my research program has been to describe the relations both among and within the subsystems that make up the integrated whole and to identify the type of nursing interventions that restore behavioral system balance.

They also found that the JBSM was more specific than NANDA (North American Nursing Diagnosis Association) diagnoses, which demonstrated considerable overlap. Poster, Dee, and Randell (1997) found the JBSM was an effective framework to use to evaluate patient outcomes.

Education

Johnson's model was used as the basis for undergraduate education at the UCLA School of Nursing. The curriculum was developed by the faculty; however, no published material is available that describes this process. Texts by Wu (1973) and Auger

(1976) extended Johnson's model and provided some idea of the content of that curriculum. Later, in the 1980s, Harris (1986) described the use of Johnson's theory as a framework for UCLA's curriculum. The Universities of Hawaii, Alaska, and Colorado also used the JBSM as a basis for their undergraduate curricula.

Loveland-Cherry and Wilkerson (1983) analyzed Johnson's model and concluded that the model could be used to develop a curriculum. The primary focus of the program would be the study of the person as a behavioral system. The student would need a background in systems theory and in the biological, psychological, and sociological sciences.

Nursing Practice and Administration

Johnson has influenced nursing practice because she enabled nurses to make statements about the links between nursing input and health outcomes for clients. The model has been useful in practice because it identifies an end product (behavioral system balance), which is nursing's goal. Nursing's specific objective is to maintain or restore the person's behavioral system balance and stability, or to help the person achieve a more optimum level of functioning. The model provides a means for identifying the source of the problem in the system. Nursing is seen as the external regulatory force that acts to restore balance (Johnson, 1980).

One of the best examples of the model's use in practice has been at the University of California, Los Angeles, Neuropsychiatric Institute (UCLA—NPI). Auger and Dee (1983) designed a patient classification system using the JBSM. Each subsystem of behavior was operationalized in terms of critical adaptive and maladaptive behaviors. The behavioral statements were designed to be measurable, relevant to the clinical setting, observable, and specific to the subsystem. The use of the model has had a major impact on all phases of the nursing process, including a more systematic assessment process, identification of patient strengths and problem areas, and an objective means for evaluating the

quality of nursing care (Dee & Auger, 1983).

The early works of Dee and Auger led to further refinement in the patient classification system. Behavioral indices for each subsystem have been further operationalized in terms of critical adaptive and maladaptive behaviors. Behavioral data is gathered to determine the effectiveness of each subsystem (Dee & Randell, 1989; Dee, 1990).

The scores serve as an acuity rating system and provide a basis for allocating resources. These resources are allocated based on the assigned levels of nursing intervention, and resource needs are calculated based on the total number of patients assigned according to levels of nursing interventions and the hours of nursing care associated with each of the levels (Dee & Randell, 1989) (Table 8-2). The development of this system has provided nursing administration with the ability to identify the levels of staff needed to provide care (licensed vocational nurse versus registered nurse), bill patients for actual nursing care services, and identify nursing services that are absolutely necessary in times of budgetary restraint. Recent research has demonstrated the importance of a model-based nursing database in medical records (Poster, Dee, & Randell, 1997) and the effectiveness of using a model to identify the characteristics of a large hospital's managed behavioral health population in relation to observed nursing care needs, level of patient functioning on admission and discharge, and length of stay (Dee, Van Servellen, & Brecht, 1998).

The work of Vivien Dee and her colleagues has demonstrated the validity and usefulness of the JBSM as a basis for clinical practice within a health care setting. From the findings of their work, it is clear that the JBSM established a systematic framework for patient assessment and nursing interventions, provided a common frame of reference for all practitioners in the clinical setting, provided a framework for the integration of staff knowledge about the clients, and promoted continuity in the delivery of care. These findings should be generalizable to a variety of clinical settings.

Table 8 • 2   Nursing Staffing Budget Unit: 2-South

Shift	Actual No. Patients	Levels of Nursing Interventions				SI	Patient Hours	—Total Cost—			—Cost per Patient—		
		I	II	III	IV			Budget	Actual	Var	Budget	Actual	Var
Night	12.3	1.5	7.1	3.5	0.1	2.49	1.65	181734	154156	27578	40.2	35.2	5.0
Day	12.0	1.2	7.3	3.4	0.2	4.24	2.91	358208	338014	20194	79.1	79.6	−0.4
Evening	12.2	1.2	7.3	3.6	0.1	3.82	2.55	183008	270855	−87847	40.4	61.9	−21.5
					Totals	10.55	7.11	722950	763025	−40075	159.7	176.7	−16.9

Source: Dee, V., & Randell, B. (1989). NPH Patient Classification System: A theory-based nursing practice model for staffing. Paper presented at the UCLA Neuropsychiatric Institute and Hospital.

Practice Exemplar

KELLY WHITE

During the change of shift report that morning, I was told that a new patient had just been wheeled onto the floor at 7:00 A.M. As a result, it was my responsibility to complete the admission paperwork and organize the patient's day. He was a 49-year-old man who was admitted through the emergency department to our oncology floor for fever and neutropenia secondary to recent chemotherapy for lung cancer.

Immediately after my initial rounds, to ensure all my patients were stable and comfortable, I rolled the computer on wheels into his room to begin the nursing admission process. Jim explained to me that he was diagnosed with small cell lung carcinoma (SCLC) 2 months ago after he was admitted to another hospital for coughing, chest pain, and shortness of breath. He went on to explain that a recent MRI showed metastasis to the liver and brain.

His past health history revealed that he irregularly visited his primary health care provider. He is 6 feet 3 inches tall and weighs 168 pounds (76.4 kg). He states that he has lost 67 pounds in the past 6 months. His appetite has significantly diminished since everything tastes like "metal." He has a history of smoking 3 packs per day of cigarettes for 30 years. He states he quit when he began his chemotherapy.

Jim, a high school graduate, is married to his high school sweetheart, Ellen. He lives with his wife and three children in their home. He and his wife are currently unemployed secondary to recent layoffs at the factory where they both worked. He explained that Ellen has been emotionally pushing him away, and from time to time disappears from the home for hours at a time without explaining her whereabouts. He informs me that before his diagnosis, they were the best of friends and were inseparable.

He has tolerated his treatments well until now, except for having frequent, burning, uncontrolled diarrhea for days at a time following his chemotherapy treatments. These episodes have caused raw, tender patches of skin around his rectal area that become increasingly more painful and irritated with each bowel movement.

Jim is exceptionally tearful this morning as he expresses concerns about his own future and the future of his family. He informs me that Ellen's mother is flying in from out-of-state to care for the children while he is hospitalized.

Assessment

Johnson's Behavioral Systems Model guided the assessment process. The significant behavioral data are as follows:

Achievement subsystem:
Jim is losing control of his life and of the relationships that matter most to him as person, his family.
He is a high school graduate.
Affiliative protective subsystem:
Jim is married but describes that his wife is distancing herself from him. He feels he is losing his "best friend" at a time when he really needs this support.
Aggressive protective subsystem:
Jim is protective of his health now (he quit smoking when he began chemotherapy), but has a long history of neglecting his health (smoking for 30 years, unexplained weight loss for 4 months, irregular visits to his primary health care provider).
Dependency subsystem:
Jim is realizing his ability to care for self and family is and will continue to diminish as his health deteriorates. He questions who he can depend on since his wife is not emotionally available to him.
Eliminative subsystem:
Jim is experiencing frequent, burning, uncontrolled diarrhea for days at a time following his chemotherapy treatments. These episodes have caused raw, tender patches of skin around his rectal area that become increasingly more painful and irritated with each bowel movement.

Continued

Ingestive subsystem:

Jim has lost 67 pounds in 6 months and has a decreased appetite secondary to the chemotherapy side effects.

Restorative subsystem:

Jim currently experiences shortness of breath, pain, and fatigue.

Sexual subsystem:

Jim has shortness of breath and possible pain on exertion, which may be leading to concerns about his sexual abilities.

Jim's wife, Ellen, is distant these days, which would be having an impact on the couple's intimacy.

The environmental assessment is as follows:

Internal/external:

After the admission process was completed, I had several concerns for my new patient. I recognized that Jim was a middle-aged man whose developmental stage was compromised regarding his productivity with family and career due to his illness. Mental and physical abilities could be impaired as this disease process advances. In addition, this may create further strain on his relationship with his wife, as she attempts to deal with her own feelings about his diagnosis. Family support would be essential as Jim's journey continued. Lastly, Jim needed to be educated on the expectations of his diagnosis, participate in a plan for treatment during his hospital stay and assist in the development of goals for his future.

Diagnostic Analysis

Jim is likely uncertain about his future as a husband, father, employee, and friend. Realizing this, I encouraged Jim to verbalize his concerns regarding these four areas of his life while I completed my physical assessment and assisted him in settling into his new environment. At first he was hesitant to speak about his family concerns, but soon opened up to me after I sat down in a chair at his bedside and simply made him my complete focus for 5 minutes. As a result of this brief interaction, together, we were able to develop short-term goals related to his hospitalization and home life throughout the rest of my shift with him that day. In addition,

he acquiesced and allowed me to order a social work consult; recognizing that he would no longer be able to adequately meet his family's needs independently at this time.

We also addressed the skin impairment issues in his rectal area. I was able to offer him ideas on how to keep the area from experiencing further breakdown. Lastly, the wound care nurse was consulted.

Evaluation

During his 10-day hospitalization, Jim and his wife agreed to speak to a counselor regarding their thoughts on Jim's diagnosis and prognosis upon his discharge. Jim's rectal area healed as he did not receive any chemotherapy/radiation during his stay. He received tips on how to prevent breakdown in that area from the wound care nurse who took care of him on a daily basis. Jim gained 3 pounds during his stay and maintained that he would continue drinking nutrition supplements daily, regardless of his appetite changes during his cancer treatment. Jim's stamina and thirst for life grew stronger as his body grew physically stronger. As he was being discharged, he whispered to me that he was thankful for the care he had received while on our floor, as he believed that the nurses had brought him and his wife closer than they had been in months. He stated that they were talking about the future and that Ellen had acknowledged her fears to him the previous evening. Jim was wheeled out of the hospital, as he continued to have shortness of breath on extended exertion. As his wife drove away from the hospital, Jim waved to me with a genuine smile and a sparkle in his eye.

Epilogue

Jim passed away peacefully three months later at home, with his wife and children at his side. His wife contacted me soon afterwards to let me know that the nursing care Jim received during his first stay on our unit opened the doors to allow them both to recognize that they needed to modify their approach to the course of his disease. In the end, they flourished as a couple and a family, creating a supportive transition for Jim and the entire family.

Summary

The Johnson Behavioral System Model captures the richness and complexity of nursing. While the perspective presented here is embedded in the past, there remains the potentiality for the theory's further development and the uncovering and shaping of significant research problems that have both theoretical and practical value. There are a variety of problem areas worthy of investigation that are suggested by the JBSM assumptions and from previous studies described on this book's website http://davisplus.fadavis.com. Some examples include examining the levels of integration (biological, psychological, and sociocultural) within and between the subsystems. For example, a study could examine the way a person deals with the transition from health to illness with the onset of asthma. There is concern with the relations between one's biological system (e.g., unstable, problems breathing), one's psychological self (e.g., achievement goals, need for assistance, self-concept), self in relation to the physical environment (e.g., allergens, being away from home), and transactions related to the sociocultural context (e.g., attitudes and values about the sick). The study of transitions (e.g., the onset of puberty, menopause, death of a spouse, onset of acute illness) also represents a treasury of open problems for research with the JBSM. Findings obtained from these studies will not only provide an opportunity to revise and advance the theoretical conceptualization of the JBSM, but will also provide information about nursing interventions. The JBSM approach leads us to seek common organizational parameters in every scientific explanation and does so using a shared language about nursing and nursing care.

References

Ainsworth, M. (1964). Patterns of attachment behavior shown by the infant in interactions with mother. *Merrill-Palmer Quarterly, 10,* 51–58.

Auger, J. (1976). *Behavioral systems and nursing.* Englewood Cliffs, NJ: Prentice-Hall.

Auger, J., & Dee, V. (1983). A patient classification system based on the Behavioral Systems Model of Nursing: Part 1. *Journal of Nursing Administration, 13*(4), 38–43.

Buckley, W. (Ed.). (1968). *Modern systems research for the behavioral scientist.* Chicago: Aldine.

Chin, R. (1961). The utility of system models and developmental models for practitioners. In: K. Benne, W. Bennis, & R. Chin (Eds.), *The planning of change.* New York: Holt.

Coward, D. D., & Wilke, D. J. (2000). Metastatic bone pain: Meanings associated with self-report and management decision making. *Cancer Nursing, 23*(2), 101–108.

Crandal, V. (1963). Achievement. In: H. W. Stevenson (Ed.), *Child psychology.* Chicago: The University of Chicago Press.

Cronbach, L. J., & Meehl, P. (1955). Construct validity in psychological tests. *Psychological Bulletin, 52,* 281–301.

Dee, V. (1990). Implementation of the Johnson Model: One hospital's experience. In: M. Parker (Ed.), *Nursing theories in practice* (pp. 33–63). New York: National League for Nursing.

Dee, V., & Auger, J. (1983). A patient classification system based on the Behavioral System Model of Nursing: Part 2. *Journal of Nursing Administration, 13*(5), 18–23.

Dee, V., & Randell, B. P. (1989). *NPH patient classification system: A theory based nursing practice model for staffing.* Paper presented at the UCLA Neuropsychiatric Institute, Los Angeles, CA.

Dee, V., Van Servellen, G., & Brecht, M. (1998). Managed behavioral health care patients and their nursing care problems, level of functioning and impairment on discharge. *Journal of the American Psychiatric Nurses Association, 4*(2), 57–66.

Derdiarian, A. K. (1983). An instrument for theory and research development using the behavioral systems model for nursing: The cancer patient. *Nursing Research, 32,* 196–201.

Derdiarian, A. K. (1988). Sensitivity of the Derdiarian Behavioral Systems Model Instrument to age, site and type of cancer: A preliminary validation study. *Scholarly Inquiring for Nursing Practice, 2,* 103–121.

Derdiarian, A. K. (1990). The relationships among the subsystems of Johnson's Behavioral System Model. *Image, 22,* 219–225.

Derdiarian, A. (1991). Effects of using a nursing model-based instrument on the quality of nursing care. *Nursing Administration Quarterly, 15*(3), 1–16.

Derdiarian, A. K., & Forsythe, A. B. (1983). An instrument for theory and research development using the behavioral systems model for nursing: The cancer patient. Part II. *Nursing Research, 3,* 260–266.

Derdiarian, A. K., & Schobel, D. (1990). Comprehensive assessment of AIDS patients using the behavioral systems model for nursing practice instrument. *Journal of Advanced Nursing, 15,* 436–446.

D'Huyvetter, C. (2000). The trauma disease. *Journal of Trauma Nursing, 7*(1), 5–12.

Gerwitz, J. (Ed.). (1972). *Attachment and dependency.* Englewood Cliffs, NJ: Prentice-Hall.

Grubbs, J. (1980). An interpretation of the Johnson behavioral system model. In: J. P. Riehl & C. Roy (Eds.), *Conceptual models for nursing practice* (pp. 217–254). New York: Appleton-Century-Crofts.

Harris, R. B. (1986). Introduction of a conceptual model into a fundamental baccalaureate course. *Journal of Nursing Education, 25,* 66–69.

Holaday, B. (1972). Unpublished operationalization of the Johnson Model. University of California, Los Angeles.

Holaday, B. (1974). Achievement behavior in chronically ill children. *Nursing Research, 23,* 25–30.

Holaday, B. (1981). Maternal response to their chronically ill infants' attachment behavior of crying. *Nursing Research, 30,* 343–348.

Holaday, B. (1982). Maternal conceptual set development: Identifying patterns of maternal response to chronically ill infant crying. *Maternal Child Nursing Journal, 11,* 47–59.

Holaday, B. (1987). Patterns of interaction between mothers and their chronically ill infants. *Maternal Child Nursing Journal, 16,* 29–45.

Holaday, B. (1997). Johnson's behavioral system model in nursing practice. In: M. Alligood & A. Marriner-Tomey (Eds.), *Nursing theory: Utilization and application* (pp. 49–70). St. Louis, MO: Mosby-Year Book.

Holaday, B., Turner-Henson, A., & Swan, J. (1997). The Johnson Behavioral System Model: Explaining activities of chronically ill children. In: P. Hinton-Walker & B. Newman (Eds.), *Blueprint for use of nursing models: Education, research, practice, and administration* (pp. 33–63). New York: National League for Nursing.

Johnson, D. E. (1956). A story of three children. *The Nursing Journal of India, XLVII*(9), 313–322.

Johnson, D. E. (1957). Nursing care of the ill child. *The Nursing Journal of India, XLVIII*(1), 12–14.

Johnson, D. E. (1959). The nature and science of nursing. *Nursing Outlook, 7,* 291–294.

Johnson, D. E. (1961). The significance of nursing care. *American Journal of Nursing, 61,* 63–66.

Johnson, D. E. (1968). *One conceptual model of nursing.* Unpublished lecture. Vanderbilt University.

Johnson, D. E. (1980). The behavioral system model for nursing. In: J. P. Riehl & C. Roy (Eds.), *Conceptual models for nursing practice* (2nd ed., pp. 207–216). New York: Appleton-Century-Crofts.

Johnson, D. E. (1990). The Behavioral System Model for Nursing. In: M. E. Parker (Ed.), *Nursing theories in practice* (pp. 23–32). New York: National League for Nursing.

Johnson, D. E., & Smith, M. M. (1963). *Crying as a physiologic state in the newborn infant.* Unpublished research report, PHS Grant NV–00055–01 (formerly GS–9768).

Kagan, J. (1964). Acquisition and significance of sex role identity. In: R. Hoffman & G. Hoffman (Eds.), *Review of child development research.* New York: Russell Sage Foundation.

Lewis, C., & Randell, R. B. (1990). Alteration in self-care: An instance of ineffective coping in the geriatric patient. In: R. M. Carroll-Johnson (Ed.), *Classification of nursing diagnosis: Proceedings of the 9th conference.* Philadelphia: J. B. Lippincott.

Loveland-Cherry, C., & Wilkerson, S. (1983). Dorothy Johnson's behavioral system model. In: J. Fitzpatrick & A. Whall (Eds.), *Conceptual models of nursing: Analysis and application.* Bowie, MD: Robert J. Brady.

Meleis, A. I. (1991). *Theoretical nursing: Development and progress.* Philadelphia: J. B. Lippincott.

Parsons, T., & Shils, E. A. (Eds.). (1951). *Toward a general theory of action: Theoretical foundations for the social sciences.* New York: Harper & Row.

Poster, E. C., Dee, V., & Randell, B. P. (1997). The Johnson Behavioral Systems Model as a framework for patient outcome evaluation. *Journal of the American Psychiatric Nurses Association, 3*(3), 73–80.

Rapoport, A. (1968). Forward to modern systems research for the behavior scientist. In: W. Buckley (Ed.), *Modern systems research for the behavioral scientist.* Chicago: Aldine.

Sears, R., Maccoby, E., & Levin, H. (1954). *Patterns child rearing.* White Plains, NY: Row & Peterson.

Stevenson, J. S., & Woods, N. F. (1986). Nursing science and contemporary science: Emerging paradigms. In *Setting the agenda for year 2000: Knowledge development in nursing* (pp. 6–20). Kansas City, MO: American Academy of Nursing.

von Bertalanffy, L. (1968). *General systems theory: Foundations, development, application.* New York: George Braziller.

Wilkie, D. (1987). Unpublished operationalization of the Johnson model. University of California, San Francisco.

Wu, R. (1973). *Behavior and illness.* Englewood Cliffs, NJ: Prentice-Hall.

Chapter **9**

Dorothea Orem's Self-Care Deficit Theory

DONNA L. HARTWEG
AND LAUREEN M. FLECK

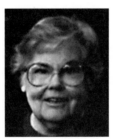

Dorothea E. Orem

Introducing the Theorist

Dorothea E. Orem (1914–2007) was a gentle, caring scholar whose life was dedicated to creation and development of a theoretical structure to improve nursing practice. As a voracious reader and extraordinary thinker, she framed her ideas in both the theoretical and the practical. She viewed nursing knowledge as theoretical with conceptual structure and elements as exemplified in her Self-Care Deficit Nursing Theory (SCDNT) and as "practically practical" with knowledge, rules, and defined roles for practice situations (Orem, 2001).

Orem's personal life experiences, formal education, and employment, as well as the influence of philosophical and logicians such as Aristotle, Thomas Aquinas, Harre (1970), and Wallace (1983) directed her thinking (Orem, 2006; Parker, 2006). She sought to understand the phenomena she observed, creating conceptualizations of nursing education, disciplinary knowledge, and finally, a general theory of nursing or SCDNT. Working independently at first, then later collaboratively, Orem continued these intellectual efforts until her death at age 93. Her insights and passion are evident throughout the world as others continue her legacy. This introduction focuses on her independent work during the early developmental period.

Orem's ability to observe and think was influenced in part by her initial nursing education at Providence Hospital School of Nursing in Washington, DC, a diploma school run by the Daughters of Charity known for their service commitment to the poor (Libster, 2008). She graduated in 1934 and quickly moved into staff/supervisory positions, including an operating room and an emergency room. After her BSN Ed (1939) from Catholic University of America, she held faculty positions at that institution and later at Provident Hospital School of Nursing, Detroit. With completion of the MSN Ed at Catholic University (1946), Orem became Director of Nursing Service and Education at Provident in Detroit (Taylor, 2007). She credits her inability to answer questions in meetings as well as a metaphysics course she took at the University of Detroit with influencing her ability to sort, structure, and understand "parts and the whole" (Taylor, 2007). These experiences did not influence specific conceptualizations of nursing, but stimulated questions and frustrations about a lack of structure for nursing knowledge.

Orem's early formulations on the nature of nursing occurred while working for the Indiana State Board of Health, 1949 to 1957 (Hartweg, 1991). She became aware of nurses' ability to "do nursing," but their inability to describe nursing to colleagues as well as administrators and physicians. Without this understanding, she knew that nurses could not improve practice. Using knowledge of science learned from biology courses in her bachelor's and master's programs, she made an initial effort to define nursing in a 1959 report to the Indiana Board, *The art of nursing in hospital service: An analysis* (Orem, 2003). Although Orem claims this publication did not influence her subsequent thinking, the language of the patient doing for himself or the nurse helping him learn to do for himself appears as antecedent language for the concept of self-care. While working for the Office of Education, Vocational Section of the Technical Division in Washington, DC, she formulated this question: "Why do people need nursing?" Orem states that after she was able to answer that question the "pieces started coming together" (Taylor, 2007). In *Guides for Developing Curriculum for the Education of Practical Nurses*, she expressed what is now her signature: the proper object of nursing. She formulated this question: "What condition exists in a person when judgments are made

that a nurse(s) should be brought into the situation (i.e., that a person should be under nursing care)?" (Orem, 2001, p. 20). The answer to the question is the "proper object":

> The condition is the inability of persons to provide continuously for themselves the amount and quality of required self-care because of situations of personal health. With children it is the inability of parents or guardians to provide the amount and quality of care required by their child because of their child's health situation. (Orem, 2001, p. 20)

From this clarity of focus, Orem's solitary thinking and writing moved to more collaborative work, a model of intellectual teamwork necessary for a practical science to inform and change nursing administration, education, research, and practice. Elaboration of her leadership within these groups and the explosion of theoretical application throughout the United States and other countries throughout the world are described within the chapter's historical section.

To recognize her contributions, Orem received honors from organizations such as Sigma Theta Tau International, the American Academy of Nursing, National League for Nursing, The Catholic University of America, and honorary doctorates from Georgetown University (1976), Incarnate Word College, San Antonio, TX (1980), Illinois Wesleyan University, Bloomington, IL (1988), and the University of Missouri–Columbia (1998) (Allison & Balmat, 2003).) To promote collaboration, the International Orem Society for Nursing Science and Scholarship was formed in 1991 with this mission: "To disseminate information related to development of nursing science and its articulation with the science of self-care" (www.scdnt.com). This has been realized through publications of the organization's newsletter (1993–2001), archived at the website. The newsletter was replaced in 2002 by a peer-reviewed journal, *Self-Care, Dependent Care & Nursing* (see www.scdnt.com/ja/jarchive.html). The scholarly articles, multiple conferences and institutes, and ten world congresses are tributes to her work and critical for continued theory development in an increasingly complex, global discipline.

Many of Orem's original papers are published in *Self-Care Theory in Nursing: Selected papers of Dorothea Orem* (Renpenning & Taylor, 2003) or available in the Mason Chesney Archives of the Johns Hopkins Medical Institutions for the Orem Collection (http://www.medicalarchives.jhmi.edu/papercollections.html#O). Audios and videos of the theorist are available through the Helene Fuld Health Trust (1988) and the National League for Nursing (1987).

Historical Evolution of Orem's Self-Care Deficit Theory

This historical section builds on Orem's independent work and continued development through committees, theory development groups, formal conferences/institutes, international exchanges or partnerships, and finally, the work of the International Orem Society for Nursing Science and Scholarship. A result was the emergence of proteges and scientists who continue SCDNT development and application to practice.

Students, colleagues, and scholars assisted Orem to refine her ideas on the structure of nursing knowledge for a practice discipline. Although Orem continued to work independently throughout the initial collaborative period, two groups reviewed her ideas and contributed to early development (Taylor, 2007). The first was the Nursing Model Committee of the nursing faculty at Catholic University of America, a group Orem chaired. When neither graduate students nor faculty were able to generate research questions in the nursing discipline, questions from a research committee provided impetus to form the Nursing Model Committee to develop ideas about nursing as a *mode of thought, as well as a mode of doing* (Helene Fuld Health Trust, 1988). In 1968, the Nursing Development Conference Group (NDCG) was formed and continued the work of the Nursing Model committee. Initially called the Improvement in Nursing Group, the 11 members, with

Orem as leader, represented nurses in practice, education, and administration. Five members were from the original Nursing Model Committee. All members came with a commitment to develop a structure for nursing knowledge for nursing as a practice discipline. The member's rich thinking, including those of Joan Backscheider, Sarah Allison, and Cora Balmat, provided additional structure to Orem's earlier work. The process and outcomes of this collaboration were published in two books edited by Orem: *Concept Formalization: Process and Product* (NDCG, 1973, 1979). Contemporary scholars continue to reference these publications to understand the foundation and application of concepts to nursing practice. Group members such as Allison (1973), Backscheider (1974), and Kinlein (1977a, 1977b) also published their unique applications and views. As theory application spread, Orem consulted in practice and in education, such as a nurse-managed clinic at The Johns Hopkins University and the nursing program at the University of Southern Mississippi (Taylor, 2007). The Center for Experimentation and Development in Nursing at The Johns Hopkins Hospital provided an opportunity for innovation and theory-driven practice. Changes in administration as well as personal tragedy resulted in a new practice direction. Two NDCG members who were involved in early development and practice applications were killed in a car accident and another seriously injured, ending the significant contribution of this unique group

Concurrent with group work, Orem published the first of six editions of *Nursing: Concepts of Practice* (1971). The title of Orem's major work reflects her clarity of purpose. Orem's conceptualizations are about nursing practice, both theoretical and scientific. The 1980 edition reflects input from the NDCG, with formalized concepts and propositions (Hartweg, 1991). The last edition in 2001 includes theoretical expansion to multiperson groups, such as family and community (Taylor & Renpenning, 2001). Other major theoretical developments are evident in books and articles such as Theory of Dependent Care (Taylor, Renpenning, Geden, Neuman, & Hart, 2001). *Nursing: Concepts of Practice* has formally been translated into Japanese, Spanish, German, Italian, and Dutch (John Scott, personal communication, April 22, 2009). Informal translations are numerous, as graduate students throughout the world (e.g., Thailand) study and apply SCDNT constructs or test the theory.

An explosion of theory in the early 1970s can be traced in part to changes in nursing education as more nurses gained graduate degrees, including many in other disciplines. However, one change that propelled development and application of nursing theory in the United States was a requirement for theory-based curriculum imposed in 1974 by the National League for Nursing accrediting arm. Educational programs across the country sought consultants, faculty with knowledge of emerging theories, and conferences to support faculty development. Susan Taylor, Professor of Nursing at the Sinclair School of Nursing, University of Missouri–Columbia, provided significant leadership resulting in development of practitioners, educators, and researchers. Beginning in earnest in the early 1980s, she facilitated theory dissemination through formation of a network, initiation and coordination of a newsletter, and the creation of summer institutes and research conferences that reached nurses throughout the world. Each semi-annual conference used work sessions, focusing on development of selected concepts. For example, the Sixth Annual Self-Care Deficit Theory Conference in 1987 explored concepts of nursing agency and nursing systems. Other countries began their own nursing development groups, most notably, Canada. By 1989, the global impact was evident when the First International Self-Care Deficit Nursing Theory (SCDNT) Conference was held in Kansas City with participants from the United States, Sweden, the Netherlands, Canada, Thailand, Australia, and Japan (Hartweg, 1991). These conferences led to collaboration among institutions and exchange of faculty such as those from Mahidol University,

Bangkok, Thailand, and Illinois Wesleyan University, Bloomington, IL. With the accrediting expectation and concurrent faculty development, exceptional theory-based curricula were developed in all types of prelicensure programs, including those leading to a diploma, ADN, and BSN. Examples include Morris Harvey College in Charleston, West Virginia, Georgetown University, University of Missouri–Columbia, and Illinois Wesleyan University (Taylor, 2007). Many educational programs used Orem's conceptualizations to frame the curriculum or to guide nursing practice (Hartweg, 2001; Ransom, 2008). Unpublished 1990s research by Taylor and Hartweg revealed Orem's conceptualization was the most frequently used of all known nursing theorists in U.S. programs.

As increasing numbers of nursing doctoral programs emerged in the 1980s, study groups and grants resulted in significant scholarship through dissertations and collaborative theory development. For example, an Orem research group was created in 1984 at Wayne State University (WSU), Detroit, MI. Faculty and doctoral students met weekly to explore theory development and testing. Publications resulted from the group's work such as those by Denyes, O'Connor, Oakley, and Ferguson (1989) or by Gast et al. (1989). Marjorie Isenberg, also at WSU, provided European leadership at the University of Limburg, Maastricht, the Netherlands. This effort led to theory testing, instrument development and testing, and a surge of development in most European countries. As international students received doctorates from WSU and other institutions, they returned home and continued theory development and dissemination in their graduate programs. An example is Thailand, with burgeoning research and development throughout the country's graduate programs and in governmental initiatives (Hanucharurnkul, Leucha, Wittya-Sooporn, & Maneesriwongul, 2001).

This international collaboration required formal organization beyond the resources of a single institution. In 1991, the International Orem Society for Nursing Science and

Scholarship was founded by scholars from the United States, Canada, Belgium, and the Netherlands. With Orem, 3 of the 11 founders were members of the Nursing Development Conference Group, continuing the legacy and expertise. Since that time, 10 biennial congresses have been held in Belgium, Canada, Germany, South Africa, Thailand, and the United States. During these congresses, scholars present theory development, research, and practice papers. As reported in the IOS journal, workgroups (e.g., Metcalfe, 2008) share ideas and develop international collaborative efforts.

Although the workgroups and congresses provided important application and development, in 1995 Orem convened a group of scholars from the United States, Germany, Belgium, and Canada. who met semiannually at her home in Savannah and independently in small groups. Scholars such as Susan Taylor and Kathryn Renpenning continue the theoretical work with extensive publications.

Changes in U.S. educational accrediting standards in the past two decades resulted in fewer graduates educated in theory-based curricula. However, scholarly curricular development continues throughout the United States (Biggs, 2008; Secrest, 2008). Biggs (2008) reported a tremendous increase in global application of Orem's SCDNT. In reviewing the literature, she compared 143 articles published between 1974 and 1999 (Taylor, Geden, Isaramalai, & Wangvatunyu, 2000) with 400 items between 1999 and 2007. Research has increased in sophistication and methodology, with use of qualitative methods, but remains focused on concepts such as self-care agency with its well-tested measurement tools. Many other concepts, such as foundational capabilities and nursing system, need development and testing.

The Theoretical Structure

Orem's general theory of nursing is correctly referred to as Self-Care Deficit Nursing Theory (SCDNT). Orem believed a general model or theory created for a practical science such as nursing encompasses not only the what and why, but also the who and how (Orem, 2006). This is an action theory with clear specifications for nurse and patient roles. The grand theory comprises three minor interrelated theories: the theory of self-care, theory of self-care deficit, and theory of nursing systems. The building blocks of these theories are six major concepts and one peripheral concept. The following is a brief overview of each of these elements. Readers are encouraged to refer to relevant sections in Orem, *Concepts of Practice* (2001) or other citations to enhance understanding.

Foundational to learning any theory is exploration of underlying assumptions, the key to conceptual understanding. Many of these principles emerged from Orem's independent work, as well as from discussions within the Nursing Development Conference Group. Five general assumptions or principles about humans provided guidance to Orem's conceptualizations (Orem, 2001, p. 140). Readings by Aristotle, Thomas Aquinas, Talcott Parsons, Pitirim Sorokin, and others influenced her thinking related to human action, human agency for deliberate action, units of action, and social interaction (Orem, 2003). When thinking about humans within the context of the theory, Orem viewed two types: those who need nursing care and those who produce it (Orem, 2006). In the simplest terms, this is the patient and the nurse, respectively. These assumptions also reveal the powers and properties of humans necessary for self-care. Consistent with most Orem writings, the term *patient* will be used to refer to the recipient of care.

Three Theories Within Self-Care Deficit Nursing Theory

Orem states the three theories "in their articulations with one another express the whole that is self-care deficit nursing theory" (Orem, 2001, p. 141). The theory of nursing system encompasses the theory of self-care deficit, which subsumes the theory of self-care. The three interlocking theories each express a central idea, presuppositions, and propositions. The central idea presents the general focus of the theory; the presuppositions are assumptions specific to this theory; the propositions are statements about the concepts and their interrelationships. The propositions have changed over time with refinement of SCDNT. These occurred in part through theory testing that validated or invalidated hypotheses generated from the relationships.

Orem uses terminology at various levels of abstraction within the three sets of theories. The reader is advised to thoroughly study SCDNT concepts, including the synonyms. For example, capabilities is also called abilities, power, and agency.

1. Theory of Self-Care (Dependent-Care)

The central idea describes self-care and dependent care in contrast to other forms of care. Self-care for one's self or for dependent care (that is, care performed by another such as a family member) must be learned and must be deliberately performed for life, human functioning, and well-being. Six presuppositions articulate Orem's notions about necessary resources, capabilities for learning, and motivation for self-care. However, there are situational variations that affect self-care such as culture.

Orem (2001) expanded two sets of propositions from previous writings. She introduced requirements necessary for life, health, and well-being and explained the complexity of a self-care system. A person performing self-care or dependent care must first *estimate or investigate what can and should be done.* This is a complex action of knowing and seeking information on specific care measures. The self-care sequence continues by *deciding what can be done,* and finally *producing the care* (see Orem, 2001, pp. 143–145).

2. Theory of Self-Care Deficit (Dependent-Care Deficit)

The central idea describes *why people need nursing* (see Orem, 2001, pp. 146–147). Requirements for nursing are health-related limitations for knowing, deciding, and producing care to self or a dependent. Orem presents two sets of presuppositions that articulate this theory with the theory of self-care (dependent care) and what she calls the idea of *social dependency.* To engage in self-care, persons must have values and capabilities to learn (to know), to decide, and to manage self (to produce and regulate care). The second set presents the context of nursing as a health service when people are in a state of social dependency.

The theory of self-care deficit includes nine propositions called principles or guides for future development and theory testing through research. These statements are essential ideas of the larger, SCDNT. Orem describes the situations that affect *legitimate nursing.* Nursing is legitimate or needed when the individual's self-care capabilities and care demands are *equal to, less than, or more than* at a point in time. With the existence of this inequity, a self-care deficit exists and nursing is needed. Legitimate nursing also occurs when a future deficit relationship is predicted such as an upcoming surgery.

Theory of Nursing Systems

The third theory encompasses the others. The central focus is the product of nursing, establishing both structure and content for nursing practice as well as the nursing role (see Orem, 2001, pp. 111, 147–149). The four presuppositions direct the nurse to major complexities of nursing practice. For example, Orem states *Nursing has results–achieving operations that must be articulated with the interpersonal and societal features of nursing* (Orem, 2001, p. 147). Although much of the theory relates to diagnosis, actions, and outcomes based on a deficit relationship between self-care capabilities (or dependent-care) and self-care demand, Orem also presents theoretical work related to the interpersonal relationship between nurse and person(s) receiving nursing and a social contract between the nurse and patient(s) (Orem, 2001, pp. 314–317). These components are often overlooked when studying the SCDNT and are important antecedents and concurrent actions in the detailed process of nursing.

The theory of nursing systems includes seven propositions related to most SCDNT concepts but adds nursing agency (capabilities of the nurse) and nursing systems (complex actions). Nursing agency and nursing systems are linked to the concepts of the person receiving care or dependent care, such as self-care capabilities (agency), self-care demands (therapeutic self-care demand), and limitations (deficits) for self-care. Through this, the general theory or SCDNT becomes concrete to the practicing nurse. Although the language is implicit, Orem proposes that nursing systems are determined by the person's (or dependent care agent's) self-care limitations (capabilities in relationship to health-related self-care demand). Nursing systems therefore vary by the amount of care the nurse must provide, such as a total care system (the unconscious critical care patient) or partial care system (patient in rehabilitation).

Theoretical work by Orem scholars continues in development as nursing practice evolves. For example, dependent care concepts within the general theory developed over time as its importance emerged and was recognized. This expansion was necessary for situations when the nurse provides care or guidance, not only to a patient, but also to a caregiver. A dependent care agent (caregiver) is a *mature or maturing person having or assuming responsibility for a dependent person* (Orem, 2001, p. 285). This may be a family member or friend providing home care or hospital care in a developing country. Factors that promote expansion of such concepts/theories vary, including an increased aging and chronically ill population, early discharge from hospitals, the global application of SCDNT, and health care cost constraints. In collaboration with Orem, significant theoretical development on dependent care resulted in a Theory of Dependent Care (Taylor, 2001). Although Orem (2001) refers to concepts such as self-care, with parenthetical concepts of dependent care and others, the reader should refer to Taylor and others for a separate theory not included in *Nursing: Concepts of Practice.*

Concepts

SCDNT is constructed from six basic concepts and a peripheral concept. Four concepts are patient related: self-care/dependent care, self-care agency/dependent care agency, therapeutic self-care demand, and self-care deficit/dependent care deficit. Two concepts relate to the nurse: nursing agency and nursing system. Basic conditioning factors, the peripheral concept, is related to both the self-care agent (person receiving care)/dependent care agent (family member/friend providing care) and also to the nurse (nurse agent). Orem defines agent as the *person who engages in a course of action or has the power to do so* (Orem, 2001, p. 514). Hence there is self-care agent, dependent care agent, and nurse agent. The unit of service is a person, whether the individual (self-care agent) or others on whom the person is socially dependent (dependent-care agent). Orem also addresses multiperson situations and multiperson units such as entire families, groups, or communities.

Each concept is defined and presented with levels of abstraction. Varied constructs within each concept allow theoretical testing at the level of middle-range theory or at the practice application level whether with the individual or multiperson situations. All build on Orem's independent work, and collaboration with the early NDCG, and the recent nursing development groups who studied with Orem. Research, including many dissertations, as well as changes in practice also contribute to understanding of concepts. A "kite-like" model provides a visual guide for the six concepts and their interrelationships (Fig. 9-1). For a model of concepts and relationships on Dependent Care Theory, the reader is referred to Taylor et al. (2001). For a model on multiperson structure, the reader should read Taylor and Renpenning (2001), *The Practice of Nursing in Multiperson Situations, Family, and Community.*

Basic Conditioning Factors

The peripheral concept, basic conditioning factors (BCFs), is related to three major concepts. For simplicity, only the patient component

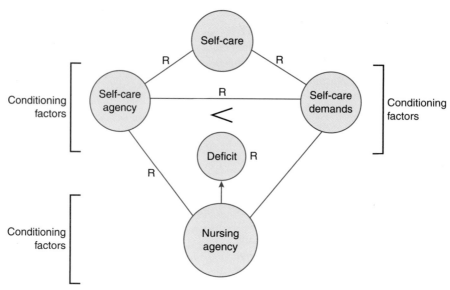

Figure 9 • 1 Structure of SCDNT.

is presented rather than the parallel dependent care components. In general, basic conditioning factors relate to the patient concepts (self-care agency and therapeutic self-care demand) and one nurse concept (nursing agency). These conditioning factors are values that affect the constructs: age, gender, developmental state, health state, sociocultural orientation, health care system factors, family system factors, pattern of living, environmental factors, resource availability, and adequacy (Orem, 2001, p. 245). For example, the family system factor such as living alone or with others may affect the person's ability (self-care agency) to care for self after hospital discharge. The self-care demand (care requirements) of a person taking insulin for type 2 diabetes will vary based on availability of resources and health system services (e.g., access to medications and care services). These same BCFs apply to nursing agency, such as health state. A nurse with recent back surgery may have limitations in nursing capabilities (nurse agency) in relationship to specific care demands of the patient.

These BCF categories have many subfactors that have not been explicitly defined. For example, sociocultural orientation refers to culture with its various components such as values and practices. Sociocultural includes economic conditions as well as others. The BCFs related to nursing agency include those such as age but expand to include nursing experience and education. A clinical specialist in diabetes has more capabilities in caring for the self-care agent with type 2 diabetes than one without such credentials. All these affect the parameters of the nurse's capability to provide care.

This list has changed over time and continues in refinement. Moore and Pichler (2000) summarized research and recommend directions for theory development related to the BCFs. Others such as Allison and McLaughlin (1999) recommend expanding BCFs related to dependent care and community. The latter include factors such as public policy and transportation.

Self-Care (Dependent Care)

Orem (2001) defined self-care as the *practice of activities that individuals initiate and perform on their own behalf in maintaining life, health, and well-being* (p. 43). Self-care is purposeful action performed in sequence and with a pattern. Although engagement in purposeful self-care may not improve health or well-being, a positive outcome is assumed. Dependent care is performed by mature, responsible persons on behalf of socially dependent individuals or self-care agents. The purpose of dependent care is to meet socially dependent persons' health-related demands (dependent care demand) or needs and/or develop their self-care capabilities (self-care agency) (Taylor et al., 2001).

Although the practice of maintaining life is self-explanatory, Orem (2001) viewed outcomes of health and well-being as related but different. Health is a state of physical–psychological, structural–functional soundness and wholeness. In contrast, well-being is preconceived as *experiences of contentment, pleasure, and kinds of happiness; by spiritual experiences; by movement toward fulfillment of one's self-ideal; and by continuing personalization* (Orem, 2001, p. 186). Self-care performed deliberately for well-being versus structural/functional health was conceptualized and developed as health promotion self-care by Hartweg (1990, 1993) and Hartweg and Berbiglia (1996). Research increasingly explores self-care to promote well-being (Matchim, Armer, & Stewart, 2008).

When persons without sufficient development or structural/functional wholeness are unable to perform self-care, dependent-care may become necessary for life, health, and well-being. This is performed by the dependent-care agent on behalf of the self-care agent, such as an infant, child, or cognitively impaired person.

Key to understanding self-care and dependent care is the concept of deliberate action, a voluntary behavior to achieve a goal. When one engages in deliberate action, it is preceded by investigating and deciding what choice to make (Orem, 2001). In practice, the nurse's attention and understanding of each of these phases of investigating, deciding, and producing self-care is essential for positive health outcomes. Take two situations: A pregnant woman must avoid alcohol for the child's health; a woman with breast cancer requires chemotherapy for life and health. Each woman must first know and understand the relationship of self-care to life, health, and well-being. Decision-making follows, such as deciding to avoid alcohol or choosing to engage in chemotherapy. Finally, the individuals must take action such as not drinking when offered alcohol and accepting of chemotherapy treatment. Without each phase, self-care does not occur. The pregnant woman may know the dangers to her fetus, decide not to drink, but deliberately engage in drinking when pressured. The woman with cancer may know the health outcome without treatment, decide to have treatment, then not follow through because of a transportation problem that disrupts her husband's employment. Because each phase of the action sequence has many components, nurses often provide partial support to patients and self-care action does not occur. If skills related to the operation to avoid alcohol when pressured or the operations necessary for transportation to a cancer center are not anticipated by the nurse for these patients, the self-care action sequences may not be completed. Then outcomes related to life, health, and well-being are affected.

Self-Care Agency (Dependent Care Agency)

Orem (2001) defined self-care agency (SCA) as "complex acquired capability to meet one's continuing requirements for care of self that regulates life processes, maintains or promotes integrity of human structure and functioning [health] and human development, and promotes well-being" (p. 254). Capability, ability, and power are all terms used to express *agency*. Self-care agency is therefore the mature or maturing individual's capability for deliberate action to care for self. Dependent care agency is the capability or power to know and meet a socially dependent person's self-care demands or limitations of self-care agency (Taylor, 2001). Viewed as the *summation of all human capabilities needed for performing self-care*, these range from very basic ability such as memory to capability for a specific action in a sequence to meet a specific self-care demand or requirement. At this concrete level, the capabilities of knowing, deciding, and acting or producing self-care are necessary. If these capabilities do not exist, then abilities of others are necessary, such as the family member or nurse. A three-part, hierarchical model of self-care agency provides a visualization of this structure (Fig. 9-2). Understanding these elements is necessary to determine the self-care agent role, dependent-care agent role, and the nurse role.

Foundational Capabilities and Dispositions

Foundational capabilities and dispositions are at the most basic level (Orem, 2001, pp. 262–263). These are capabilities for all types of *deliberate action*, not just self-care. Included are abilities related to perception, memory, and orientation. One example is the deliberate act of repairing a car. One must have perception of the concept of the car and its parts, memory of methods of repair, and orientation of self to the equipment and vehicle. If these foundational abilities are not present, then those related to performing self-care cannot occur. If there is no memory, then one cannot learn to care for self.

Power Components

At the midlevel of the hierarchy are the power components, or 10 powers or types of abilities necessary for *self care*. Examples are the valuing of health, ability to acquire knowledge about self-care resources, and physical energy for self-care. At a very general level, these capabilities relate to knowledge, motivation, and skills to produce self-care. If a mature person becomes comatose, the abilities to maintain attention, to reason, to make decisions, to physically carry out the actions are not functioning. The self-care actions necessary for life, health, and well-being must then be performed by the dependent care agent or the nurse agent.

Capabilities for Estimative, Transitional, and Productive Operations

The most concrete level of self-care agency is one specific to the individual's detailed components of self-care demand or requirements. Capabilities related to estimative operations are those necessary to determine what self-care actions are needed in a specific nursing situation at one point in time, that is, capabilities of investigating and estimating what needs to be done. This includes capabilities of learning in situations related to health and well-being. For example, does the newly diagnosed person with asthma have the capability to learn about regular exercise activities and rescue medication? Does the person know how to obtain the necessary resources? Transitional operations relate to abilities necessary for decision-making, such as reflecting on the course of action and making the decision. The patient may have capabilities to learn and obtain resources, but not the ability to make the decision. The asthma patient has the capability to learn about the exercise and medication, but not the capability to make the decision to follow through on directions. Capabilities for productive operations are those necessary for preparing the self for the action, carrying out the action, monitoring the effects, and evaluating the action's effectiveness. If the person decides to use the inhaler, does the person have the ability to take time to engage in the necessary self-care, to monitor the changes, and determine the effectiveness of the action? Just as the action sequence is important in the self-care concept, these types of capabilities reveal the complexity of human capability.

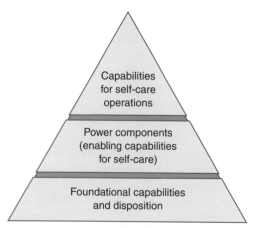

Figure 9 • 2 Structure of Self-Care Agency.

At the concrete practice level, self-care agency also varies by development and operability. For example, the nurse must determine if capabilities for learning are fully developed at the level necessary to understand and retain information about the required actions. For example, a mature adult with late stage Alzheimer's disease is not able to retain new information. The self-care agency is therefore *developed but declining*, creating the possible need for dependent care agency or nursing agency. A second determination is the operability of agency. Is agency not operative, partially operative, or fully operative? A comatose patient may have fully developed capabilities before a motor vehicle accident, but the trauma results in inoperable cognitive functioning. SCA is therefore *developed, but not operative* at that moment in time. In this situation, the nurse agent or dependent care agent (or both) will provide all care.

These important classifications were developed by the NDCG (1979).

Therapeutic Self-Care Demand

Therapeutic self-care demand (TSCD) is a complex theoretical concept that summarizes all actions that should be performed over time for life, health, and well-being. When first developed, the concept was referred to as *action demand* or *self-care demand* (Orem, 2001). Readers will therefore see these terms used in Orem's writings and in the literature. The word *therapeutic* is essential to one's understanding. Consideration is always on a therapeutic outcome of life, health, and well-being. A Pakistani mother in a remote village may expect to apply horse or cow dung to the severed umbilical cord to facilitate drying, a culturally adjusted self-care measure for a newborn. With horse/cow dung as the major carrier of *Clostridium tetanus*, this dependent care action may lead to disease and infant death, not a *therapeutic* outcome.

Constructing or calculating a TSCD requires extensive nursing knowledge of evidenced-based practice, communication, and interpersonal skills. Both scientific nursing knowledge and knowledge of the person and environment are merged to formulate *what needs to be done* in a particular nursing situation (NDCG, 1979). The process of calculating the TSCD includes adjusting values by the basic conditioning factors. For example, a mental health patient will have different needs based on the type of mental health condition (health state), family system factors, and health care resources.

Self-Care Requisites

To provide the framework for determining the TSCD, three types of self-care requisites (or requirements) for action were developed: universal, developmental, and health deviation. These are the *purposes or goals* for which actions are performed for life, health, and well-being. The individual sleeps once each day and engages in daily activities to meet the requisite or goal of *maintaining a balance of activity and rest*. Without rest, a human cannot survive. Therefore, these are general statements within a three-part framework that provide a level of abstraction similar to the power components of self-care agency. Denyes, Orem, and Bekel (2001) presented an explication of the self-care requisite to *maintain an adequate intake of water*. This example demonstrates the complexity of actions necessary to meet a very basic human need. Yet, without consideration of this complexity, analysis and diagnosis of patient requirements is not complete.

Universal self-care requisites: The eight universal self-care requisites (USCR) are necessary for all human beings of all ages and in all conditions, such as air, food, activity and rest, solitude, and social interaction. The BCFs influence the quality and quantity of the action necessary to achieve the purpose. Actions to be performed over time that meet the requisite, *prevention of hazards to human life, human functioning, and human well-being (the purpose)*, will vary for an infant (e.g., keeping crib rails up) versus an adult (e.g., ambulation safety). Some requisites are very general yet provide important concepts necessary for all humans. One example is the concept of normalcy, the eighth USCR. The goal is *promotion of human functioning and development within social groups in accord with human potential, human limitations, and the human desire to be normal* (Orem, 2001, p. 225). Practice examples in the literature have emerged, such as the importance of normalcy to individuals with learning disabilities (Horan, 2004). These two requisites, prevention of hazards and promotion of normalcy, also relate to the other six USCRs. For example, when maintaining a sufficient intake of food, one must consider hazards to ingestion of food. Avoiding pesticides is one example.

Developmental self-care requisites: Orem (2001) identified three types of developmental self-care requisites (DSCRs). The first refers to actions necessary for general human developmental processes throughout the lifespan. These requisites are often met by dependent care agents when caring for developing infants and children or when disaster and serious physical or mental illness affects adults. Engagement in self-development, the second DSCR, refers to demands for action by individuals in positive roles and in positive mental health. Examples include self-reflection, goal-setting, and responsibility in one's roles. The third DSCR, interferences with development, express goals achieved by actions that are necessary in situational crises such as loss of friends and relatives, loss of job, or terminal illness. Originally subsumed under USCRs, Orem created the developmental self-care requisite types to indicate the importance of human development to life, health, and well-being.

Health deviation self-care requisites: Health deviation self-care requisites (HDSCR) are situation-specific requisites or goals when people have disease, injuries, or are under professional medical care. These six often underused requisites guide actions when pathology exists or when medical interventions are prescribed. The first HDSCR refers in part to a patient purpose: *to seek and secure appropriate medical assistance for genetic, physiological, or psychological conditions known to produce or be associated with human pathology* (Orem, 2001, p. 235). For a person with history of breast cancer, seeking regular diagnostic tests is a goal to preserve life, health, and well-being. A teenager in treatment for severe acne takes action to meet HDSCR 5: to modify *the self-concept (and self-image) in accepting oneself as being in a particular state of health and in need of a specific form of health care* (Orem, 2001, p. 235).

Each TSCD, through the three types of self-care requisites, is individualized and adjusted by the basic conditioning factors (BCFs) such as age, health state, and sociocultural orientation. Once adjusted to the specific patient in a unique situation, the purposes are specific for the patient or type of patient. These are called "particularized self-care requisites." Dennis and Jesek-Hale (2003) proposed a list of particularized self-care requisites for a nursing population of newborns. Although created for nursery newborns, that is, a group particularized by age, the individual patient adjustments are then made. For example, a newborn's sucking needs may vary, necessitating variation in feeding methods.

Self-Care Deficit (Dependent–Care Deficit)

As a theoretical concept, self-care deficit expresses the value of the relationship between two other concepts: self-care agency and therapeutic self-care demand (Orem, 2001). When the person's self-care agency is not adequate to meet all self-care requisites (TSCD), a self-care deficit exists. This qualitative and quantitative relationship at the conceptual level of abstraction is expressed as "equal to," "more than," or "less than" (see Fig. 9-1). A deficit relationship is also described as complete or partial; a complete deficit suggests no capability to engage in self-care or dependent care. An example of a complete deficit may exist in a premature infant in a neonatal intensive care unit. A partial self-care deficit may exist in a patient recovering from a routine bowel resection one day after surgery. This person is able to provide some self-care.

Understanding self-care deficit is necessary to appreciate Orem's concept of *legitimate nursing*. If a nurse determines a patient has self-care agency (estimative, transitional, and productive capabilities) to carry out a sequence of actions to meet the self-care requisites, then nursing is not necessary. A self-care deficit or anticipated self-care deficit must exist before a nursing system is designed and implemented. The nurse reflects with the patient: Is self-care agency (and/or dependent care agency) adequate to meet the therapeutic self-care demand, comprising of all the three requisite types? If adequate, there is no need for nursing.

A dependent-care deficit may occur when two or more persons provide care to the socially dependent person, the self-care agent. This occurs when an actual or potential deficit relationship exists between the dependent care demand and the capabilities (agency) of the dependent care agent and the self-care agent (Taylor et al., 2001). When this deficit occurs, then a need for nursing exists. When a parent has the capabilities to meet all health-related self-care requisites of an ill child, then no nursing is needed.

As the presence of an existing or potential self-care deficit is identified and legitimate nursing is needed, an analysis by the nurse/patient/dependent care agents results in identification of types of limitations in relationship to the particularized self-care requisites. These are generally described as limitations of knowing, limitations or restrictions of decision-making, and limitations in ability to engage in result-achieving courses of action. Orem classified these into sets of limitations (see Orem, 2001, pp. 279–282).

Nursing System

Orem describes a nursing system as an "action system," or actions and sequence of actions performed for a purpose. This is a composite of all the nurse's concrete actions completed or to be completed for or with a self-care agent to promote life, health, and well-being. The composite of actions and their sequence produced by the dependent-care agent to meet the therapeutic dependent self-care demand is termed a dependent-care system (Taylor et al., 2001). These actions relate to three types of subsystems: interpersonal, social/contractual, and professional-technological.

The interpersonal subsystem includes all necessary actions or operations such as entering into and maintaining effective relationships with the patient and/or family or others involved in care. The social/contractual subsystem relates to all nursing actions/operations to reach agreements with the patient and others related to information necessary to determine the therapeutic self-care demand and self-care agency of an individual and caregivers. Within this subsystem, the nurse, in collaboration with the patient or dependent-caregiver, determine roles for all care participants (Orem, 2001). These are based on social norms and other variables such as basic conditioning factors. Although other nursing theories emphasize interpersonal interactions, Orem's general theory clearly specifies details of interpersonal and contractual operations as necessary antecedents and concurrent components of care. This element of Orem's model is often overlooked and clarifies the decision-making process and collaborative relationship within the nurse–patient–family/multiperson roles.

The professional–technological subsystem comprises actions/operations that are diagnostic, prescriptive, regulatory, evaluative, and case management. The latter involves placing all operations within a system that uses resources effectively and efficiently with a positive patient outcome. Orem views the professional–technological subsystem as the process of nursing, a nonlinear one that integrates all operations of this subsystem with those of the interpersonal and the social–contractual. This involves collecting data to determine existing and projected universal, developmental, and health-deviation self-care requisites, and methods to meet these requisites as adjusted by the basic conditioning factors. Using the interpersonal and social–contractual subsystems, the nurse incorporates modifications of her or his diagnosis and prescriptions in collaboration with the patient and family on *what is possible.* The nurse also identifies the patient's usual self-care practices and assesses the person's estimative, transitional, and productive capabilities for knowledge, skills, and motivation in relationship to the known self-care requisites. That is, are the capabilities (self-care agency/dependent care agency) needed to meet the self-care requisites developed, operable, and adequate? Are there limitations in knowing, deciding, or producing self-care? If so, there is no need for nursing and no nursing system is developed. If there is a self-care deficit or dependent-care deficit, then the nurse and patient or caregivers reach agreement about the patient's role, the family's role, and the nurse's role. Orem (2001) charted the progression of these steps by subsystems (pp. 311, 314–317).

With determination of a real or potential self-care deficit or dependent-care deficit, the nurse develops one of three types of nursing systems: wholly compensatory, partly compensatory, or supportive-educative (developmental). The nurse then continues the query: *Who can or should perform actions that require movement in space and controlled manipulation?* (Orem, 2001, p. 350). If the answer is only the nurse, then a wholly compensatory system is designed. If the patient has some capabilities to perform operations or actions, then the nurse and patient share responsibilities. If the patient can perform all actions that control movement in space and controlled manipulation, but nurse actions are required for support (physical or psychological), then the system is supportive–educative. Note, in all systems, the self-care deficit is the necessary element that leads to the design of a nursing system. Using the interpersonal and social–contractual operations, the nurse first enters into an interpersonal relationship and an agreement to determine a real or potential self-care deficit, prescribe roles, and implement productive operations of self-care and/or dependent-care. Regulation or treatment operations are designed or planned and then produced or performed. Control operations are used to appraise and evaluate the effectiveness

of nursing actions and if adjustments should be made. These emphasize validity of operations or actions in relationship to standards. Selecting valid operations in the plan and in evaluation incorporate evidence-based practices. These processes, including diagnosis, prescription, designing, planning, regulating, and controlling, can be viewed as elements of Orem's steps in the process of nursing (Fig. 9-3).

Orem's language of the nursing process varies from the standard language of assessment, diagnosis, planning, implementation,

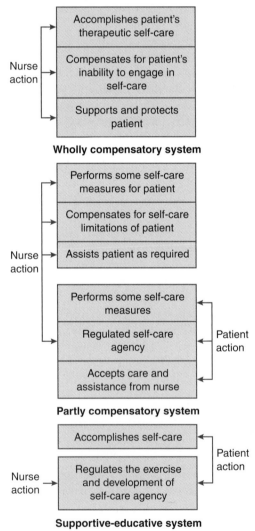

Figure 9 • 3 Basic Nursing System.

and evaluation. The interaction of the three aforementioned subsystems creates a model for true collaboration with the recipient of care or the caregiver.

The three steps of Orem's process of nursing are as follows: (1) diagnosis and prescription; (2) design and plan; and (3) produce and control. For example, Orem considers the term "assessment" too limiting. Within Orem's process, assessments are made throughout the iterative social–contractual and professional-technological operations. During the first step of diagnosis, data are collected on the basic conditioning factors and a determination is made about their relationship to the self-care requisites and to self-care agency. How does health state (e.g., type 2 diabetes) affect the individual's universal, developmental, and health-deviation self-care requirements? How does the basic conditioning factor, health state, affect the individual's self-care agency (capabilities)? What, if any, are limitations for deliberate action related to the estimative (investigative–knowing), transitional (decision-making), and productive (performing) phases of self-care? (Orem, 2001, p. 312). The nurse collects information and analyzes and makes judgments about the information within the limits of nursing agency (capabilities to nurse, such as expertise).

Orem describes nursing as a specialized helping service and identifies five helping methods to overcome self-care limitations or regulate functioning and development of patients or their dependents. Nurses employ one or more of these methods throughout the process of nursing, including acting for or doing for another, guiding another; supporting another; providing for a developmental environment, and teaching another (Orem, 2001, pp. 56–60). Acting for or doing for another includes physical assistance such as positioning the patient. Assuming self-care agency that is developed and operable, the nurse replaces this method with others that focus on cognitive development, such as guiding and teaching. These methods are not unique to nursing, but are used by most health professionals. Through their unique role functions, nurses perform a specific sequence of actions in relationship to the identified patient and/or dependent care agent's self-care limitations in combination with other health professionals to meet the self-care requirements.

Although comparisons are made between these steps and those of the general nursing process, Orem's complexity is unique in addressing an integration of interpersonal, social–contractual, and professional–technological subsystems. The intricacy of her steps is also evident in the complexity of the diagnostic and prescriptive components. The exemplar in this chapter provides one simplified example of this process.

Nursing Agency

Nursing agency is the power or ability to nurse. The agency or capabilities are necessary to *know and meet patients' therapeutic self-care demands and to protect and to regulate the exercise of development of patient's self-care agency* (Orem, 2001, p. 290). Nursing agency is analogous to self-care agency, but with capabilities performed on behalf of "legitimate patients." Similar to self-care agency, nursing agency is affected by basic conditioning factors. The nurse's family system, as well as nursing education and experience, may affect his or her ability to nurse.

Orem categorizes nursing capabilities (agency) as interpersonal, social–contractual, and professional-technological. That is, the nurse must have capabilities within each of the subsystems described in the nursing system. Capabilities that result in desirable interpersonal nurse characteristics include effective communication skills and ability to form relationships with patients and significant others. Social–contractual characteristics require the ability to apply knowledge of variations in patients to nursing situations and to form contracts with patients and others for clear role boundaries. Desirable professional–technologic characteristics require abilities to perform techniques related to the process of nursing: diagnosis of therapeutic self-care demand of an assigned patient with consideration of all self-care requisites (universal, developmental, and health deviation) and a concomitant diagnosis of a patient's self-care agency. Others include the ability to prescribe roles: Assuming a self-care deficit (and therefore legitimate patient), what are the roles and related responsibilities of the nurse, the patient, the aide, and the family? Nurses must also have the ability to know and apply care measures such as general helping techniques (teaching, guiding) and specialized interventions and technologies such as those identified with evidence-based practice. These nursing capabilities also have implications for design of undergraduate curricula as nursing agency is developed in prelicensure students.

Multiperson Situations and Units

The concepts just presented relate to care for an individual. The focus is on the person's therapeutic self-care demand or self-care agency. When a dependent care agent provides care, the primary focus is still the person with the deficit, not the dependent care agent. Nursing care to groups and to communities requires an expanded model.

Taylor and Renpenning (2001) extended application to families, groups, and communities, where the recipient of nursing care is more than a single individual with a self-care deficit. They distinguish among types of multiperson units, such as community groups and family or residential group units. These authors present categories of multiperson care systems, create family and community as basic conditioning factors, and present a model of community as aggregate. This model appropriately incorporates additional basic conditioning factors such as public policy, health care system changes, and community development. Other frameworks such as a community participation model have been developed (Isaramalai, 2002).

Community groups have a selected number of common self-care requisites and or limitations of knowledge, decision-making, and producing care. This can be directed to entire communities, to groups within the communities, or to other situations when groups have common needs. For example, the focus of a student health nurse at a university may be a group of first-year students and the self-care requisite, prevention of the hazards of alcohol poisoning. The self-care limitations of the group may be knowledge of binge drinking outcomes and the skills to resist peer pressure at parties. This environment and situation, the college milieu and new independence, creates the common set of self-care requisites. The action system designed by the college health nurse is to develop the knowledge, decision-making, and result-producing skills of new students collectively so life, health, and well-being are enhanced for the group, as well as the college community.

Family or others in a communal living arrangement are another type of multiperson unit of service. Because of the interrelationship of the individuals in the living unit, the purpose of nursing varies from that for a community group. In this situation, the focus is often an individual, as well as the family as a unit. The health-related requirements of one individual trigger the need for nursing, but also affect the unit as a whole. In one situation, an elderly parent moves into the family home. Not only is the therapeutic self-care demand of the parent involved, but also the needs of all family members as it affects the self-care requisites of all members. These models continue in development as nursing expands to populations.

Practice Applications

Much has been written about application of Orem's Self-Care Deficit Nursing Theory (SCDNT) to nursing practice. Nursing scholars investigated the practice application during the theory's development and others expanded its use throughout the United States and international nursing arena. Biggs (2008) conducted the most recent review of the nursing literature from 1999 to 2007. The results revealed more than 400 articles, including those in *International Orem Society Newsletters* and *Self-Care, Dependent-Care, and Nursing,* the official journal of the International Orem

Society. Although Biggs noted a tremendous increase in publications during the last 10 years, the author observed that SCDNT research has not always contributed to theory progression and development. She identified deficient areas such as those related to concepts such as therapeutic self-care demand, self-care deficit, nursing systems, and the methods of helping or assisting. These limitations of development have restricted SCDNT's applicability to specific nursing situations or use in varied nursing roles.

For this chapter a literature review was conducted to provide diverse examples of SCDNT's utility for nursing practice in a variety of settings and situations. Evidence-based research studies were also reviewed for examples valuable to practitioners. Between 2000 and 2009 more than 700 citations of SCDNT in nursing practice were identified through CINAHL, OVID, and Medline search engines. Key terms were self-care deficit theory in nursing practice, self-care, Orem, and evidence-based nursing practice. This search was further restricted to Orem nursing practice and evidence-based nursing practice. The resulting 127 citations, including five books and chapters, were subsequently reviewed. Although a Proquest dissertation search revealed 300 citations using the theory, they were not included in this review.

Selected practice and evidence-based research publications are presented in two tables, one on application to nursing practice using case studies or nursing process examples, the second on evidence-based research. Table 9-1 appears in this chapter and Table 9-2 within the ancillary materials on http://davisplus.fadavis.com. Domestic and international examples are included as well as a range of clinical settings and types of nursing situations. This narrative provides an extension of the tables to encourage the reader to explore the bibliography for additional resources applicable to relevant practice situations.

Examples in Table 9-1 demonstrate the practical utility across age groups, health states, and settings. For example, Dennis and Jesek-Hale (2003) focus on the normal infant in a newborn nursery. This relates to a therapeutic self-care demand as conditioned by age. The article provides the practitioner with a foundation for application with healthy infants in the nursery setting before further particularizing to the individual infant. Oliver (2003) describes the use of SCDNT as the nurse collaborates with the dependent-care agents to develop self-care agency in autistic preschoolers. This example demonstrates the nurses' role in collaborating with all key care providers to strengthen the child's capabilities. Others, such as Schmidt (2008), exemplify development of a nursing system as therapeutic self-care demand and self-care agency are diagnosed and prescribed and nursing agency is determined.

Schmidt (2008) presented a case study using SCDNT for a specific patient within a dependent-care nursing situation. The author created a unique nursing system using guided imagery to manage pain of a 10-year-old child with vaso-occlusive sickle cell anemia. This school-aged child presented with years of hospitalizations and chronic care treatment. The presence of pain conditioned his self-care requisites, thereby increasing his therapeutic self-care demand and decreasing his ability care for self, that is, limiting his self-care agency. A self-care deficit was determined. Consistent with the theory and development of a nursing system, the capabilities of the nurse in relationship to the specific deficit were also considered to promote a positive outcome, in this case reduction of pain and ability to care for self. In this situation, nursing agency of the assigned practitioner includes expertise from 5 years of experience and certification in guided imagery beyond the general pediatric staff nurse knowledge and skills. With the mother as a dependent care agent providing most of the physical care, the nurse determines the "legitimate" nursing in this specific situation – the addition of guided imagery. Because the child provides some self-care and participates in dependent care, a partially compensatory nursing system is needed. The nurse's method of assisting is to teach him self-management of pain using

Table 9 · 1 Examples of Practice Applications

Author/Year Country	Health or Illness Focus	Settings	SCDNT Concept(s)	Patient or Practice Focus (Selected Examples)
Conway, McMillan, & Solman (2006) Australia	Cardiac rehabilitation: Adult	Cardiac step-down unit	Nurse agency	Knowledge of nurses' responses to patient's needs; nursing actions from acute care to discharge
Dennis & Jesek-Hale (2003) United States	Normal newborn basic needs	Newborn nursery	Therapeutic self-care demand	Therapeutic self-care demand: Feeding/elimination/activity and rest/prevention of hazards for normal newborns
Grando (2005) United States	Mental health situations: Personal crisis, relationship abuse and psychosis	Outpatient psychiatric clinic	Self-care agency	Nurse practitioner's exploration: Inabilities to manage self-care requirements
Herber, Schnepp, & Rieger (2008) Germany	Leg ulcers management: Adult	Outpatient wound clinic	Therapeutic self-care demand and self-care agency	Nurse-led program for patients and dependents: Determination of therapeutic self-care demands: Health deviation self-care; Self-care agency: Decision-making operations
Kumar (2007) United States	Type 2 diabetes management: Adult	Outpatient vascular office; clinical nurse specialist	Self-care agency	Knowledge: Impaired learning and functioning: Imbalanced nutrition influencing weight loss success and control of peripheral vascular pain Diabetes management: Adequate nutrition (for weight loss), pain control, and health beliefs of powerlessness and coping
Martinez (2005) United States	Rectal cancer: Adult	Home care	Self-care agency	Knowledge; determination and promotion of self-care agency to meet therapeutic self-care demand related to severe anxiety, stress, and body image disturbance. Interventions identified
Oliver (2003) United States	Autism in preschool child	Preschool setting	Self-care agency	Self care agency enhancement through collaboration between dependent care agents (multidisciplinary management) Case management
Sampaio, Aquino, de Araujo, & Galvo (2007) Brazil	Chagas disease: Adult	Home care	Self-care agency	Knowledge of stoma care, control of complications and access to health services
Schmidt (2009) United States	Sickle cell anemia: School-age child	Acute care setting: Inpatient	Self-care agency; Nursing agency	Self-care agency enhancement through guided imagery and teaching for pain management Nursing certification related to abilities;

guided imagery. After each session, the child reports feeling "a little bit better" with pain ratings decreasing from 8 to 6 to 3 over several sessions. Concomitantly, he uses less pain medication, increases ambulation, and is soon discharged, meeting all outcomes objectives.

In contrast to the partly compensatory system, Herber (2008) developed a supportive-educative nursing system within a dependent care situation. The health state of leg ulcers conditions the therapeutic self-care demand and self-care agency. With the illness or disability emphasis, Herber focuses on the health-deviation self-care requisites. As the reader considers the various examples, the complexity of Orem's concepts become apparent, revealing SCDNT's

pragmatic adequacy in multiple situations, cases, and nursing preparation.

A concept more recently described by Orem (2001) is the notion of self-management. She defines this as the *ability to manage self in stable or changing environments and ability to manage one's personal affairs* (p. 111). This definition relates to the extent and continuity of contacts and interactions one would expect over time with nursing. For example, chronic conditions are collaboratively managed with the self-care agent, dependent-care agent by nurse practitioners, home health nurses, or telenurses. However, neither the theory nor extensive research guides the practitioner on an extended model of care.

Practice Exemplar

Marion W. presents to a primary care office seeking care for recent fatigue. She is assigned to the nurse practitioner. The nurse explains the need for information to determine *what needs to be done and by whom* to promote Marion's life, health, and well-being. Information regarding Marion is gathered in part using Orem's conceptualizations as a guide. First, the nurse introduces herself and then describes the information she will seek to help her with the health situation. Marion agrees to provide information to the best of her knowledge. As the nurse and Marion have entered into a professional relationship and agreed to the roles of nurse and patient, the nurse initiates the three steps of Orem's process of nursing:

Step 1: Diagnosis and Prescription
I. Basic Conditioning Factors

As basic conditioning factors affect the value of therapeutic self-care demand and self-care agency, the nurse seeks information regarding the following: age, gender, developmental state, patterns of living, family system factors, sociocultural factors, health state, health care system factors, availability of resources, and

external environmental factors such as the physical or biological.

Marion is 42, female, in a developmental stage of adulthood where she carries out tasks of family and work responsibilities as a productive member of society. The history related to patterns of living and family system reveals employment as a school crossing guard, a role that allows time after school with her children, ages 5, 7, and 9. Her husband works for "the city," but recently had hours cut to 4 days per week. Therefore money is very tight. They pay bills on time, but no money remains at the end of the month. She has learned to stretch their money by shopping at the local discount store for clothes and food and cooking "one-pot meals" so they have leftovers to stretch throughout the week. As an African American, she worships in a community-based Black church, a source of spiritual strength and social support. Marion has a high-school education.

Questions about her health state and health system reveal Marion has type 2 diabetes and was diagnosed more than 5 years ago. Except for periodic fatigue, she believes she has managed this chronic condition by following the

Continued

Practice Exemplar cont.

treatment plan, faithfully taking oral medication, and checking blood sugar once per day. The morning reading is 230 mg/dL. Although the family has no health insurance, Marion has access to the community health care clinic and free oral medications. There is a small co-pay for her blood glucose testing strips, which is now a concern. The children receive health care through the State Children's Health Insurance Program. The neighborhood Marion lives in has a safe, outdoor environment. The latter has been a comfort because she works as a crossing guard and walks her children to school. Although she enjoys this exercise, her increasing fatigue discourages additional exercise.

When asked about her perception of her current condition, Marion expressed concern for her weight and considers this a partial explanation for the fatigue. She desires to lose weight but admits she has no will power, snacks late at night, and finds "healthy foods" too expensive. At 205 lbs (93 kg) and 5 feet 3 inches (1.6 m), Marion is classified as obese with a body mass index of 38 kg/m².

II. Calculating the Therapeutic Self-Care Demand

With Marion, the nurse identifies many actions that *should be performed* to meet the universal, developmental, and health deviation self-care requisites. Her health state and health system factors (including prior treatment modalities) are major conditioners of two universal self-care requisites: *maintain a sufficient intake of food* and *maintain a balance between activity and rest.* Throughout the interview, the nurse determines that Marion is clear about her chronic condition and has accepted herself in need of continued monitoring and care.

Two health deviation self-care requisites also emerge as the primary focus for seeking helping services: *being aware and attending to effects and results of pathological conditions;* and *effectively carrying out medically prescribed diagnostic and therapeutic measures.* Without

additional self-care actions beyond the prescribed medication, short walks, and daily blood glucose testing, the risks of uncontrolled diabetes may lead to diabetic retinopathy, nephropathy, and coronary artery disease (American Diabetes Association [ADA], 2009).

One particularized self-care requisite (PSCRs) is presented as an example, with the related actions Marion should perform to improve her health and well-being. Once the *actions to be performed* and concomitant methods are identified, then the nurse determines Marion's self-care agency: the capabilities of knowing (estimative operations), deciding (transitional operations), and performing these actions (productive operations).

PSCR: Reduce and maintain blood glucose level within normal parameters through increased blood glucose monitoring, appropriate healthy food choices, and increased activity. **If this PSCR is achieved, Marion's weight will be decreased, a related purpose that provides motivation to engage in self-care.** The methods to achieve the PSCR include detailed actions:

A. Increase blood glucose monitoring to twice per day; 100–110 mg/dL fasting and <140 mg/dL at 2 hours after a main meal.

1. Obtain discounted glucose monitoring strips from ABC drug company.
2. Obtain assistance from community clinic for monthly replacement request to ABC drug company.
3. Monitor glucose level through testing two times per day, with one test before breakfast and one test 2 hours after a main meal. Add more testing when needed for symptoms of high or low blood sugar (ADA, 2009).
4. Seek assistance from health professional when levels are below 60 mg/dL and not responsive to sugar intake or higher than 300 mg/dL with feelings of fatigue, thirst, or visual disturbances.
5. Adjust activity and meal planning/portion sizes when levels are not within parameters.

B. Make healthy food choices.

6. Seek knowledge of healthy food choices for family meal planning from dietician at clinic.
7. Review family expenses with health professional to adjust grocery budget to purchase affordable but healthy foods.
8. Eat three balanced meals per day including midmorning, afternoon, and evening snack as desired. These meals and snacks will have portion sizes established between Marion and the nurse.
9. All meals will have a selection of protein, fats, and carbohydrates and the snacks will be limited to 15 grams of carbohydrate or less.

C. Increase physical activity to 150 minutes/week.

10. Gain knowledge regarding step walking program to increase activity. Discuss community options for safe walking areas.
11. Explore budget to include properly fitting foot wear. Tennis shoes with socks are to be worn for each walk. Obtain free pedometer from clinic to measure performance of steps and walking.
12. Review pedometer measures three times a week. Increase steps by 10% each week if natural increase in steps has not occurred. For example, if walking 2000 steps/walk increase next walk by 200 steps as a goal. Maintain goals until 10,000 step/day is achieved (ADA, 2009).

III. Determining Self-Care Agency

The nurse and Marion then seek information about self-care agency or the capabilities related to knowledge, decision-making, and performance necessary to meet this PSCR. This includes the ability to seek and obtain required resources important to each action. What capabilities are necessary to increase blood glucose testing? Does Marion have the knowledge about access to drug company resources (testing strips) available to persons with their income level? Does she have the communication skills to seek resources from the community center? Does she have the knowledge regarding blood glucose parameters and methods to adjust exercise and diet to maintain the levels? The nurse and Marion together determine capabilities for each of these components of each action necessary to meet her particularized self-care requisite.

After collecting and analyzing data about her abilities in relationship to the required actions, the nurse determines the absence or existence of a self-care deficit, that is, is self-agency adequate to meet the therapeutic self-care demand? The nurse quickly determines throughout the data collection period that Marion's foundational and disposition capabilities (necessary for any deliberate action) and the power components (necessary for self-care) are developed and operable. The question is the adequacy of self-care agency in relationship to this PSCR.

1. Blood glucose monitoring: The nurse learns that Marion possesses necessary capabilities of knowing, deciding, and performing to obtain additional testing strips from ABC drug company and to increase her blood glucose testing to two times per day. After questioning, the nurse determines Marion is aware of norms and in general the effect of food and exercise. In addition to verbalizing available time for testing, Marion also recalls that the school nurse where she works agreed to be a resource if blood glucose readings are not within the required range. She agreed to seek out this resource if adjustment in exercise or food intake is needed. The nurse practitioner concludes Marion's self-care capabilities of knowing, deciding, and performing the necessary actions is intact to meet the particularized self-care requisite, maintain blood glucose level at 100–110 mg/dL fasting and <140 mg/dL at 2 hours after a main meal.
2. Dietary practices: The nurse seeks information from Marion on her knowledge of effective dietary practices and healthy foods, including flexibility in the family

Continued

Practice Exemplar cont.

budget, shopping practices, and family cultural practices that may influence her food purchases. The nurse learns Marion has misinformation about her selected foods and is aware of resources, such as the local health department that offers free classes by a registered dietician. However, transportation to dietary classes is not possible as her husband uses the only car to drive to work. Although Marion understands the relationship of her high blood glucose levels to the resulting fatigue, she seems to focus on losing weight, a possible motivational asset. Marion maintains the ability to shop, cook, use the stove safely, and ingest all food types.

3. The nurse assesses that Marion enjoys walking and generally feels safe in the surrounding environment. She also possesses time while the children are at school to take walks. The nurse discovers that Marion is not aware of proper foot care or the step program for increasing exercise. Marion does not believe the family budget can manage both changes in food purchases as well as the purchase of good walking shoes.

IV. Self-Care Limitations

Marion has self-care limitations in the area of knowledge and decision-making about required dietary actions. The limitations of knowing are related to healthy dietary practices. This includes the use of carbohydrate counting. She lacks knowledge about purchasing options for healthier foods and methods to incorporate these into her meal effort. Although interested, she is unable to enroll in dietary classes at the health department due to transportation issues. Marion has knowledge and decision-making authority for managing the family budget, but has no experience incorporating healthier foods into the planning. Marion also has self-care limitations in relationship to knowledge of the step program, proper footware, and related foot care. No resources exist to purchase the necessary walking shoes. Major capabilities include

Marion's ability to learn, availability of time, and her motivation to lose weight, and hence have less fatigue. If Marion decides to make healthier food choices that are affordable and also increase her general activity, she will need monitoring, counseling, and support from a health professional related to the blood glucose levels, access to resources for classes, budgeting, and purchase of equipment.

With analysis of self-care agency in relationship to the particularized self-care requisite, the nurse and patient establish the presence of a self-care deficit. Now that legitimate nursing has been established, a nursing system is designed.

Step 2: Design and Plan of Nursing System

Now that the self-care limitations of knowing are identified, the nurse will use helping methods of guiding and supporting by designing a supportive-educative nursing system. The design involves planning Marion's activities to meet the particularized self-care requisite with nurse guidance and monitoring and also to establishing the nurse's role. Together they agree on communication methods to work together, to monitor progress as Marion attends classes to learn healthy dietary practices and increase activity. Marion agrees to share information related to blood glucose testing with the school nurse and the pharmacist at the community clinic when refilling medication and supplies.

The nurse agrees to seek out resources for transportation to the health department for dietary classes, purchase of footwear, assistance to fill out forms, and also to meet with Marion every 2 weeks to review food consumption and activity records. Although the goal is to maintain blood glucose levels at 100–110 mg/dL fasting and <140 mg/dL at 2 hours after a main meal, the priority actions relate to dietary changes, followed by slow, incremental changes in activity. The nurse expects it will take 1 month to obtain the necessary footwear. Objectives will be reviewed at

1 month. Marion knows that weight loss is her objective, but she must start changes in dietary practices. The goal for weight loss will be set at the first month's meeting after attendance at the dietary sessions and initial experience with changing the family's food purchases and meal planning. Marion and the nurse practitioner begin implementing their roles as prescribed.

Step 3: Treatment, Regulation, Case Management, Control/Evaluation

Marion and the nurse begin implementing their agreed upon actions as they collaborate within the nursing system. The nurse practitioner maintains contact via phone with Marion as she completes actions, such as seeking resources for the dietary classes and footwear. Marion contacts the school nurse where she works to see if she will be a resource for weekly reports on blood glucose levels. She also seeks out additional testing strips and calls the clinic to obtain the routine forms for monthly renewal requests. They proceed through each of these actions as agreed upon as social–contractual operations. Throughout this step, the interpersonal operations are essential as the nurse evaluates Marion's progress and new roles are determined and agreed upon. This continues over time, with continued review of the design, the role prescriptions, until Marion's therapeutic self-care demand is decreased or self-care agency is developed so no self-care deficit exists, and nursing is no longer required.

Throughout the process, nursing agency was evident. The capabilities related to interpersonal, social-contractual, and professional-technological operations were evident.

◾ Summary

This chapter provided an overview of Orem's Self-Care Deficit Nursing Theory. Orem created this general theory of nursing to address the proper objective of nursing through the question, "What condition exists in a person when judgments are made that a nurse(s) should be brought into the situation (i.e., that a person should be under nursing care)?" (Orem, 2001, p. 20). The grand theory comprises three minor interrelated theories: the theory of self-care, theory of self-care deficit, and theory of nursing systems. The building blocks of these theories are six major concepts and one peripheral concept. Orem's SCDNT has been applied extensively in nursing practice throughout the United States and internationally. It is applicable to nursing in diverse settings and with diverse populations.

References

Allison, S. E. (1973). A framework for nursing action in a nurse-conducted diabetic management clinic. *Journal of Nursing Administration, 3*(4), 53–73.

Allison, S. E., & Balmat, C. S. (2003). Foreword. In: K. Mc Renpenning & S. G. Taylor (Eds.), *Self-Care Theory in Nursing: Selected papers of Dorothea Orem* (pp. xvi–xvii). New York: Springer.

Allison, S. E., & McLaughlin, K. (1999). *Nursing administration in the 21st century: A self-care approach.* Newbury Park, CA: Sage.

American Diabetes Association (ADA). (2009). Clinical practice recommendations 2009. *Diabetes Care 32*(1), 13.

Artinian, N. T., Magnan, M., Sloan, M., & Lange, M. P. (2002). Self-care behaviors among patients with heart failure. *Heart and Lung, 31*(3), 161–172.

Backscheider, J. E. (1974). Self-care requirements, self-care capabilities and nursing systems in the diabetic nurse management clinic. *American Journal of Public Health, 64*(12), 1138–1146.

Biggs, A. J. (2008). Orem's Self-Care Deficit Nursing Theory: Update on the state of the art and science. *Nursing Science Quarterly, 21*(3), 200–206.

Callaghan, D. M. (2006). The influence of growth on spiritual self-care agency in an older population. *Journal of Gerontological Nursing, 9*, 43–51.

Chang, S. H., Crogan, N. L., & Shu-Fen, W. (2007). The self-care self-efficacy enhancement program for Chinese nursing home elders. *Geriatric Nursing, 28*(1), 31–36.

Conway, J., McMillan, M., & Solman, A. (2006). Enhancing cardiac rehabilitation nursing through aligning practice to theory: Implications for nursing education. *The Journal of Continuing Education in Nursing, 37*(5), 233–238.

DeBruin, M. P., Hospers, H. J., Van den Borne, H. W., & Kok, G. (2005). Theory and evidence-based intervention to improve adherence to antiretroviral therapy among HIV-infected patients in the Netherlands: A pilot study. *AIDS, Patient Care and STD, 19*(6), 384–394.

Dennis, C. M., & Jesek-Hale, S. M. (2003). Calculating the therapeutic self-care demand for a nursing population of nursery newborns' particularized self-care requisites. *Self-Care, Dependent-Care, & Nursing, 11*(1), 3–10.

Denyes, M. J., O'Connor, N. A., Oakley, D., & Ferguson, S. (1989). Integrating nursing theory, practice and research throughout collaborative practice. *Journal of Advanced Nursing, 14,* 141-145.

Denyes, M. J., Orem, D. E., & Bekel, G. (2001). Self-care: A foundational science. *Nursing Science Quarterly, 14*(2), 48–54.

Fan, L. (2008). Self-care behaviors of school-age children with heart disease. *Pediatric Nursing, 34*(2), 131–140. Continuing Nursing Education Series.

Fawcett, J. (2003). Orem's self-care deficit nursing theory: actual and potential sources for evidence based practice. *Self-Care, Dependent Care, & Nursing, 11*(1), 11–16.

Fowler, C., Kirschner, M., Van Kuiken, D., & Bass, L. (2007). Promoting self-care through system management: A theory-based approach for nurse practitioners. *Journal of the American Academy of Nurse Practitioners, 19,* 221–227.

Gary, R. (2006). Self-care practices in women with diastolic heart failure. *Heart and Lung, 35*(1), 9–18.

Gast, H., Denyes, M. J., Campbell, J. C., Hartweg, D. L., Schott-Baer, D., & Isenberg, M. (1989). Self-care agency: Conceptualizations and operationalizations. *Advances in Nursing Science, 12*(1), 26–38.

Geden, E. A., Isaramalai, S., & Taylor, S. G. (2001). Self-care Deficit Nursing Theory and the nurse practitioner's practice in primary care settings. *Nursing Science Quarterly, 14*(1), 29–33.

Glasson, J., Chang, E., Chenoweth, L., & Hancock, K. (2006). Evaluation of a model of nursing care for older patients using participatory action research in an acute medical ward. *Journal of Clinical Nursing, 15,* 588–598.

Grando, V. T. (2005). A Self-Care Deficit Nursing Theory practice model for advanced practice psychiatric/mental health nursing. *Self-Care, Dependent Care, & Nursing, 13*(1), 4–8.

Hanucharurnkul, S., Leucha, Y., Wittya-Sooporn, J. & Maneesriwongul, W. (2001). An integrative review and meta-analysis of self-care research in Thailand: 1988–1999. *Thai Journal of Nursing Research, 5*(2), 119–132.

Harre, R. (1970). *The principles of scientific thinking.* Chicago: University of Chicago Press.

Hartweg, D. L. (1990). Health promotion self-care within Orem's general theory of nursing. *Journal of Advanced Nursing, 15*(1), 35–41.

Hartweg, D. L. (1991). *Dorothea Orem: Self-Care Deficit Nursing Theory.* Newbury Park, CA: Sage.

Hartweg, D. L. (1993). Self-care actions of healthy, middle-aged women to promote well-being. *Nursing Research, 42*(4), 221–227.

Hartweg, D. L. (2001). Use of Orem's conceptualizations in a baccalaureate nursing program (1980–2000). *International Orem Society Newsletter, 8*(1), 5–7.

Hartweg, D. L., & Berbiglia, V. A. (1996). Determining the adequacy of a health promotion self-care interview guide with healthy, middle-aged Mexican-American women: A pilot study. *Health Care for Women International, 17*(1), 57–68.

Helene Fuld Health Trust (1988). *The nurse theorists: Portraits of excellence: Dorothea Orem.* Oakland, CA: Studio III.

Herber, O. R., Schnepp, W., & Rieger, M. (2008). Developing a nurse-led education program to enhance self-care agency in leg ulcer patients. *Nursing Science Quarterly, 21*(2), 150–155.

Hines, S. H., Sampselle, C. M., Ronis, D. L., & Yeo, S. (2007). Women's self-care agency to manage urinary incontinence: The impact of nursing agency and body experience. *Advances in Nursing Science, 30*(2), 175–187.

Horan, P. (2004). Exploring Orem's self-care deficit nursing theory in learning disability nursing: Philosophical parity paper, part 1. *Learning Disability Practice, 7*(4), 28–33.

Isaramalai, S. (2002). *Developing a cross-cultural measure of the self-as-career inventory questionnaire for the Thai population.* Unpublished doctoral dissertation, University of Missouri.

Kinlein, M. L. (1977a). *Independent nursing practice with clients.* Philadelphia: J. B. Lippincott.

Kinlein, M. L. (1977b). The self-care concept. *American Journal of Nursing, 77,* 598–601.

Kumar, C. (2007). Application of Orem's self-care deficit theory and standardized nursing languages in a case study of a woman with diabetes. *International Journal of Nursing Terminologies and Classifications, 18*(3), 103–110.

Libster, M. (2008). Perspectives on the history of self-care. *Self-Care, Dependent-Care, & Nursing, 16*(2), 8–17.

Martinez, L. (2005). Self-care for stoma surgery: mastering independent stoma self-care skills in an elderly woman. *Nursing Science Quarterly, 18*(1), 66–69.

Matchim, Y. M., Armer, J. M., & Stewart, B. R. (2008). A qualitative study of participants' perceptions of effect of mindfulness meditation practice on self-care and overall well-being. *Self-Care, Dependent-Care, & Nursing, 16*(2), 45–53.

Metcalfe, S. A. (2008). Report from SCDNT in nursing education workgroup. *Self-Care, Dependent-Care, & Nursing, 16*(2), 7.

Moore, J. B., & Pichler, V. H. (2000). Measurement of Orem's Basic Conditioning Factors: A review of published literature. *Nursing Science Quarterly, 13*(2), 137–142.

National League for Nursing. (1987). *Nursing theory: A circle of knowledge.* New York: Author.

Oliver, C. J. (2003). Triage of the autistic spectrum child utilizing the congruence of case management concepts and Orem's nursing theories. *Lippincott's Case Management, 8*(2), 66–82.

Nursing Development Conference Group [NDCG] (1973). *Concept formalization: Process and product.* Boston: Little Brown.

Nursing Development Conference Group [NDCG] (1979). *Concept formalization: Process and product* (2nd Ed.). Boston: Little Brown.

Orem, D. E. (1987). Orem's general theory of nursing. In: R. Parse (Ed.), *Nursing science: Major paradigms, theories, and critiques* (pp. 67–89). Philadelphia: W. B. Saunders.

Orem, D. E. (2001). *Nursing: Concept of practice* (6th Ed.). St. Louis: Mosby.

Orem, D. E. (2003). Development of the Self-Care Deficit Theory of nursing: Events and circumstances. In: K. Mc.Renpenning & S. G. Taylor (Eds.). *Self-care Theory in Nursing. Selected Papers of Dorothea Orem* (pp. 254–266), New York: Springer.

Orem, D. E. (2006). Dorothea E. Orem's Self-Care Nursing Theory. In: M. E. Parker(Ed.) *Nursing theories and nursing practice* (2nd ed., pp. 141–149). Philadelphia: F. A Davis.

Parker, M. E. (2006). *Nursing theories & nursing practice.* (2nd Ed). Philadelphia: F. A.Davis.

Ransom, J. E. (2008). Facilitating emerging nursing agency in undergraduate nursing students. *Self-Care, Dependent Care, & Nursing, 16*(2), 39–45.

Renpenning, K. Mc., & Taylor, S. G. (Eds.). (2003). *Self-care theory in nursing: Selected papers of Dorothea Orem.* New York: Springer.

Sampaio, F., Aquino, P., deAraujo, T., & Galvo, M. T. (2008). Nursing care to an ostomy patient: application of the Orem's theory. *Acta Paul Enferm, 21*(1), 94–100.

Schmidt, N. A. (2008). Guided imagery as internally oriented self-care: A nursing case. *Self-Care, Dependent-Care, & Nursing, 16*(2), 41–48.

Scott, J. (April 22, 2009). Personal email communication on foreign translations of *Nursing: Concepts of Practice.*

Secrest, J. (2008). The role of tool development in an Orem-based curriculum. *Self-Care, Dependent-Care, & Nursing, 16*(2), 25–33.

Swanlund, S. L., Scherck, K. A., Metcalfe, S. A., & Jesek-Hale, S. R. (2008). Keys to successful self-management of medications. *Nursing Science Quarterly, 21*(3), 238–246.

Taylor, S. G. (2001). Orem's general theory of nursing and families. *Nursing Science Quarterly, 14*(1), 7–9.

Taylor, S. G. (2007). The development of Self-Care Deficit Nursing Theory: A historical analysis. *Self-Care, Dependent Care, & Nursing, 15*(1), 22–25.

Taylor, S. G., Geden, E., Isaramalai, S., & Wongvatunyu, S. (2000). Orem's self-care deficit nursing theory: Its philosophic foundation and the state of the science. *Nursing Science Quarterly, 13*, 104–111.

Taylor, S. G., & Renpenning, K. Mc. (2001). The practice of nursing in multiperson situations, family and community. In: D. E. Orem (Ed.), *Nursing: Concepts of practice* (6th ed., pp. 394–433). St. Louis, MO: C. V. Mosby.

Taylor, S. G., Renpenning, K. Mc., Geden, E. A., Neuman, B. M., & Hart, M. A. (2001). A theory of dependent-care: A corollary theory to Orem's Theory of Self-Care. *Nursing Science Quarterly, 14*(1), 39–47.

Wallace, W. A. (1983). *From a realist point of view: Essays on the philosophy of science.* Washington, D. C.: University Press of America.

Wilson, F. L., Baker, L. M., Nordstrom, C. K., & Legwand, C. (2008). Using the teach-back and Orem's self-care deficit nursing theory to increase childhood immunization communication among low-income mothers. *Issues in Comprehensive Pediatric Nursing, 31*, 7–22.

Chapter 10

Imogene King's Theory of Goal Attainment

IMOGENE KING, CHRISTINA L. SIELOFF, MARY B. KILLEEN, AND MAUREEN A. FREY

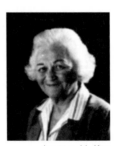

Imogene M. King

Introducing the Theorist: The Nightingale Tribute to Imogene King[1]

Imogene M. King was born on January 30, 1923 in West Point, Iowa, and died on December 24, 2007 in St. Petersburg, Florida and is buried in Fort Madison, Iowa. She received a diploma in Nursing from St. John's Hospital School of Nursing, St. Louis, Missouri in 1945. While working in a variety of staff nurse roles, King completed a Bachelor of Science in Nursing Education, which she received from St. Louis University in 1948; she completed a Master of Science in Nursing from St. Louis University in 1957. From 1947 to 1958, King worked as an instructor in medical–surgical nursing and served as assistant director at St. John's Hospital School of Nursing. She went on to study with Mildred Montag as her dissertation chair at Teachers College, Columbia University, New York, receiving a Doctor of Education (EdD) in 1961.

From 1968 to 1972, King was the director of the School of Nursing at Ohio State University in Columbus. During this time, her book, *Toward a Theory for Nursing: General Concepts of Human Behavior* (1971), was published. In this early work, King concluded,

---

[1]This tribute has been modified slightly from the original version that was reproduced, with permission, from C. L. Sieloff & P. R. Messmer. (2009). Conceptual systems framework and middle range theory of goal attainment. In: A. Marriner-Tomey & M. R. Alligood (Eds.), *Nursing theorists and their work* (7th ed.). St. Louis, MO: Mosby-Elsevier.

"a systematic representation of nursing is required ultimately for developing a science to accompany a century or more of art in the everyday world of nursing" (1971, p. 129). The book was awarded the *American Journal of Nursing* Book of the Year Award in 1973 (King, 1995).

From 1961 to 1966, King was an assistant and associate professor of nursing at Loyola University in Chicago, where she developed a master's degree program in nursing based on a nursing conceptual framework. Her first theory article appeared in 1964 in the *Nursing Science* journal edited by Martha Rogers.

Between 1966 and 1968, King served as Assistant Chief of Research, Grants Branch, Division of Nursing, in the United States Department of Health, Education, and Welfare under Jessie Scott. While she was in Washington, DC, her article "A Conceptual Frame of Reference for Nursing" was published in *Nursing Research* (King, 1968).

From 1968 to 1972, King served as Director of the Nursing Department at Ohio State University. She returned to Chicago in 1972 as a professor in the Loyola University graduate program, and served as the Coordinator of Research in Clinical Nursing at the Loyola Medical Center, Department of Nursing, from 1978 to 1980. In May, 1998, King received an honorary doctorate from Loyola University, where her collection is housed.

From 1972 to 1975, King was a member of the Defense Advisory Committee on Women in the Services for the United States Department of Defense. She was also elected alderman for a 4-year term (1975–1979) in Ward 2, Wood Dale, Illinois, in 1975.

In 1980, King was appointed professor at the University of South Florida, College of Nursing in Tampa, Florida (Houser & Player, 2007). In 1981, the manuscript for her second book, *A Theory for Nursing: Systems, Concepts, Process*, was published. In addition to her first two books, she authored multiple book chapters and articles in professional journals, and a third book, *Curriculum and Instruction in Nursing: Concepts and Process*, was published in 1986. King retired in 1990, and was named

professor emeritus at the University of South Florida, and continued to guest lecture there.

King continued to provide community service and helped plan care through her conceptual system and theory at various health care organizations, including Tampa General Hospital (Messmer, 1995). King never really retired, as she continued to collaborate with students, faculty, and colleagues who were using her theory, and even went "round the clock" to implement her theory at Tampa General Hospital.

In 1948, King joined the American Nurses Association (ANA) as a member of the Missouri Nurses Association and was active in Illinois and Ohio as well. On her move to Tampa, Florida, she became very active member in the Florida Nurses' Association (FNA) and FNA District 4, Tampa. King held offices in various organizations including president of the Florida Nurses Foundation, served on the FNA and the FNA District IV boards, and frequently was a delegate from the FNA to the ANA House of Delegates. In 1997, King received a gold medallion from Governor Chiles for advancing the nursing profession in the state of Florida. King was inducted into the FNA Hall of Fame and the ANA Hall of Fame in 2004. In 1994, King was also inducted into the American Academy of Nursing (AAN), served on the AAN Theory-Guided Practice Panel, and was honored as a Living Legend in 2005. In 1996, King received the Jessie M. Scott Award at the ANA convention. King was thrilled when Jessie Scott attended the presentation.

King was inducted into the Teachers College, Columbia University Hall of Fame in 1999. The King International Nursing Group (K. I. N. G.) was created to facilitate the dissemination and utilization of King's conceptual system, Theory of Goal Attainment, and related theories. Even after the organization became inactive, King consulted with members of the organization on an individual basis regarding her theory. The K. I. N. G. has been reactivated to honor Dr. King.

King was one of the original Sigma Theta Tau International (STTI) Virginia Henderson

Fellows, and received the STTI Elizabeth Russell Belford Founders Award for Excellence in Education in 1989 (Messmer, 2007). King was keynote speaker at two STTI theory conferences in 1992, and presented at multiple regional, national, and international STTI conferences on application of her theory.

King's theory books were translated into Japanese, Spanish, and German. In addition, she authored numerous articles on her theory and served on the editorial board of *Nursing Science Quarterly*. King authored several chapters in various books, for example, Frey and Sieloff's *Advancing King's Systems Framework and Theory of Nursing* (1995), and Sieloff and Frey's *Middle Range Theory Development Using King's Conceptual Systems* (2007). She served as an advisor for Sieloff's (2003) development of an instrument to measure the power of a nursing group within an organization, Killeen's (2007) instrument to measure patient satisfaction with professional nursing care, and Frey's (1995) seminal work on adolescent patients diagnosed with type 1 diabetes.[1]

King's Conceptual System and Theory of Goal Attainment: In Her Own Words

My first theory publication pronounced the problems and prospect of knowledge development in nursing (King, 1964). Over 30 years ago, the problems were identified as: (1) lack of a professional nursing language; (2) a theoretical nursing phenomena; and (3) limited concept development. Today, theories and conceptual frameworks have identified theoretical approaches to knowledge development and utilization of knowledge in practice. Concept development is a continuous process in the nursing science movement (King, 1988).

My rationale for developing a schematic representation of nursing phenomena was influenced by the Howland Systems Model (Howland, 1976) and the Howland and McDowell conceptual framework (Howland & McDowell, 1964). The levels of interaction

in those works influenced my ideas relative to organizing a conceptual frame of reference for nursing. Because concepts offer one approach to structure knowledge for nursing, a comprehensive review of nursing literature provided me with ideas to identify five comprehensive concepts as a basis for a conceptual system for nursing. The overall concept is a human being, commonly referred to as an "individual" or a "person." Initially, I selected abstract concepts of perception, communication, interpersonal relations, health, and social institutions (King, 1968). These ideas forced me to review my knowledge of philosophy relative to the nature of human beings (ontology) and to the nature of knowledge (epistemology).

Philosophical Foundation

In the late 1960s, while auditing a series of courses in systems research, I was introduced to a philosophy of science called General System Theory (Von Bertalanffy, 1968). This philosophy of science gained momentum in the 1950s, although its roots date to an earlier period. This philosophy refuted logical positivism and reductionism and proposed the idea of isomorphism and perspectivism in knowledge development. Von Bertalanffy, credited with originating the idea of General System Theory, defined this philosophy of science movement as a "general science of wholeness: systems of elements in mutual interaction" (von Bertalanffy, 1968, p. 37).

My philosophical position is rooted in General System Theory, which guides the study of organized complexity as whole systems. This philosophy gave me the impetus to focus on knowledge development as an information-processing, goal-seeking, and decision-making system. General System Theory provides a holistic approach to study nursing phenomena as an open system and frees one's thinking from the parts-versus-whole dilemma. In any discussion of the nature of nursing, the central ideas revolve around the nature of human beings and their interaction with internal and external environments. During this journey, I began to conceptualize a theory for nursing. However, because a manuscript was due in the publisher's office, I organized my ideas into a conceptual system (formerly called a "conceptual framework"), and the result was the publication of a book entitled *Toward a Theory of Nursing* (King, 1971).

Design of a Conceptual System

A conceptual system provides structure for organizing multiple ideas into meaningful wholes. From my initial set of ideas in 1968 and 1971, my conceptual framework was refined to show some unity and relationships among the concepts. The conceptual system consists of individual systems, interpersonal systems, and social systems and concepts that are important for understanding the interactions within and between the systems (Fig. 10-1).

The next step in this process was to review the research literature in the discipline in which the concepts had been studied. For example, the concept of perception has been studied in psychology for many years. The literature indicated that most of the early studies dealt with sensory perception. Around the 1950s, psychologists began to study interpersonal perception, which related to my ideas about interactions. From this research literature, I identified the characteristics of perception and defined the concept for my framework. I continued searching literature for knowledge of each of the concepts in my framework. An update on my conceptual system was published in 1995 (King, 1995).

Process for Development Concept

"Searching for scientific knowledge in nursing is an ongoing dynamic process of continuous identification, development, and validation of relevant concepts" (King, 1975, p. 25). What is a concept? A concept is an organization of reference points. Words are the verbal symbols used to explain events and things in our environment and relationships to past experiences. Northrop (1969) noted: "[C]oncepts fall into different types according to the different sources of their meaning. … A concept is a term to which meaning has been assigned." Concepts are the categories in a theory.

The concept development and validation process is as follows:

1. Review, analyze, and synthesize research literature related to the concept.
2. From the above review, identify the characteristics (attributes) of the concept.
3. From the characteristics, write a conceptual definition.
4. Review literature to select an instrument or develop an instrument.
5. Design a study to measure the characteristics of the concept.
6. Decisions are made on selection of the population to be sampled.
7. Collect data.
8. Analyze and interpret data.
9. Write results of findings and conclusions.
10. State implications for adding to nursing knowledge.

Concepts that represent phenomena in nursing are structured within a framework and theory to show relationships.

Multiple concepts were identified from my analysis of nursing literature (King, 1981). The concepts that provided substantive knowledge about human beings (self, body image, perception, growth and development, learning, time,

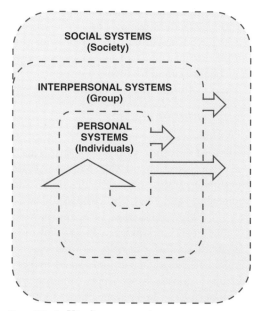

Figure 10 • 1 King's conceptual system.

and personal space) were placed within the personal system, those related to small groups (interaction, communication, role, transactions, and stress) were placed within the interpersonal system, and those related to large groups that make up a society (decision making, organization, power, status, and authority) were placed within the social system (King, 1995). However, knowledge from all of the concepts is used in nurses' interactions with individuals and groups within social organizations, such as the family, the educational system, and the political system. Knowledge of these concepts came from my synthesis of research in many disciplines. Concepts, when defined from research literature, give nurses knowledge that can be applied in the concrete world of nursing. The concepts represent basic knowledge that nurses use in their role and functions either in practice, education, or administration. In addition, the concepts provide ideas for research in nursing.

One of my goals was to identify what I call the essence of nursing. That brought me back to the question, What is the nature of human beings? A vicious circle? Not really! Because nurses are first and foremost human beings who give nursing care to other human beings, my philosophy of the nature of human beings has been presented along with assumptions I have made about individuals (King, 1989a). Recognizing that a conceptual system represents structure for a discipline, the next step in the process of knowledge development was to derive one or more theories from this structure. Lo and behold, a theory of goal attainment was developed (King, 1981, 1992). More recently, others have derived theories from my conceptual system (Frey & Sieloff, 1995).

Theory of Goal Attainment

Generally speaking, nursing care's goal is to help individuals maintain health or regain health (King, 1990). Concepts are essential elements in theories. When a theory is derived from a conceptual system, concepts are selected from that system. Remember my question: What is the essence of nursing?

The concepts of self, perception, communication, interaction, transaction, role, growth and development, stress, time, and personal space were selected for the Theory of Goal Attainment.

Transaction Process Model

A transaction model, shown in Figure 10-2, was developed that represented the process whereby individuals interact to set goals that result in goal attainment (King, 1981, 1995). The model is a human process that can be observed in many situations when two or more people interact, such as in the family and in social events (King, 1996). As nurses, we bring knowledge and skills that influence our perceptions, communications, and interactions in performing the functions of the role. In your role as a nurse, after interacting with a patient, sit down and write a description of your behavior and that of the patient. It is my belief that you can identify your perceptions, mental judgments, mental action, and reaction (negative or positive). Did you make a transaction? That is, did you exchange information and set a goal with the patient? Did you explore the means for the patient to use to achieve the goal? Was the goal achieved? If not, why? It is my opinion that most nurses use this process but are not aware that it is based in a nursing theory. With knowledge of the concepts and of the process, nurses have a scientific base for practice that can be clearly articulated and documented to show quality care. How can a nurse document this transaction model in practice?

Documentation System

A documentation system was designed to implement the transaction process that leads to goal attainment (King, 1984). Most nurses use the nursing process of assess, diagnose, plan, implement, and evaluate, which I call a method. My transaction process provides the theoretical knowledge base to implement this method. For example, as one assesses the patient and the environment and makes a nursing diagnosis, the concepts of perception, communication, and interaction represent

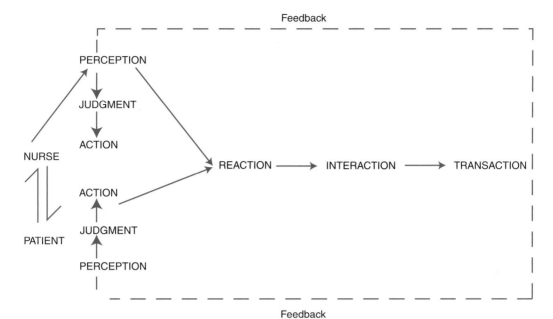

Figure 10 • 2 Transaction process model. *(From King, I. M. [1981]. A theory for nursing: Systems, concepts, process [p. 145]. New York: John Wiley & Sons.)*

knowledge the nurse uses to gather information and make a judgment. A transaction is made when the nurse and patient decide mutually on the goals to be attained, agree on the means to attain goals that represent the plan of care, and then implement the plan. Evaluation determines whether or not goals were attained. If not, you ask why, and the process begins again. The documentation is recorded directly in the patient's chart. The patient's record indicates the process used to achieve goals. On discharge, the summary indicates goals set and goals achieved. One does not need multiple forms when this documentation system is in place, and the quality of nursing care is recorded. Why do nurses insist on designing critical paths, various care plans, and other types of forms when, with knowledge of this system, the nurse documents nursing care directly on the patient's chart? Why do we use multiple forms to complicate a process that is knowledge-based and also provides essential data to demonstrate outcomes and to evaluate quality nursing care?

Federal laws have been passed that indicate that patients must be involved in decisions about their care and about dying. This transaction process provides a scientifically based process to help nurses implement federal laws such as the Patient Self-Determination Act (Federal Register, 1995).

Goal Attainment Scale

Analysis of nursing research literature in the 1970s revealed that very few instruments were designed for nursing research. In the late 1980s, the faculty at the University of Maryland, experts in measurement and evaluation, applied for and received a grant to conduct conferences to teach nurses to design reliable and valid instruments. I had the privilege of participating in this two-year continuing education conference, where I developed a Goal Attainment Scale (King, 1989b). This instrument may be used to measure goal attainment. It may also be used as an assessment tool to provide patient data to plan and implement nursing care.

Vision for the Future

My vision for the future of nursing is that nursing will provide access to health care for all citizens. The United States' health care system will be structured using my conceptual system. Entry into the system will be via nurses' assessment so individuals are directed to the right place in the system for nursing care, medical care, social services information, health teaching, or rehabilitation. My transaction process will be used by every practicing nurse so that goals can be achieved to demonstrate quality care that is cost-effective. My conceptual system, Theory of Goal Attainment, and Transaction Process Model will continue to serve a useful purpose in delivering professional nursing care. The relevance of evidence theory–based practice, using my theory, joins the art of nursing of the twentieth century to the science of nursing in the twenty-first century.

Concept and Middle Range Theory Development within King's Conceptual System or Theory of Goal Attainment

Concept development within a conceptual framework is particularly valuable, as it often explicates concepts more clearly than a theorist may have done in his or her original work. Concept development may also demonstrate how other concepts of interest to nursing can be examined through a nursing lens. Such explication further assists the development of nursing knowledge by enabling the nurse to better understand the application of the concept within specific practice situations. Examples of concepts developed from within King's work include the following: collaborative alliance relationship (Hernandez, 2007); decision making (Ehrenberger, Alligood, Thomas, Wallace, & Licavoli, 2007), empathy (May, 2007), and patient satisfaction with nursing care (Killeen, 2007) (see http://davisplus.fadavis.com).

Practice Applications

Since the first publication of Dr. Imogene King's work (1971), nursing's interest in the application of her work to practice has grown. The fact that she was one of the few theorists who generated both a framework and a mid-range theory further expanded her work. Today, new publications related to Dr. King's work are a frequent occurrence. Additional middle-range theories have been generated and tested, and applications to practice have expanded. Following her retirement, Dr. King continued to publish and examine new applications of her work. The purpose of this part of the chapter is to provide an updated review of the state of the art in terms of the application of King's Conceptual System (KCS) and mid-range theory in a variety of areas: practice, administration, education, and research. Publications, identified from a review of the literature, are summarized and briefly discussed. Finally, recommendations are made for future knowledge development in relation to King's conceptual system and mid-range theory, particularly in relation to the importance of their application within an evidence-based practice environment.

In conducting the literature review, the authors began with the broadest category of application—application within King's Conceptual System to nursing care situations. Because a conceptual framework is, by nature, very broad and abstract, it can only serve to guide, rather than prescriptively direct, nursing practice.

King's Conceptual System has been used to guide nursing practice in multiple settings and with multiple populations. For example, Frey and colleagues (2007) used intervention research in a population of adolescents with poorly controlled type 1 diabetes. Whelton (2007) described the nursing act as a human act in an application of KCS using philosophical analysis. For additional information, please visit DavisPlus at http://davisplus.fadavis.com.

Development of middle-range theories is a natural extension of a conceptual framework. Middle-range theories, clearly developed from within a conceptual framework, accomplish two goals: (1) Such theories can be directly applied to nursing situations, whereas a conceptual framework is usually too abstract for such direct application; and (2) validation of middle-range theories, clearly developed within a particular conceptual framework, lends validation to the conceptual framework itself.

In addition to the mid-range Theory of Goal Attainment (King, 1981), several other mid-range theories have been developed from within King's Interacting Systems framework. In terms of the personal system, Brooks and Thomas (1997) used King's framework to derive a theory of perceptual awareness. The focus was to develop the concepts of judgment and action as core concepts in the personal system. Other concepts in the theory included communication, perception, and decision-making.

In relation to the interpersonal system, several middle-range theories have been developed regarding families. Doornbos (2007), using her Family Health Theory, addressed family health in terms of families with adults with persistent mental illness. Wicks, Rice, and Talley (2007) further explored their middle-range theory regarding the broader concept of family health in the context of chronic obstructive pulmonary disease. In relation to social systems, Sieloff (2007) developed the Theory of Group Power within Organizations to assist in explaining the power of groups within organizations. For additional information please visit DavisPlus at http://davisplus.fadavis.com.

Instrument development in nursing continues to be needed in order to measure relevant nursing concepts. However, instruments developed for a research study rarely undergo the rigor of research undertaken for the purpose of instrument development.

However, review of the literature identified instruments specifically designed within King's framework. King (1988) developed the Health Goal Attainment instrument, designed to detail the level of attainment of health goals by individual clients. The Nurse Performance Goal Attainment (NPGA) was developed by Kameoka, Funashima, and Sugimori (2007).

Practice

King's mid-range theory has found great application to nursing practice, since the theory focuses on concepts relevant to all nursing situations—the attainment of client goals. The application of the mid-range Theory of Goal Attainment (King, 1981) is documented in several categories: (1) general application of the theory, (2) exploring a particular concept within the context of the Theory of Goal Attainment, (3) exploring a particular concept related to the Theory of Goal Attainment, and (4) application of the theory in nonclinical nursing situations. For example, King (1997) described the use of the Theory of Goal Attainment in nursing practice. Alligood (1995) applied the theory to orthopedic nursing with adults. Short-term group psychotherapy was the focus of theory application for Laben, Sneed, and Seidel (1995). In contrast, Benedict and Frey (1995) examined the use of the theory within the delivery of emergency care.

The mid-range Theory of Goal Attainment (King, 1981) is also used when nurses wish to explore a particular concept within a theoretical context. Palmer (2006) examined anxiety with short-term memory loss while patients' awareness of their illness was explored by Wang and Yang (2006).

Nurses also use the Theory of Goal Attainment (King, 1981) to examine concepts related to the theory. This application was demonstrated by Smith (2003), and Jones and Bugge (2006).

Finally, the theory has been applied in nonclinical nursing situations. Secrest, Iorio, and Martz (2005) used the theory in examining the empowerment of nursing assistants. Kameoka, Funashima, and Sugimori (2007) explored the relationship of nurse goal attainment and work satisfaction using the theory. For additional information, please visit DavisPlus at http://davisplus.fadavis.com.

Nursing Process and Nursing Terminologies, Including Standardized Nursing Languages

Within the nursing profession, the nursing process has consistently been used as the basis for nursing practice. King's framework and mid-range Theory of Goal Attainment

(1981) have been clearly linked to the process of nursing. Although many published applications have broad reference to the nursing process, several deserve special recognition. First, Dr. King herself (1981) clearly linked the Theory of Goal Attainment to nursing process as theory, and to nursing process as method. Application of King's work to nursing curricula further strengthened this link.

In addition, the steps of the nursing process have long been integrated within the KCS and the mid-range Theory of Goal Attainment (Daubenmire & King, 1973; Husband, 1988; Woods, 1994). In these process applications, assessment, diagnosis, and goal-setting occur, followed by actions based on the nurse–client goals. The evaluation component of the nursing process consistently refers back to the original goal statement(s). In related research, Frey and Norris (1997) also drew parallels between the processes of critical thinking, nursing, and transaction.

Over time, nursing has also developed nursing terminologies that are used to assist the profession to improve communication both within, and external to, the profession. These terminologies include the nursing diagnoses, nursing interventions, and nursing outcomes. With the use of these standardized nursing languages (SNLs), the nursing process is further refined. Standardized terms for diagnoses, interventions, and outcomes also potentially improve communication among nurses.

Using SNLs also enables the development of middle-range theory by building on concepts unique to nursing, such as those concepts of King that can be directly applied to the nursing process: action, reaction, interaction, transaction, goal-setting, and goal attainment. Biegen and Tripp-Reimer (1997) suggested middle-range theories be constructed from the concepts in the taxonomies of the nursing languages focusing on outcomes. Alternatively, King's framework and theory may be used as a theoretical basis for these phenomena, and may assist in knowledge development in nursing in the future.

With the advent of SNLs, "outcome identification" is identified as a step in the nursing process following assessment and diagnosis (McFarland & McFarland, 1997, p. 3). King's (1981) concept of mutual goal-setting is analogous to the outcomes identification step, because King's concept of goal attainment is congruent with the evaluation of client outcomes.

In addition, King's concept of perception (1981) lends itself well to the definition of client outcomes. Johnson and Maas (1997) defined a nursing-sensitive client outcome as "a measurable client or family caregiver state, behavior, or perception that is conceptualized as a variable and is largely influenced and sensitive to nursing interventions" (p. 22). This is fortuitous since the development of nursing knowledge requires the use of client outcome measurement. The use of standardized client outcomes as study variables increases the ease with which research findings could be compared across settings and contributes to knowledge development. Therefore, King's concept of mutually set goals could be studied as "expected outcomes." Also, by using SNLs, King's (1981) mid-range Theory of Goal Attainment could be conceptualized as the "attainment of expected outcomes" as the evaluation step in the application of the nursing process.

In summary, although these terminologies, including SNLs, were developed after many of the original nursing theorists had completed their works, nursing frameworks such as the KCS (1981) can still find application and use within the terminologies. In addition, it is this type of application that further demonstrates the framework's utility across time. For example, Chaves and Araujo (2006), Ferreira De Sourza, Figueiredo De Martino and Daena De Morais Lopes (2006), Goyatá, Rossi, and Dalri (2006), and Palmer (2006) implemented nursing diagnoses within the context of King's framework. (See http://davisplus.fadavis.com for Table 10-4.)

Applications with Clients Across the Life Span

Additional evidence of the scope and usefulness of King's framework and theory is its use with clients across the life span. Several applications have targeted high-risk infants (Frey & Norris, 1997; Norris & Hoyer, 1993; Syzmanski, 1991). Frey (1993, 1995, 1996) developed and tested relationships among multiple systems with children, youth, and young adults. Interestingly, these studies considered personal systems (infants), interpersonal systems (parents, families), and social systems (the nursing staff and hospital environment). Clearly, a strength of King's framework and theory is their utility in encompassing complex settings and situations.

The Conceptual System (KCS) and mid-range Theory of Goal Attainment have also been used to guide practice with adults (young adults, adults, mature adults) with a broad range of concerns. Goyatá et al. (2006) used King's work in their study of adults experiencing burns. Additional examples of applications focusing on adults include women with breast cancer (Funghetto, Terra, & Wolff, 2003) and women with weight problems (Jewell, 2007). Gender-specific work included Sharts-Hopko's (2007) use of a middle-range Theory of Health Perception to study the health status of women during menopause transition and Martin's (1990) application of the framework toward cancer awareness among males.

Several of the applications with adults have targeted the mature adult, thus demonstrating contributions to the nursing specialty of gerontology. Reed (2007) used a middle-range theory to examine the relationship of social support and health in older adults. Zurakowski (2007) also used a middle-range theory to examine the relationship between social and interpersonal influences in older adults living in nursing homes. Clearly, these applications, and others, show how the complexity of King's framework and mid-range theory increases its usefulness for nursing. For additional information, please visit DavisPlus at http://davisplus.fadavis.com.

Applications in Client Systems

In addition to discussing client populations across the life span, client populations can be identified by focus of care (client system) and/or focus of health problem (phenomenon of concern). The focus of care, or interest, can be an individual (personal system) or group (interpersonal or social system). Thus, application of King's work, across client systems, would be divided into the three systems identified within the KCS (1981): personal (the individual), interpersonal (small groups), and social (large groups/society).

Use with personal systems has included both patients and nurses. Patients as personal systems were the focus of applications to nursing students (May, 2007). Brooks and Thomas (1997) considered critical care nurses as the personal system of interest.

When the focus of interest moves from an individual to include interaction between two people, the interpersonal system is involved. Interpersonal systems often include clients and nurses. An example of an application to a nurse-client dyad and larger groups is Campbell-Begg's (2000) approach to "animal-assisted therapy to promote abstinence from the use of chemicals by groups" (p. 31).

In relation to interpersonal systems, or small groups, many publications focus on the family. Gonot (1986) proposed the Conceptual System (KCS) as a model for family therapy. Frey and Norris (1997) used both the Conceptual System (KCS) and Theory of Goal Attainment in planning care with families of premature infants.

King's Conceptual System (KCS) and mid-range Theory of Goal Attainment have a long history of application with large groups or social systems (organizations, communities). The earliest applications involved the use of the framework and theory to guide continuing education (Brown & Lee, 1980) and nursing curricula (Daubenmire, 1989; Gulitz & King, 1988). More contemporary applications address a variety of organizational settings. For example, the framework served as the basis for the development of a middle range theory relating to practice in a nursing home (Zurakowski, 2007). In addition, applications proposed the Theory of Goal Attainment as the practice model for case management (Hampton, 1994; Tritsch, 1996). These latter applications are especially important, as they may be the first use of the framework by other disciplines.

Applicable to administration and management in a variety of settings, a mid-range theory of group power within organizations has been developed (Sieloff, 1995, 2003, 2007). Educational settings, also considered as social systems, have been the focus of application of King's work (Bello, 2000). (See http://davisplus.fadavis.com for Table 10-8.)

Focus on Phenomena of Concern to Clients

Within King's work, it is critically important for the nurse to focus on, and address, the phenomenon of concern to the client. Without this emphasis on the client's perspective, mutual goal-setting cannot occur. Hence, a client's phenomena of concern was selected as neutral terminology that clearly demonstrated the broad application of King's work to a wide variety of practice situations. For additional information, please visit DavisPlus at http://davisplus.fadavis.com.

Health is one area that certainly binds clients and nurses. Improved health is clearly the desired end point, or outcome, of nursing care and something to which clients aspire. Review of the outcome of nursing care, as addressed in published applications, tends to support the goal of improved health directly and/or indirectly, as the result of the application of King's work. Health status is explicitly the outcome of concern in practice applications by Smith (1988). Several applications used health-related terms. For example, Kohler (1988) focused on increased morale and satisfaction, and DeHowitt (1992) studied well-being.

Health promotion has also been an emphasis for the application of King's ideas. Sexual counseling was the focus of work by Villeneuve and Ozolins (1991). The experi-

ence of parenting was studied by Norris and Hoyer (1993), and health behaviors were Hanna's (1995) focus of study.

King (1981) stated that individuals act to maintain their own health. Although not explicitly stated, the converse is probably true as well: Individuals often do things that are not good for their health. Accordingly, it is not surprising that the Conceptual System (KCS) and related mid-range theory are often directed toward patient and group behaviors that influence health. Frey (1997), Frey and Denyes (1989), and Frey and Fox (1990) looked at both health behaviors and illness management behaviors in several groups of children with chronic conditions. In addition, Frey (1996) expanded her research to include risky behaviors.

As stated previously, diseases or diagnoses are often identified as the focus for the application of nursing knowledge. Hernandez (2007) conducted research with patients with type 1 diabetes, while women with breast cancer were the focus of the work of Funghetto et al. (2003). In addition, clients with chronic obstructive pulmonary disease were involved in research by Wicks and colleagues (2007).

Clients experiencing a variety of psychiatric concerns have also been the focus of work, using King's conceptualizations (Murray & Baier, 1996; Schreiber, 1991). Clients' concerns ranged from psychotic symptoms (Kemppainen, 1990) to families experiencing chronic mental illness (Doornbos, 2007), to clients in short-term group psychotherapy (Laben, Sneed, & Seidel, 1995). For additional information, please visit DavisPlus at http://davisplus.fadavis.com.

Application within Nursing Specialties

A topic that frequently divides nurses is their area of specialty. However, by using a consistent framework across specialties, nurses would be able to focus more clearly on their commonalities, rather than highlighting their differences. A review of the literature clearly demonstrates that Dr. King's framework and related theories have application within a variety of nursing specialties. (See http://davisplus.fadavis.com for Table 10-10.) This application is evident whether one is reviewing a "traditional" specialty, such as surgical nursing (Khowaja, 2006; Palmer, 2006; Susleck, Secrest, Holweger, & Myhan, 2007), or in the nontraditional specialties of forensic nursing (Laben, Dodd, & Sneed, 1991) and/or nursing administration (Secrest, Iorio, & Martz, 2005).

Application in Varied Work Settings

An additional potential source of division within the nursing profession is the work sites where nursing is practiced and care is delivered. As the delivery of health care moves from the more traditional site of the acute care hospital to community-based agencies and clients' homes, it is important to highlight commonalities across these settings, and it is important to identify that King's framework and mid-range Theory of Goal Attainment continue to be applicable. Although many applications tend to be with nurses and clients in traditional settings, successful applications have been shown across other, including newer and nontraditional, settings. From hospitals (Hessig, Arcand, & Frost, 2004; Kameoka, Funashima, & Sugimori, 2007) to nursing homes (Zurakowski, 2007), King's framework and related theories provide a foundation on which nurses can build their practice interventions. In addition, the use of the KCS and related theories are also evident within quality improvement projects (Anderson & Mangino, 2006; Durston, 2006; Khowaja, 2006). For additional information, please visit DavisPlus at http://davisplus.fadavis.com.

Multicultural Applications

Multicultural applications of King's Conceptual System (KCS) and related theories are many. Such applications are particularly critical as many theoretical formulations are limited by their culture-bound nature. Several authors specifically addressed the utility of King's framework and theory for transcultural nurs-

ing. Spratlen (1976) drew heavily from King's framework and theory to integrate ethnic cultural factors into nursing curricula and to develop a culturally oriented model for mental health care. Key elements derived from King's work were the focus on perceptions and communication patterns that motivate action, reaction, interaction, and transaction. Rooda (1992) derived propositions from the mid-range Theory of Goal Attainment as the framework for a conceptual model for multicultural nursing.

Cultural relevance has also been demonstrated in reviews by Frey, Rooke, Sieloff, Messmer, and Kameoka (1995) and Husting (1997). Although Husting identified that cultural issues were implicit variables throughout King's framework, particular attention was given to the concept of health, which, according to King (1990), acquires meaning from cultural values and social norms.

Undoubtedly, the strongest evidence for the cultural utility of King's conceptual framework and mid-range Theory of Goal Attainment (1981) is the extent of work that has been done in other cultures. Applications of the framework and related theories have been documented in the following countries beyond the United States: Canada (Coker et al., 1995), Japan (Kameoka et al., 2007), Portugal (Chauves & Araujo, 2006; Goyatá et al., 2006; Pelloso & Tavares, 2006), and Sweden (Rooke, 1995a, 1995b). In Japan, a culture very different from the United States with regard to communication style, Kameoka (1995) used the classification system of nurse-patient interactions identified within the Theory of Goal Attainment (King, 1981) to analyze nurse-patient interactions. In addition to research and publications regarding the application of King's work to nursing practice internationally, publications by and about Dr. King have been translated into other languages, including Japanese (King, 1976, 1985; Kobayashi, 1970). Therefore, perception and the influence of culture on perception were identified as strengths of King's theory.

Multidisciplinary Applications

When originally developing the Conceptual Systems Framework, King (1981) borrowed from knowledge external to nursing and used a systems framework perspective to assist in explaining nursing phenomena. This use of knowledge across disciplines occurs frequently and can be very appropriate if both disciplines' perspectives are similar and reformulation occurs. Because of King's emphasis on the attainment of goals and the relevancy of goal attainment to many disciplines, both within and external to health care, it is reasonable to expect that King's work could find application beyond nursing-specific situations. Two specific examples of this include the application of King's work to case management (Hampton, 1994; Sowell & Lowenstein, 1994) and to managed care (Hampton, 1994). Both case management and managed care incorporate multiple disciplines as they work to improve the overall quality and cost efficiency of the health care provided. These applications also address the continuum of care, a priority in today's health-care environment. Specific researchers (Khowaja, 2006; Fewster-Thuente & Velsor-Friedrich, 2008) detailed their research related to multidisciplinary activities and interdisciplinary collaborations, respectively. (See http://davisplus.fadavis.com for Table 10-14.)

Relationship to Evidence-Based Practice

A nursing definition of evidence-based practice (EBP) is "A problem-solving approach to clinical practice that integrates a systematic search for and critical appraisal of the most relevant evidence to answer a burning clinical question, one's own clinical expertise and patients' preferences and values" (Melnyk & Fineout-Overholt, 2005, p. 6). Nursing, as a discipline, has continued to evolve in the use of scientific evidence.

Finding and applying relevant evidence requires good clinical judgment (Melnyk & Fineout-Overholt, 2005). The validity of the best evidence is important in EBP. In addition to research, Fawcett (2008) maintains that nursing theory is evidence. Research and theory must be examined using rigorous research and theoretical evaluation.

From an evidence-based practice *and* King perspective, the profession must implement three strategies to apply theory-based research findings effectively. First, nursing as a discipline must agree on rules of evidence in evaluation of quality research that reflect the unique contribution of nursing to health care. Second, the nursing rules of evidence must include heavier weight for research that is derived from, or adds to, nursing theory. Third, the nursing rules of evidence must reflect higher scores when nursing's central beliefs are affirmed in the choice of variables. This third strategy, for the use of concepts central to nursing, has clear relevance for evidence-based practice when using King's (1981) concepts as reformulated within interventions or outcomes. Outcomes, as in King's concept of goal attainment, provide data for evidence-based practice.

Currently, safety and quality initiatives in organizations, with evidence-based practice as the innovation, use many concepts initially defined by King and found in middle-range theories (Sieloff & Frey, 2007). King's (1981) work on the concepts of client and nurse perceptions, and the achievement of mutual goals has been assimilated and accepted as core beliefs of the discipline of nursing. Research conducted with a King theoretical base is well positioned for application by nurse caregivers (Durston, 2006), nurse administrators (Sieloff, 2007), and client-consumers (Killeen, 2007) as part of evolving evidence-based nursing practice. (See http://davisplus.fadavis.com for Table 10-12.)

Recommendations for Future Applications Related to King's Framework and Theory

Obviously, new nursing knowledge has resulted from applications of King's framework and theory. However, nursing, as are all sciences, is evolving. Additional work continues to be needed. Based on a review of the applications previously discussed, recommendations for future applications focus on: (1) the need for evidence-based nursing practice that is theoretically derived; (2) the integration of King's work in evidence-based nursing practice; (3) the integration of King's concepts within standardized nursing language (SNLs); (4) analyzing the future impact of managed care, continuous quality improvement, and technology on King's concepts; (5) identification, or development and implementation, of additional relevant instruments; and (6) clarification of effective nursing interventions, including identification of relevant NICs, based on King's work.

Practice Exemplar

Application of the Theory of Goal Attainment to Interdisciplinary teams, Quality Improvement and Evidence-Based Practice

Claire Smith RN, BSN is a recent nursing graduate in her first position on a medical ICU in a suburban community hospital. Claire's manager suggests Claire join the unit's interdisciplinary quality improvement committee for development of her leadership on the unit. The goal of the committee is to improve patient care by using the best available evidence to develop and implement practice protocols.

At the first meeting, Claire was asked if she had any burning clinical questions as a new graduate. She stated that she was taught to avoid use of normal saline for tracheal suctioning. However, she noticed many respiratory therapists and some nurses routinely using normal saline with suctioning. When asked about this practice, she was told that normal saline was useful to break up secretions and aid in their removal. The committee affirmed Claire's observation of contradictory practices between what is taught and what is done in practice. After discussion, the group formulated the following clinical question: *Does instilling normal saline decrease favorable patient outcomes among patients with endotracheal tubes or tracheostomies?*

Claire suggests to the committee that King's Theory of Goal Attainment might be useful as a theoretical guide for this project because the normal saline clinical question is focused on patient outcomes, or according to King's theory, *goals*. The nursing members are familiar with King's theory and all members value using theory to guide practice. Claire's proposal is accepted. Claire experienced working on EBP group projects as a student so she feels comfortable volunteering to develop a draft of the theoretical foundation for the project. Two other committee members agree to work on the plan and present it at the next meeting.

These are the questions Claire and her colleagues discussed and their conclusions.

1. *How does King's Theory of Goal Attainment help the unit's QI committee?*

Goal attainment theory is derived from King's conceptual system which includes personal, interpersonal, and social systems. The QI committee is a type of interpersonal system. An interpersonal system encompasses individuals in groups interacting to achieve goals. The QI committee is engaged in the committee's goal attainment for the benefit of patients. "Role expectations and role performance of nurses and clients influence transactions" (King, 1981, p. 147). When used in interdisciplinary teams, the transaction process in King's theory facilitates mutual goal-setting with nurses, and ultimately patients, based on each member of the team's specific knowledge and functions.

Multidisciplinary care conferences, an example of a situation where goal-setting among professionals occurs, is a label for an indirect nursing intervention within the Nursing Interventions Classification (NIC)

Continued

Practice Exemplar cont.

(Dochterman & Bulechek, 2000). Some of the activities listed under this NIC reflect King's (1981) concepts: "establish mutually agreeable goals; solicit input for client care planning; revise client care plan, as necessary; discuss progress toward goals; and provide data to facilitate evaluation of client care plan" (p. 460).

2. *How does King define goals and goal attainment and how are these related to quality patient outcomes?*

According to King's Theory of Goal Attainment (1981), goals are mutually agreed upon, and through a transaction process, are attained. Goals are similar to outcomes that are achieved after agreement on the definitions and measurement of the outcomes. Quality improvement has shown agreement that evaluation of care must include process and outcomes. Outcomes are the results of interventions or processes. The term "outcome" assumes a process is central to effective care. Outcome is defined as a change in a patient's health status. Effectiveness of care

can be measured by whether or not the patient goals, i.e., outcomes, have been attained. The QI Committee engages in goal attainment through communication by setting goals, exploring means and agreeing on means to achieve goals. In this example, members will gather information, examine data and evidence, interpret the information and participate in developing a protocol for patients to achieve quality patient outcomes, that is, goals.

3. *How does King's Theory of Goal Attainment provide a theoretical foundation for the clinical problem of normal saline with suctioning?*

First, use of King's theory will help guide the literature search to include studies that address interventions or processes that lead to favorable patient outcomes or goals among patients similar to the population on the unit. Claire's subgroup enlisted the help of the hospital librarian in searching the literature using the elements of the clinical question and the theoretical concepts

Clinical problem elements	King's concepts	Application to the project
Population: *patients with endotracheal tubes or tracheostomies*	Clients and nurses	Members of the Interdisciplinary Committee
Intervention: normal saline with suctioning	Transaction process: Disturbance	Clinical problem formulated and relevance to unit discussed.
Outcomes	Goals explored	Evidence sought and examined to select measurable goals/ outcomes.
Outcomes	Explore means to achieve goals	Implementation plan devised.
Outcomes	Agree on means to achieve goals	Implementation plan accepted by members.

Figure 10 • 3 Theoretical foundation for a quality improvement project using Imogene King's Theory of Goal Attainment derived from King's Conceptual System (1981).

as key words. Second, the theoretical formulation of the study helps organize the implementation and evaluation plans so they are attainable.

4. *What key words would you use for the search considering the clinical question and King's theory?*

Key words used are: *endotracheal tubes, tracheostomies, normal saline, suctioning, outcomes, King's theory of goal attainment,* and *goal attainment.*

5. *How does a theoretical foundation, such as King's Theory of Goal Attainment, apply to a quality improvement or EBP project?*

Claire used these criteria from her nursing program to develop a theoretical foundation for the project.

The theoretical foundation for the project was presented to the committee and accepted (Fig. 10-3).

6. What were the results of the committee's work?

The search strategy included MEDLINE, CINAHL, Cochrane Library, Joanna Briggs Institute, and TRIP databases. All types of evidence (nonexperimental, experimental, qualitative studies, systematic reviews) were included. The evidence was evaluated by the QI committee and determined that the evidence included physiological and psychological effects of instillation of normal saline. The collective evidence, relevant to their unit's practice problem, supported against the routine use of normal saline with suctioning (similar to Halm & Kriski-Hagel, 2008). From the evidence, the committee selected the specific outcomes to track for the project: sputum recovery, oxygenation, and subjective symptoms of pain, anxiety, and dyspnea. Owing to anticipated small samples, hemodynamic alterations and infections were not selected as outcomes. The committee devised a theory-based implementation plan to discontinue normal saline for suctioning using the 5 Ws (who, what, where, when, why) and how as the outline for the plan. Change processes were employed in the plan. Evaluation of the attainment of outcomes will address the effectiveness of the plan using the measurable outcomes and the degree to which they were attained.

■ Summary

An essential component in the analysis of conceptual frameworks and theories is the consideration of their adequacy (Ellis, 1968). Adequacy depends on the three interrelated characteristics of scope, usefulness, and complexity. Conceptual frameworks are broad in scope and are sufficiently complex to be useful for many situations. Theories, on the other hand, are narrower in scope, usually addressing less abstract concepts, and are more specific in terms of the nature and direction of relationships and focus.

King fully intended her conceptual system for nursing to be useful in all nursing situations. Likewise, the mid-range Theory of Goal Attainment (King, 1981) has broad scope because interaction is a part of every nursing encounter.

Although evaluation of the scope of King's framework and mid-range theory has resulted in mixed reviews (Austin & Champion, 1983; Carter & Dufour, 1994; Frey, 1996; Jonas, 1987; Meleis, 1985), the nursing profession has clearly recognized their scope and usefulness. In addition, the variety of practice applications evident in the literature clearly attests to the complexity of King's work. As researchers continue to integrate King's theory and framework with the dynamic health-care environment, future applications involving evidence-based practice will continue to demonstrate the adequacy of King's work in nursing practice.

References

Alligood, M. R. (1995). Theory of goal attainment: Application to adult orthopedic nursing. In: M. A. Frey & C. L. Sieloff (Eds.), *Advancing King's systems framework and theory of nursing* (pp. 209–222). Thousand Oaks, CA: Sage.

Anderson, C. D., & Mangino, R. R. (2006). Nurse shift report: Who says you can't talk in front of the patient? *Nursing Administration Quarterly, 30*(2), 112–122.

Austin, J. K., & Champion, V. L. (1983). King's theory for nursing: Explication and evaluation. In: P. L. Chinn (Ed.), *Advances in nursing theory development* (pp. 49–61). Rockville, MD: Aspen.

Bello, I. T. R. (2000). Imogene King's theory as the foundation for the set of a teaching-learning process with undergraduation [sic] students [Portuguese]. *Texto & Contexto Enfermagem, 9*(2 part 2), 646–657.

Benedict, M., & Frey, M. A. (1995). Theory-based practice in the emergency department. In: M. A. Frey & C. L. Sieloff (Eds.), *Advancing King's systems framework and theory of nursing* (pp. 317–324). Thousand Oaks, CA: Sage.

Biegen, M. A., & Tripp-Reimer, T. (1997). Implications of nursing taxonomies for middle-range theory development. *Advances in Nursing Science, 19*(3), 37–49.

Bigony, M. D. (2007). Perceptions of the nurse-caregiver relationship and its influence on the utilization of respite care services by spousal caregivers of patients diagnosed with dementia. *Dissertation Abstracts International, 68-04B*, 2243.

Brooks, E. M., & Thomas, S. (1997). The perception and judgment of senior baccalaureate student nurses in clinical decision making. *Advances in Nursing Science, 19*(3), 50–69.

Brown, S. T., & Lee, B. T. (1980). Imogene King's conceptual framework: A proposed model for continuing nursing education. *Journal of Advanced Nursing, 5*, 467–473.

Bulechek, G. M., Butcher, H. K. & Dochterman, J. M. (2008). *Nursing Interventions Classification (NIC)* (5th ed.). St. Louis, MO: C. V. Mosby.

Campbell-Begg, T. (2000). A case study using animal-assisted therapy to promote abstinence in a group of individuals who are recovering from chemical addictions. *Journal of Addictions Nursing, 12*(1), 31–35.

Carter, K. F., & Dufour, L. T. (1994). King's theory: A critique of the critiques. *Nursing Science Quarterly, 7*(3), 128–133.

Chaves, E. S., & Araujo, T. L. (2006). Nursing care for an adolescent with cardiovascular risk [Portuguese]. *Ciencia Cuidado e Saude, 5*(1), 82–87.

Coker, E., Fradley, T., Harris, J., Tomarchio, D., Chan, V., & Caron, C. (1995). Implementing nursing diagnoses within the context of King's conceptual framework. In: M. A. Frey & C. L. Sieloff (Eds.), *Advancing King's systems framework and theory of nursing* (pp. 161–176). Thousand Oaks, CA: Sage.

Daubenmire, M. J. (1989). A baccalaureate nursing curriculum based on King's conceptual framework. In: J. P. Riehl-Sisca (Ed.), *Conceptual models for nursing practice* (3rd ed., pp. 167–178). Norwalk, CT: Appleton & Lange.

Daubenmire, M. J., & King, I. M. (1973). Nursing process models: A systems approach. *Nursing Outlook, 21*, 512–517.

DeHowitt, M. C. (1992). King's conceptual model and individual psychotherapy. *Perspectives in Psychiatric Care, 28*(4), 11–14.

Doornbos, M. M. (2007). King's conceptual system and family health theory in the families of adults with persistent mental illness—An evolving conceptualization. In: C. L. Sieloff & M. A. Frey (Eds.), *Middle range theory development using King's conceptual system* (pp. 31-49). New York: Springer.

Durston, P. (2006, April). Partners in caring: a partnership for healing. *Nursing Administration Quarterly, 30*(2), 105–111. Retrieved August 22, 2008, from CINAHL with Full Text database.

Ehrenberger, H. E., Alligood, M. R., Thomas, S. P., Wallace, D. C., & Licavoli, C. M. (2007). Testing a theory of decision making derived from King's systems framework in women eligible for a cancer clinical trial. In: C. L. Sieloff & M. A. Frey (Eds.), *Middle range theory development using King's conceptual system* (pp. 75–91). New York: Springer.

Ellis, R. (1968). Characteristics of significant theories. *Nursing Research, 17*, 217–222.

Fawcett, J. (2008). The added value of nursing conceptual model-based research, *Journal of Advanced Nursing, 61*(6), 583.

Federal Register (1995). Final Revisions: 60(123), Tuesday. June 27, 1995, p. 33294 forward.

Ferreira De Souza, E., Figueiredo De Martino, M. M., & Daena De Morais Lopes, M. H. (2006, Jan–Mar). Analyzing nursing diagnoses in chronic renal clients using Imogene King's Conceptual System. *International Journal of Nursing Terminologies & Classifications, 17*(1), 53–54. Retrieved August 22, 2008, from CINAHL with Full Text database.

Fewster-Thuente, L., & Velsor-Friedrich, B. (2008). Interdisciplinary collaboration for healthcare professionals. *Nursing Administration Quarterly, 32*(1), 40–48.

Frey, M. A. (1993). A theoretical perspective of family and child health derived from King's conceptual framework of nursing: A deductive approach to theory building. In S. L. Feetham, S. B. Meister, J. M. Bell, & C. L. Gillis (Eds.), *The nursing of families: Theory/research/education/practice* (pp. 30–37). Newbury Park, CA: Sage.

Frey, M. A. (1995). Toward a theory of families, children, and chronic illness. In M. A. Frey & C. L. Sieloff (Eds.), *Advancing King's systems framework and theory of nursing* (pp. 109–125). Thousand Oaks, CA: Sage.

Frey, M. A. (1996). Behavioral correlates of health and illness in youths with chronic illness. *Advanced Nursing Research, 9*(4), 167–176.

Frey, M. A. (1997). Health promotion in youth with chronic illness: Are we on the right track? *Quality Nursing, 3*(5), 13–18.

Frey, M. A., & Denyes, M. J. (1989). Health and illness self-care in adolescents with IDDM: A test of Orem's theory. *Advances in Nursing Science, 12*(1), 67–75.

Frey, M. A., Ellis, D. A., & Naar-King, S. (2007). Testing nursing theory with intervention research: The congruency between King's conceptual system and multisystemic therapy. In C. L. Sieloff & M. A. Frey (Eds.), *Middle range theory development using King's conceptual system* (pp. 273–286). New York: Springer.

Frey, M. A., & Fox, M. A. (1990). Assessing and teaching self-care to youths with diabetes mellitus. *Pediatric Nursing, 16,* 597–599.

Frey, M. A., & Norris, D. M. (1997). King's systems framework and theory in nursing practice. In A. Marriner-Tomey (Ed.), *Nursing theory utilization and application* (pp. 71–88). St. Louis, MO: C. V. Mosby.

Frey, M. A., Rooke, L., Sieloff, C. L., Messmer, P., & Kameoka, T. (1995). King's framework and theory in Japan, Sweden, and the United States. *Image: Journal of Nursing Scholarship, 27*(2), 127–130.

Frey, M. A., & Sieloff, C. L. (1995). *Advancing King's systems framework and theory of nursing.* Thousand Oaks, CA: Sage.

Funghetto, S. S., Terra, M. G., & Wolff, L. R. (2003). Woman [sic] with breast cancer: Perception about the disease, family and society [Portuguese]. *Revista Brasileira de Enfermagem, 56*(5), 528–532.

Gonot, P. J. (1986). Family therapy as derived from King's conceptual model. In: L. Whall (Ed.), *Family therapy for nursing: Four approaches* (pp. 33–48). Norwalk, CT: Appleton-Century-Crofts.

Gorski, M. S., & Hackbarth, D. (2005). Quality of care in nursing homes. *Online Journal of Clinical Innovations, 8*(4), 1–61.

Goyatá, S., Rossi, L., & Dalri, M. (2006, Jan–Feb). Nursing diagnoses for family members of adult burned patients near hospital discharge [Portuguese]. *Revista Latino-Americana de Enfermagem, 14*(1), 102–109. Retrieved August 22, 2008, from CINAHL with Full Text database.

Gulitz, E. A., & King, I. M. (1988). King's general systems model: Application to curriculum development. *Nursing Science Quarterly, 1,* 128–132.

Halm, M. A., & Kriski-Hagel, K. (2008). Instilling normal saline with suctioning: Beneficial technique or potentially harmful sacred cow? *American Journal of Critical Care, 17*(5), 469–472.

Hampton, D. C. (1994). King's theory of goal attainment as a framework for managed care implementation in a hospital setting. *Nursing Science Quarterly, 7*(4), 170–173.

Hanna, K. M. (1995). Use of King's theory of goal attainment to promote adolescents' health behavior. In: M. A. Frey & C. L. Sieloff (Eds.), *Advancing King's systems framework and theory of nursing* (pp. 239–250). Thousand Oaks, CA: Sage.

Hernandez, C. A. (2007). The theory of integration: Congruency with King's conceptual system. In: C. L. Sieloff & M. A. Frey (Eds.), *Middle range theory development using King's conceptual system* (pp. 105–124). New York: Springer.

Hessig, R., Arcand, L., & Frost, M. (2004). The effects of an educational intervention on oncology nurses' attitude, perceived knowledge, and self-reported application of complementary therapies. *Oncology Nursing Forum, 31*(1), 71–78. Retrieved August 22, 2008, from CINAHL with Full Text database.

Houser, B. P. & Player, K. N. (2007). Imogene King. In: *Pivotal moments in nursing* (vol. 2., pp. 106–131). Sigma Theta Tau International Honor Society of Nursing. Indianapolis, IN.

Howland, D. (1976). An adaptive health system model. In: H. H. Werley & J. C. Abbey (Eds.), *Health research: The systems approach* (p. 109). New York: Springer.

Howland, D., & McDowell, W. (1964). A measurement of patient care: A conceptual framework. *Nursing Research, 13*(4), 320–324.

Husband, A. (1988). Application of King's theory of nursing to the care of the adult with diabetes. *Journal of Advanced Nursing, 13,* 484–488.

Husting, P. M. (1997). A transcultural critique of Imogene King's theory of goal attainment. *Journal of Multicultural Nursing & Health, 3*(3), 15–20.

Jewell, D. A. (2007). Perceptions of dyspnea, physical activity, and functional status in obese women. *Dissertation Abstracts International, 68-11B,* 7248.

Johnson, M., & Maas, M. (1997). *Nursing outcomes classification (NOC).* St. Louis, MO: Mosby-Year Book.

Jonas, C. M. (1987). King's goal attainment theory: Use in gerontological nursing practice. *Perspectives: Journal of the Gerontological Nursing Association, 11*(4), 9–12.

Jones, A., & Bugge, C. (2006, September). Improving understanding and rigour through triangulation: an exemplar based on patient participation in interaction. *Journal of Advanced Nursing, 55*(5), 612-621. Retrieved August 22, 2008, from CINAHL with Full Text database.

Jones, S., Clark, V. B., Merker, A., & Palau, D. (1995). Changing behaviors: Nurse educators and clinical nurse specialists design a discharge planning program. *Journal of Nursing Staff Development, 11*(6), 291–295.

Kameoka, T. (1995). Analyzing nurse-patient interactions in Japan. In M. A. Frey & C. L. Sieloff (Eds.), *Advancing King's systems framework and theory of goal attainment* (pp. 251–260). Thousand Oaks, CA: Sage.

Kameoka, T., Funashima, N., & Sugimori, M. (2007). If goals are attained, satisfaction will occur in nurse-patient interaction: An empirical test. In: C. L. Sieloff & M. A. Frey (Eds.), *Middle Range Theory Development Using King's Conceptual System* (pp. 261-272). New York: Springer.

Kemppainen, J. K. (1990). Imogene King's theory: A nursing case study of a psychotic client with human immunodeficiency virus infection. *Archives of Psychiatric Nursing, 4*(6), 384–388.

Khowaja, D. (2006). Utilization of King's interacting systems framework and theory of goal attainment with new multidisciplinary model: Clinical pathway. *Australian Journal of Advanced Nursing, 24*(2), 44–50.

Killeen, M. B. (2007). Development and initial testing of a theory of patient satisfaction with nursing care. In: C. L. Sieloff & M. A. Frey (Eds.), *Middle range theory development using King's conceptual system* (pp. 138–163). New York: Springer.

King, I. M. (1964). Nursing theory: Problems and prospect. *Nursing Science Quarterly, 2,* 294.

King, I. M. (1968). A conceptual frame of reference for nursing. *Nursing Research, 17,* 27–31.

King, I. M. (1971). *Toward a theory for nursing: General concepts of human behavior.* New York: John Wiley & Sons.

King, I. M. (1975). A process for developing concepts for nursing through research. In P. J. Verhonick (Ed.), *Nursing research* (p. 25). Boston: Little, Brown.

King, I. M. (1976). *Toward a theory of nursing: General concepts of human behavior* (Sugimori, M., trans.). Tokyo: Igaku-Shoin.

King, I. M. (1981). *A theory of goal attainment: Systems, concepts, process.* New York: John Wiley & Sons.

King, I. M. (1984). Effectiveness of nursing care: Use of a goal oriented nursing record in end stage renal disease. *American Association of Nephrology Nurses and Technicians Journal, 11*(2), 11–17, 60.

King, I. M. (1985). *A theory for nursing: Systems, concepts, process* (Sugimori, M., trans.). Tokyo: Igaku-Shoin.

King, I. M. (1986). *Curriculum and instruction in nursing: Concepts and process.* Norwalk, CT: Appleton-Century-Crofts.

King, I. M. (1988). Concepts: Essential elements of theories. *Nursing Science Quarterly, 1*(1), 22–24.

King, I. M. (1989a). King's general systems framework and theory. In J. P. Riehl-Sisca (Ed.), *Conceptual models for nursing practice* (p. 149). Norwalk, CT: Appleton & Lang.

King, I. M. (1989b). King's systems framework for nursing administration. In: B. Henry (Ed.), *Dimensions of nursing administration: Theory, research, education* (p. 35). Cambridge, UK: Blackwell Scientific.

King, I. M. (1990). Health as a goal for nursing. *Nursing Science Quarterly, 3,* 123–128.

King, I. M. (1992). King's theory of goal attainment. *Nursing Science Quarterly, 5,* 19.

King, I. M. (1995). The theory of goal attainment. In: M. A. Frey & C. L. Sieloff (Eds.), *Advancing King's systems framework and theory of goal attainment* (p. 23). Thousand Oaks, CA: Sage.

King, I. M. (1996). The theory of goal attainment in research and practice. *Nursing Science Quarterly, 9,* 61.

King, I. M. (1997). King's theory of goal attainment in practice. *Nursing Science Quarterly, 10*(4), 180–185.

Kobayashi, F. T. (1970). A conceptual frame of reference for nursing. *Japanese Journal of Nursing Research, 3*(3), 199–204.

Kohler, P. (1988). Model of shared control. *Journal of Gerontological Nursing, 14*(7), 21–25.

Laben, J. K., Dodd, D., & Sneed, L. (1991). King's theory of goal attainment applied in group therapy for inpatient juvenile offenders, maximum security state offenders, and community parolees, using visual aids. *Issues in Mental Health Nursing, 12*(1), 51–64.

Laben, J. K., Sneed, L. D., & Seidel, S. L. (1995). Goal attainment in short-term group psychotherapy settings: Clinical implications for practice. In: M. A. Frey & C. L. Sieloff (Eds.), *Advancing King's systems framework and theory of nursing* (pp. 261–277). Thousand Oaks, CA: Sage.

Martin, J. P. (1990). Male cancer awareness: Impact of an employee education program. *Oncology Nursing Forum, 17,* 59–64.

May, B. A. (2007). Relationships among basic empathy, self-awareness, and learning styles of baccalaureate prenursing students within King's personal system. In: C. L. Sieloff & M. A. Frey (eds). *Middle range theory development using King's conceptual system* (pp. 164–177). New York: Springer.

McFarland, G. K., & McFarland, E. A. (1997). *Nursing diagnosis and intervention: Planning for patient care.* St. Louis, MO: Mosby-Year Book.

Meleis, A. (1985). *Theoretical nursing: Developments and progress* (2nd ed.). Philadelphia: J. B. Lippincott.

Melnyk, B. M., & Fineout-Overholt, E. (2005). *Evidence-based practice in nursing and healthcare: A guide to best practice.* Philadelphia: Lippincott, Williams & Wilkins.

Messmer, P. R. (1992). Implementing theory based nursing practice. *Florida Nurse, 40*(3), 8.

Messmer, P. R. (1995). Implementation of theory-based nursing practice. In M. A. Frey & C. L. Sieloff (Eds.), *Advancing King's systems framework and theory of nursing* (pp. 294–304). Thousand Oaks, CA: Sage.

Messmer, P. R. (2007). Tribute to the theorists: Imogene M. King over the years. *Nursing Science Quarterly, 20*(3), 198.

Murray, R. L. E., & Baier, M. (1996). King's conceptual framework applied to a transitional living program. *Perspectives in Psychiatric Care, 32*(1), 15–19.

Norris, D. M., & Hoyer, P. J. (1993). Dynamism in practice: Parenting within King's framework. *Nursing Science Quarterly, 6*(2), 79–85.

Northrop, F. C. S. (1969). *The logic of the sciences and the humanities.* Cleveland, OH: Meridian.

Palmer, J. A. (2006). Nursing implications for older adult patient education. *Plastic Surgical Nursing, 26*(4), 189–194.

Pelloso, S. M., & Tavares, M. S. G. (2006). Family problems and mother's death [Portuguese]. *Ciencia Cuidado e Saude, 5*(Suppl), 19–25.

Reed, J. E. F. (2007). Social support and health of older adults. In: C. L. Sieloff & M. A. Frey (Eds.), *Middle range theory development using King's conceptual system* (pp. 92–104). New York: Springer.

Rooda, L. A. (1992). The development of a conceptual model for multicultural nursing. *Journal of Holistic Nursing, 10*(4), 337–347.

Rooke, L. (1995a). The concept of space in King's systems framework: Its implications for nursing. In M. A. Frey & C. L. Sieloff (Eds.), *Advancing King's systems framework and theory of nursing* (pp. 79–96). Thousand Oaks, CA: Sage.

Rooke, L. (1995b). Focusing on King's theory and systems framework in education by using an experiential learning model: A challenge to improve the quality of nursing care. In M. A. Frey & C. L. Sieloff (Eds.), *Advancing King's systems framework and theory of nursing* (pp. 278–293). Thousand Oaks, CA: Sage.

Schreiber, R. (1991). Psychiatric assessment— "A la King." *Nursing Management, 22*(5), 90, 92, 94.

Secrest, J., Iorio, D. H., & Martz, W. (2005). The meaning of work for nursing assistants who stay in long-term care. *International Journal of Older People Nursing, 14*(8b), 90–97.

Sharts-Hopko, N. C. (2007). A theory of health perception: Understanding the menopause transition. In: C. L. Sieloff & M. A. Frey (Eds.), *Middle range theory development using King's conceptual system* (pp. 178–195). New York: Springer.

Sieloff, C. L. (1995). Development of a theory of departmental power. In: M. A. Frey & C. L. Sieloff (Eds.), *Advancing King's systems framework and theory of nursing* (pp. 46–65). Thousand Oaks, CA: Sage.

Sieloff, C. L. (2003). Measuring nursing power within organizations. *Journal of Nursing Scholarship, 35*(2), 183–187.

Sieloff, C. L. (2007). The theory of group power within organizations—Evolving conceptualization within King's conceptual system. In: C. L. Sieloff & M. A. Frey (Eds.), *Middle range theory development using King's conceptual system* (pp. 196–214). New York: Springer.

Sieloff, C. L., & Frey, M. (2007). *Middle range theories for nursing practice using King's interacting systems framework.* New York: Springer.

Sieloff, C. L., & Messmer, P. R. (2010). Conceptual systems framework and middle range theory of goal attainment. In: M. R. Alligood (Ed.), *Nursing theorists and their work* (7th ed., pp. 286-308). St. Louis, MO: Mosby-Elsevier.

Smith, L. (2003, October). Image counts: Greeting cards mail it in when it comes to accurately portraying nurses. *Nursing Spectrum (Midwest), 4*(10), 18–21. Retrieved August 22, 2008, from CINAHL with Full Text database.

Smith, M. C. (1988). King's theory in practice. *Nursing Science Quarterly, 1,* 145–146.

Sowell, R. L., & Lowenstein, A. (1994). King's theory: A framework for quality; linking theory to practice. *Nursing Connections, 7*(2), 19–31.

Spees, C. M. (1991). Knowledge of medical terminology among clients and families. *Image: Journal of Nursing Scholarship, 23*(4), 225–229.

Spratlen, L. P. (1976). Introducing ethnic-cultural factors in models of nursing: Some mental health care applications. *Journal of Nursing Education, 15*(2), 23–29.

Susleck, D., Secrest, J., Holweger, J., & Myhan, G. (2007). The perianesthesia experience from the patient's perspective. *Journal of PeriAnesthesia Nursing, 22*(1), 10–20.

Syzmanski, M. E. (1991). Use of nursing theories in the care of families with high-risk infants: Challenges for the future. *Journal of Perinatal and Neonatal Nursing, 4*(4), 71–77.

Tritsch, J. M. (1996). Application of King's theory of goal attainment and the Carondelet St. Mary's case management model. *Nursing Science Quarterly, 11*(2), 69–73.

Villeneuve, M. J., & Ozolins, P. H. (1991). Sexual counselling in the neuroscience setting: Theory and practical tips for nurses. *AXON, 12*(3), 63–67.

Von Bertalanffy, L. (1968). *General system theory.* New York: Braziller.

Wang, S., & Yang, T. Applying King's theory to establish psychotic patients' awareness of illness [Chinese]. *Tzu Chi Nursing Journal, 5*(1), 120–130.

Whelton, B. J. B. (2007). The nursing act is an excellent human act: A philosophical analysis derived from classical philosophy and the conceptual system and theory of Imogene King. In: C. L. Sieloff & M. A. Frey (Eds.), *Middle range theory development using King's conceptual system* (pp. 12–28). New York: Springer.

Wicks, M. N., Rice, M. C., & Talley, C. H. (2007). Further exploration of family health within the context of chronic obstructive pulmonary disease. In: C. L. Sieloff & M. A. Frey (Eds.), *Middle range theory development using King's conceptual system* (pp. 215–236). New York: Springer.

Woods, E. C. (1994). King's theory in practice with elders. *Nursing Science Quarterly, 7*(2), 65–69.

Zurakowski, T. L. (2007). Theory of social and interpersonal influences on health. In: C. L. Sieloff & M. A. Frey (Eds.), *Middle range theory development using King's conceptual system* (pp. 237–257). New York: Springer.

Chapter # 11

Sister Callista Roy's Adaptation Model

CALLISTA ROY AND LIN ZHAN

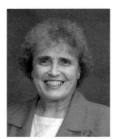

Sister Callista Roy

Introducing the Theorist

Sister Callista Roy is a highly respected nurse theorist, writer, lecturer, researcher, teacher, and member of a religious community. She currently holds the position of professor and nurse theorist at Boston College Connell School of Nursing. Roy's name is one of the most recognized in the field of nursing today worldwide. She is considered among nursing's great living thinkers. However, she notes that her best work is yet to come and will likely be done by one of her students. As a theorist, Roy often emphasizes her primary commitment to define and develop nursing knowledge. She regards her work with the Roy Adaptation Model as a rich source of knowledge for improving nursing practice for individuals and groups. In the first decade of the 21st century, Roy has provided an expanded, values-based concept of adaptation based on insights related to the place of the person in the universe and in society. She hopes these developments: the redefinition of adaptation; enhanced philosophical, scientific and cultural assumptions; theoretical understanding of life processes of the adaptive modes; and processes described for individuals and for groups, will become the basis for developing knowledge that will make nursing a major social force in this century.

In her personal and professional growth, Roy credits the major influences of her family, her religious commitment, and her teachers and mentors. Roy was born in Los Angeles, California, on October 14, 1939. Her middle name, Callista, came from St. Callistus, the saint of the day from the Roman Catholic calendar. She is the oldest daughter of a family of seven boys and seven girls. A deep spirit of faith, hope, love, commitment to God, and service to others was central in the family. Her mother was a licensed vocational nurse and instilled the values of always seeking to know more about people, as well as their care, and of selfless giving as a nurse. Roy noted that she also had excellent teachers in parochial schools, high school, and college. At age 14 she began working at a large general hospital, first as a pantry girl, then as a maid, and finally as a nurse's aide. After a soul-searching process of discernment, she entered the Sisters of Saint Joseph of Carondelet, of which she has been a member for 50 years. Her college education began with a bachelor of arts degree with a major in nursing at Mount St. Mary's College, Los Angeles, followed by master's degrees in pediatric nursing and sociology at the University of California, Los Angeles, and a Ph.D. in sociology at the same school. Later, Roy had the opportunity to be a clinical nurse scholar in a 2-year postdoctoral program in neuroscience nursing at the University of California at San Francisco. Important mentors in her life have included Dorothy E. Johnson, Ruth Wu, Connie Robinson, and Barbara Smith Moran.

Roy is best known for developing and continually updating the Roy Adaptation Model as a framework for theory, practice, and research in nursing. Books on the model have been translated into many languages, including French, Italian, Spanish, Finnish, Chinese, Korean, and Japanese. Two recent publications that Roy considers significant are *The Roy Adaptation Model* (2009) and *Nursing Knowledge Development and Clinical Practice* (with D. Jones, 2007). Another important work is *The Roy Adaptation Model-based Research: Twenty-five Years of Contributions to Nursing Science*, published as a research monograph by Sigma Theta Tau. The latter is a critical analysis of the 25 years of model-based literature, which includes 163 studies published in 46 English-speaking journals, and dissertations and theses. This project was completed by the Boston-Based Adaptation Research in Nursing Society (BBARNS), a group of scholars founded by Roy in the interest of advancing nursing practice by developing basic and clinical nursing knowledge based on the Roy Adaptation Model. This group later became the Roy Adaptation Association. The executive committee continues the work of synthesizing research based on the model and other projects in research, education, and practice. The research publications in English now identified number more than 350.

One of Roy's major activities has been planning New England Knowledge Conferences from 1996 to 2001 and a collaborative nursing knowledge conference with the International Philosophy of Nursing Society in 2008. Roy has been a major speaker throughout North America and 31 other countries over the past 40 years on topics related to nursing theory, research, curriculum, clinical practice, and professional trends for the future. She was a Senior Fulbright Scholar in Australia and her visiting faculty appointments include La Sabana University, Colombia; Autonomous University in Nuevo Leon, Mexico; St. Mary's College, Fukuoka, Japan; University of Lund, Sweden; and University of Conception, Chile as well as invited scholar of the Ministry of University Affairs, Bangkok, Thailand for educators from 19 schools. Roy served on the Board of the International Network for Doctoral Education from 2003 to 2006 and is Faculty Senior Nurse Scientist at the Yvonne L. Munn Center for Nursing Research at Massachusetts General Hospital. She was a Charter Member of the Nursing Research Study Section, Division of Research Grants, National Institutes of Health and has received 42 research and training grants covering a wide range of topics including neuroscience.

Roy was honored as a Living Legend by both the American Academy of Nursing and the Massachusetts Association of Registered Nurses. She has received many other awards, including the National League for Nursing Martha Rogers Award for advancing nursing science; the Sigma Theta Tau International Founders Award for contributions to professional practice; and honorary doctorates from

Eastern Michigan University, Alverno College in Milwaukee, St. Joseph's College in Standish, Maine, and St. Anselm's College in Manchester, New Hampshire. Roy holds several teaching awards, two institution-wide from Mount St. Mary's College in Los Angeles and Boston College. She has received Massachusetts State House recognition for her volunteer work with women in prison. Roy has also received the outstanding Alumna Award and Carondelet Medal from Mount St. Mary's, where she holds a concurrent position as research professor in nursing at her alma mater.

The Roy Adaptation Model has been in use for 40 years, providing direction for nursing practice, education, and research. Extensive implementation efforts around the world, and continuing philosophical and scientific developments by the theorist, have contributed to model-based knowledge for nursing practice. The purpose of this chapter is to describe the model as the foundation for a knowledge-based practice. The developments of the model, including assumptions and major concepts are described. The reader is introduced to the knowledge that the model provides as the basis for planning nursing care. We provide an overview of applications in practice and a practice exemplar that views a family through the lens of one adaptive mode, the group identify mode.

Overview of the Roy Adaptation Model

The Roy Adaptation Model (Roy, 1970, 1984, 1988a, 1988b, 2009; Roy & Andrews, 1991, 1999; Roy & Roberts, 1981) provides a framework for nursing practice with individuals and groups as well as for designing nursing care systems in health care organizations. The model can be understood by looking at the historical development, assumptions, and major concepts. These elements provide the basis for showing how the model provides both theoretical knowledge and guidance for the process of nursing care. Organizational applications of the model in practice are described. Finally, the self-identity adaptive

mode is described in greater detail as background for a specific exemplar that describes nursing care for a Chinese family dealing with a parent diagnosed with dementia.

Historical Development

Under the mentorship of Dorothy E. Johnson, Roy first developed a description of the adaptation model while a masters' nursing student at the University of California at Los Angeles. The first publication on the Model appeared in 1970 (Roy, 1970) while Roy was on the faculty of the baccalaureate nursing program of a small liberal arts college. There, she had the opportunity to lead the implementation of this model of nursing as the basis of the nursing curriculum. During the next decade, more than 1500 faculty and students at Mount St. Mary's College helped to clarify, refine, and develop this approach to nursing. The constant influence of practice was important during this development. One example of data from practice used in model development was to derive four adaptive modes from 500 samples of patient behavior described by nursing students. At a conference held at Mount St. Mary's College in 1981, an evaluation noted that the model met the criteria of significance, usefulness, and completeness.

The mid-1970s to the mid-1980s saw the expansion of the use of the model in nursing education. Roy and the faculty at her home institution consulted on curriculum in more than 30 schools. By 1987 it was estimated that more than 100,000 students had graduated from curricula based on the Roy model. Theory development was also a focus during this time, and 91 propositions based on the model were identified. These described relationships between and among the regulator and cognator and the four adaptive modes (Roy & Roberts, 1981). In the 1980s, Roy also was influenced by postdoctoral work in neuroscience nursing and an increasing number of commitments in other countries. During the 1990s, as a faculty member and nurse-theorist at Boston College, Roy found that working with PhD students challenged and deepened her thinking. She focused on contemporary movements in nursing knowledge and the continued integration of spirituality with an understanding of nursing's role in promoting adaptation. The first decade of the 21st century included a greater focus on philosophy, knowledge for practice, and global concerns.

Philosophical, Scientific, and Cultural Assumptions

Assumptions provide the beliefs, values, and accepted knowledge that form the basis for the work. For the Roy Adaptation Model, the concept of adaptation rests on scientific and philosophic assumptions that Roy has developed over time. The scientific assumptions initially reflected von Bertalanffy's (1968) general systems theory and Helson's (1964) adaptation-level theory. Later beliefs about the unity and meaningfulness of the created universe were included (Young, 1986). Early identification of the philosophic assumptions for the model named humanism and veritivity. In 1988, Roy introduced the concept of veritivity as an option to total relativity. Veritivity was a term coined by Roy, based on the Latin word *veritas*. For Roy, the word offered the notion of the rootedness of all knowledge

being one. Veritivity is the principle of human nature that affirms a common purposefulness of human existence, within the Roy Adaptation Model. Veritivity affirms people in society viewed in the context of the purposefulness of human existence, unity of purpose of humankind, activity and creativity for the common good, and the value and meaning of life.

Currently, Roy views the 21st century as a time of transition, transformation, and need for spiritual vision. The further development of the philosophic assumptions focuses on people's mutuality with others, the world, and a God-figure. The development and expansion of the major concepts of the model show the influence of the theorist's scientific and philosophic background and global experiences. For nursing in the 21st century, Roy (1997) provided a redefinition of adaptation and a restatement of the assumptions that are the foundations of the model, which led expanded philosophical and scientific assumptions in contemporary society and to adding cultural assumptions. These assumptions are listed in Table 11-1 and further described in the basic work on the model (Roy, 2009). Roy also uses the idea of cosmic unity that stresses

Table 11 · 1   Assumptions of the Roy Adaptation Model for the 21st Century

Philosophic Assumptions

Persons have mutual relationships with the world and the God-figure.
Human meaning is rooted in an omega point convergence of the universe.
God is intimately revealed in the diversity of creation and is the common destiny of creation.
Persons use human creative abilities of awareness, enlightenment, and faith.
Persons are accountable for entering the process of deriving, sustaining, and transforming the universe.

Scientific Assumptions

Systems of matter and energy progress to higher levels of complex self organization.
Consciousness and meaning are consistent of person and environment integration.
Awareness of self and environment is rooted in thinking and feeling.
Human decisions are accountable for the integration of creative processes.
Thinking and feeling mediate human action.
System relationships include acceptance, protection, and fostering interdependence.
Persons and the Earth have common patterns and integral relations.
Person and environment transformations created human consciousness.
Integration of human and environment meanings result in adaptation.

Table 11 · 1	**Assumptions of the Roy Adaptation Model for the 21st Century—cont'd**
Cultural Assumptions	
Experiences within a specific culture will influence how each element of the RAM model is expressed.	
Within a culture, there may be a concept that is central to the culture and will influence some or all of the elements of the RAM to a greater or lesser extent.	
Cultural expressions of the elements of the RAM may lead to changes in practice activities such as nursing assessment.	
As RAM elements evolve within a cultural perspective, implications for education and research may differ from experience in the original culture.	

her vision for the future and emphasizes the principle that people and Earth have common patterns and integral relationships. Rather than the system acting to maintain itself, the emphasis shifts to the purposefulness of human existence in a creative universe.

Model Concepts

The underlying assumptions of the Roy Adaptation Model are the basis for and are evident in the specific description of the major concepts of the model. The major concepts include people as adaptive systems (both individuals and groups), the environment, health, and the goal of nursing.

People as Adaptive Systems

Roy describes people, both individually, and in groups, as holistic adaptive systems, complete with coping processes acting to maintain adaptation and to promote person and environment transformations. As with any type of system, people have internal processes that act to maintain the integrity of the individual or group. These processes have been broadly categorized as a regulator subsystem and a cognator subsystem for the person and stabilizer and innovator for the group. The regulator uses physiologic processes such as chemical, neurologic, and endocrine responses to cope with the changing environment. For example, when an individual sees a sudden threat, such as an oncoming car approaching when stepping off the curb, an increase of adrenal hormones provides immediate energy enabling

him or her to escape harm. The cognator subsystem involves the cognitive and emotional processes that interact with the environment. In the example of the individual who escapes from an oncoming car, the cognator acts to process the emotion of fear. The person also processes perceptions of the situation and comes to a new decision about where and how to cross the street safely.

The coping processes for the group relate to stability and change. The stabilizer subsystem has structures, values, and daily activities to accomplish the primary purpose of the group. Thus a family group is structured to earn a living and to provide for the nurturance and education of children. Family values also influence how the members respond to the environment to fulfill their responsibilities to maintain the family. Groups also have processes to respond to the environment with innovation and change by way of the innovator subsystem. For example, organizations use strategic planning activities and team building sessions. When the innovator is functioning well, the group creates new goals and growth, achieving new mastery. Nurses can use innovator subsystems to create organizational change in practice.

Both the cognator-regulator and stabilizer-innovator coping processes are manifested in four particular ways in each individual and in groups of people. These four ways of categorizing the effects of coping activity are called adaptive modes. These four modes, initially developed for human systems as individuals, were expanded to encompass groups.

These are termed the physiologic–physical, self-concept–group identity, role function, and interdependence modes. These four major categories describe responses to and interaction with the environment and are how adaptation can be observed.

For individuals, the physiologic mode in the Roy Adaptation Model is associated with the way people as individuals interact as physical beings with the environment. Behavior in this mode is the manifestation of the physiologic activities of all the cells, tissues, organs, and systems comprising the human body. The physiologic mode has nine components: the five basic needs of oxygenation, nutrition, elimination, activity and rest, and protection and four complex processes that are involved in physiologic adaptation, including the senses; fluid, electrolyte, and acid–base balance; neurologic function; and endocrine function. The underlying need for the physiologic mode is physiologic integrity.

The category of behavior related to the personal aspects of individuals is termed the self-concept. The basic need underlying the self-concept mode has been identified as psychic and spiritual integrity; one needs to know who one is in order to be or exist with a sense of unity. Self-concept is defined as the composite of beliefs and feelings that a person holds about him- or herself at a given time. Formed from internal perceptions and perceptions of others, self-concept directs one's behavior. Components of the self-concept mode are the physical self, including body sensation and body image; and the personal self, including self-consistency, self-ideal, and moral–ethical–spiritual self. Processes in the mode are the developing self, perceiving self, and focusing self.

Behavior relating to positions in society is termed the role function mode for both the individual and the group. From the perspective of the individual, the role function mode focuses on the roles that the individual occupies in society. A role, as the functioning unit of society, is defined as a set of expectations about how a person occupying one position behaves toward a person occupying another position. The basic need underlying the role function mode for the individual has been identified as social integrity, the need to know who one is in relation to others in order to act. The underlying processes include developing roles and role taking.

Behavior related to interdependent relationships of individuals and groups is the interdependence mode, the final adaptive mode Roy describes. For the individual, the mode focuses on interactions related to the giving and receiving of love, respect, and value. The basic need of this mode is termed relational integrity, the feeling of security in nurturing relationships. Two specific relationships are the focus within the interdependence mode for the individual: significant others, persons who are the most important to the individual, and support systems, others contributing to meeting interdependence needs. Interdependence processes include affectional adequacy and developmental adequacy.

For people in groups it is more appropriate to use the term physical in referring to the first adaptive mode. At the group level, this mode relates to the manner in which the human adaptive system of the group manifests adaptation relative to basic operating resources, that is, participants, physical facilities, and fiscal resources. The basic need associated with the physical mode for the group is resource adequacy, or wholeness achieved by adapting to change in physical resource needs. Processes in this mode for groups include resource management and strategic planning.

Group identity is the relevant term used for the second mode related to groups. Identity integrity is the need underlying this group adaptive mode. The mode comprises interpersonal relationships, group self-image, social milieu, and culture.

A nurse can have a self-concept of seeing self as physically capable of the work involved. In addition, the nurse feels comfortable meeting self expectations of being a caring professional. In a social system, such as a nursing care unit, an associated culture can be described. There is a social environment experienced by the nurses, administrators, and other staff that is reflected by those who are part of the nursing care group. The group feels shared values and counts on each other. As such, the self-concept–group identity mode can reflect adaptive or ineffective behaviors associated with an individual nurse or the nursing care unit as an adaptive system. As we note below, two processes identified in this mode are group shared identity and family coherence.

Roles within a group are the vehicle through which the goals of the social system are actually accomplished. They are the action components associated with group infrastructure. Roles are designed to contribute to the accomplishment of the group's mission, or the tasks or functions associated with the group. The role mode includes the functions of administrators and staff, the management of information, and systems for decision making and maintaining order. The basic need associated with the group role function mode is termed role clarity, the need to understand and commit to fulfill expected tasks, in order to achieve common goals. Processes involve socializing for role expectations, reciprocating roles, and integrating roles.

For groups, the interdependence mode pertains to the social context in which the group operates. It involves private and public contacts both within the group and with those outside the group. The components of group interdependence include context, infrastructure, and resources. The processes for group interdependence include relational integrity, developmental adequacy, and resource adequacy.

The four adaptive modes are interdependent, which can be illustrated by drawing the modes as overlapping circles. The physiologic–physical mode is intersected by each of the other three modes. Behavior in the physiologic–physical mode can have an effect on or act as a stimulus for one or all of the other modes. In addition, a given stimulus can affect more than one mode, or a particular behavior can be indicative of adaptation in more than one mode. Such complex relationships among

modes further demonstrate the holistic nature of humans as adaptive systems. The adaptive modes and coping processes for individuals and groups of individuals are described by the Roy model (Roy, 2009). One example is described in this chapter as the basis for practice, the group identity mode.

Environment

The Roy model defines environment as all the conditions, circumstances, and influences surrounding and affecting the development and behavior of individuals and groups. Given the model's view of the place of the person in the evolving universe, environment is a biophysical community of beings with complex patterns of interaction, feedback, growth and decline, constituting periodic and long-term rhythms. Individual and environmental interactions are input for the individual or group as adaptive systems. This input involves both internal and external factors. Roy used the work of Helson (1964), a physiologic psychologist, to categorize these factors as focal, contextual, and residual stimuli. A specific internal input stimulus is an adaptation level that represents the individual's or group's coping capacities. This changing level of ability has an internal effect on adaptive behaviors. Roy defined three levels of adaptation: integrated, compensatory, and compromised. Integrated adaptation occurs when the structures and functions of the adaptive modes are working as a whole to meet human needs. The compensatory adaptation level occurs when the cognator and regulator or stabilizer and innovator are activated by a challenge. Compromised adaptation occurs when integrated and compensatory processes are inadequate, creating an adaptation problem.

Health

Roy's concept of health is related to the concept of adaptation and the idea that adaptive responses promote integrity. Individuals and groups are viewed as adaptive systems that interact with the environment and grow, change, develop, and flourish. Health is the reflection of personal and environmental interactions that are adaptive. According to the Roy Adaptation model, health is defined as (1) a process, (2) a state of being, and (3) becoming whole and integrated in a way that reflects individual and environment mutuality.

Goal of Nursing

When Roy began her theoretical work, the goal of nursing was the first major concept of her nursing model to be described. She began by attempting to identify the unique function of nursing in promoting health. As a number of health care workers have the goal of promoting health, it seemed important to identify a unique goal for nursing. While she was working as a staff nurse in pediatric settings, Roy noted the great resiliency of children in responding to major physiologic and psychological changes. Yet nursing intervention was needed to support and promote this positive coping. It seemed then that the concept of adaptation, or positive coping, might be used to describe the goal or function of nursing. From this initial notion, Roy developed a description of the goal of nursing: the promotion of adaptation for individuals and groups in each of the four adaptive modes, thus contributing to health, quality of life, and dying with dignity.

Practice Applications

The assumptions and concepts of the model provide the basis for theory building for nursing practice, as well as a specific approach to the nursing process. As early as the 1970s, human life processes and patterns were identified as the common focus of nursing knowledge (Donaldson & Crowley, 1978). Adaptation is a significant life process that leads to health. To lead to middle range theories within the model, Roy identified the major life processes within each adaptive mode. For example, in the physiological mode there are processes and patterns for the need for oxygenation that include ventilation, patterns of gas exchange, transport of gases, and compensation for inadequate oxygenation. Similarly, the self-concept mode has three processes identified to meet the person's need for psychic and spiritual integrity: the developing self, the perceiving self, and the focusing self. On the group level, two examples of processes identified to meet the need for a shared self image are group shared identity and family coherence.

To develop knowledge for practice from the grand theory, Roy described a five-step process for developing middle or practice level theory and nursing knowledge:

1. Select a life process.
2. Study the life process in the literature and in people.
3. Develop an intervention strategy to enhance the life process.
4. Derive a proposition for practice.
5. Test the proposition in research.

Processes can also be identified by using qualitative research to identify and describe human experiences.

The nursing process based on the model stems from the assumptions and concepts of the model. First-level assessment of behavior involves gathering data about the behavior of the person or group as an adaptive system in each of the adaptive modes. Second-level assessment is the assessment of stimuli, that is, the identification of internal and external stimuli that influence the person's adaptive behaviors. Stimuli are classified as focal, contextual, and residual. Focal refers to those factors most immediately confronting the person, contextual are all other stimuli affecting the situation, and residual stimuli are those whose effect on the situation are unclear. The nurse uses the first- and second-level assessment to make a nursing judgment called a nursing diagnosis. In collaboration with the person or group, the data are interpreted in statements about the adaptation status of the person, including behavior and most relevant stimuli. The adaptation level is then classified as integrated, compensatory, or compromised.

Also, in collaboration with the person or group, the nurse sets goals, establishing clear statements of the behavioral outcomes for nursing care. Interventions then involve the determination of how best to assist the person in attaining the established goals. These may involve changing stimuli or strengthening coping ability. The aim is to promote an integrated adaptation level. Evaluation involves judging the effectiveness of the nursing intervention in relation to the resulting behavior in comparison with the goal established. The steps of the nursing process have been given in sequential order; however, the process is ongoing and the steps can be simultaneous. For example, the nurse may be intervening in one adaptive mode and assessing in another at the same time.

Senesac (2003) reviewed published projects that have implemented the Roy Adaptation Model in institutional practice settings and identified seven distinct projects ranging from an ideology basis for a single unit to hospital-wide projects. In some cases the published project developed from a unit implementation to a full agency implementation, as in one of the early projects reported by Mastal, Hammond, and Roberts (1982). Gray (1991) discussed involvement in five projects. She reported that not all implementation projects were completed due to changes in hospital management, philosophy, or direction. Gray's initial work was at a 132-bed acute care, not-for-profit children's hospital. Other projects varied from a 100-bed proprietary hospital to a 248-bed nonprofit, community-owned hospital. The main focus of the implementation projects was to improve patient care through quality nursing care plans and in some cases to develop performance standards. Two implementation projects in Colombia were reported on by Moreno (2007). One project was in an ambulatory rehabilitation service (Moreno, 2001) and the other a pediatric intensive care unit of a cardiology institute (Monroy et al., 2003). As hospitals in the United States work toward certification of Magnet Status, more nursing groups are requesting information about application of the Roy Adaptation Model in institutional health care settings.

Theoretical Basis for Practice Exemplar

Within a general understanding of the Roy Adaptation Model for practice, a specific practice exemplar is presented. As theoretical background for discussion of this exemplar, the group identity mode is discussed in greater detail. It reflects how people in groups perceive themselves based on environmental feedback about the group. Persons in a group have perceptions about their shared relations, goals, and values. The social milieu and the culture provide feedback for the group. "Milieu" is another word for environment, while "social" relates to human societies, therefore "social milieu" refers to the human-made environment of the group in which the group is embedded. The economic, political, religious, family, and other structures are included. Each structure has established beliefs. Social culture is a specific part of the milieu or environment of the group. Ethnicity and socioeconomic status in particular make up the social culture. The belief systems of the milieu and social culture are particularly significant for a group. They act as stimuli for the group, which affects other groups with which the group interacts. The group self-image and shared responsibility for goal achievement is central to group identity. Identity integrity is the basic need underlying the group identity mode. Identity integrity implies the honesty, soundness, and completeness of the group members' identification with the group at large. As noted, according to the Roy Adaptation Model, groups have basic life processes in each adaptive mode. Nursing care uses the understanding of these processes to evaluate the adaptation level and to provide care to promote integrated processes at the highest level of adaptation possible. There may be many basic processes for the shared identity mode. As examples, two processes have been identified and developed to date: the group's shared identity process and family coherence. A significant consideration is the family, which most often is the first group with which a person identifies.

Practice Exemplar

Family coherence is an indicator of positive adaptation and refers to a state of unity or a consistent sequence of thought that connects family members who share group identity, goals, and values (Roy, 2009). This section presents an exemplar case about family coherence involving a Chinese American family (Zhan, 2003).

Introduction to the Practice Exemplar: The Wang Family

The Wang family includes David Wang, his wife Teresa, and their 7-year-old daughter, Vivian. When David moved to a metropolitan area of the United States with his parents at the age of 10, his father was 38 and his mother 35. On their arrival, the parents worked in a local Chinese restaurant. Ten years later, they opened a small Chinese restaurant in the city's Chinatown. David's father retired at the age of 75, and David continued managing the restaurant. After retirement, David's parents regularly participated in activities organized by Chinatown's Council on Aging. They are currently 78 (father) and 75 (mother) years old.

David's extended family includes his uncle, Frank Wang, and his cousin, Lisa Wang, a 32-year-old social worker in a community hospital, Lisa's husband, and their 5-year old son. As David grew up in the family with his parents, they had a *shared self-image* as Chinese immigrants, and a shared *group identity* as the Wang family. The Wang family shares a strong cultural commitment to *filial piety* as a virtue to be cultivated. To the family members, this means to be good to one's parents; to take care of one's parents; to engage in good conduct not just toward the parents, but also outside the home in order to bring a good name to one's parents and ancestors; to perform the duties of one's job well in order to obtain the material means to support the parents; offer sacrifices to the ancestors; and to show love, respect, and support. The term *filial*, meaning "of a child,"

denotes the respect and obedience that a child, primarily a son, should show to his parents, especially to his father. David, along with his family, visits his parents regularly and, if needed, helps with their house chores. David's parents were happy that they were able to keep the family together, see their son graduate from college, marry, and work a decent job. At Chinese New Year, all the Wang family members—Frank Wang, Lisa Wang, David's parents, and his wife and daughter—get together to celebrate. The Wang family visit and help each other regularly throughout the year. Family coherence exists as evidenced by shared group identity, values, relations, and goals of building a good life in the United States.

At the age of 78, David's father suffered a stroke and later died. David's mother, age 75, began to show decline in memory by often repeating herself, being unable to find her way in familiar places, misplacing objects in the house, and becoming easily irritated. Several times, she burned cooking pots and began to confuse the time of day. David thought his mother's loss of memory was a sign of aging. As her condition grew worse, David finally took his mother for a physical examination. She was diagnosed with dementia and referred to a specialist for further evaluation that confirmed her diagnosis. David recognized that his mother was unable to live independently and sold his parents' condominium. He arranged for his mother to come to live with his family in their three-bedroom house where David and his wife could care for her. Lisa Wang, David's cousin, visited them regularly on weekends and helped with house chores. David was glad that he was able to keep the family together despite the passing of his father and cognitive impairment of his mother. David and his wife took on the family caregiver role while trying to keep their respective jobs.

As David's mother's cognitive function deteriorated, David was virtually overwhelmed by caring for his mother while keeping his responsibility of managing the restaurant. As he was the one who provided primary financial support for his family, his wife had to quit a full-time job as an administrative assistant to attend to her mother-in-law's care when David was not available. When David and his wife tried to find someone in the Chinese community who could provide respite care to their mother, they heard some strong negative reactions. Some considered his mother's dementia as "insanity" or "a mental disorder"; some talked about dementia as contagious; some noted his mother's dementia being caused by a bad *Feng Shui*.[1] The perception of dementia triggered a strong negative response from the Chinese community, and as a result, his mother's friends stopped visiting her. One day David received a phone call from his daughter's elementary school. The teacher told David that his daughter Vivian did not come to the school twice last week and her grades were declining. Both David and his wife Teresa were feeling overwhelmed and depressed.

Analysis of the Practice Exemplar

In the case of the Wang family, the focus of nursing practice is on the relational system of the family. The family is addressed as an adaptive system to begin planning nursing care.

Assessment of Behaviors

The nurse first meets with David and Teresa to assess family structure, function, relationships, and consistency. The nurse collects data on members of the Wang family; the division of chores such as housekeeping, shopping, and/or repairs; their employment status; the living arrangement and space allocation for family members; and division of family caregiving responsibilities. The nurse assesses how decisions are made in the family, from small daily decisions to larger, health care–related decisions. The nurse observes that David and his wife show love, respect, and loyalty to David's mother and to each other. Although the mother's needs for care are met, individual needs of both David and his wife Teresa are unmet. As they alternate care for their ill mother, they find it quite challenging to maintain their own jobs and attend to their daughter, Vivian's, elementary schoolwork and her growth needs. An increase in demand for care of David's mother lessens the time the parents have for their daughter. They struggle to find alternatives for family caregiving responsibilities and both feel stressed from time to time. The nurse discovers that the Wang family holds a strong Chinese tradition of *filial piety*, and they feel a moral obligation to take care of their elderly mother. However, a strong stigma attached to dementia in the Chinese community takes an emotional toll on them.

Assessment of Stimuli

The nurse conducts a second level of assessment by meeting with the Wang family, including Frank Wang and his daughter Lisa, to identify influencing factors or stimuli, related to group identity and family coherence. Roy (2009) explained that families are constantly interpreting changes in the reactions of others toward them. Accordingly, the nurse notes that the major stimuli for the Wang family are the demands they face and the problems posed for them to solve. David's mother with dementia requires attendant medical and personal care. Although David Wang and Teresa need to work to support the family, ensure their own health insurance coverage, and pay for the cost of personal care, they find it quite difficult to care for David's mother while maintaining full-time jobs. They are trying to find Chinese-speaking home health aides from

---

[1]*Feng Shui* refers to an ancient Chinese belief in which *Feng*, the force of wind, and *Shui*, the flow of water, are viewed as living energies that flow around one's home and workplace, and that affect one's life and well-being. If *Feng Shui* flows gently and peacefully, it brings happiness and health to one's family. *Feng Shui* can stagnate according to the location, shape, and forms of one's environment. As it occurs, one can be ill, poor, and unfortunate (Beattie, 2000).

Continued

their community, as David's mother has limited English language skills. However, with the strong social stigma toward dementia, it becomes very challenging to find someone from the Chinese community. The Wang family agrees that stigma and reaction from the external social environment are stressors to their family caregiving. The strong negative responses to dementia from groups outside the family have brought shame to the Wang family and isolated David's mother from her ethnic community.

Nursing Diagnosis

After the initial assessment, the nurse arrives at three *tentative* diagnoses. First, the Wang family has shared values and goals based on a strong ethnic heritage related to the group responsibility to maintain values and goals. Second, family conflict exists as the demand of family caregiving for David's mother increases. Third, strong stigma attached to dementia from an out-group in the social milieu (in this case, the Chinese community) creates prejudice against the Wang family and causes some members of the Wang family to feel distressed and ambivalent.

The nurse calls a meeting with the Wang family and again includes David's extended family: Uncle Frank Wang and Lisa Wang. After several attempts to coordinate everyone's schedule, finally the family meeting time is set. At the family meeting, the nurse continues to assess behaviors of shared identity and cohesion in the Wang family. What are common perceptions, feelings, and experiences of caring for the loved one with dementia? What are shared understandings of dementia? What are emotional, cognitive, and motivational responses to family caregiving for the loved one with dementia? The nurse observes the family dynamics, listens to reports from David and his wife, and Lisa and her father. The nurse's focus is on patterns of family behavior.

At this meeting, the nurse learns that David considers family caregiving solely his

responsibility because he is the only son and, according to traditional Chinese culture, has a moral responsibility to care for his mother. The nurse asks each member of the Wang family group to find common orientations by sharing their thinking and feelings. The Wang family reflects on questions that Chinn (2008) posed: Do I know what I do, and do I do what I know? (*Praxis*) Am I expressing of my own will in the context of love and respect for others? (*Empowerment*) Am I fully aware of others and myself, and do I bring such awareness to discussion? (*Awareness*) Do I honor and encourage everyone's opinions, skills, and contributions? (*Cooperation*) and Do I welcome practices that encourage growth and change for others, the group, and myself? (*Evolvement*) (Chinn, 2008, p. 13). David and Teresa openly share their feelings and frustrations. Lisa and her father, Frank Wang, express their willingness to share responsibility and help out.

The nurse helps the Wang family set up short-term goals based on shared cognitive and emotional orientations and common values. They all want to maintain quality of life for their loved one and to share family caregiving responsibilities together with Frank and Lisa Wang. Lisa arranges for two home health aides to alternately provide personal care to David's mother during weekdays and one day on weekends. This arrangement allows David to attend to his management work and his wife to spend more time with their daughter. Lisa also uses her social worker skill to triage family caregiving activity which helps David greatly. Frank Wang helps with some shopping. David's wife spends more time attending to her daughter's schoolwork and personal needs. The Wang family coherence is evident and strengthened.

Goal Setting

After hearing everyone, the nurse knows the Wang family better as individuals and as a group. At the following meeting, the nurse works with the Wang family to set attainable goals. Goals and values determine the actions of the Wang family. Attaining goals requires shared responsibilities and some division of labor. The Wang family values their commitment and caring for their loved one and set a goal to find ways to sustain family coherence while providing quality care arrangement for their loved one.

Setting goals includes (1) working together with home health aides to provide the best care for their loved one; (2) supporting each other through not only shared feelings and thoughts, but also shared responsibilities of family caregiving based on each family member's desire, skill, and availability; (3) communicating with the Chinese community about their perception of dementia and finding ways to demystify dementia. The Wang family decides to have Lisa Wang, a social worker, lead in searching for home health aides; David Wang convenes family meetings as needed; and Frank Wang plans to talk with Chinese community key players. At the end of this meeting, despite stressors they have encountered, the Wang family members, again, feel a sense of unity through compensatory adaptation process.

Intervention

Nursing intervention in the case of the Wang family involves focusing on the stimuli affecting the behavior and managing the stimuli by altering, increasing, or decreasing, removing, or maintaining stimuli as proposed by the Roy Adaptation Model. The nurse (1) assesses the Wang family with respect to shared values, shared goals, shared relations, group identity, and social environment and stimuli; (2) works with the Wang family to write down shared goals, values, and expectations; (3) encourages the family to explore additional resources. The nurse also helps the Wang family use effective coping strategies to strengthen compensatory processes by acknowledging how good the family is at transcending the crisis; by working with the family to identify additional

resources in support of family caregiving; and by reinforcing their shared goals, values, relations, and group identity.

Evaluation

The nurse follows up and evaluates the effectiveness of the nursing intervention in relation to the group's adaptive behaviors in agreement with the stated goals as described by the model. The nurse attends the Wang family's biweekly meetings and learns that Lisa Wang used her social worker network and found appropriate home health aides for David's mother, allowing Teresa more time to attend to Vivian's schoolwork. Vivian has not had an absence from school since the meeting. Frank Wang, an activist in the Chinese community, began to talk with other Chinese about dementia, although there is still a strong stigma attached to the disease. David Wang hired another manager to sustain the restaurant business which brings a stable income to support the family and his mother's personal care and leaves him time to take his mother for clinical appointments. David's mother's old friend stopped and visited her briefly.

A particular factor influencing an adaptation problem in the Wang family is related to strong stigma attached to dementia in the Chinese community. Stigma can be socially pervasive and distort the perceptions of individuals. It can impact how the disease is perceived and conceptualized, how caregiving for persons with dementia is supported, and how dementia diagnosis and services are sought. To reduce stigma in promotion of effective adaptation of individual family caregivers and health care providers, families and the community need to work together toward a better understanding of dementia, its diagnosis, treatment, and care options. Educational and service outreach is the first step to reduce stigmatizing in the Chinese community. Educational materials and services need to be linguistically appropriate and adaptable to Chinese patients and their families. Publishing information on dementia

Continued

Practice Exemplar cont.

and related educational articles in widely circulated Chinese newspapers helps reach out to Chinese families, particularly elderly Chinese immigrants who often read Chinese newspapers as a way to connect them to their culture and people. Bilingual professional staff and linguistically appropriate oral and written instructions on dementia are helpful (Valle, 1998).

When interacting with the Chinese family, or families of other cultures, health care providers need to assess cultural norms and beliefs. These norms determine patterns of interaction with the health and social services system, health care decision-making, the extent to which social support is available to caregivers. In addition, these cultural beliefs and values have implications for the psychosocial experience of family caregivers and the clients. Roy's Group Identity Model provides a useful conceptual framework that guides health care providers for working with families of diverse ethnic backgrounds.

■ Summary

This chapter focused on the Roy Adaptation Model as a foundation for knowledge-based practice. The backgound of the theorist and the historical development of the model were presented briefly. The most recent theoretical developments by Roy were the main focus of the description of the model assumptions and major concepts. The process for theory becoming the basis for developing knowledge for practice was introduced by outlining how to develop middle- and practice-level theory that is tested in research. In particular, the effects of the Roy Adaptation Model on practice were articulated from a general summary of major practice projects and by the use of the self-identity adaptive mode as an example of using theory-based knowledge to provide care for a Chinese family dealing with a parent diagnosed with dementia.

References

Beattie, A (2000). *Using Feng Shui.* Raincoast Book Dist. Ltd.

Boston-Based Adaptation Research in Nursing Society. (1999). *Roy adaptation model-based research: 25 years of contributions to nursing science.* Indianapolis, IN: Centre Nursing Press.

Chinn, P. L. (2008). *Peace and power: Creative leadership for building community* (7th ed.). Sudbury, MA: Jones and Bartlett.

Donaldson, S. K., & Crowley, D. (1978). The discipline of nursing. *Nursing Outlook, 26*, 113–120.

Gray, J. (1991). The Roy Adaptation Model in nursing practice. In C. Roy & H. A. Andrews (Eds.), *The Roy Adaptation Model: The definitive statement* (pp. 429–443). Norwalk, CT: Appleton & Lange.

Helson, H. (1964). *Adaptation level theory.* New York: Harper & Row.

Mastal, M. F., Hammond, H., & Roberts, M. P. (1982). Theory into Hospital Practice: A Pilot Implementation. *The Journal of Nursing Administration, 12*, 9–15.

Monroy, P. (2003). Aproximación a la experiencia de aplicación del Modelo de Callista Roy en la Unidad de cuidado intensivo pediátrico. *Enfermería Hoy, 1*(1), 17–20.

Moreno-Ferguson, M. E. (2001). Rehabilitation ambulatory service in Clínica Puente del Común-Teletón, Chía, Colombia. From Moreno-Ferguson, M. E. (2007). *Application of the Roy Adaptation Model in Latin America: Literature review.* Roy Adaptation Association Conference 2007, Los Angeles, CA.

Moreno-Ferguson, M. E. (2007). *Application of the Roy Adaptation Model in Latin America: Literature review.* Roy Adaptation Association Conference 2007, Los Angeles, CA.

Roy, C. (1970). Adaptation: A conceptual framework for nursing. *Nursing Outlook, 18*, 42–45.

Roy, C. (1984). *Introduction to nursing: An adaptation model* (2nd ed.). Englewood Cliffs, NJ: Prentice-Hall.

Roy, C. (1988a). Altered cognition: An information processing approach. In: P. H. Mitchell, L. C. Hodges, M. Muwaswes, & C. A. Walleck (Eds.), *AANN's neuroscience nursing, phenomenon and practice: Human responses to neurological health problems* (pp. 185–211). Norwalk, CT: Appleton & Lange.

Roy, C. (1988b). Human information processing. In: J. J. Fitzpatrick. R. L. Taunton, & J. Q. Benoliel (Eds.), *Annual review of nursing research* (pp. 237–261). New York: Springer.

Roy, C. (1997). *Knowledge as universal cosmic imperative. Proceedings of nursing knowledge impact conference 1996* (pp. 95–118). Chestnut Hill, MA: Boston College Press.

Roy, C. (2009). T*he Roy adaptation model* (3rd ed.). Upper Saddle River, NJ: Prentice-Hall Health.

Roy, C., & Andrews, H. A. (1991). *The Roy Adaptation Model: The definitive statement.* East Norwalk, CT: Appleton & Lange.

Roy, C., & Andrews, H. A. (1999). *The Roy adaptation model* (2nd ed.). Stamford, CT: Appleton & Lange.

Roy, C., & Jones, D. (Eds.) (2007). *Nursing knowledge development and clinical practice.* New York: Springer.

Roy, C., & Roberts, S. (1981). *Theory construction in nursing: An adaptation model.* Englewood Cliffs, NJ: Prentice-Hall.

Senesac, P. (2003). Implementing the Roy Adaptation Model: From theory to practice. *Roy Adaptation Association Review, 4*(2), 5.

Valle, R. (1998). C*aregiving across cultures: Working with dementing illness and ethnically diverse populations.* Boca Raton, FL: Taylor & Francis.

von Bertalanffy, L. (1968). *General system theory: Foundations, development, applications.* New York: George Braziller

Young, L. B. (1986). *The unfinished universe.* New York: Simon & Schuster.

Zhan, L. (2003). *Asian Americans: Vulnerable population, model intervention, and clarifying agendas.* Sudbury, MA: Jones and Bartlett.

Chapter 12

Betty Neuman's Systems Model

PATRICIA DEAL AYLWARD

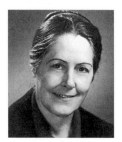

Betty Neuman

Introducing the Theorist

Betty Neuman developed the Neuman Systems Model (NSM) in 1970 to "provide unity, or a focal point, for student learning" (Neuman, 2002b, p. 327) at the School of Nursing, University of California at Los Angeles (UCLA). Neuman recognized the need for educators and practitioners to have a framework to view nursing comprehensively within various contexts. Although she developed the model strictly as a teaching aid, it is now used globally as a nursing conceptual model and as a guide for clinical practice in the full array of health care disciplines.

Betty Neuman's autobiography is presented in her latest book edition (Neuman, 2002b). Neuman was born in southeastern Ohio on a 100-acre family farm on September 11, 1924. Her father died at age 37 when she was 11, and she, her mother, and two brothers worked hard to keep the farm.

Neuman idealized nursing because her father had praised nurses during his 6 years of intermittent hospitalizations. In gratitude, she developed a strong commitment to become an excellent bedside nurse. She also attributed her decisions about her life's work to the very important influence of her mother's charity experiences as a self-taught rural midwife.

Betty Neuman graduated from high school soon after the onset of World War II. Although she had dreamed of attending nearby Marietta College, she lacked the financial means, and instead became an aircraft instrument repair technician. After the Cadet Nurse Corps Program became available, she entered the 3-year diploma nurse program at People Hospital, Akron, Ohio (currently General Hospital Medical Center).

During her career, Neuman worked in a variety of nursing positions including communicable disease nurse, school nurse, industrial nurse, and private duty nurse, developing a broad base of knowledge and skills in critical care. Later she worked as an office nurse in her husband's obstetrical practice.

She completed her baccalaureate degree in nursing and master's degree, with a major in public health nursing from UCLA. During her master's program at UCLA, she worked on special education projects, as a relief psychiatric head nurse, and as a volunteer crisis counselor. Because of this experience Neuman became one of the first California Nurse Licensed Clinical Fellows of the American Association of Marriage and Family Therapy.

Neuman became a UCLA faculty member in January 1967, assuming chairmanship of the program from which she had graduated. She expanded the master's program for students in the psychiatric specialty, focusing it on interdisciplinary practice in community mental health.

In 1970, she developed the Neuman Systems Model. The model was first published in the May–June 1972 issue of *Nursing Research*. Since 1980, several important changes have enhanced the model. A nursing process format was designed, and in 1989 Neuman introduced the concepts of the created environment and the spiritual variable. In collaboration with Dr. Audrey Koertvelyessy, Neuman developed a Theory of Client System Stability. She continues to clarify concepts and components of the model.

Neuman completed a doctoral degree in clinical psychology in 1985 from Pacific Western University in Los Angeles and has received honorary doctorates from Neumann College in Aston, Pennsylvania in 1992 and Grand Valley State University in Allendale, Michigan, in 1998. She is an honorary fellow in the American Academy of Nursing.

Neuman has expressed her hope that "through continued nurturance, the Neuman Systems Model will live well into the twenty-first century to benefit nursing, and other health disciplines, at all levels, and across all cultural boundaries" (Neuman, personal communication, August 1, 2008; Neuman, 2002b, p. 331).

Overview of the Neuman Systems Model

The philosophic base of the Neuman Systems Model encompasses wholism, a wellness orientation, client perception and motivation, and a dynamic systems perspective of energy and variable interaction with the environment to mitigate possible harm from internal and external stressors, while caregivers and clients form a partnership relationship to negotiated desired outcome goals for optimal health retention, restoration, and maintenance. This philosophic base pervades all aspects of the model.

—BETTY NEUMAN (2002c, p. 12)

As its name suggests, the Neuman Systems Model is classified as a systems model or a systems category of knowledge. Neuman (1995) defined "system" as a pervasive order that holds together its parts. With this definition in mind, she writes that nursing can be readily conceptualized as a complete whole, with identifiable smaller wholes or parts. The complete whole structure is maintained by interrelationships among identifiable smaller wholes or parts through regulations that evolve out of the dynamics of the open system. In the system there is dynamic energy exchange, moving either toward or away from stability. Energy moves toward negentropy or evolution as a system absorbs energy to increase its organization, complexity, and development when it moves toward a steady or wellness state. An open system of energy exchange is never at rest. The open system tends to move cyclically toward differentiation and elaboration for further growth and survival of the organism. With the dynamic energy exchange, the system can also move away from stability. Energy can move toward extinction (entropy) by gradual disorganization, increasing randomness, and energy dissipation.

The Neuman Systems Model illustrates a client–client system and presents nursing as a discipline concerned primarily with defining appropriate nursing actions in stressor-related situations or in possible reactions of the client–client system. The client and environment may be positively or negatively affected by each other. There is a tendency within any system to maintain a steady state or balance among the various disruptive forces operating within or upon it. Neuman has identified these forces as stressors, and suggests that possible reactions and actual reactions with identifiable signs or symptoms may be mitigated through appropriate early interventions (Neuman, 1995).

Unique Perspectives of the Neuman Systems Model

Neuman (2002c, p. 14) has identified 10 unique perspectives inherent within her model. They describe, define, and connect concepts essential to understanding the conceptual model that is presented in the next section of this chapter.

1. Each individual client or group as a client system is unique; each system is a composite of common known factors or innate characteristics within a normal, given range of response contained within a basic structure.

2. The client as a system is in a dynamic, constant energy exchange with the environment.

3. Many known, unknown, and universal environmental stressors exist. Each differs in its potential for disturbing a client's usual stability level, or normal line of defense. The particular interrelationships of client variables—physiological, psychological, sociocultural, developmental, and spiritual—at any point in time can affect the degree to which a client is protected by the flexible line of defense against possible reaction to a single stressor or a combination of stressors.

4. Each individual client–client system has evolved a normal range of response to the environment that is referred to as a normal line of defense, or usual wellness/ stability state. It represents change over time through coping with diverse stress encounters. The normal line of defense can be used as a standard from which to measure health deviation.

5. When the cushioning, accordion-like effect of the flexible line of defense is no longer capable of protecting the client– client system against an environmental stressor, the stressor breaks through the normal line of defense. The interrelationships of variables—physiological, psychological, sociocultural, developmental, and spiritual—determine the nature and degree of system reaction or possible reaction to the stressor.

6. The client, whether in a state of wellness or illness, is a dynamic composite of the interrelationships of variables— physiological, psychological, sociocultural, developmental, and spiritual. Wellness is on a continuum of available energy to support the system in an optimal state of system stability.

7. Implicit within each client system are internal resistance factors known as lines of resistance, which function to stabilize and return the client to the usual wellness state (normal line of defense) or possibly to a higher level of stability following an environmental stressor reaction.

8. Primary prevention relates to general knowledge that is applied in client assessment and intervention in identification and reduction or mitigation of possible or actual risk factors associated with environmental stressors to prevent possible reaction. The goal of health promotion is included in primary prevention.

9. Secondary prevention relates to symptomatology following a reaction to stressors, appropriate ranking of intervention priorities, and treatment to reduce their noxious effects.

10. Tertiary prevention relates to the adaptive processes taking place as reconstitution begins and maintenance factors move the client back in a circular manner toward primary prevention.

The Conceptual Model

Neuman's original diagram of her model is illustrated in Figure 12-1. The conceptual model was developed to explain the client–client system as an individual person for the discipline of nursing. Neuman chose the term "client" to show respect for collaborative relationships that exist between the client and the caregiver in Neuman's model, as well as the wellness perspective of the model. The model can be applied to an individual, a group, a community, or a social issue and is appropriate for nursing and other health disciplines (Neuman, 1995, 2002c).

The Neuman Systems Model provides a way of looking at the domain of nursing: humans, environment, health, and nursing.

Client–Client System

The client–client system (see Fig. 12-1) consists of the flexible line of defense, the normal line of defense, lines of resistance, and the basic structure energy resources (shown at the core of the concentric circles in Fig. 12-2). Five client variables—physiological, psychological, sociocultural, developmental, and spiritual—occur and are considered simultaneously in each concentric circle that makes up the client–client system (Neuman, 1995, 2002c).

Flexible Line of Defense

Stressors must penetrate the flexible line of defense before they are capable of penetrating the rest of the client system. Neuman described this line of defense as accordionlike in function. The flexible line of defense acts like a protective buffer system to help prevent stressor invasion of the client system and protects the normal line of defense. The client has more protection from stressors when the flexible line expands away from the normal line of defense. The opposite is true when the

flexible line moves closer to the normal line of defense. The effectiveness of the buffer system can be reduced by single or multiple stressors. The flexible line of defense can be rapidly altered over a relatively short time period by states of emergency, or short-term conditions, such as loss of sleep, poor nutrition, or dehydration (Neuman, 1995, 2002c). Consider the latter examples. What are the effects of short-term loss of sleep, poor nutrition, or dehydration on a client's normal state of wellness? Will these situations increase the possibility for stressor penetration? The answer is that the possibility for stressor penetration may be increased. The actual response depends on the accordionlike function previously described, along with the other components of the client system.

Normal Line of Defense

The normal line of defense represents what the client has become over time, or the usual state of wellness. The nurse should determine the client's usual level of wellness in order to recognize a change. The normal line of defense is considered dynamic, because it can expand or contract over time. The usual wellness level or system stability can decrease, remain the same, or improve following treatment of a stressor reaction. The normal line of defense is dynamic because of its ability to become and remain stabilized, with life stressors over time protecting the basic structure and system integrity are protected (Neuman, 1995, 2002c).

Lines of Resistance

Neuman identified the series of concentric broken circles that surround the basic structure as lines of resistance for the client. When the normal line of defense is penetrated by environmental stressors, a degree of reaction, or signs and/or symptoms, will occur. Each line of resistance contains known and unknown internal and external resource factors. These factors support the client's basic structure and the normal line of defense, resulting in protection of system integrity. Examples of the factors that support the

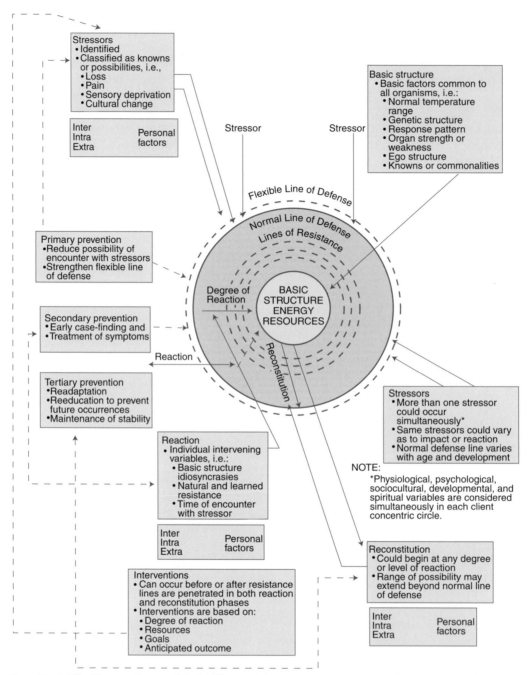

Figure 12 • 1 The Neuman Systems Model. (Original diagram copyright 1970 by Betty Neuman. A holistic view of a dynamic open client–client system interacting with environmental stressors, along with client and caregiver collaborative participation in promoting an optimum state of wellness.) *(From Neuman, 1995, p. 17, with permission.)*

Basic Structure

The basic structure or central core consists of factors that are common to the species. Neuman offered the following examples of basic survival factors: temperature range, genetic structure, response pattern, organ strength or weakness, ego structure, and knowns or commonalities (Neuman, 1995, 2002c).

Five Client Variables

Neuman (1995, p. 28; 2002c, p. 17) identified five variables that are contained in all client systems: physiological, psychological, sociocultural, developmental, and spiritual. These variables are considered simultaneously in each client concentric circle. They are present in varying degrees of development and in a wide range of interactive styles and potential. Neuman offers the following definitions for each variable:

Physiological: Refers to bodily structure and function

Psychological: Refers to mental processes and relationships

Sociocultural: Refers to combined social and cultural functions

Developmental: Refers to life-developmental processes

Spiritual: Refers to spiritual beliefs and influence

Neuman elaborated that the spiritual variable is an innate component of the basic structure. While it may or may not be acknowledged or developed by the client or client system, Neuman views the spiritual variable as being on a continuum of development that penetrates all other client system variables and supports the client's optimal wellness. The client–client system can have a complete lack of awareness of the spiritual variable's presence and potential, deny its presence, or have a conscious and highly developed spiritual understanding that supports the client's optimal wellness.

Neuman explained that the spirit controls the mind, and the mind consciously or unconsciously controls the body. She used an analogy of a seed to clarify this idea.

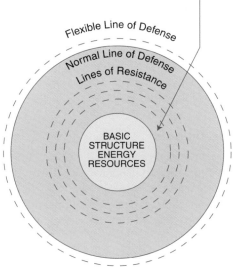

Basic structure
• Basic factors common to all organisms, i.e.:
  • Normal temperature range
  • Genetic structure
  • Response pattern
  • Organ strength or weakness
  • Ego structure
  • Knowns or commonalities

Flexible Line of Defense
Normal Line of Defense
Lines of Resistance

BASIC STRUCTURE ENERGY RESOURCES

NOTE:
Physiological, psychological, sociocultural, developmental, and spiritual variables occur and are considered simultaneously in each client concentric circle.

Figure 12 • 2 Client–client system. The structure of the client-client system, including the five variables that are occurring simultaneously in each client concentric circle. *(From Neuman, 1995, p. 26, with permission.)*

basic structure and normal line of defense include the body's mobilization of white blood cells and activation of the immune system mechanisms. There is a decrease in the signs or symptoms, or a reversal of the reaction to stressors, when the lines of resistance are effective. The system reconstitutes itself and system stability is returned. The level of wellness may be higher or lower than it was before the stressor penetration. When the lines of resistance are ineffective, energy depletion and death may occur (Neuman, 1995, 2002c).

It is assumed that each person is born with a spiritual energy force, or "seed," within the spiritual variable, as identified in the basic structure of the client system. The seed or human spirit with its enormous energy potential lies on a continuum of dormant, unacceptable, or undeveloped to recognition, development, and positive system influence. Traditionally, a seed must have environmental catalysts, such as timing, warmth, moisture, and nutrients, to burst forth with the energy that transforms into a living form that then, in turn, as it becomes further nourished and develops, offers itself as sustenance, generating power as long as its own source of nurture exists. (Neuman, 2002c, p. 16)

The spiritual variable affects or is affected by a condition and interacts with other variables in a positive or negative way. Neuman gave the example of grief or loss (psychological state), which may inactivate, decrease, initiate, or increase spirituality. There can be movement in either direction of a continuum (Neuman, 1995, 2002c). Neuman believes that spiritual variable considerations are necessary for a truly wholistic perspective and for a truly caring concern for the client–client system.

Fulton (1995) has studied the spiritual variable in depth. She elaborated on research studies that extend our understanding of the following aspects of spirituality: spiritual well-being, spiritual needs, spiritual distress, and spiritual care. She suggested that spiritual needs include (1) the need for meaning and purpose in life; (2) the need to receive love and give love; (3) the need for hope and creativity; and (4) the need for forgiving, trusting relationships with self, others, and God or a deity, or a guiding philosophy.

Environment

A second concept identified by Neuman is the environment, as illustrated in Figure 12-3. She defined *environment* broadly as "all internal and external factors or influences surrounding the identified client or client

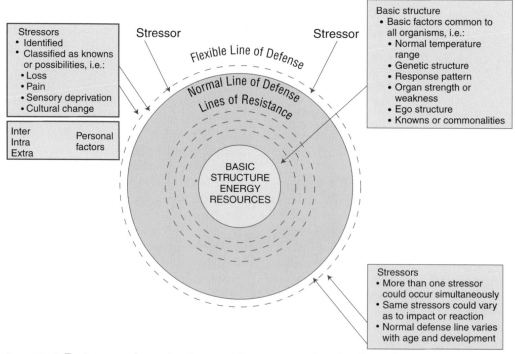

Figure 12 • 3 Environment. Internal and external factors surrounding the client–client system. *(From Neuman, 1995, p. 27, with permission.)*

system" (Neuman, 1995, p. 30; 2002c, p. 18), including:

- Internal environment: Intrapersonal factors
- External environment: Inter- and extrapersonal factors
- Created environment: Intra-, inter-, and extrapersonal factors (Neuman, 1995, p. 31; 2002c, pp. 18–19)

The internal environment consists of all forces or interactive influences contained within the boundaries of the client–client system. Examples of intrapersonal forces are presented for each variable.

- Physiological variable: Autoimmune response, degree of mobility, range of body function.
- Psychological and sociocultural variables: Attitudes, values, expectations, behavior patterns, coping patterns, conditioned responses
- Developmental variable: Age, degree of normalcy, factors related to the present situation
- Spiritual variable: Hope, sustaining forces (Neuman, 1995, 2002c)

The external environment consists of all forces or interactive influences existing outside the client–client system. Interpersonal factors in the environment are forces between people or client systems. These factors include the relationships and resources of family, friends, or caregivers. Extrapersonal factors include education, finances, employment, and other resources (Neuman, 1995, 2002c).

Neuman (1995, 2002c) identified a third environment as the "created environment." The client unconsciously mobilizes all system variables, including the basic structure of energy factors toward system integration, stability, and integrity to create a safe environment. This safe, created environment, offers a protective perceptive coping shield that helps the client to function. A major objective of this environment is to stimulate the client's health. Neuman pointed out that what was originally created to safeguard the health of the system may have a negative effect because of the binding of available energy. This environment represents an open system that exchanges energy with the internal and external environments. The created environment supersedes or goes beyond the internal and external environments while encompassing both; it provides an insulating effect to change the response or possible response of the client to environmental stressors. Neuman (1995, 2002c) gave the following examples of responses: use of denial or envy (psychological), physical rigidity or muscle constraint (physiological), life-cycle continuation of survival patterns (developmental), required social space range (sociocultural), and sustaining hope (spiritual).

Neuman believes the caregiver, through assessment, will need to determine (1) what has been created (nature of the created environment), (2) the outcome of the created environment (extent of its use and client value), and (3) the ideal that has yet to be created (the protection that is needed or possible, to a lesser or greater degree). This assessment is necessary to best understand and support the client's created environment (Neuman, 1995, 2002c). Neuman suggested that further research is needed to understand the client's awareness of the created environment and its relationship to health. Neuman believes that as the caregiver recognizes the value of the client-created environment and purposefully intervenes, the interpersonal relationship can become one of important mutual exchange (Neuman, 1995, 2002c).

Health

Health is a third concept in Neuman's model. She believes that health, or wellness, and illness are on opposite ends of the continuum. *Health* is equated with optimal system stability (the best possible wellness state at any given time). Client movement toward wellness exists when more energy is built and stored than expended. Client movement toward illness and death exists when more energy is needed than is available to support life. The degree of wellness depends on the amount of energy required to return to and maintain system stability. The system is stable when more energy is available than is being used. Health is seen as varying levels within a normal range, rising and falling throughout the lifespan. These changes are in response to basic structure factors and reflect satisfactory or unsatisfactory adjustment by the client system to environmental stressors (Neuman, 1995, 2002c).

Nursing

Nursing is a fourth concept in Neuman's model and is depicted in Figure 12-4. Nursing's major concern is to keep the client system stable by (1) accurately assessing the effects and possible effects of environmental stressors and (2) assisting client adjustments required for optimal wellness. Nursing actions, which are called prevention as intervention, are initiated to keep the system stable. Neuman created a typology for her prevention as intervention nursing actions that includes primary prevention as intervention, secondary prevention as intervention, and tertiary prevention as intervention. All of

these actions are initiated to best retain, attain, and maintain optimal client health or wellness. Neuman (1995, 2002c) believes the nurse creates a linkage among the client, the environment, health, and nursing in the process of keeping the system stable.

Prevention as Intervention

The nurse collaborates with the client to establish relevant goals. These goals are derived only after validating with the client and synthesizing comprehensive client data and relevant theory to determine an appropriate nursing diagnostic statement. With the nursing diagnostic statement and goals in mind, appropriate interventions can be planned and implemented (Neuman, 1995, 2002c).

Primary prevention as intervention involves the nurse's actions that promote client wellness by stress prevention and reduction of risk factors. These interventions can begin at any point a stressor is suspected or identified, before a reaction has occurred. They protect

Primary prevention
• Reduce possibility of encounter with stressors
• Strengthen flexible line of defense

Secondary prevention
• Early case-finding and
• Treatment of symptoms

Tertiary prevention
• Readaptation
• Reeducation to prevent future occurrences
• Maintenance of stability

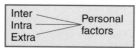

Interventions
• Can occur before or after resistance lines are penetrated in both reaction and reconstitution phases
• Interventions are based on:
   • Degree of reaction
   • Resources
   • Goals
   • Anticipated outcome

Figure 12 • 4 Nursing. Accurately assessing the effects and possible effects of environmental stressors (inter-, intra-, and extrapersonal factors) and using appropriate prevention by interventions to assist with client adjustments for an optimal level of wellness. *(From Neuman, 1995, p. 29, with permission.)*

the normal line of defense by reducing the possibility of an encounter with a stressor and strengthen the flexible lines of defense. Health promotion is a significant intervention. The goal of primary prevention as intervention is to *"retain"* optimal stability or wellness. Ideally, the nurse should consider primary prevention along with secondary and tertiary preventions as interventions when actual client problems exist.

Once a reaction from a stressor occurs, the nurse can use secondary prevention as intervention to treat the symptoms within the nurse's scope of practice, reduce the degree of reaction to the stressors, and protect the basic structure by strengthening the lines of resistance. The goal of secondary prevention as intervention is to "attain" optimal client system stability or wellness and energy conservation. The nurse uses as much of the client's existing internal and external resources (lines of resistance) as possible to stabilize the system.

Reconstitution represents the return and maintenance of system stability following nursing intervention for stressor reaction. The state of wellness may be higher, the same, or lower than the state of wellness before the system was stabilized. Death occurs when secondary prevention as intervention fails to protect the basic structure and thus fails to reconstitute the client (Neuman, 1995, 2002c).

Tertiary prevention as intervention can begin at any point in the client's reconstitution. This includes interventions that promote (1) readaptation, (2) reeducation to prevent further occurrences, and (3) maintenance of stability. These actions are designed to "maintain" an optimal wellness level by supporting existing strengths and conserving client system energy. Tertiary prevention tends to lead back toward primary prevention in a circular fashion. Neuman pointed out that one or all three of these prevention modalities give direction to or may be used simultaneously for nursing actions with possible synergistic benefits (Neuman, 1995, 2002). These interventions may be planned and carried out at the same time.

Nursing Tools for Model Implementation

Neuman designed the Neuman Systems Model Nursing Process format and the Neuman Systems Model Assessment and Intervention Tool: Client Assessment and Nursing Diagnosis to facilitate implementation of the Neuman model. These tools are presented in the fourth edition of *The Neuman Systems Model* (Neuman, 2002a, pp. 347–359).

The Neuman Systems Model Nursing Process format reflects a process that guides information processing and goal-directed activities. Neuman uses the nursing process within three categories: nursing diagnosis, nursing goals, and nursing outcomes. In 1982, the Neuman nursing process format was validated by doctoral students. The format's validity and social utility have been supported in a wide variety of nursing education and practice areas.

The Neuman Systems Model Assessment and Intervention Tool

Client Assessment and Nursing Diagnosis is used to guide the nursing process. The nurse collects wholistic comprehensive data to determine the impact or possible impact of environmental stressors on the client system, then validates the data with the client before formulating a nursing diagnosis. Selected nursing diagnoses are prioritized and related to relevant knowledge. Nursing goals are determined mutually with the caregiver–client–client system, along with mutually agreed on prevention as intervention strategies. Mutually agreed on goals and interventions are consistent with current mandates within the health care system for client rights related to health care issues.

The Client Assessment and Nursing Diagnosis tool with primary, secondary, and tertiary prevention as intervention was developed to convey appropriate nursing actions with each typology of prevention. There are clear instructions for writing appropriate nursing actions (Neuman, 2002a, p. 354), which students are encouraged to review before writing these nursing actions. Keep in mind that the nature of stressors and their threat to the client–client system are first determined for each type of prevention before any other nursing actions are initiated. The same stressors could produce variable impacts or reactions. Nursing outcomes are determined by the accomplishment of the interventions and evaluation of goals after intervention.

Applications

Because the model is flexible and adaptable to a wide range of groups and situations, people have used it globally for more than three decades. Neuman's first book, *The Neuman Systems Model: Application to Nursing Education and Practice,* was published in 1982 as a response to requests for data and support in applying the model. The fourth edition was published in 2002 to clearly reflect the broad, cross-cultural applications of the Neuman Systems Model and is used as a primary resource for global applications highlighted in this chapter (Neuman & Fawcett, 2002).

Application of the Neuman Systems Model to Nursing Practice

"The function of a conceptual model in nursing practice is to provide a distinctive frame of reference that guides approaches to patient care" (Amaya, 2002, p. 43). There is a critical need for meaningful definitions and conceptual frames of reference for nursing practice if the profession is to be established as a science (Neuman, 2002c). "Nurses who conduct their practice from a nursing theory base, while assisting individuals and families to meet their health needs are more likely to provide comprehensive, individualized care that exemplifies best practices" (Ume-Nwangbo, DeWan, & Lowry, 2006, p. 31).

Amaya (2002) asserted that the value of the Neuman Systems Model is supported by the substantial body of literature related to its applications that has emerged since its inception. She conducted an integrative review of literature addressing application of the model to clinical practice, including practice applications of Neuman variables and intra-, inter-, and extrapersonal stressors, and identified 115 publications with practice-related titles through May 2000. An additional 12 articles have been published to date. These numbers do not include doctoral dissertations and master's theses.

The Neuman Systems Model is being used in diverse practice settings. The model is used in critical care nursing, psychiatric mental health nursing, gerontological nursing, perinatal nursing, community nursing, occupational health nursing, rehabilitation, and advanced nursing practice (Amaya, 2002; Bueno & Sengin, 1995; Chiverton & Flannery, 1995; McGee, 1995; Peirce & Fulmer, 1995; Russell, Hileman, & Grant, 1995; Stuart & Wright, 1995; Trepanier, Dunn, & Sprague, 1995; Ware & Shannahan, 1995).

In the United States, the model is used to guide practice with clients with acute and chronic health care problems (e.g., hypertension, chronic obstructive pulmonary disease, renal disease, cardiac surgery, cognitive impairment, mental illness, multiple sclerosis, pain, grief, pediatric cancers, perinatal stressors); meet family needs of clients in critical care; provide stable support groups for parents with infants in neonatal intensive care units; and meet the needs of home caregivers, with emphasis on clients with cancer, HIV/AIDS, and head traumas.

Internationally, the model is being used in Canada, the United Kingdom, Sweden, the Netherlands, New Zealand, Australia, Jordan, Israel, Slovenia, Japan, Korea, and Taiwan (Betty Neuman, personal communication, January 10, 1999; Crawford & Tarko 2002; Beddome, 1995; Beynon, 1995; Craig, 1995a; Damant, 1995; Davies & Proctor, 1995; Engberg, Bjalming, & Bertilson, 1995; Felix, Hinds, Wolfe, & Martin, 1995; Vaughan & Gough, 1995; Verberk, 1995).

Practice Exemplar

A nurse guided by the Neuman Systems Model met Gloria Washington while providing care for her mother in Gloria's home. Gloria's 74-year-old mother has Alzheimer's disease and Gloria has been her caregiver for 4 years. The nurse was aware that, according to Neuman, the family client system includes Gloria and her mother. This nurse uses practice-based research to guide her work (best practice). She recently read Jones-Cannon and Davis's (2005) research study that examined the coping strategies of African American daughters who have functioned as caregivers. In their study, African American caregivers of a family member with dementia or a stroke believed that attending support groups and knowing that their parent needed them influenced their caregiving experience positively. Most caregivers identified that religion gave them a strong tolerance for the caregiving situation and served to mediate strain. Caregivers who voiced a lack of support from family, especially siblings, had much anger and resentment.

The nurse used this new knowledge to enhance the nursing process with Gloria. Through using the Neuman Systems Model Assessment and Intervention Tool she learned that Gloria is a 52-year-old divorced African American woman who is employed full-time by a company for which she enjoys working. She also has a teenage daughter who lives with her, and a grown son who lives away from home. Gloria attends the Baptist church in her neighborhood 2 or 3 times a week, and attributes this experience to her ability to care for her mother.

The nurse assessed for stressors as they were perceived by Gloria and by herself. The nurse assessed for discrepancies between their perceptions and found none. She identified the intrapersonal, interpersonal, and extrapersonal factors that made up Gloria's environment. To ensure the assessment was wholistic and comprehensive she identified the physiological, psychological, sociocultural, developmental, and spiritual variables for

each of these factors. Gloria identified caring for her mother with Alzheimer's disease as her major stressor.

Assessment

The nurse's assessment of Gloria's environmental factors is identified below. Examples of assessment data for each variable are included.

Intrapersonal factors

Physiological: Gloria experiences occasional signs and symptoms of increased anxiety such as rapid heart rate and increased blood pressure.

Psychological: Gloria occasionally worries about the future, but she tries to focus on the present and prides herself on her sense of humor.

Sociocultural: Gloria values her belief that African American families take care of their elderly.

Developmental: Gloria is in Erickson's (1959) developmental stage of middle adulthood with its crisis of generativity versus stagnation. She strives to look outside of herself to care for others.

Spiritual: Gloria reports that religion, faith, and prayer help her cope with caregiving demands.

Interpersonal factors

Physiological: Gloria occasionally has interrupted sleep when her mother awakens and wanders during the night.

Psychological: Gloria reminds herself when physically caring for her mother that this is an expected part of her mother's aging.

Sociocultural: Gloria is the full-time caregiver of her mother who has Alzheimer's disease. She works full-time with supportive people, but does not attend an Alzheimer's support group because she didn't know anything about them.

Developmental: Gloria has significant relationships with her co-workers.

Spiritual: Gloria is supported by her pastor and friends at church.

Continued

Practice Exemplar cont.

Extrapersonal factors

Physiological: Gloria received the gift of a comfortable bed mattress from a co-worker that promotes her sleep.

Psychological: Gloria shared that reading her Bible helps her think positive thoughts.

Sociocultural: Gloria earns $35,000/year.

Developmental: Gloria can feel "in charge of the situation" with a comfortable house for her mom.

Spiritual: Gloria attends church services in her neighborhood 2 to 3 times per week

The nurse applied the Neuman Systems Model nursing process format focusing on: (1) nursing diagnosis (based on valid database), (2) nursing goals negotiated with the client including appropriate levels of prevention as interventions, and (3) nursing outcomes.

The nurse prepared a comprehensive list of nursing diagnoses based on her wholistic and comprehensive assessment and then prioritized the list. She validated her findings with Gloria to ensure that their perceptions were in agreement.

The nurse and Gloria identified Gloria's full-time role as a caregiver for her mother with Alzheimer's disease as a significant stressor. The nurse considered the research study by Jones-Cannon and Davis (2005) that reported that caregivers of a family member with dementia believed attendance at a support group influenced their caregiving in a positive way. One of the nursing diagnoses they determined was *"risk for* caregiver role strain." While this was identified as a risk, they both agreed there was not a supporting sign or symptom to validate the existence of caregiver role strain at this time. However, it was very important to prevent this strain in the future.

The nurse recognized that their observations provided a glimpse of Gloria's normal line of defense, then they identified an immediate goal to strengthen her flexible line of defense.

The goal is that Gloria will report that she has participated in a monthly Alzheimer support group session by (date). They could have identified intermediate and future goals at that time. Together they planned nursing actions for primary prevention as intervention.

The nurse also used the tool and nursing process to provide wholistic comprehensive care for Gloria's mother, and the family client system was strengthened. By strengthening Gloria's lines of defense, the nurse helped strengthen Gloria's mother's lines of defense. The model is dynamic as the individual and family client systems are assessed continuously, leading to new diagnoses, goals, and interventions that promote optimal wholistic comprehensive nursing care. The desired outcome goal for Gloria in the case example was optimal health retention.

If this had been an actual problem of "caregiver role strain," they would have identified secondary prevention as interventions and tertiary prevention as interventions that would activate resource factors (lines of resistance) to protect Gloria's basic structure (organ strength or ability to cope). An example of each follows.

Secondary prevention as intervention: Assist Gloria to schedule respite care for a determined period of time

Tertiary prevention as intervention: Provide ongoing education at each visit about practical resources that will provide caregiver support.

The nurse would have continued to use the nursing process by implementing and evaluating their plan; reassessing, as part of evaluation, for a reduction or elimination of caregiver role strain; and maintenance of system stability. Neuman refers to this as "reconstitution."

Reconstitution represents the return and maintenance of system stability, following treatment of a stressor reaction, which may result in a higher or lower level of wellness than previously. It represents successful mobilization of energy resources (Neuman, 2002c, p. 324).

The desired outcome goals are for optimal health retention, restoration, and maintenance. In Neuman's model high importance is placed on validating nurse and client perceptions, validating data, in Neuman's model.

Application of the Neuman Systems Model to Nursing Education

Lowry (2002) discussed the history of the Neuman Systems Model implementation in educational programs using the model. The acceptance and use of the Neuman Systems Model accelerated in the mid-1970s in the United States when the National League for Nursing (NLN) mandated the use of a conceptual model for the nursing curriculum. Other schools of nursing adapted the model, including schools in Canada and San Juan, Puerto Rico. Over the next 10 years other schools followed in Scandinavian countries, England, Australia, Holland, Kuwait, Taiwan, and Thailand. The NLN eliminated their requirement for a specific conceptual framework for curriculum development in the early 1990s. Some faculties have adapted eclectic frameworks that retain some of the model's concepts.

In the United States, practical nursing, associate degree, diploma, baccalaureate, and graduate and multilevel nursing programs have chosen to use the Neuman Systems Model as a curriculum framework or for selected courses. Schools chose the Neuman model for the model's consistency with the school's philosophy related to the metaparadigm concepts of humans, environment, health, and nursing.

Lowry (2002) conducted a study to determine the current use of the model. Thirty-four programs in the United States and two programs in other countries responded. The following schools returned a survey and continue to use the model: Athens Area Technical College, Athens, GA, California State University, Fresno, CA; Cecil Community College, North East, MD; Central Florida Community College, Ocala, FL; Douglas College, Vancouver, British Columbia, Canada; Dutch Reformed College for Higher Education in the Netherlands; Gulf Coast Community College, Panama City, FL; Fitchburg State College, Fitchburg, MA; Holy Name College, Oakland, CA; Indiana University—Purdue University, Ft. Wayne, IN; Lander University, Greenwood, SC; Loma Linda University, Loma Linda, CA; Los Angeles County Medical Center, Los Angeles, CA; Louisiana College, Pineville, LA; Mansfield College, Mansfield, PA; Milligan College, Milligan, TN; Minnesota Intercollegiate Consortium, St. Olaf, MN; Neumann College, Aston, PA; Santa Fe Community College, Gainesville, FL; Seattle Pacific College, WA; Southern Adventist University, Collegedale, TN; St. Anselm's College, Manchester, NH; Texas Woman's University, Houston, TX; University of Nevada, Las Vegas, NV; and the University of Tennessee, Martin, TN.

Additional nursing programs have been identified in the literature as users of the model. Practical nursing programs using the model include Gulf Coast Community College, Panama City, FL; and Santa Fe Community College, Gainesville, FL. Other associate degree nursing programs that have used the model include Los Angeles Valley College, Van Nuys, California; and Yakima Valley Community College, Yakima, Washington (Glazebrook, 1995; Hilton & Grafton, 1995; Klotz, 1995; Lowry, 2002; Lowry & Newsome, 1995; Stittich, Flores, & Nuttall, 1995; Strickland-Seng, 1995).

Educational programs in the United States reported benefits with using the model. The model (1) facilitated cultural considerations in the curriculum related to the populations the schools and graduates served (Stittich, Flores, & Nuttall, 1995); (2) provided a nursing focus as opposed to medical focus (Lowry & Newsome, 1995); (3) included the concept of clients as holistic beings (Lowry & Newsome, 1995); (4) allowed flexibility in arrangement of content and conceptualization of program needs (Lowry & Newsome, 1995); (5) was comprehensive and facilitated seeing the person as composites of the five variables; (6) provided a framework to study individual illness and reaction to stressors; (7) was broad enough to allow educational programs to consider family as the context within which individuals live or as the unit of care; (8) was a guide for comprehensive nursing practice with individuals, families, and groups (Cammuso & Wallen, 2002); and (9) considered the created environment.

Education programs have developed evaluation instruments to determine the effects of using the model as a framework for nursing knowledge. The curriculum evaluation instrument cited in the literature is the Lowry–Jopp Neuman Model Evaluation Instrument, which was developed to examine the efficacy of using the model at Cecil Community College (Lowry & Newsome, 1995). The results of a 5-year longitudinal study showed that the graduates used the model most of the time when fulfilling roles of care provider and teacher. All classes in the study claimed colleagues rarely knew, accepted, or encouraged model use. Therefore, colleagues in work settings tended to have a negative effect on the use of models.

International educational programs have used the model. Craig (1995b) reported on the experiences of 10 educational institutions in Canada in six Canadian provinces: the University of Saskatchewan, University of Prince Edward Island, University of Calgary, Brandon University of New Brunswick, Université de Moncton, University of Western Ontario, University of Windsor, Okanagan College, University of Toronto, and University of Ottawa. Reported model strengths included the holistic approach, which addressed levels of prevention that guided the student to focus on the client in his or her own environment. The model also assisted students to perform in-depth assessments, to categorize comprehensive data, and to plan specific interventions with the client. Students reported some difficulty in understanding the complexity of the model and the developmental and spiritual variables. In addition, they noted that it was not always easy to differentiate between the lines of defense and resistance or to assess the degree of stressor penetration. The Neuman Model is also being used in educational institutions in Holland, South Australia, the United Kingdom, Sweden, and Turkey (Eileen Gigliotti, personal communication,

July 25, 2008; de Kuiper, 2002; Engberg, 1995; McCulloch, 1995; Vaughan & Gough, 1995).

De Kuiper (2002) described the use of the Neuman Systems Model at the Dutch Reformed University in Holland. A new curriculum was needed that would combine a clear philosophy of nursing and a clear statement about the Christian identity of the school. After serious study, the Neuman Systems Model was selected. In Holland the 19 schools of nursing are rated numerically based on quality of education. Before the introduction of the model, the university fell in 12th place. After implementation, the university topped the list for 3 consecutive years. McCulloch (1995) reported that a survey of all Australian university programs showed that 4 undergraduate programs used the model as the major organizational curriculum framework, and another 16 programs introduced undergraduate and postgraduate students to the Neuman Model as one of several models.

Vaughan and Gough (1995) found that many nursing and midwifery students chose to use the model in their own practice in the United Kingdom. They also reported that Avon and Gloucestershire College of Health used the model as the guiding principle behind curriculum development for child care.

Engberg (1995) reported on colleges in Sweden. Most colleges throughout Sweden use the Neuman Systems Model as the theoretical framework in the module of primary health in nursing education.

Nursing Administration and the Neuman Systems Model

The Neuman Systems Model has been used to guide nursing administration in the United States. These settings include an interdisciplinary collaborative team across nine agencies, adult and children's hospitals; a community nursing center, a psychiatric hospital, a continuing care retirement community, and Oklahoma State Public Health Nursing (Frioux,

Roberts, & Butler, 1995; Lowry, Burns, Smith, & Jacobson, 2000; Rodriguez, 1995; Sanders & Kelley, 2002; Scicchitani, Cox, Heyduk, Maglicco, & Sargent, 1995; Torakis, 2002; Walker, 1995).

Sanders and Kelley (2002) acknowledge the changes in administrative practice and the work environment to an integrated health care system in a managed care market, along with changes in expectations for health professionals. They maintain that the primary role of the nurse administrator is to maintain system integrity by realigning the nursing or organizational system to its internal and external environments. Sanders and Kelley believe that problems and issues identified in this complex system require multidimensional, comprehensive, and collaborative interventions to maintain, restore, or revive the health of complex systems. An integrated framework with a more comprehensive approach to assessing and resolving problems in nursing administration and to evaluate the total system's response to stressors should be used by nurse administrators.

Sanders and Kelley (2002) conducted an integrative review of the literature regarding the Neuman Systems Model and administration of nursing. As part of the review they looked at published reports of administrative research. They found studies on examination of the effects of environmental stressors on autonomy, stress, and burnout of staff nurses; and the effect of an educational program on nurses' attitudes.

Lowry, Burns, Smith, and Jacobson (2000) reported on a demonstration project in one south Florida county designed to develop interdisciplinary collaborative teams for delivery of health care across a continuum of nine agencies, settings, and a hospital that serves a predominately rural population that included farm workers and used the Neuman Systems Model as the clinical practice model.

Hinton-Walker (1995) identified three categories of roles the nurse administrator must assume and be able to make shifts in focus: patient/client as consumer, organization as consumer, and employee/staff as consumer. She included a blending of the concepts and principles for total quality management and continuous quality improvement to strengthen the collaboration between the health care provider and the client system toward achieving mutual goals. Her work shows that a nursing framework is effective in guiding an interdisciplinary approach to preparing nursing and health care administrators.

Poole and Flowers (1995) reported on care management. They demonstrated how the Neuman Systems Model is used in case management of pregnant substance abusers. Kelley and Sanders (1995) used an assessment tool that intertwined the management process, the Neuman Systems Model, and environmental dimensions.

The Neuman Systems Model has been used in diverse nursing administration settings in other countries. Sanders and Kelley (2002) reported that these settings included public health in Canada and Wales, primary health care in Sweden, and psychiatric nursing in the Netherlands. De Munck and Merks (2002) reported that the Neuman Systems Model is being used to guide the administration of nursing services at Emergis, Institute for Mental Health Care in Holland and described the way in which it is being used.

Value for the Future

Neuman and Reed (2007) dialogued about projected applications of the Neuman Systems Model in the year 2050. "The value of the model is its wholistic perspective, which is timeless and expansive in being adaptable to all client care situations" (p. 112). Neuman speculated that the ideal nurse role will be one of coordinating client health care toward optimal wellness within an identified interactive client system. Greater emphasis on in-depth assessment of client needs for appropriate interventions will be required. An organizing framework is imperative to categorize and highlight gaps in knowledge, and to maintain continuity of care over multiple venues and disciplines due to the increase in the amount of available data. With the increased technical aspects of care, special consideration needs to be given to client intra- and interpersonal needs to offset possible depersonalization. Evidence-based practice and middle-range theory development will increase. With the identification of best practices there will be a need for a comprehensive description of practice that allows for critique and interpretation of evidence. According to Neuman and Reed, "a great need exists for unification, integration, and validation of client healthcare processes on a continuing basis into the future for wholistic care" (p. 113).

Networking to Enhance Applications of the Model

There are opportunities to network with others using the model in a variety of applications and settings. One way is to attend a Neuman Systems Model International Symposium, which is held every 2 years. International scholars gather to share ideas, insights, innovations, practice, and research from the model. The Neuman Systems Model Web site provides the latest information: http://neumansystemsmodel.org/.

The Neuman Archives were established to preserve and protect the work of Betty Neuman and others working with the model. The archives are located at Neumann College, Aston, Pennsylvania, and can be accessed through contacts by telephone (610-361-5206; 610-558-5545) or e-mail (CARRM@neumann.edu).

■ Summary

The Neuman Systems Model has been used for more than three decades, first as a teaching tool and later as a conceptual model to observe and interpret the phenomena of nursing and health care globally. The model is well accepted by the nursing profession. "The concept of client wholeness, the goal of optimal health and utilization of primary prevention strategies to maintain wellness, and popular thinking in the lay literature all catapulted the Neuman systems model into acceptance by the nursing profession. These same values are very much alive in today's world. If anything, there is more emphasis on wholistic health and wholistic nursing today than there was 37 years ago" (Neuman & Reed, 2007, p. 111). Additional citations compiled by Fawcett (2002, pp. 364–400) may be helpful to the reader.

References

Amaya, M. A. (2002). The Neuman Systems Model and clinical practice: An integrative review 1974–2000. In: B. Neuman & J. Fawcett, *The Neuman Systems Model* (4th ed., pp. 216–243). Upper Saddle River, NJ: Prentice-Hall.

Beddome, G. (1995). Community-as-client assessment. A Neuman-based guide for education and practice. In: B. Neuman, *The Neuman Systems Model* (3rd ed., pp. 567–579). Norwalk, CT: Appleton & Lange.

Beynon, C. E. (1995). Neuman-based experiences of the Middlesex-London Health Unit. In: B. Neuman, *The Neuman Systems Model* (3rd ed., pp. 537–547). Norwalk, CT: Appleton & Lange.

Breckenridge, D. M. (1995). Nephrology practice and directions for nursing research. In B. Neuman, *The Neuman Systems Model* (3rd ed., pp. 499–507). Norwalk, CT: Appleton & Lange.

Bueno, M. M., & Sengin, K. K. (1995). The Neuman Systems Model for critical care nursing. A framework for practice. In: B. Neuman, *The Neuman Systems Model* (3rd ed., pp. 275–291). Norwalk, CT: Appleton & Lange.

Cammuso, B. S., & Wallen, A. J. (2002). Using the Neuman Systems Model to guide nursing education in the United States. In: B. Neuman & J. Fawcett, *The Neuman Systems Model* (4th ed., pp. 244–253). Upper Saddle River, NJ: Prentice-Hall.

Chiverton, P., & Flannery J. C. (1995). Cognitive impairment. Use of the Neuman Systems Model. In: B. Neuman, *The Neuman Systems Model* (3rd ed., pp. 249–259). Norwalk, CT: Appleton & Lange.

Craig, D. M. (1995a). Community/public health nursing in Canada. Use of the Neuman Systems Model in a new paradigm. In: B. Neuman, *The Neuman Systems Model* (3rd ed., pp. 529–535). Norwalk, CT: Appleton & Lange.

Craig, D. M. (1995b). The Neuman Systems Model Examples of its use in Canadian educational programs. In: B. Neuman, *The Neuman Systems Model* (3rd ed., pp. 521–527). Norwalk, CT: Appleton & Lange.

Crawford, J. A., & Tarko, M. A. (2002). Using the Neuman Systems Model to guide nursing practice in Canada. In: B. Neuman & J. Fawcett, *The Neuman Systems Model* (4th ed., pp. 90–110). Upper Saddle River, NJ: Prentice-Hall.

Damant, M. (1995). Community nursing in the United Kingdom. A case for reconciliation using the Neuman Systems Model. In: B. Neuman, *The Neuman Systems Model* (3rd ed., pp. 607–620). Norwalk, CT: Appleton & Lange.

Davies, P., & Proctor, H. (1995). In Wales: Using the model in community mental health. In B. Neuman, *The Neuman Systems Model* (3rd ed., pp. 621–627). Norwalk, CT: Appleton & Lange.

De Kuiper, M. (2002). Using the Neuman Systems Model to guide nursing education in Holland. In: B. Neuman & J. Fawcett, *The Neuman Systems Model* (4th ed., pp. 254–262). Upper Saddle River, NJ: Prentice-Hall.

De Munck, R., & Merks, A. (2002). Using the Neuman Systems Model to guide administration of nursing services in Holland: The case of Emergis, Institute for Mental Health Care. In: B. Neuman & J. Fawcett, *The Neuman Systems Model* (4th ed., pp. 300–315). Upper Saddle River, NJ: Prentice-Hall.

Engberg, I. B. (1995). Brief abstracts. Use of the Neuman Systems Model in Sweden. In B. Neuman, *The Neuman Systems Model* (3rd ed., pp. 653–656). Norwalk, CT: Appleton & Lange.

Engberg, I. B., Bjalming, E., & Bertilson, B. (1995). A structure for documenting primary health care in Sweden using the Neuman Systems Model. In: B. Neuman, *The Neuman Systems Model* (3rd ed., pp. 637–651). Norwalk, CT: Appleton & Lange.

Erikson, E. H. (1959). *Identity and the life cycle.* New York: International Universities Press.

Fawcett, J. (1995). Constructing conceptual-theoretical-empirical structures for research. Future implications for use of the Neuman Systems Model. In: B. Neuman, *The Neuman Systems Model* (3rd ed., pp. 459–471). Norwalk, CT: Appleton & Lange.

Fawcett, J. (1999). *Relationship of theory and research* (3rd ed.). Philadelphia: F. A. Davis.

Fawcett, J. (2002). Neuman Systems Model bibliography. In: B. Neuman & J. Fawcett, *The Neuman Systems Model* (4th ed., pp. 364–400). Upper Saddle River, NJ: Prentice-Hall.

Fawcett, J., & Giangrande, S. K. (2002). The Neuman Systems Model and research: An integrative review. In: B. Neuman & J. Fawcett, *The Neuman Systems Model* (4th ed., pp. 120–149). Upper Saddle River, NJ: Prentice-Hall.

Felix, M., Hinds, C., Wolfe, C., & Martin, A. (1995). The Neuman Systems Model in a chronic care facility: A Canadian experience. In: B. Neuman, *The Neuman Systems Model* (3rd ed., pp. 549–566). Norwalk, CT: Appleton & Lange.

Frioux, T. D., Roberts, A. G., & Butler, S. J. (1995). Oklahoma State public health nursing. In: B. Neuman, *The Neuman Systems Model* (3rd ed., pp. 407–414). Norwalk, CT: Appleton & Lange.

Fulton, R. A. (1995). The spiritual variable. In: B. Neuman, *The Neuman Systems Model* (3rd ed., pp. 77–91). Norwalk, CT: Appleton & Lange.

Gigliotti, E. (1997). Use of Neuman's lines of defense and resistance in nursing research: Conceptual and empirical considerations. *Nursing Science Quarterly, 10,* 136–143.

Gigliotti, E., & Fawcett, J. (2002). The Neuman Systems Model and research instruments. In: B. Neuman & J. Fawcett, *The Neuman Systems Model* (4th ed., pp. 150–175). Upper Saddle River, NJ: Prentice-Hall.

Glazebrook, R. S. (1995). The Neuman Systems Model in cooperative baccalaureate nursing education: The Minnesota Intercollegiate Nursing Consortium Experience. In: B. Neuman, *The Neuman Systems Model* (3rd ed., pp. 227–230). Norwalk, CT: Appleton & Lange.

Hilton, S. A., & Grafton, M. D. (1995). Curriculum transition based on the Neuman Systems Model. Los Angeles County Medical Center School of Nursing. In: B. Neuman, *The Neuman Systems Model* (3rd ed., pp. 163–174). Norwalk, CT: Appleton & Lange.

Hinton-Walker, P. (1995). TQM and the Neuman Systems Model: Education for health care administration. In: B. Neuman & J. Fawcett, *The Neuman Systems Model* (4th ed., pp. 365–376). Upper Saddle River, NJ: Prentice-Hall.

Jones-Cannon, S., & Davis, B. (2005). Coping among African-American daughters caring for aging parents. *The ABNF Journal*, November-December, 118–123.

Kelley, J. A., & Sanders, N. F. (1995). A systems approach to the health of nursing and health care organizations. In: B. Neuman, *The Neuman Systems Model* (3rd ed., pp. 347–364). Norwalk, CT: Appleton & Lange.

Klotz, L. C. (1995). Integration of the Neuman Systems Model into the BSN curriculum at the University of Texas at Tyler. In: B. Neuman, *The Neuman Systems Model* (3rd ed., pp. 183–195). Norwalk, CT: Appleton & Lange.

Louis, M., Neuman, B., & Fawcett, J. (2002). Guidelines for Neuman Systems Model-based nursing research. In: B. Neuman & J. Fawcett, *The Neuman Systems Model* (4th ed., pp. 113–119). Upper Saddle River, NJ: Prentice-Hall.

Lowry, L. (2002). The Neuman Systems Model and education. An integrative review. In: B. Neuman & J. Fawcett, *The Neuman Systems Model* (4th ed., pp. 216–237). Upper Saddle River, NJ: Prentice-Hall.

Lowry, L. W., Burns, C. M., Smith, A. A., & Jacobson, H. (2000). An interdisciplinary approach to training health professionals. *Nursing and Health Care Perspectives, 21*(2), 76–81.

Lowry, L. W., & Newsome, G. G. (1995). Neuman-based associate degree programs: Past, present, and future. In: B. Neuman, *The Neuman Systems Model* (3rd ed., pp. 197–214). Norwalk, CT: Appleton & Lange.

McCulloch, S. J. (1995). Utilization of the Neuman Systems Model: University of South Australia. In: B. Neuman, *The Neuman Systems Model* (3rd ed., pp. 591–597). Norwalk, CT: Appleton & Lange.

McGee, M. (1995). Implications for use of the Neuman Systems Model in occupational health nursing. In: B. Neuman, *The Neuman Systems Model* (3rd ed., pp. 657–667). Norwalk, CT: Appleton & Lange.

Neuman, B. (1995). *The Neuman Systems Model* (3rd ed.). Norwalk, CT: Appleton & Lange.

Neuman, B. (1996). The Neuman Systems Model in research and practice. *Nursing Science Quarterly, 9,* 67–70.

Neuman, B. (2002a). Assessment and intervention based on the Neuman Systems Model. In B. Neuman & J. Fawcett, *The Neuman Systems Model* (4th ed., pp. 347–359). Upper Saddle River, NJ: Prentice-Hall.

Neuman, B. (2002b). Betty Neuman's autobiography and chronology of the development and utilization of the Neuman Systems Model. In: B. Neuman & J. Fawcett, *The Neuman Systems Model* (4th ed., pp. 325–346). Upper Saddle River, NJ: Prentice-Hall.

Neuman, B. (2002c). The Neuman Systems Model. In: B. Neuman & J. Fawcett, *The Neuman Systems Model* (4th ed., pp. 3–33). Upper Saddle River, NJ: Prentice-Hall.

Neuman, B., & Fawcett, J. (Eds.). (2002). *The Neuman Systems Model.* Upper Saddle River, NJ: Prentice-Hall.

Neuman, B., & Reed, K. S. (2007). A Neuman Systems Model perspective on nursing in 2050. *Nursing Science Quarterly, 20*(2), 111–113.

Peirce, A. G., & Fulmer, T. T. (1995). Application of the Neuman Systems Model to gerontological nursing. In: B. Neuman, *The Neuman Systems Model* (3rd ed., pp. 293–308). Norwalk, CT: Appleton & Lange.

Poole, V. L., & Flowers, J. S. (1995). Care management of pregnant substance abusers using the Neuman Systems Model. In: B. Neuman, *The Neuman*

Systems Model (3rd ed., pp. 377–386). Norwalk, CT: Appleton & Lange.

Rodriguez, M. L. (1995). The Neuman Systems Model adapted to a continuing care retirement community. In: B. Neuman, *The Neuman Systems Model* (3rd ed., pp. 431–442). Norwalk, CT: Appleton & Lange.

Russell, J., Hileman, J. W., & Grant, J. S. (1995). Assessing and meeting the needs of home caregivers using the Neuman Systems Model. In: B. Neuman, *The Neuman Systems Model* (3rd ed., pp. 331–341). Norwalk, CT: Appleton & Lange.

Sanders, N. F., & Kelley, J. A. (2002). The Neuman Systems Model and administrative nursing services: An integrative review. In: B. Neuman & J. Fawcett, *The Neuman Systems Model* (4th ed., pp. 271–287). Upper Saddle River, NJ: Prentice-Hall.

Scicchitani, B., Cox, J. G., Heyduk, L. J., Maglicco, P. A., & Sargent, N. A. (1995). Implementing the Neuman model in a psychiatric hospital. In: B. Neuman, *The Neuman Systems Model* (3rd ed., pp. 387–395). Norwalk, CT: Appleton & Lange.

Smith, M. C., & Edgil, A. E. (1995). Future directions for research with the Neuman Systems Model. In: B. Neuman, *The Neuman Systems Model* (3rd ed., pp. 509–517). Norwalk, CT: Appleton & Lange.

Stittich, E. M., Flores, F. C., & Nuttall, P. (1995). Cultural considerations in a Neuman-based curriculum. In: B. Neuman, *The Neuman Systems Model* (3rd ed., pp. 147–162). Norwalk, CT: Appleton & Lange.

Strickland-Seng, V. (1995). The Neuman Systems Model in clinical evaluation of students. In: B. Neuman, *The Neuman Systems Model* (3rd ed., pp. 215–225). Norwalk, CT: Appleton & Lange.

Stuart, G. W., & Wright, L. K. (1995). Applying the Neuman Systems Model to psychiatric nursing practice. In: B. Neuman, *The Neuman Systems Model* (3rd ed., pp. 263–273). Norwalk, CT: Appleton & Lange.

Torakis, M. L. (2002). Using the Neuman Systems Model to guide administration of nursing services in the United States: Redirecting nursing practice in a freestanding pediatric hospital. In: B. Neuman & J. Fawcett, *The Neuman Systems Model* (4th ed., pp. 288–299). Upper Saddle River, NJ: Prentice-Hall.

Trepanier, M., Dunn, S. I., & Sprague, A. E. (1995). Application of the Neuman Systems Model to perinatal nursing. In: B. Neuman, *The Neuman Systems Model* (3rd ed., pp. 309–320). Norwalk, CT: Appleton & Lange.

Ume-Nwagbo, P. N., DeWan, S. A., & Lowry, L. (2006). Using the Neuman Systems Model for best practices. *Nursing Science Quarterly, 19*(1), 31–35.

Vaughan, B., & Gough, P. (1995). Use of the Neuman Systems Model in England. In: B. Neuman, *The Neuman Systems Model* (3rd ed., pp. 599–605). Norwalk, CT: Appleton & Lange.

Verberk, F. (1995). In Holland: Application of the Neuman model in psychiatric nursing. In: B. Neuman, *The Neuman Systems Model* (3rd ed., pp. 629–636). Norwalk, CT: Appleton & Lange.

Walker, P. H. (1995). Neuman-based education, practice, and research in a community nursing center. In: B. Neuman, *The Neuman Systems Model* (3rd ed., pp. 415–430). Norwalk, CT: Appleton & Lange.

Ware, L. A., & Shannahan, M. K. (1995). Using Neuman for a stable parent support group in neonatal intensive care. In: B. Neuman, *The Neuman Systems Model* (3rd ed., pp. 321–330). Norwalk, CT: Appleton & Lange.

Chapter 13

Helen Erickson, Evelyn Tomlin, and Mary Ann Swain's Theory of Modeling and Role Modeling

HELEN L. ERICKSON

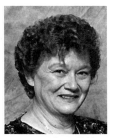

Helen L. Erickson

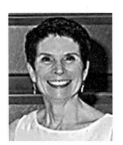

Mary Ann Swain

Introducing the Theorist

My life journey, filled with challenges, opportunities, and choices, has helped me discover the essence of my Self, to understand my Reason for Being, and uncover my Life Purpose (Erickson, H., 2006a). The essence of my Self is reflected in my values and beliefs; my Reason for Being is to learn that unconditional acceptance is a key component of human relationships; and my Life Purpose is to facilitate growth in others. These understandings emerged as I wandered the pathways of my life, sometimes joined with others and sometimes connected only to God. The following paragraphs offer snippets of my journey and an occasional glimpse into my Self and the underlying philosophy of Modeling and Role-Modeling.

Born and raised in a north-central Michigan town with one older brother and two younger sisters, I grew up knowing that family relations are essential. My father worked for the highway department, often spending 12- to 24-hour days building roads during the summer and keeping them open in the winter. During my early years, our mother took care of the family, sewed clothes, and canned food needed to last throughout the cold Michigan winter. Later, she worked part-time as a retail clerk. My sisters and I learned that women can do whatever they choose. Family recreation consisted of evening croquet games, a Sunday afternoon drive, picnics at one of the lakes, berry picking, an occasional movie, family board games, and reading. I learned that family connections, caring about others, positive attitudes, respect for the environment, and hard work are basic essentials of life.

I was 5 when World War II was declared. Although too young to understand the full implications of the war, I learned that it was important to stand up for our beliefs and life principles. I remember sending letters to family members fighting overseas; our family gathering around the radio for the news; rationing; and the sirens that notified us when we needed to go into a blackout. I also remember the evening the siren declared the end of the war. Our family immediately went to town to join the street celebrations. Everyone was excited and hopeful about the future. That evening I knew that nearly anything is possible if we are persistent, our goals have integrity, and we are honest with others and ourselves.

From the time I was a preteen until I graduated from high school, I worked to earn my own money. Some of my jobs included babysitting, keeping house for a family in need, waitressing, and clerking. Each job was an opportunity to learn about myself and each was a step toward nursing school. Although I was one of only four who took advanced math courses, no one suggested that I should go to a college or university. Instead, I enrolled in a nursing diploma program at Saginaw General Hospital.

I loved nursing and knew I had been wise in my choice of life work. I decided to become a missionary after I graduated, perhaps to go to Africa or some place where I might help people! In my junior year I met my future husband and his family. His father, Milton Erickson, well known for his work with hypnosis and mind–body healing, taught me that people know more about themselves than health care providers did, that their inner-knowing is essential to healing, and that we can help them by facilitating them to reveal their own view of the world. My projected life course changed; instead of moving to Africa, I committed to married life, moved to Texas and accepted the position of head nurse in the emergency room of the Midland Memorial Hospital, Midland, Texas. Little did I know that I was on a mission of my own!

For the next 2 years, I worked 6 days a week and often did double shifts, floating to other units in the hospital, working in every unit except the labor room. My appetite for learning seemed insatiable. I learned about blind prejudice, discrimination, and the importance of staying true to one's values and beliefs while negotiating a health care system. I also learned that people have their own stories about their lives, stories that provide insight into their needs and how we can help them.

When we left Texas in 1959 with our first-born daughter, we returned to Michigan and extended family. I worked in a small community hospital and then in a home for the handicapped for 2 years. I learned that people often considered unworthy or inadequate due to liabilities acquired through birth or accident were honest, loving people with integrity often exceeding that of the more fortunate members of society. In 1960, we added one more child to our family, deepening my understanding of human nature and the uniqueness of people.

In 1961, we moved to San German, Puerto Rico, where I worked as a dorm nurse for 3 months. Then, frustrated with the inefficiency of the system, I designed a health care system for Inter-American University (IAU). The president responded positively and named me the director of the IAU Health Care System for students, faculty, and families. In 1963 we enhanced our family with our third child, first son.

We moved to Ann Arbor, Michigan in 1964 so my husband could earn a PhD. I worked as a staff nurse part time for a few months at St. Joseph's Hospital, and then resigned so we could add yet one more member to our family. In 1967, I resumed part-time staff nursing at the University of Michigan Hospital, primarily on medical–surgical units, but sometimes floating to other units, often working extra shifts.

During my years of clinical experience I had developed a practice model that guided my professional activities. Determined to label and articulate what I had learned, to be *true* about human nature and nursing, I entered the University of Michigan's RN-BSN program in 1972. Although I had nearly 16 years of experience, no credit was awarded for past learning. However, we were allowed to earn credit by examination, and clinical practice was acknowledged for experienced nurses. Two years later I had earned a BSN, but realized that this credential did not validate me as an expert. Although I had been recruited to work as a faculty member in the RN-BSN program and to consult at the University Hospital, I knew that I had to continue my education to be able to articulate my ideas further and to validate myself as an expert.

I entered the master's program in nursing at the University of Michigan, enrolling in both the medical–surgical and psychiatric programs in 1974, and graduated in 1976. During this time, affirmed and supported by Evelyn Tomlin, I talked freely about the nursing model I had derived from practice. I also labeled and articulated it, theorized and tested the Adaptive Potential Assessment Model, and worked with Mary Ann Swain testing some of my hypotheses (Erickson & Swain, 1982). I continued my faculty position, advancing to chairman of the undergraduate program and assistant dean. After earning my master's degree, I maintained these roles, while expanding my research activities, consulting, speaking, supervising graduate students, and continuously working to merge theory, practice, and research.

Over the next 10 years, my model of nursing acquired a life of its own. By the early 1980s, I had received several speaking invitations, yet little had been written (Erickson, 1976; Erickson & Swain, 1982). Together Evelyn, Mary Ann, and I further elaborated and articulated some of the concepts. The title Modeling and Role-Modeling (MRM), first coined by Milton Erickson, was selected as the best way to describe this work. The original edition was printed in November, 1982 (Erickson, Tomlin, & Swain, 2009), has had eight reprints, and is now considered a classic by the Society for the Advancement of Modeling and Role-Modeling (SAMRM).

I left Michigan in 1986, spent 2 years at the University of South Carolina School of Nursing as associate dean of academic affairs and then moved to the University of Texas where I assumed the role of professor of nursing and chair of adult health nursing. During my tenure at The University of Texas, I served as vice-chair of the Faculty Senate, assistant dean for graduate affairs in the School of Nursing, chair of Adult Holistic Nursing, conducted research on MRM, taught numerous courses, and chaired several doctoral dissertations. When I retired in 1997, the Helen L. Erickson Endowed Lectureship on Holistic Nursing was established at the University of Texas in Austin.

Since 1997, I have served on the Board of Directors, the American Holistic Nurses Certification Corporation (AHNCC), first as a member and co-chair and then as chair of the board. During this period of time we launched AHNCC, developed two national certification processes—including an examination for certification at the Basic Level and another for certification at the Advanced Level—and an Endorsement Program for schools of nursing that offer curricula in holistic nursing. I have authored or co-authored various chapters on MRM and/or holistic nursing (Clayton & Erickson, 2006; Erickson, 1996, 2002, 2006b–e, 2007, 2008; Erickson, Erickson, & Jensen, 2006; Walker & Erickson, 2006), some of which are included in the second book on Modeling and Role-Modeling. I anticipate continued involvement in the movement of holistic nursing, recently recognized by ANA as a nursing specialty.

Overview of Modeling and Role-Modeling Theory

Modeling and Role-Modeling (MRM) is based in several nursing principles that guide the assessment, intervention, and evaluation aspects of professional nursing. These principles are reflected in the data collection categories (Erickson, Tomlin, & Swain, 2009, pp. 148–168), and linked to *intervention aims* and *goals* (Erickson et al., 2009, pp. 168–201). Although both intervention aims and intervention goals involve nursing actions, the difference between them is based in their purpose. Nursing interventions should have intent; nurses should *aim to make something happen when they interact with clients.* At the same time, there should be general markers that help us evaluate the efficacy of our interventions; these are called *intervention goals.* Table 13-1 shows the relations among MRM principles of nursing, types of data needed to practice this model, the aims of nursing actions, and specific goals.

Modeling

The *modeling* process involves an assessment of a client's situation. It starts when we initiate an interaction with an individual and concludes with an understanding of that person's perspective of their circumstances. We aim to learn how that individual describes the situation, what he expects will happen, and his perceived resources and life goals. As we listen and observe, we interpret the information based on the constructs embedded in the theory. Simplistically stated, *modeling is the process we use to build a mirror image of an individual's worldview. This worldview helps us understand what that person perceives to be important, what has caused his problems, what will help him, and how he wants to relate to others.*

Table 13-2 shows the categories of data and the type of information needed in the modeling process.

Table 13 · 1 Relations Among MRM Principles, Categories of Data, Intervention Goals, and Aims

Principles	Categories of Data	Goals	Aims
The nursing process requires that a trusting and functional relationship exist between nurse and client.	Description of the situation	Develop a trusting and functional relationship between self and your client.	Build trust.
Affiliated-individuation is contingent on the individual's perceiving that he or she is an acceptable, respectable, and worthwhile human being.	Expectation	Facilitate a self-projection that is futuristic and positive.	Promote client's positive orientation.
Human development is dependent on the individual's perceiving that he or she has some control over life while concurrently sensing a state of affiliation.	(External) Resource potential	Promote affiliated-individuation with the minimum degree of ambivalence possible.	Promote client's control.
There is an innate drive toward holistic health that is facilitated by consistent and systematic nurturance.	(Internal) Resource potential	Promote a dynamic, adaptive, and holistic state of health.	Affirm and promote client's strengths.
Human growth is dependent on satisfaction of basic needs and is facilitated by growth-need satisfaction.	(Internal) Resource potential	Promote (and nurture) coping mechanisms that satisfy basic needs and permit growth-need satisfaction.	Set mutual goals that are health directed.
	Goal and life tasks	Facilitate congruent actual and chronological development stages.	

Adapted with permission from Erickson, H., Tomlin, E., & Swain, M. A. (Eds.). (2009). *Modeling and role-modeling: A theory and paradigm for nursing* (p. 171). Cedar Park, TX: EST.

Table 13 · 2 **Categories of Data and Purpose for Obtaining Data**	
Categories of Data Collection	**Purpose of Data Is to Obtain**
Description of the Situation	1. An overview of client's perception of the problem 2. The etiology of the problem including stressors and destressors 3. Client's perceived therapeutic needs
Expectations	1. Immediate expectations 2. Long-term expectations
Resource Potential	1. External: Social network, support system, and health care system. 2. Internal: Self-strengths, adaptive potential, feeling states, physiological states
Goal and Life Tasks	1. Current goals 2. Plans for future

Adapted with permission from Erickson, H., Tomlin, E., & Swain, M. A. (Eds.). (2009). *Modeling and role-modeling: A theory and paradigm for nursing* (p. 119). Cedar Park, TX: EST.

Table 13-3 shows the priority given to the information we collect. Primary data include information acquired directly from the client; secondary data include the nurse's observations and information collected from the family. Tertiary data include all information collected from medical records and other sources. Primary and secondary data are essential for professional practice while tertiary data are added as needed.

Role-Modeling

The *role-modeling* process requires both objective and artistic actions. First we analyze the data using theoretical *propositions* in the

Table 13 · 3 **Sources of Information**	
Primary Source	Client's self-care knowledge
Secondary Source	Information from family and nurses' observations
Tertiary Source	Medical records and other information related to client's case

MRM model (Table 13-4; Erickson et al., 2009, pp. 148–167). We interpret the meaning of what has been provided and search for linkages among the data that will help us understand the client's worldview. As we analyze the data, implications for nursing actions emerge (Erickson et al., 2009, pp. 168–220). Nursing actions are then artistically designed with *intent* (i.e., the aims of interventions) and specific *outcomes* (i.e., intervention goals). Our overall objectives are to help people find meaning in their experiences and to enhance their sense of well-being.

The following sections elaborate each of these objectives. The first section addresses the philosophical assumptions that underlie this model; theoretical underpinnings follow with implications for practice. Finally, the global applications of MRM are presented.

Philosophical Assumptions

Nursing has a metaparadigm that includes four extant constructs: person, environment, health, and nursing; sometimes social justice is added as a fifth construct (Schim, Benkert, Bell, Walker, & Danford, 2007). The operational definitions of these constructs provide the context necessary to clarify how an individual's actions are unique to nursing as

Table 13 · 4   Selected Theoretical Propositions in MRM Theory

1. Developmental task resolution is related to basic need status.
2. Growth depends on basic need status and is facilitated by growth need satisfaction.
3. Basic need satisfaction leads to object attachment.
4. Object loss leads to basic need deficits.
5. Affiliated-individuation is dependent on one's perception of acceptance and worth.
6. Feelings of worth result in a sense of futurity.
7. Development of self-care resources is related to basic need satisfaction.
8. Ability to mobilize coping resources is related to need satisfaction.
9. Responses to stressors are mediated by internal and external resources.
10. Ability to mobilize appropriate and adequate resources determines resultant health status.

opposed to the actions of another profession. Although all nursing theories are developed and articulated within this context, our personal philosophy impacts how we define and operationalize the constructs of nursing, and therefore how we articulate our models (Erickson, 2010). For this reason, it is important to be clear about our own philosophical beliefs and how they impact our conceptual definitions and our theoretical models. Nurses can use clear philosophical statements to determine if the underpinnings of a theoretical model are consistent with their own belief systems (Erickson, 2010). When they are not, discrepancies among nursing's philosophical beliefs, the nurse's personal belief system, and the theoretical propositions often create dissonance that impedes the nurses' ability to use the model (Erickson et al., 2009).

The philosophical assumptions underlying the MRM theory and paradigm are described in the text that follows. The first section presents MRM's orientation toward two of nursing's metaparadigm constructs: person and environment. Health, nursing, and social justice are described in the following sections.

Person and Environment

Humans are inherently holistic. This means that the parts are interconnected and dynamically interactive; what affects one part affects another. This is different from the wholistic person wherein the parts are associated but not necessarily interconnected or interactive (Fig. 13-1). When we approach people as

though they are wholistic, we can break them down into systems, organs, and other parts. When we view them as holistic, we understand that all the dimensions of the human being are interconnected; what affects one part has the potential to affect other parts. Our holistic nature is manifested through our innate instincts and drives: instincts and drives necessary for *humans* to maneuver through the pathways of their life journey. Table 13-5 provides examples of each of these.

While some might argue that all animals have an *innate instinct* to cope, and some have an innate ability to receive and interpret stimuli, most would agree that not all animals have an *innate drive* to receive stimuli in a cognitive form, acquire skills necessary to perceive and understand stimuli, to give and receive feedback, or the freedom to speak, or the freedom to choose. These latter characteristics are unique to *the human species, are innate, and often motivate our behavior* (Maslow, 1968, 1982). I have added one instinct—an inherent instinct for holistic well-being—and two human drives: the drive for healthy affiliated-individuation and the drive for self-actualization. These instincts and drives affect how we function as *holistic beings*. The holistic person is one in whom the whole is greater than the sum of the parts, while a wholistic person is one in whom the whole is *equal to the sum of the parts* (Erickson, Tomlin, & Swain, 2009, pp. 45-46).

As holistic beings, our mind, body, and spirit are inextricably interrelated with continuous

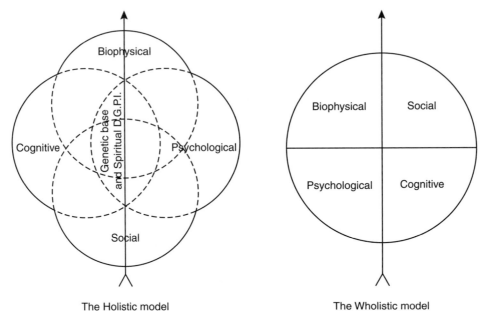

The Holistic model   The Wholistic model

Figure 13 • 1 Holism versus wholism.

feedback loops. Cells in each dimension can produce stimuli affecting responses in cells of other dimensions. Cellular responses have the potential to become new stimuli, moving the chain reaction around and among the dimensions of the human being. These interactions are dynamic and ongoing. Because we have an internal environment (i.e., within the confines of our physical being) and an external environment (i.e., outside the confines of the biopsychosocial being), external stimuli have the potential to create multiple internal responses, and vice versa. To agree that we are holistic is to believe that we are human beings, living in a context that includes all that is within us and within our external environment—holistic beings, constantly in process both internally and externally. These dynamically interactive dimensions cannot be separated without a loss of information about the person, a loss that diminishes our ability to fully understand the person's situation. There are three strategies that facilitate a trusting-functional relationship. Consider, for example, the student who

Table 13 • 5 **Selected List of Human Instincts and Drives**	
Instincts Inherent in Human Nature	To receive and interpret stimuli To cope and adapt to stressors To experience mind–body–spirit intraconnectedness, or holistic well-being
Drives that Motivate Our Behavior	To cognitively interpret stimuli To acquire skills necessary to perceive and interpret stimuli To give and receive feedback To communicate freely To choose and act freely To experience balanced affiliated-individuation To be self-actualized

states that she has the flu because she is too stressed; she had three exams, work, and no time to sleep. Although we all know influenza is caused by a virus, we also know that our ability to resist a virus depends on the status of our immune system at any given time. Couple that with an understanding of how the mind and body interact (i.e., psychoneuroimmunology) and we can appreciate how influenza and stress are related (Walker & Erickson, 2006).

Humans are also inherently intuitive. We know (at some level) what we need. We know what has made us sick, and what will help us get well, grow, develop, and heal. We have *instinctual* information about our own personhood and our mind–body–spirit linkages. This information is called *self-care knowledge*. Our perceptions of what we have available to help us are called *self-care resources*. Self-care resources are both internal and external. We have resources within ourselves as well as resources within our external environment. Our actions, thoughts, biophysical responses, and behavior, that help us get our needs met are our *self-care* actions.

We are *inherently* social beings with an innate drive to grow and develop, to become the most that we can be, find meaning in our lives, fulfill our potential, and self-actualize. However, we are very vulnerable. Our ability to grow and develop is dependent upon *repeated satisfaction* of our needs. We want and *need* to be connected or *affiliated* to others in some way. Simultaneously, we also need to perceive ourselves as unique and *individuated* from these same people. We call this affiliated-individuation (Acton, 1992; Erickson et al., 2009, p. 47; 2006, pp. 182–207).

Our drive to be both affiliated and individuated at the same time mandates a balance between being connected while perceiving a sense of one's self as a unique human being, separate from others. We achieve our drive for a balanced affiliated-individuation through our interactions with others. How well we achieve this balance at any point in our life will determine how we relate to others in the following years.

While we are social beings with a drive for affiliated-individuation with others, we are also spiritual beings with an inherent drive to be connected spiritually with our soul (Erickson et al., 2009; Erickson, Erickson, & Jensen, 2006). More specifically, our drive for individuation is to fulfill our psychosocial needs while doing soul-work unique to our life journey.

Health

Health is a matter of perception. It is a state of well-being in the whole person, not just a part of the person. It is not the presence, absence or control of disease; one's ability to adapt; or one's ability to perform social roles. Instead, it is a *eudemonistic health* that incorporates all of these and more. It is a *sense of well-being* in the holistic, social being. It includes one's perceptions of her life quality, her ability to find meaning in her existence, and a capacity to enjoy a positive orientation toward the future. As a result, personal perceptions of health may differ from those of others. It is possible for persons with no obvious physical problem to perceive a low level of health, while at the same time others, taking their last mortal breath, may perceive themselves as very healthy. The perception of health status is always related to perceived balance of affiliated-individuation.

Nursing

Nursing is the unconditional acceptance of the inherent worth of another human being. When we have unconditional acceptance for another person, we recognize that all humans have an innate need to be loved, to belong, to be respected, and to feel worthy. Unconditional acceptance of a person as a worthwhile being is not the same as accepting all behaviors without conditions. It does mean, however, that we recognize that behaviors are motivated by unmet needs. Our work, then, is to help people find ways to get their needs met without hurting or harming themselves or others.

We do this through nurturance and facilitation of the holistic person. Our goal is to help people grow, develop, and when necessary, to heal. We use all of our skills acquired through formal education as well as our own innate ability to connect with others to help them recover from illnesses and to live meaningful lives. We do this from the beginning of physical life to the end, even as people are taking their last breath. Within this context, our *intent,* or what we aim to facilitate when we interact with another human being, is important.

Social Justice

As professional nurses, we are committed to live by the ethics of our profession, to serve as advocates for our clients, and to serve the public as defined by our professional standards. For nurses who use the MRM theory, this means that we are committed to recognize the individual's worldview as valid information, to act on that information with the intent of nurturing and facilitating growth and well-being in our clients, and to practice within the context of the Standards of Holistic Nursing as defined by the American Holistic Nurses Association (AHNA, 2007) and recognized by the American Nurses Association (ANA, 2008).

Theoretical Constructs

People have an innate instinct to *cope* and *adapt* to stressors and related stress responses that confront us constantly. We adapt as much as we are able to, given our life situation.

We need oxygen, glucose, protein, to maintain our physical systems; we also need to feel safe and to be loved. When these needs are perceived to be unmet, they create stressors; stressors produce the stress response. Stress responses can become new stressors mandating still more responses, and so on (Benson, 2006, pp. 240–266; Erickson, 1976; Erickson et al., 2009). Many of our stress responses are instinctual, a part of our human makeup; however, some have to be learned and developed. As our needs are met, the stressors decrease and we are able to work through the stress response.

Adaptive Potential

Our ability to mobilize resources at any moment in time can be identified as our

Adaptive Potential. The Adaptive Potential Assessment Model (APAM; Fig. 13-2), first labeled in 1976 (Erickson, 1976; Erickson & Swain, 1982; Erickson et al., 2009), was derived by synthesizing Selye's (1974, 1976, 1980, 1985) work with that of George Engel (1964). Our Adaptive Potential has three states: equilibrium, arousal, and impoverishment. Equilibrium, a state of nonstress or eustress, represents maximum ability to mobilize resources. The individual in equilibrium is in a healthy balance between need demands and need resources.

Arousal and impoverishment are both stress states; needs are unmet, creating stressors and the related stress responses. However, people in arousal are temporarily able to mobilize their resources while those in impoverishment are not. Persons in the first group (arousal) need help solving their problem, finding alternatives. They tend to be tense and anxious, but do not demonstrate depleted resources through the expression of fatigue and sadness. On the other hand, impoverished people show the wear and tear of prolonged stress. They have diminished physical resources and are fatigued and sad. People in arousal are at risk for becoming impoverished and impoverished people are at risk for depleting their resources, getting sick, developing complications, and even dying (Barnfather, 1987; Barnfather & Ronis, 2000; Benson, 2006, pp. 242–254; Erickson, 1976; Erickson et al., 2009, pp. 75–83; Erickson & Swain, 1982). As indicated, a person's ability

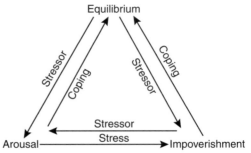

Figure 13 • 2 The adaptive potential assessment model.

to cope is related to how well his or her needs are met at any given point in time.

Human Needs

Human needs, classified as basic, social, and growth needs, *drive* our behavior. They provide motivation for our self-care actions and emerge in a quasi-hierarchical order. Physiological needs must be met to some degree before social needs emerge. Growth or higher-level needs emerge after the basic and social needs have been met to some degree. Table 13-6 provides examples of each. For a more detailed taxonomy of human needs, see Erickson, H., 2006a, pp. 484–485.

Basic needs are related to survival of the species. When they are unmet, tension rises, motivating behavioral response(s) necessary to decrease the tension. When self-care actions decrease the tension, the need dissipates. When the need is completely satisfied, the tension disappears. When needs are met

repeatedly, need assets are built. Conversely, when the need is not met, the tension rises, and need deficits emerge. When the tension continues, need deprivation exists. Need status can be classified on a 0–5 scale ranging from deprivation to asset status (Fig. 13-3).

Growth needs are different. Because people have an innate drive for self-actualization, growth needs emerge when basic needs are met (to some degree). Unmet growth needs do not create tension unless they are related to a basic need. Instead, *satisfaction* of growth needs creates tension. The need increases in intensity. Until one feels satiated, the need to *continue to behave in ways that will meet growth needs continues.*

Need Satisfaction and the Object Attachment Process

Objects that repeatedly meet humans needs become *attachment objects*. These objects take on significance unique to the individual, are

Table 13 · 6 Basic and Growth Needs Inherent to the Human Being

Hierarchical Level	Classification of Need	Type of Need	Purpose	Examples
Basic Needs	Physiological needs	1. Survival	Required for biological homeostasis.	Food, water, oxygen, temperature control, etc.
		2. Stimulation	Required for physical and emotional growth	Activity, manipulation, exploration.
	Social needs	1. Safety and security	Required for healthy growth	Fair and predictable world, safety from harm, nurturing care.
		2. Love and belonging	Required for healthy growth/development	Affection, kindness, mutual trust, identity
		3. Esteem and self-esteem	Required for healthy growth/development	Confidence, respect, dignity, attention, adequacy.
Growth Needs		Required for continuous development		Meaningfulness in life Playfulness Simplicity Goodness and truth Beauty

Adapted with permission from Erickson, H. (Ed.). (1975). An operational taxonomy of human needs. In: Erickson H. (Ed.). (2006) *Modeling and role-modeling: A view from the client's world.* Cedar Park, TX: Unicorns Unlimited.

Deprivation	Deficit	Unmet	Met	Satisfied	Assets
0	1	2	3	4	5

Figure 13 • 3 The needs status scale, 0–5.

both human and nonhuman, have a physical form (so they stimulate one of the five senses) or are abstract (such as an idea) and are necessary throughout life. When a person perceives that the object is or will be lost, a grieving response occurs. Loss is a subjective experience known by the individual; it can be real, threatened, or perceived. Any loss produces a grieving process. One's difficulty in resolving the loss depends on the significance of the lost object.

The grieving response is normal, occurs in a predetermined sequence, and is self-limited. Normal grieving processes take about 1 year

(Fig. 13-4). Grief resolution occurs as the individual finds new ways to view the lost object or finds alternative objects that meet their needs. Commonly accepted processes of grief include sequential phases of shock/disbelief, anger, bargaining, sadness, and acceptance (Kübler-Ross). Other models (Engel, Bowlby) indicate slightly different phases (Erickson, M., 2006, p. 229). Table 13-7 compares three of these models. I believe that their differences are based in the nature of the lost object, its meaning to the individual, and the resources accrued before the experienced loss. Resources are based upon one's ability to work through the normal developmental tasks encountered during the human journey. This issue is discussed further in the text that follows.

Attachment to new objects is necessary for continued growth and grief resolution. The

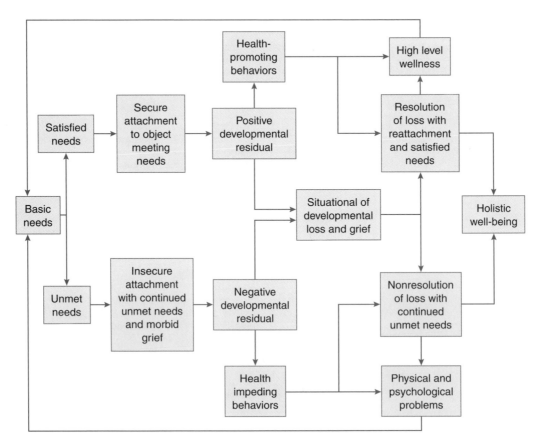

Figure 13 • 4 The needs–attachment–development–loss–reattachment model.

Table 13 · 7	**Stages of Grief According to Contributing Authors**	
Engel	**Kübler-Ross**	**Bowlby**
Shock/disbelief	Denial/shock	
Awareness	Anger/hostility	Protest
Resolution	Bargaining	
Loss resolution	Depression	*Despair*
Idealization	Acceptance	*Detachment*

Italicized stages indicate unresolved loss with movement toward morbid grief.
Reprinted with permission from Erickson, H. (Ed.). (2006). *Modeling and role-modeling: A view from the client's world* (p. 229). Cedar Park, TX: Unicorns Unlimited.

new object can be the *same* object, perceived in a new way, or a completely new object. Sometimes *transitional objects* are used to facilitate this process. Transitional objects are those that symbolize the lost object, and are never human, but are almost always concrete. For example, mothers attached to their children as preschoolers often experience a loss when their children start school and become increasingly independent. It is common to see these mothers attach to their child's baby shoes, pictures, or some other symbol of who they were in their previous life stage.

Morbid grief emerges when the individual is unable to find alternative objects that will repeatedly meet their needs. Because we are holistic beings, morbid grief has the potential to result in physical symptoms, illness, and over the long period, disease. What happens in one part of the holistic person has the potential of creating disease in another part, disease that becomes distressful, mandates mobilization of resources often not available, and therefore producing alternative biophysical responses, depleting psychoneuroimmunological resources (Erickson & Walker, 2006).

Behaviors that indicate emergence of morbid grief include an inability to move on and let go of the lost object, combined with vacillation between *anger* and *sadness* (Erickson, M., 2006, pp. 209–239; Lindeman, 1944, pp. 141–148). Initially individuals are able to focus their anger and sadness, but with time, anger grows into hostility and sadness into depression. When this happens, people are less able to articulate the focus of their feelings or recognize the loss that produced the grieving response in the beginning. They often use language that describes giving-up rather than letting go, and sometimes express nostalgia for the lost object. In contrast, those who have let go of the lost object, worked through the normal grief response, and reattached to a new object can usually describe the importance of *moving on.*

Need Satisfaction and Life Orientation

The degree to which a person's needs are met repeatedly determines how he or she relates to others; it *effects* their *life orientation.* When needs are met repeatedly, people are able to grow and develop, to integrate mind–body–spirit, perceive themselves as worthy human beings, and to experience a healthy balance of affiliated-individuation. When this happens, they are interested in others as individuals who are unique and worthwhile. They enjoy both a sense of connectedness and a sense of individuation. Their life orientation is called a *being orientation* because they are interested in becoming all they can be and in participating in the same way with others.

However, when needs are repeatedly unmet, growth is limited and people have difficulty with their developmental processes. Their relationships with others *exist within a context of what can be obtained from the other.* They are not interested in the well-being of the other, might be threatened by growth in significant others, and are intolerant of the uniqueness of others. More interested in what they can get from someone than what they can give, *these people often view others as a source of getting their basic needs met. As a result, often unable to meet the needs of significant others, they are perceived as "needy people."* Their life orientation is called a *deficit orientation.* Being and deficit orientations exist on a scale; most people have some of both. The balance between the two is what determines one's overriding traits or personal attributes, one's values and virtues, and one's ways of interacting with others.

Developmental Processes

People have an inherent drive for self-actualization. This requires that they pass through predetermined chronological developmental stages—stages with *task*s that mandate attention as they emerge. Our ability to work on these *developmental tasks* depends on our ability to mobilize resources. Resources are derived by getting our needs met at any given time as well as our past experiences. Since our experiences are always contextual, how we resolve our developmental tasks will determine the resources we have to work on current tasks. As we work through a stage-related task, a *developmental residual* is produced. This residual includes positive *and* negative attributes, strengths, and virtues. In our original work, we followed Erik Erikson's work to define eight stages, their tasks, and the associated residual. Our more recent work has modified work, expanding the stages to include one pre-birth and another at the time of death (Erickson, M., 2006, pp. 121–181; Table 13-8).

Table 13 · 8	**Developmental Stages, Residual, Virtues, and Strengths**		
Stages/Age	**Residual**	**Virtue**	**Strength(s)**
Integration of Spirit (Pre–post birth)	Unity vs. duality	Groundedness	Awareness
Building Trust (Birth–15 months)	Trust vs. mistrust	Hope	Drive toward future
Acquiring Autonomy (12–36 months)	Autonomy vs. introspection	Will power	Self-control
Taking Initiative (2–7 years)	Initiative vs. responsibility	Purpose	Drive
Developing Industry (5–13 years)	Competency vs. inferiority	Competence	Methodological problem-solving
Developing Identity (11–30 years)	Self-identity vs. role confusion	Fidelity	Devotion
Building Intimacy (20–50 years)	Intimacy vs. isolation	Love	Affiliation with individuation
Developing Generativity (midlife to 60s)	Generativity vs. stagnation	Caring	Production
Ego Integrity (60s to transformation)	Ego integrity vs. despair	Wisdom	Renunciation
Transformation (end of physical life)	Reconnecting vs. disconnecting	Oneness	Peace, cosmic understanding, compassion

Adapted with permission from Erickson, H. (Ed.). (2006). *Modeling and role-modeling: A view from the client's world* (Table 5.1, pp. 128–129). Cedar Park TX: Unicorns Unlimited.

Sequential Development

Development occurs as a series of predetermined stages with specific tasks in each stage. It is also chronological: unique, sequential stages, and their related tasks emerge during a specific time frame in our lives. During that time, the task becomes predominate in our life journey, drawing resources, focusing attention, and motivating behaviors.

Epigenisis

Development is also epigenetic. Although we have specific tasks that focus our attention at specific times in life, we also rework earlier life tasks and set the framework for later tasks at the same time. This later work is done *within the context of the appointed life task.* Simply stated, we repeatedly work on all of the developmental tasks at every stage of life, although we have a key task that dominates at any given time. Our ability to manage these multiple tasks is dependent on the residual we have produced throughout the process and our current ability to have our needs met.

Linkages

Several major theoretical linkages exist in the MRM model. Relations exist between/among:

1. Adaptive potential and need status
2. Need status, object attachment, loss, and new attachment status.
3. Developmental task resolution and need satisfaction.

Several theoretical propositions are derived from these major linkages (see Table 13-4). Many others exist, too numerous to list individually.

Practice Applications

We cannot cure people, but we can help them heal and grow, even as they are taking their first or last breath. When people heal they become more fully connected with the multiple dimensions of their mind, body, and spirit, and as a result, they become more fully actualized. A caring-healing environment, created by the nurses' *intent,* fosters growth and well-being in their clients.

Because people have inherent instincts and drives to grow, develop, and heal, when necessary, *all nursing actions* focus on facilitation and nurturance of these innate abilities. We *use ourselves to connect* with our clients in such a way that we can create *trusting functional relationships* with them, relationships that have a *purpose* or are *aimed* at some outcome. In the MRM model, these relationships aim to affirm their worth; help them mobilize and build resources needed to cope with their stressors/stress; foster a hope for the future; and promote a sense of affiliated-individuation. When people have these experiences, a sense of well-being follows. While we use every professional skill we have acquired, these are secondary to using *ourselves* as healing agents. As nurses, we nurture and facilitate people to become the most that they can be. We help them actualize their life roles and find meaning in their existence. When this happens, it affects not only our clients, but it also affects those who are significant in their lives.

As nurses, every interaction with our clients and their loved ones provides us with opportunities to affect the future; I call this the "long-arm affect" (Erickson, H., 2006b, p. 390). How we perceive our roles as nurses will determine our intent. This in turn affects what we do, how we interact, the focus of our work, and the *outcomes* of our relationships. While we cannot always change what will happen in our lives or those of others, we can set the intent to help people grow, heal, and move on. J. M.'s letter suggests that not only did I help his family deal with a life tragedy, but I also helped them discover ways to find meaning in the experience. I helped them grow, heal, and to move on.

Practice Exemplar

A man who was the strong, dominant member of his family was lying in bed, incontinent, riddled with cancer and feeling hopeless. When I learned that he no longer allowed his family to visit, I gently took his hand and told him I was happy to be his nurse that evening. He "...looked at me with very sad eyes...[and said] that he didn't want his family to see him in this condition. ...he had always taken care of his family, and now...he couldn't take care of himself" (Erickson, H., 2006a, p. 325). I rephrased his words, and then told him that although he had been the bread-winner in the past and that his family members had enjoyed that, all they wanted now was to be with him, to share his life, that he was important because he loved them and they loved him. He agreed and for the next few days his family members took turns *just being with him.* On the third day when he quietly passed, he and his family were able to grieve with dignity and peace.

Eight years later I received a letter from his son (only 16 at the time of his father's death) notifying me that his mother had died. He *knew* I would want to know that because of what they had learned from me, she was able to pass at home with her family at her side, singing her favorite songs and strumming on the guitar. He went on to state:

In the year my Dad was with you people in Ann Arbor, you were of incalculable aid and comfort to both my parents—you gave them confidence in you and your staff, and the dignity and respect which makes life worth living; no one else could, or did, more genuinely have their gratitude and respect. When I would come down and all seemed to be lost, the one bright spot was that Mrs. Erickson would be coming on, and we could breathe a little more easily as Dad's anxiety visibly receded. Your kindness and humanity made the world a better place at that time and without you the experience would have been more difficult than you probably believe. Thank you, J. M.

Initiating the Relationship

I have found three sequential strategies, important for those using the MRM model: Establishing a Mind-Set, Creating a Nurturing Space, and Facilitating the Story (Erickson, H., 2006b, pp. 309–317; Table 13-9). Each can be done in seconds once the essence of the strategy is understood. However, before you can start, it is necessary to explore your own beliefs about human nature and nursing, and to consider how these affect your practice. This helps you clarify *how to get your needs met*—a prerequisite to meeting the needs of others. Unless we know how to initiate our own self-care, we have difficulty mobilizing the energy necessary to focus on the needs of our clients. Finally, we have to open ourselves to the worth of each individual, to *unconditionally accept that each human has an inherent need to be valued, to be treated with respect, and to live with dignity.*

Establishing a Mind-Set

Establishing a mind-set involves three strategies: centering, focusing, and opening. *Centering* helps to organize our resources so that we can connect energetically with our client. It requires that we temporarily put aside other thoughts, worries, or concerns, and *believe* that at *some level* we can discover what we need to know to help our clients, and to focus on the other with the *intent* of nurturing their growth and facilitating their healing. When we *focus on our client's needs,* we initiate an energetic connection, necessary for a caring–healing environment.

Creating a Nurturing Space

Creating a nurturing space follows naturally when we have established a mind-set. Our goal is to create a caring–healing environment. Although one cannot force growth in others, we can create environments that

Table 13 · 9　**Three Strategies that Facilitate a Trusting–Functional Relationship**

Establish a Mind-Set	Self-care preliminaries Moving forward	Enhance sense-of-self. Center self. Focus intent. Open self to the essence of other.
Create a Nurturing Space	Reduce distracting stimuli. Respect client's space. Connect spirit to spirit.	Attend to sounds, lights, smells, and other stimuli that are distracting and. discomforting Recognize and respect client's physical/energetic space. Use eye contact, soft tones, and gentle touch to connect with client.
Facilitate the Client's Story	Tap self-care knowledge.	Address stimuli, encourage focus on nurse–client linkage. Relate to beliefs about client's self-care knowledge as primary. Encourage client's perceptions of the situation.

Adapted with permission from Erickson, H. (Ed.). (2006). *Modeling and role-modeling: A view from the client's world* (pp. 307–317). Cedar Park, TX: Unicorns Unlimited.

nurture growth. We do this by decreasing adverse stimuli while increasing positive ones. It is important to remember that you are *entering the client's space* and to respect it. Even though you may think it is important to close the door, turn on the radio, fluff pillows, you will want to assess whether your actions serve to comfort the client or not. Each of these processes helps you connect with your client in such a way that you will initiate a trusting relationship and create a caring–healing environment.

Any stimuli that affects the five senses has the possibility of being comforting, uncomfortable, or discomforting. We can influence these by our actions in the milieu and by our interactions with our client. For example, a noisy hallway or bright lights shining in our eyes are stimuli that seem to *drain* energy from us, and no doubt our clients experience the same thing. Or consider a beautiful picture, the glimpse of a fully leafed tree swaying in a gentle breeze, soft music of our choice, clean sheets against our skin, or the gentle touch of a loving person. In thinking about how you respond to these stimuli you will understand that these have the possibility of

comforting another human being. You will also understand that how you touch, look, or speak to someone conveys a message about your intent to comfort or *not to comfort.*

Facilitating the Story

Facilitating the story is the third strategy that MRM nurses use. Disclosure of our clients' self-care knowledge provides basic information needed before we can decide what nursing actions are required—information that provides insight into their worldview. We learn about their perceptions and beliefs, what they believe about their current situation, what they expect will happen, what resources they believe they have, and what they would like to do to alter the situation. It also allows them to "... *contextualize* life experiences and present them in a way that softens associated feelings" (Erickson, H., 2006b, p. 315).

Our clients' self-care knowledge is best obtained by allowing them to tell their story in their own way. We use *active listening* to facilitate them. This can be done very quickly by initiating the discussion with statements such as, "Tell me about your situation" followed by "Why do *you* think this has happened?" or "What do *you* think has caused it?" and "How do you *feel about that?*" and so forth (Erickson et al., 2009, pp. 153–167). The data are then organized into four distinct but interrelated categories: description of the situation, expectations, resource potential, and goals (see Table 13-2). Information provided by our clients has to be *interpreted, aggregated, and analyzed* before we can use it to plan interventions (Erickson et al., 2009, pp. 153–168).

Understanding the Data

In *data interpretation,* we use the philosophical and theoretical underpinnings discussed earlier as we attend to words, affects, and nonverbal language, searching for evidence of coping potential (i.e., adaptive potential), needs status, and developmental residual. Sometimes it is necessary to clarify what we observe to avoid superimposing our own interpretations on these data. For example, clients might have a spouse or significant other, but not perceive this individual as supportive. When this happens, they often describe them as "draining" rather than invigorating. We cannot always make these distinctions without asking the client how they perceive their relationship with their significant other (Erickson et al., 2009, pp. 160–163).

A person's story usually includes information about interactions among the dimensions of the holistic person, but nurses often have trouble understanding the significance of what they have heard. For example, when people say they are sick because they are too stressed, our first response might be to think about the *cause and effect of disease*—for example, bacteria (not stress) causes infections. However, the MRM model supports a *holistic perspective;* we know that mind and body are inextricably interactive. Therefore, we recognize that psychosocial stress stimulates the hypothalamic–pituitary–adrenal axis interactions, compromising the immune system. When this happens, we have more difficulty fighting bacterial invasions. As a result, we know that psychosocial stress has the potential of causing signs and symptoms of physical illness and/or disease.

Practice Exemplar

Most data are easy to understand although there are some that are symbolic of earlier losses. A middle-aged man I worked with a number of years ago had just been admitted to the hospital for a "work-up." Mr. S. had complained of chronic fatigue for the past 6 months. An hour or so before I saw him, he had learned that he had acute leukemia. When I asked him to tell me about his situation he told me about his leukemia and then launched into a story about his childhood. He described a time when he was about 16 years old, had been told to watch his younger sister, and had let her ride a horse without supervision. She fell off and was killed. He remembered that his father told him that he had not been responsible and that he needed to grow-up and be a man.

Mr. S. looked surprised and said that he didn't know what had made him think of that event and that he hadn't thought about it for years. When I asked him what he expected would happen, he said that he guessed this meant that he was going to die. He went on to say that he thought *he had developed leukemia because he hadn't been responsible, and when he wasn't responsible, people died.* As we explored his resources he explained that he had been promoted about 9 months ago and that his new job required skills he didn't think he had. His conclusions were that he was sick because he had "worried himself to death." He also stated that he didn't want his wife to come see him, that he needed to decide what he wanted to do first, and how he could take care of her now that he was sick. When I asked if she or someone else could help him consider options, he said no, that it was his responsibility to take care of himself. To understand these data I needed to recognize that:

- People who link new stressful experiences to past experiences are usually dealing with a *loss related to the past experience*. In his case, it was not only the loss of his sister, but also the *meaning of the loss*. As a 16-year-old boy, he was learning about his ability to make sound decisions, to be independent, to determine who he was as a unique human being in society. He had learned that "when he wasn't responsible, people died."
- While he identified his wife as his significant other, he was over-individuated. He needed to decide how to "tell" his wife about his problem—his problem of not being responsible, not being a "man." He did not perceive that it was appropriate to seek comfort from her or others.

The second phase, *data aggregation,* sometimes occurs as we are interpreting data derived from the *primary source* (i.e., the client), but not always. To aggregate the data accurately, we need to consider data derived from the *secondary* and *tertiary* sources as well as the data derived from the client. Although data can be aggregated with only the client's story and the nurse's clinical knowledge, it is helpful to hear the family's perspective also. Sometimes it is also important to include the information collected from tertiary sources.

When aggregating data, we consider all the information and look for consistencies as well as inconsistencies across the sources of information. Additional information may be necessary to clarify perspectives. Usually, this phase helps in determining what needs to be done when moving into the intervention phase of the nursing process.

Data analysis is the next step. Again, you may be doing all three—interpreting, aggregating, and analyzing—simultaneously. During the analysis phase you look for theoretical linkages among the data, make diagnoses. An example that follows the case described earlier would be:

- Mr. S. is in arousal with unmet safety and belonging needs, unresolved loss with morbid grief, and both positive and negative residual from adolescence on. Strong positive residual from early childhood provides some resources that could be mobilized with assistance.

- Although Mr. S. is chronologically in the stage of Intimacy versus Isolation, his stressors are related to residuals from the stage of Competency versus Limitations.
- Mr. S's healthy affiliated–individuation has been threatened due to over-individuation.
- Mr. S. wished to be "responsible" to "take care of his wife."

Proactive Nursing Care

Often *the process of assessing our clients' worldview* serves as a therapeutic intervention. People in arousal commonly state that they feel much better after talking. Some will ask for minimal help, but some require more sophisticated help. In any case, based on our diagnoses, nursing care is planned within the context of the MRM principles of care, aimed at facilitating well-being in our clients, and designed specifically to meet intervention goals. We do this as we manage technical care such as wound management, intravenous insertion, and so forth. We use nonjudgmental language, caring tones, and direct statements that relay information needed to feel safe and cared about. We also use Ericksonian hypnotherapeutic techniques to promote growth and facilitate healing (Erickson et al., 2009, pp. 84–85, 145–147; Erickson, H., 2006b, pp. 315–317; 372–374; Zeig, 1982).

We can also do this without ever touching the person because *we use ourselves as conduits of healing energy*. Sometimes knowing that someone cares about us and our life helps us grow and heal. We project these messages through our actions when we *unconditionally accept* the worth of another human being. Watzlawick (1967) states that "we cannot not communicate." Our attitudes, nonverbal behaviors, and touch are often more important than what we say when we convey our *intent* to help others heal and grow; words are not always necessary. Our demeanor, the way we look at the person, what we focus on first, and how we touch our clients relays our *intent*. When we enter a relationship with the *intent to comfort and nurture the other person,* our energy field connects with his; we convey *presence* and initiate a caring–healing environment (Erickson, H., 2006b, pp. 300–324).

Global Applications of the Model

The MRM theory and paradigm have been recognized by AHNA as one of the extant holistic nursing theories. It is used in a variety of settings including educational institutions as a framework for entire programs or specific courses, hospitals to guide practice, and for independent practice (Table 13-10). The Society for the Advancement of Modeling and Role-Modeling (mrmnursingtheory.org) was established in 1985 under the supervision of Carolyn Kinney and 32 others. Members meet biennially with retreats in the alternate year to achieve four major goals shown in Table 13-11.

Several articles, chapters, and books have been published reporting the use of MMR across populations from pediatrics to the

Table 13 · 10	Agencies Using/Teaching MRM	
Academic Programs	East Carolina University, Greenville, North Carolina	Theoretical foundation for transition from RN to graduate student
	Harding University, School of Nursing, Searcy, Arkansas	Theoretical foundation for pediatric clinical course
	Humboldt State University, School of Nursing, Eureka, California	Theoretical foundation, BSN and RN–BSN programs
	Metro State University, School of Nursing, St. Paul, Minnesota	Theoretical foundation, and student advising
	The College of St. Catherine's, School of Nursing, St. Paul, Minnesota	Theoretical foundation, ADN Program
	The University of Texas at Austin, School of Nursing	Theoretical foundation, the Alternate Entry Program
	Washtenaw Community College, School of Nursing, Ypsilanti, Michigan	Theoretical foundation, ADN Program
Health Care Agencies	Contemporary Health Care, Austin, Texas	Theoretical foundation for nursing practice
	Oregon Health & Science University, Portland, Oregon	Theoretical foundation for nursing practice
	Salina Regional Health Center, Salina, Kansas	Theoretical foundation for nursing practice
	The University of Texas Health System, San Antonio, Texas	Theoretical foundation for nursing practice
	The University of Tennessee Medical Center, Knoxville, Tennessee	Theoretical foundation for nursing practice

Table 13 · 11 Goals Set by SAMRM, 1985

1. Promote the continuous study and integration of the theoretical propositions and philosophical foundations through research, practice, and continuous education.
2. Develop a network for the support, stimulation, and growth of the membership through newsletters, conferences, and membership meetings
3. Disseminate knowledge and information through conferences and publication of conference proceedings
4. Address societal needs by contributing to improvement of health care through proactive promotion of holistic health.

Table 13 · 12 Practice/Intervention Studies Related to MRM Theory and Paradigm

Author	Tested	Source
Erickson, H., & Swain, M. (1982)	MRM and well-being	*Research in Nursing & Health, 5*, 93–101
Walsh, K., van den Bosch, T., & Boehm, S. (1989)	MRM applied to two clinical cases	*Journal of Advanced Nursing, 14*(9), 755–761
Finch, D. (1987)	Clinical assessment of developmental residual	Unpublished master's thesis, the University of Michigan
Erickson, H., & Swain, M. (1990)	MRM and hypertension reduction	*Issues in Mental Health Nursing, 11*(3), 217–235
Finch, D. (1990)	MRM nursing assessment model	*Modeling and Role-Modeling: Theory, Practice and Research, 1*(1), 203–213
Kinney, C. (1990)	Long-term effect of MRM on growth and development	*Issues in Mental Health Nursing, 11*, 375–395
Erickson, H. (1990)	MRM with mind–body problems	*In Brief Therapy,* J. Zeig & S. Gilligan
Barnfather, J. (1991)	MRM and school nurse role	*Public Health Nursing, 8*(4), 234–238
Holl, R. (1992)	MRM vs. contracting and well-being	*Dissertation Abstracts International, 53*, 4030B
Holl, R. (1993)	MRM vs. restricted visiting	*Critical Care Nursing Quarterly, 16*(2), 70–82
Webster, D., Vaughn, K., Webb, M., & Player, A. (1995)	MRM and brief solution-focused therapy	*Issues in Mental Health Nursing, 16*(6), 505–518
Erickson, M. (1996)	EMBAT and maternal well-being	*Issues in Mental Health Nursing, 17*, 185–200
Sappington, J., & Kelly, J. (1996)	A case study	*Journal of Holistic Nursing, 14*(2), 130–141
Jensen, B. (1999)	Caregiver responses to MRM	*Dissertation Abstracts International, B 56/06*, 3127
Scheela, R. (1999)	Remodeling sex offenders	*Journal of Psychosocial Nursing and Mental Health Services, 37*(9), 25–31
Mayhew, P., Acton, G., Yauk, S., & Hopkins, B. (2001)	Communication, dementia, and well-being	*Gerontological Nursing, 22*, 106–110

elderly (Table 13-12). Some describe MRM in various settings ranging from critical care units, home health care, and independent practice. In addition, some (such as Noreen Frisch, Jane Kelly, Gloria Weber, and Janet Barnfather) have written about the use of MRM in particular types of nursing, such as with clients with psychiatric concerns, employed mothers with preschool children, and undereducated adult learners. The MRM Web site provides a selected listing of these publications (mrmnursingtheory.org).

References

Acton, G. (1992). The relationships among stressors, stress, affiliated-individuation, burden, and well-being in caregivers of adults with dementia: A test of the theory and paradigm for nursing, modeling and role-modeling. Doctoral dissertation, the University of Texas at Austin. *Dissertation Abstracts International*, AAT 9323314.

American Holistic Nurses Association (AHNA). (2007). *Holistic nursing: Scope and standards of practice*. Silver Spring, MD: American Holistic Nurses Association, American Nurses Association.

American Nurses Association (ANA). Retrieved from http://www.ahna.org/AboutUs/ANASpecialtyRecognition/tabid/1167/Default.aspx (Accessed June 3, 2008).

Barnfather, J. (1987). Mobilizing coping resources related to basic need status in healthy, young adults. Doctoral dissertation, the University of Texas at Austin. *Dissertation Abstract International*, 49-02B (AAF8801275).

Barnfather, J., & Ronis, D. (2000). Test of a model of psychosocial resources, stress, and health among undereducated adults. *Research in Nursing & Health*, *23*(1), 55–66.

Benson, D. (2006). Adaptation: Coping with stress. In: H. Erickson (Ed.), *Modeling and role-modeling: A view from the client's world* (pp. 240–274). Cedar Park, TX: Unicorns Unlimited.

Bowlby, J. (1973). *Separation*. New York: Basic Books.

Clayton, D., Erickson, H., & Rogers, S. (2006). Finding meaning in our life journey. In: H. Erickson (Ed.), *Modeling and role-modeling: A view from the client's world* (pp. 391–410). Cedar Park, TX: Unicorns Unlimited.

Engel, G. (1964). Grief and grieving. *American Journal of Nursing, 64*, 93.

Erickson, H. C. (1976). *Identification of states of coping utilization physiological and psychological data*. Unpublished master's thesis, University of Michigan, Ann Arbor, MI.

Erickson, H. (1990). Theory based nursing. In: C. Kinney & H. Erickson (Eds.), *Modeling and role-modeling: Theory, practice and research* (vol. 1, pp. 1–27). Cedar Park, TX: Society for Advancement of Modeling and Role-Modeling.

Erickson, H. (1996). Holistic healing: Intra/inter relations of person and environment. (Guest Editor). *Issues of Mental Health Nursing, 17*(3), vii–viii.

Erickson, H. (2002). Facilitating generativity and ego integrity: Applying Ericksonian methods to the aging population. In: B. B. Geary & J. K. Zeig (Eds.), *The Handbook of Ericksonian Psychotherapy*. Phoenix, AZ: Zeig Tucker Publications.

Erickson, H. (Ed.). (2006a). *Modeling and role-modeling: A view from the client's world*. Cedar Park, TX: Unicorns Unlimited.

Erickson, H. (2006b). Connecting. In: H. Erickson (Ed.), *Modeling and role-modeling: A view from the client's world* (pp. 300–322). Cedar Park, TX: Unicorns Unlimited.

Erickson, H. (2006c). Facilitating development. In: H. Erickson (Ed.), *Modeling and role-modeling: A view from the client's world* (pp. 346–390). Cedar Park, TX: Unicorns Unlimited.

Erickson, H. (2006d). Nurturing growth. In: H. Erickson (Ed.), *Modeling and role-modeling: A view from the client's world* (pp. 324–345). Cedar Park, TX: Unicorns Unlimited.

Erickson, H. (2006e). The healing process. In: H. Erickson (Ed.), *Modeling and role-modeling: A view from the client's world* (pp. 411–434). Cedar Park, TX: Unicorns Unlimited.

Erickson, H. (2007). Philosophy and theory of holism. *Nursing Clinics of North America, 42*, 140.

Erickson, H. (2008). Nursing of the body, mind & spirit? *Advance for Nurses, 6*(20), 31–32.

Erickson, H. (2010). Paradigm choices: Implications for nursing knowledge. In: H. Erickson (Ed.), *Exploring the context and essence of holistic nursing: Modeling and role-modeling for nurse educators*. Cedar Park, TX: Unicorns Unlimited. In press.

Erickson, H., Tomlin, E., & Swain, M. A. (2009). *Modeling and role-modeling: A theory and paradigm for nursing*. Cedar Park, TX: EST.

Erickson, H. C., & Swain, M. A. (1982). A model for assessing potential adaptation to stress. *Research in Nursing and Health, 5*, 93–101.

Erickson, M. (2006). Attachment, loss and reattachment. In: H. Erickson (Ed.), *Modeling and role-modeling: A view from the client's world* (pp. 208–237). Cedar Park, TX: Unicorns Unlimited.

Erickson, M., Erickson, H., & Jensen, B. (2006). Affiliated-individuation and self-actualization: Need satisfaction as prerequisite. In: H. Erickson (Ed.), *Modeling and role-modeling: A view from the client's world* (pp. 182–207). Cedar Park, TX: Unicorns Unlimited.

Kübler-Ross, E. (1969). *On death and dying.* London: Tavistock.

Lindeman, E. (1944). Symptomatology and management of acute grief. *American Journal of Psychiatry, 101,* 141–148.

Maslow, A. (1968). *Toward a psychology of being* (2nd ed.). New York: D. Van Nostrand.

Maslow, A. (1982). *The farthest reaches of human nature.* New York: D. Van Nostrand.

Schim, S., Benkert, R., Bell, S., Walker, D., & Danford, C. (2007). Social justice: Added metaparadigm concept for urban health nursing. *Public Health Nursing, 24*(1), 73–80.

Selye, H. (1974). *Stress without distress.* Philadelphia: J. B. Lippincott.

Selye, H. (1976). *The stress of life* (rev. ed.). New York: McGraw-Hill.

Selye, H. (1980). *Selye's guide to stress research* (vol. 1). New York: Van Nostrand Reinhold.

Selye, H. (1985). History and present status of the stress concept. In: A. Monat & R. S. Lazarus (Eds.), *Stress and coping: An anthology* (pp. 17–29). New York: Columbia University Press.

Walker, M., & Erickson, H. (2006). Mind, body and spirit relations. In: H. Erickson (Ed.), *Modeling and role-modeling: A view from the client's world* (pp. 67–91). Cedar Park, TX: Unicorns Unlimited.

Wazlawick, P. (1967). *Pragmatics of human communication: A study of interactional patterns, pathologies, and paradoxes.* New York: W. W. Norton.

Zeig, J. (Ed.) (1982). *Ericksonian approaches to hypnosis and psychotherapy.* New York: Brunner/Mazel.

Chapter # 14

Barbara Dossey's Theory of Integral Nursing

BARBARA MONTGOMERY DOSSEY

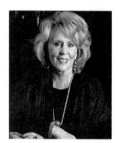

Barbara Montgomery
Dossey

Introducing the Theorist

Barbara Montgomery Dossey, PhD, RN, AHN-BC, FAAN, is internationally recognized as a pioneer in the holistic nursing movement. She is International Co-Director and board member of the Nightingale Initiative for Global Health (NIGH), Washington, DC and Ottawa, Ontario, Canada, and Director, Holistic Nursing Consultants in Santa Fe, New Mexico. She is a Florence Nightingale scholar and an author or co-author of 23 books. Her most recent books include *Holistic Nursing: A Handbook for Practice* (5th ed., 2008), *Being with Dying: Compassionate End-of-Life Care Training Guide* (2007), *Florence Nightingale Today: Healing, Leadership, Global Action* (2005), and *Florence Nightingale: Mystic, Visionary, Healer* (Commemorative Edition, 2010).

Dossey's *Theory of Integral Nursing* (2008) is considered a grand theory that presents the science and art of nursing. Her collaborative global nursing project, the Nightingale Declaration Campaign (NDC), has developed a UN Resolution proposal for adoption—recognizing the contributions of nurses globally as they engage in the promotion of world health, including the United Nations Millennium Development Goals (MDGs). Barbara Dossey is a Fellow of the American Academy of Nursing. She is certified in holistic nursing. She is an nine-time recipient of the prestigious *American Journal of Nursing* Book of the Year Award. She was named the 1985 Holistic Nurse of the Year by the American Holistic Nurses' Association and the 1998 Healer of the Year by the Nurse Healers Professional Associates International, Inc.; she received the 1999 Pioneering Spirit Award from the American Association of Critical Care Nurses and the 1999 Scientific and Medical Network Book of the Year award from the Scientific and Medical Network, United Kingdom. In 2001, she was recognized as TWU 100 Great Nursing Alumni, Texas Woman's University, Denton, Texas. In 2003, she received the Distinguished Alumna Award from Baylor University, Waco, Texas. With her husband, Larry, she received the 2003 Archon Award from Sigma Theta Tau International, the international honor society of nursing, honoring the contributions that they have made to promote global health. In 2004, Barbara and Larry also received the Pioneer of Integrative Medicine Award from the Aspen Center for Integrative Medicine, Aspen, Colorado.

Barbara Dossey is a Nightingale scholar and advocate. For the 72nd General Episcopal Church Convention in Philadelphia July 1997, Barbara wrote three of five documents to accompany the Resolution Proposal to request the reconsideration of Nightingale's commemoration and for her name to be placed on the church calendar list of *Lesser Feasts and Fasts* in the *Book of Common Prayer*. The official vote to accept Nightingale into the church calendar occurred in July 2000. The inaugural Florence Nightingale Commemorative Service was held on August 12, 2001, at the Washington National Cathedral, Washington, DC. To commemorate the 100th year since Nightingale's death in 1910, a Florence Nightingale Centennial Service will be held at the Cathedral April 25, 2010, 4-5 PM.

Overview of the Theory

As you begin to explore the Theory of Integral Nursing, I invite you to reflect on the following questions: Why am I here? What is my life's purpose? How can I strengthen my passion in nursing and in my life? Are my personal and professional actions sourced from my soul's purpose and wisdom? What am I currently doing to become more aware of my personal health and the health of my home and workplace? What am I doing locally that can impact the health and well being of humanity and our Earth? How am I connected to my nursing colleagues and concerned citizens in my community, in other cities and nations? What is my calling?

The Theory of Integral Nursing is a grand theory that guides the science and art of integral nursing practice, education, research, and health care policy. It invites nurses to think widely and deeply about an individual's personal health, as well as that of the local community and the global village. This theory recognizes the philosophical foundation and legacy of Florence Nightingale (1820–1910), (Dossey, 2010; Dossey et al., 2005) healing and healing research, the metaparadigm of nursing (nurse, person(s), health, and environment [society]), six patterns of knowing (personal, empirics, aesthetics, ethics, not knowing, sociopolitical), and several nonnursing theories. It builds on existing theoretical work in nursing and on our solid holistic and multidimensional theoretical nursing foundation of other nurse theorists (see Acknowledgments); it is not a freestanding theory. It incorporates concepts from various philosophies and fields that include holistic, multidimensionality, integral, chaos, spiral dynamics, complexity, systems, and many other paradigms. See Acknowledgments. [***Note:*** *Concepts specific to the Theory of Integral Nursing are in italics throughout this chapter. Please consider these words as a frame of reference and a way to explain what you have observed or experienced with yourself and others.*]

Integral nursing is a comprehensive integral worldview and process that includes holistic theories and other paradigms; holistic nursing is included (embraced) and transcended (goes beyond); this integral process and integral worldview enlarges our holistic nursing knowledge and understanding of body–mind–spirit connections and our knowing, doing, and being to more comprehensive and deeper levels. To delete the word integral or to substitute the word holistic diminishes the impact of the expansiveness of the integral process and integral worldview and its implications.

The Theory of Integral Nursing includes an integral process, integral worldview, and integral dialogues that is *praxis*—theory in action (Dossey, 2008a,b). An *integral process* is defined as a comprehensive way to organize multiple phenomena of human experience and reality from four perspectives: (1) the individual interior (personal/intentional); (2) individual exterior (physiology/behavioral); (3) collective interior (shared/cultural); and (4) collective exterior (systems/structures). An *integral worldview* examines values, beliefs, assumptions, meaning, purpose, and judgments related to how individuals perceive reality and relationships from the four perspectives. *Integral dialogues* are transformative and visionary exploration of ideas and possibilities across disciplines where these four perspectives are considered as equally important to all exchanges, endeavors, and outcomes. With an increased integral awareness and an integral worldview, we are more likely to raise our collective nursing voice and power to engage in social action in our role and work of service for society—local to global.

As you read this chapter, 15 million nurses and midwives are engaged in nursing and health care around the world (NIGH, 2007). Together, we are collectively addressing human health—of individuals, of communities, of environments (interior and exterior) and the world as our first priority. We are educated and prepared—physically, emotionally, socially, mentally, and spiritually—to accomplish the required activities effectively—on the ground—to create a healthy world. Nurses are key in mobilizing new approaches in health education and health care delivery in all areas of the profession and society as a whole. Theories, solutions, and evidence-based practice protocols can be shared and implemented around the world through dialogues, the Internet, and publications.

We are challenged to "act locally and think globally" and to address ways to create healthy environments (Dossey et al., 2005). For example, we can address global warming in our personal habits at home as well as in our workplace (using green products, turning off lights when not in the room, using water efficiently) and simultaneously address our personal health and the health of the communities where we live. In 2000, the United Nations Millennium Goals were recommended to articulate clearly how to achieve health and decrease health disparities (United Nations, 2000). As we expand our awareness of individual and collective states of healing consciousness and integral dialogues, we are able to explore integral ways of knowing, doing, and being. We can unite 15 million nurses, midwives, and concerned citizens through the Internet to create a healthy world through many endeavors such as the Nightingale Declaration (Dossey et al., 2007; NIGH, 2007). You are invited to sign the Nightingale Declaration at http://www.nightingaledeclaration.net. Our Nightingale nursing legacy, as discussed in the next section, is foundational to the Theory of Integral Nursing and to understanding our important roles as 21st-century nurses.

Philosophical Foundation: Florence Nightingale's Legacy

Florence Nightingale (1820–1910), the philosophical founder of modern secular nursing and the first recognized nurse theorist, was an *integralist*. Her worldview focused on the individual and the collective, the inner and outer, and human and nonhuman concerns. She identified environmental determinants (clean air, water, food, houses, etc.) and social determinants (poverty, education, family relationships, employment), from local to global. She also experienced and recorded her personal understanding of the connection with the Divine, the awareness that something greater than she, the Divine, was present in all aspects of her life.

Nightingale's work was *social action* that clearly articulated the science and art of an integral worldview for nursing, health care, and humankind. Her social action was also *sacred activism* (Harvey, 2007), the fusion of the deepest spiritual knowledge with radical action in the world. Nightingale was ahead of her time; her dedicated and focused 50 years of work and service still inform and impact the nursing profession and our global mission of health and healing. In the 1880s, Nightingale began to write in letters that it would take 100 to 150 years before sufficiently educated and experienced nurses would arrive to change the health care system. We are that generation of 21st-century Nightingales who can transform health care and carry forth her vision to create a healthy world.

Personal Journey Developing the Theory of Integral Nursing

As a young nurse attending my first nursing theory conference in the late 1960s, I was captivated by nursing theory and the eloquent visionary words of these theorists as they spoke about the science and art of nursing. This opened my heart and mind to the exploration and necessity to understand and use nursing theory. Thus, I began my professional commitment to address theory in all endeavors as well as to increase my knowledge of other disciplines that could inform a deeper understanding about the human experience. I realized that nursing was not an either "science" or "art", but both. From the beginning of my critical care and cardiovascular nursing focus, I learned how to combine science and technology with the art of nursing. For example, for patients with severe pain after an acute myocardial infarction, I gave pain medication while simultaneously guiding them in a relaxation or imagery practice to enhance relaxation and release anxiety. I also experienced a difference in myself when I used this approach to combine the science and art of nursing.

In the late 1960s, I began to study and attend workshops on holistic and mind–body-related ideas as well as read in other disciplines such as systems theory, quantum physics, integral theory, and Eastern and Western philosophy and mysticism. I was reading theorists from nursing and other disciplines that informed my knowing, doing, and being in caring, healing, and holism. My husband, an internist, who was caring for critically ill patients and their families, was with me on this journey of discovery. As we cared for patients and families, some of our greatest teachers, we reflected on how to blend the art of caring–healing modalities with the science of technology and traditional modalities. I discussed these ideas with a critical care and cardiovascular nursing soulmate, Cathie Guzzetta, PhD, RN, AHN-BC, FAAN. We began writing teaching protocols and presenting in critical care courses as well as writing textbooks and articles with other contributors.

My husband and I both had health challenges—mine was postcorneal transplant rejection, and my husband's challenge was blinding migraine headaches. We both began to take courses related to body–mind–spirit therapies (biofeedback, relaxation, imagery, music, meditation, and other reflective practices) and begin to incorporate them into our daily lives. As we strengthened our capacities with self-care and self-regulation modalities, our personal and professional philosophies and clinical practices changed. We took teaching seriously and integrated these modalities into the traditional health care setting that today is called integrative and integral health care.

As a founding member in 1980 of the American Holistic Nurses Association (AHNA), and with my AHNA colleagues, our collective holistic nursing endeavors were recognized as the specialty of holistic nursing by the American Nurses Association (ANA) in November 2006. The *AHNA and ANA Holistic Nursing: Scope and Standards of Practice* were published in June 2007 (AHNA & ANA, 2007). I believe that this important holistic specialty can now be expanded by using an integral lens.

Beginning in 1992 in London, my Florence Nightingale primary, historical research of studying and synthesizing her original letters, army and public health documents, manuscripts, and books, deepened my understanding of her relevance for nursing as Nightingale was indeed an integralist that is discussed later. This led to my Nightingale authorship (Dossey, 2010; Dossey et al., 2005, 2008) and my collaborative Nightingale Initiative for Global Health and the Nightingale Declaration

(NIGH, 2007), the first global nursing internet signature campaign. My professional mission now is to articulate and use the integral process and integral worldview in my nursing and health care endeavors and to explore rituals of healing with many. My sustained nursing career focus with nursing colleagues on wholeness, unity and healing and my Florence Nightingale scholarship have resulted in numerous protocols and standards for practice, education, research, and health care policy. My integral focus since 2000, and my many conversations with Ken Wilber and the integral team and other interdisciplinary integral colleagues, has led to my development of the Theory of Integral Nursing at this time.

Theory of Integral Nursing Developmental Process and Intentions

The Theory of Integral Nursing advances the evolutionary growth processes, stages, and levels of human development and consciousness toward a comprehensive integral philosophy and understanding. It can assist nurses to map human capacities that begin with healing and evolve to the transpersonal self in connection with the Divine, however defined or identified, in their endeavors to create a healthy world.

The intention (purpose) in a nursing theory is the aim of the theory. The Theory of Integral Nursing has three intentions: (1) to embrace the unitary whole person and the complexity of the nursing profession and health care; (2) to explore the direct application of an integral process and integral worldview that includes four perspectives of realities—the individual interior and exterior and the collective interior and exterior; and (3) to expand nurses' capacities as 21st-century Nightingales, health diplomats, and integral nurse coaches for integral health, from local to global.

Integral Foundation and the Integral Model

The Theory of Integral Nursing adapts the work of Ken Wilber, one of the most significant

American new-paradigm philosophers, to strengthen the central concept of healing. His elegant, four-quadrant model was developed over 35 years. In the eight-volume *The Collected Works of Ken Wilber* (Wilber, 1999, 2000), Wilber synthesizes the best known and most influential thinkers to show that no individual or discipline can determine reality or lay claim to all the answers. Many concepts within this integral nursing theory have been researched or are in very formative stages of development within integral medicine, integral health care administration, integral business, integral health care education, and integral psychotherapy (Wilber, 2000a,b, 2005a). Within the nursing profession, other nurses are exploring integral and related theories and ideas. When nurses use an integral lens, they are more likely to expand nurses' roles in transdisciplinary dialogues and to explore commonalities and differences across disciplines (Baye, 2007a,b; Clark, 2006; Fiandt et al., 2003; Frisch, 2008; Jarrin, 2007; Quinn et al., 2003; Watson, 2005; Zahourek, 2008).

Content, Context, and Process

To present the Theory of Integral Nursing, Barbara Barnum's (Barnum, 2004) framework to critique a nursing theory—content, context, and process—provides an organizing framework that is most useful. The philosophical assumptions of the Dossey Theory of Integral Nursing are as follows:

1. An integral understanding recognizes the individual as an energy field connected to the energy fields of others and the wholeness of humanity; the world is open, dynamic, interdependent, fluid, and continuously interacting with changing variables that can lead to greater complexity and order.

2. An integral worldview is a comprehensive way to organize multiple phenomena of human experience from four perspectives of reality: (a) individual interior (subjective, personal); (b) individual exterior (objective, behavioral); (c) collective interior (interobjective, cultural); and (d) collective

exterior (interobjective, systems/ structures).

3. Healing is a process inherent in all living things; it may occur with curing of symptoms, but it is not synonymous with curing.

4. Integral health is experienced by a person as wholeness with development toward personal growth and expanding states of consciousness to deeper levels of personal and collective understanding of one's physical, mental, emotional, social, and spiritual dimensions.

5. Integral nursing is founded on an integral worldview using integral language and knowledge that integrates integral life practices and skills each day.

6. Integral nursing is broadly defined to include knowledge development and all ways of knowing.

7. An integral nurse is an instrument in the healing process and facilitates healing through her or his knowing, doing, and being.

8. Integral nursing is applicable in practice, education, research, and health care policy.

Content Components

Content of a nursing theory includes the subject matter and building blocks that give a theory its form. It comprises the stable elements that are acted on or that do the acting. In the Theory of Integral Nursing the subject matter and building blocks are (1) healing; (2) the metaparadigm of nursing; (3) patterns of knowing; (4) the four quadrants that are adapted from Wilber's (2000b) integral theory (individual interior [subjective, personal/ intentional], individual exterior [objective, behavioral], collective interior [intersubjective, cultural], and collective exterior [interobjective, systems/structures]); and (5) Wilber's (2000b) "all quadrants, all levels, all lines" (Wilber, 2006).

Content Component 1: Healing. The first content component in a Theory of Integral Nursing is *healing*, illustrated as a diamond shape in Figure 14-1A. The Theory of Integral Nursing enfolds from the central core concept of healing. Healing includes knowing, doing,

Figure 14 • 1 *A*, Healing.

and being, and is a lifelong journey and process of bringing together aspects of oneself at deeper levels of harmony and inner knowing leading toward integration. This healing process places us in a space to face our fears, to seek and express self in its fullness where we can learn to trust life, creativity, passion, and love. Each aspect of healing has equal importance and value that leads to more complex levels of understanding and meaning.

Healing capacities are inherent in all living things. No one can take healing away from life; however, we often get "stuck" in our healing or forget that we possess it due to life's continuing challenges and perceived barriers to wholeness. Healing can take place at all levels of human experience, but it may not occur simultaneously in every realm. In truth, healing will most likely not occur simultaneously or even in all realms, and yet, the person may still have a perception of healing having occurred (Gaydos, 2005).

Healing embraces the individual as an energy field that is connected with the energy fields of all humanity and the world. Healing is transformed when we consider four perspectives of reality in any moment: (1) the individual interior (personal/intentional), (2) individual exterior (physiology/behavioral), (3) collective interior (shared/cultural), and (4) collective exterior (systems/structures). Using our reflective integral lens of these four perspectives of reality assists us to more likely experience a unitary grasp on the complexity that emerges in healing.

Healing is not predictable; it may occur with curing of symptoms, but it is not synonymous with curing. Curing may not always occur, but the potential for healing is always present even until one's last breath. Intention and intentionality are key factors in healing (Engebretson, 1998; Zahourek,

2004). Intention is the conscious determination to do a specific thing or to act in a specific manner; it is the mental state of being committed to, planning to, or trying to perform an action. Intentionality is the quality of an intentionally performed action.

Content Component 2: Metaparadigm of Nursing. The second content component in the Theory of Integral Nursing is the recognition of the *metaparadigm* in a nurse theory: nurse, person/s, health, and environment (society) (Fig. 14-1B). Starting with healing at the center, a Venn diagram surrounds healing and implies the interrelation, interdependence, and impact of these domains as each informs and influences the others; a change in one will create a degree(s) of change in the other(s), thus impacting healing at many levels. These concepts are important to the Theory of Integral Nursing because they are encompassed within the quadrants of human experience as seen in Content Component 4.

An *integral nurse* is defined as a 21st-century Nightingale. Using terms coined by Patricia Hinton Walker, PhD, RN, FAAN (Walker, 2007) nurses' endeavors of social action and sacred activism engage "nurses as health diplomats" and "integral nurse coaches" that are "coaching for integral health." As nurses

strive to be integrally informed, they are more likely to move to a deeper experience of a connection with the Divine or Infinite, however defined or identified. *Integral nursing* provides a comprehensive way to organize multiple phenomena of human experience in the four perspectives of reality as previously described. The nurse is an instrument in the healing process, bringing her or his whole self into relationship to the whole self of another or a group of significant others and thus reinforcing the meaning and experience of oneness and unity.

A *person(s)* is defined as an individual (patient/client, family members, significant others) who engages with a nurse in a manner that is respectful of a person's subjective experiences about health, health beliefs, values, sexual orientation, and personal preferences. It also includes an individual nurse who interacts with a nursing colleague, other health care team members, or a group of community members or other groups.

Integral health is the process through which we reshape basic assumptions and worldviews about well-being and see death as a natural process of the cycle of life. Integral health may be symbolically seen as a jewel with many facets that is reflected as a "bright gem" or a "rough stone" depending on one's situation and personal growth that influence states of health, health beliefs, and values. The jewel may also be seen as a spiral or as a symbol of transformation to higher states of consciousness to more fully understand the essential nature of our beingness as energy fields and expressions of wholeness. This includes evolving one's state of consciousness to higher levels of personal and collective understanding of one's physical, mental, emotional, social, and spiritual dimensions. It acknowledges the individual's interior and exterior experiences and the shared collective interior and exterior experiences with others where authentic power is recognized within each person. Disease and illness at the physical level may manifest for many reasons and variables. It is important *not* to equate physical health, mental health, and spiritual health, as they are not the same

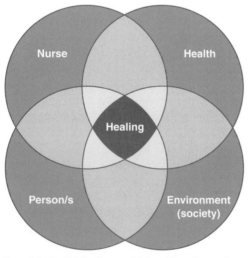

Figure 14 • 1 *B,* Healing and Meta-Paradigm of Nursing.

thing. They are facets of the whole jewel of integral health.

An *integral environment(s)* has both interior and exterior aspects. The *interior* environment includes the individual's mental, emotional, and spiritual dimensions including feelings and meanings as well as the brain and its components that constitute the internal aspect of the exterior self. It includes patterns that may not be understood or may manifest related to various situations or relationships. These patterns may be related to living and nonliving people and things, for example, a deceased relative, pet, lost precious object(s) that surface through flashes of memories stimulated by a current situation (e.g., a touch may bring forth past memories of abuse, suffering). Insights gained through dreams and other reflective practices that reveal symbols, images, and other connections also influence one's internal environment. The *exterior* environment includes objects that can be seen and measured that are related to the physical and social in some form in any of the gross, subtle, and causal levels that are expanded later in Content Component 4.

Content Component 3: Patterns of Knowing. The third content component in a Theory of Integral Nursing is the recognition of the patterns of knowing in nursing (Fig. 14-1C). These six patterns of knowing are personal, empirics, aesthetics, ethics, not-knowing, and sociopolitical. As a way to organize nursing knowledge Carper (1978) in her now classic 1978 article, identified the four fundamental patterns of knowing (personal, empirics, ethics, aesthetics) followed by the introduction of the pattern of not-knowing by Munhall (1993), and the pattern of sociopolitical knowing by White (1995). All of these patterns continue to be refined and reframed with new applications and interpretations (Averill & Clements, 2007; Barnum, 2003; Burhardt, 2008; Chinn & Kramer, 2004; Cowling, 2004; Fawcett et al., 2001; Halifax et al., 2007; Koerner, 2007; McKivergin, 2008; Meleis, 2005; Newman, 2003). These patterns of knowing assist nurses in bringing themselves into a full presence in the moment, to integrate aesthetics with science, and to develop the flow of ethical experience with thinking and acting.

Personal knowing is the nurse's dynamic process of being whole that focuses on the synthesis of perceptions and being with self. It may be developed through art, meditation, dance, music, stories, and other expressions of

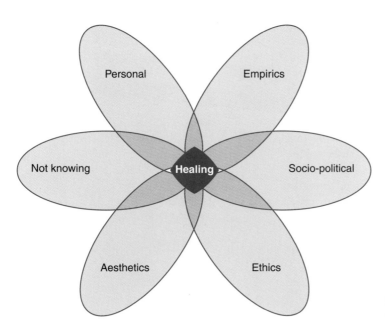

Figure 14 • 1 *C,* Healing and patterns of knowing in nursing.

the authentic and genuine self in daily life and nursing practice.

Empirical knowing is the science of nursing that focuses on formal expression, replication, and validation of scientific competence in nursing education and practice. It is expressed in models and theories and can be integrated into evidence-based practice. Empirical indicators are accessed through the known senses that are subject to direct observation, measurement, and verification.

Aesthetic knowing is the art of nursing that focuses on how to explore experiences and meaning in life with self or another that includes authentic presence, the nurse as a facilitator of healing, and the artfulness of a healing environment (Gaydos, 2004). It calls forth resources and inner strengths from the nurse to be a facilitator in the healing process. It is the integration and expression of all the other patterns of knowing in nursing praxis. By combining knowledge, experience, instinct, and intuition, the nurse connects with a patient/client to explore the meaning of a situation about the human experiences of life, health, illness, and death.

Ethical knowing is the moral knowledge in nursing that focuses on behaviors, expressions, and dimensions of both morality and ethics. It includes valuing and clarifying situations to create formal moral and ethical behaviors intersecting with legally prescribed duties. It emphasizes respect for the person, the family, and the community that encourages connectedness and relationships that enhance attentiveness, responsiveness, communication, and moral action.

Not knowing is the capacity to use healing presence, to be open spontaneously to the moment with no preconceived answers or goals to be obtained. It engages authenticity, mindfulness, openness, receptivity, surprise, mystery, and discovery with self and others in the subjective space and the intersubjective space that allows for new solutions, possibilities, and insights to emerge.

Sociopolitical knowing addresses the important contextual variables of social, economic, geographic, cultural, political, historical, and other key factors in theoretical, evidence-based practice and research. This pattern includes informed critique and social justice for the voices of the underserved in all areas of society along with protocols to reduce health disparities. [*Note: As all patterns of knowing in the Theory of Integral Nursing are superimposed on Wilber's four quadrants these patterns will be primarily positioned as seen; however, they may also appear in one, several, or all quadrants and inform all other quadrants.*]

Content Component 4: Quadrants. The fourth content component in the Theory of Integral Nursing examines four perspectives for all known aspects of reality, or expressed another way, it is how we look at and/or describe anything (Fig. 14-1D). Healing, the core concept in the Theory of Integral Nursing, is transformed by adapting Ken Wilber's integral model (Wilber, 2000b). Starting with healing at the center to represent our integral nursing philosophy, human capacities, and global mission, dotted horizontal and vertical lines illustrate that each quadrant can be understood as permeable and porous, with each quadrant experience(s) integrally informing and empowering all other quadrant experiences. Within each quadrant we see "I," "We," "It," and "Its" to represent four perspectives of realities that are already part of our everyday language and awareness.

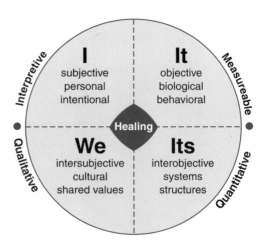

Figure 14 • 1 *D,* Healing and the four quadrants (I, We, It, Its).

Virtually all human languages use first-person, second-person, and third-person pronouns to indicate three basic dimensions of reality (Wilber, 2000b). First-person is "the person who is speaking," which includes pronouns like I, me, mine in the singular, and we, us, ours in the plural (Wilber, 2000b, 2005a). Second-person means "the person who is spoken to," which includes pronouns like you and yours. Third-person is "the person or thing being spoken about," such as she, her, he, him, or they, it, and its. For example, if I am speaking about my new car, "I" am first-person, and "you" are second-person, and the new car is third-person. If you and I are communicating, the word "we" is used to indicate that we understand each other. "We" is technically first person plural, but if you and I are communicating, then you are second person and my first person is part of this extraordinary

"we." So we can simplify first-, second- and third-person as: "I", "we," "it and its."

These four quadrants show the four primary dimensions or perspectives of how we experience the world; these are represented graphically as the upper-left (UL), upper-right (UR), lower-left (LL), and lower-right (LR) quadrants. It is simply the inside and the outside of an individual and the inside and outside of the collective. It includes expanded states of consciousness where one feels a connection with the Divine and the vastness of the universe, the infinite that is beyond words. Integral nursing considers all of these areas in our personal development and any area of practice, education, research, and health care policy—local to global. Each quadrant, which is intricately linked and bound to each other, carries its own truths and language (Wilber, 2000b). The specifics of the quadrants are provided in Figure 14-1E.

Integral Model

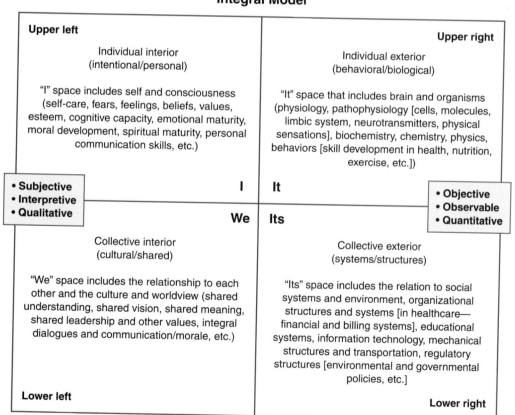

Figure 14 • 1 *E*, Integral Model and quadrants.

- **Upper-left (UL)**. In this "I" space (subjective) can be found the world of the individual's interior experiences. These are the thoughts, emotions, memories, perceptions, immediate sensations, and states of mind (imagination, fears, feelings, beliefs, values, esteem, cognitive capacity, emotional maturity, moral development, and spiritual maturity). Integral nursing starts with "I". (*Note: When working with various cultures, it is important to remember that within many cultures, the "I" comes last or is never verbalized or recognized as the focus is on the "We" and relationships. However, this development of the "I" and an awareness of one's personal values is critical.*)
- **Upper-right (UR)**. In this "It" (objective) space can be found the world of the individual's exterior. This includes the material body (physiology [cells, molecules, neurotransmitters, limbic system], biochemistry, chemistry, physics), integral patient care plans, skill development (health, fitness, exercise, nutrition etc.), behaviors, leadership skills, and integral life practices (see Process and Integral Nursing Principles), and anything that we can touch or observe scientifically in time and space. Integral nursing with our nursing colleagues and health care team members includes the "It" of new behaviors, integral assessment and care plans, leadership and skills development.
- **Lower-left (LL)**. In this "We" (intersubjective) space can be found the interior collective of how we can come together to share our cultural background, stories, values, meanings, vision, language, relationships, and to form partnerships to achieve a healing mission. This can decrease our fragmentation and enhance collaborative practice and deep dialogue around things that really matter. Integral nursing is built upon "We."
- **Lower-right (LR)**. In this "Its" space (interobjective) can be found the world of the collective, exterior things. This includes social systems/structures, networks, organizational structures, and systems (including financial and billing systems in health care), information technology, regulatory structures (environmental and governmental

policies, etc.), any aspect of the technological environment, and the natural world. Integral nursing identifies the "Its" in the structure that can be enhanced to create more integral awareness and integral partnerships to achieve health and healing—local to global.

We see that the left-hand quadrants (UL, LL) describe aspects of reality as interpretive and qualitative (see Fig. 14-1D). In contrast, the right-hand quadrants (UR, LR) describe aspects of reality as measurable and quantitative. When we fail to consider these subjective, intersubjective, objective, and interobjective aspects of reality our endeavors and initiatives become fragmented and narrow, inhibiting our ability to reach meaningful outcomes and goals. The four quadrants are a result of the differences and similarities in Wilber's investigation of the many aspects of identified reality. The model describes the territory of our own awareness that is already present within us and an awareness of things outside of us. These quadrants help us connect the dots of the actual process to more deeply understand who we are, and how we are related to others and all things.

Content Component 5: AQAL (All Quadrants, All Levels). The fifth content component in the Theory of Integral Nursing is the exploration of Wilber's "all quadrants, all levels, all lines, all states, all types" or A-Q-A-L (pronounced ah-qwul), as seen in Figure 14-1F. These levels, lines, states, and types are important elements of any comprehensive map of reality. The integral model simply assists us in further articulating and connecting all areas, awareness, and depth in these four quadrants. Briefly stated, these levels, lines, states, and types are as follows.

- **Levels**: Levels of development that become permanent with growth and maturity (e.g., cognitive, relational, psychosocial, physical, mental, emotional, spiritual) that represent a level of increased organization or level of complexity. These levels are also referred to as waves and stages of development. Each individual possesses both the masculine and the feminine voice or energy. One is not

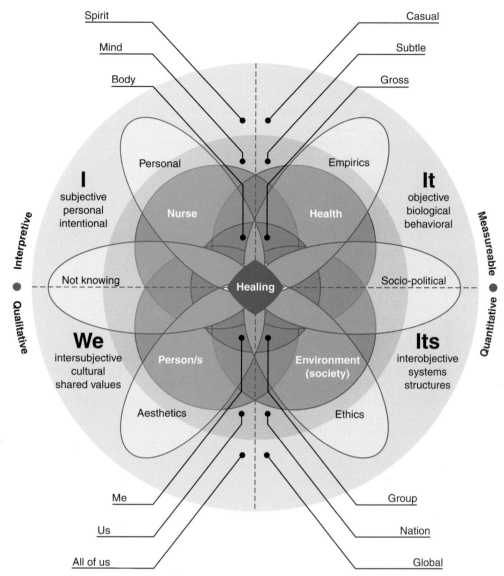

Figure 14 • 1 *F*, Healing and AQAL (all quadrants, all levels).

superior to the other; they are two equivalent types at each level of consciousness and development.

- **Lines**: Developmental areas that are known as multiple intelligences (e.g., cognitive line [awareness of what is]; interpersonal line [how I relate socially to others]; emotional/affective line [the full spectrum of emotions]; moral line [awareness of what should be]; needs line [Maslow's hierarchy of needs]; aesthetics line [self-expression of art,

beauty, and full meaning]; self-identity line [who am I?]; spiritual line [where "spirit" is viewed as its own line of unfolding, and not just as ground and highest state], and values line [what a person considers most important; studied by Clare Graves and brought forward by Don Beck (Beck, 2007) in his Spiral Dynamics Integral that is beyond the scope of this article].

- **States**: Temporary changing forms of awareness (e.g., waking, dreaming, deep sleep, altered meditative states [due to meditation, yoga, contemplative prayer, etc.]; altered states [due to mood swings, physiology and pathophysiology shifts with disease/illness, seizures, cardiac arrest, low or high oxygen saturation, drug-induced]; peak experiences [triggered by intense listening to music, walks in nature, love-making, mystical experiences such as hearing voice of God or voice of a deceased person, etc.].

- **Types**: Differences in personality and masculine and feminine expressions and development (e.g., cultural creative types, personality types, enneagram).

This part of the Theory of Integral Nursing (see Fig. 14-1F) starts with healing at the center surrounded by three increasing concentric circles with dotted lines of the four quadrants. This part of the integral theory moves to higher orders of complexity through personal growth, development, expanded stages of consciousness (permanent and actual milestones of growth and development), and evolution. These levels or stages of development can also be expressed as being self-absorbed (such as a child or infant) to ethnocentric (centers on group, community, tribe, nation) to worldcentric (care and concern for all peoples regardless of race or national origin, color, sex, gender, sexual orientation, creed, and to the global level).

In the UL, the "I" space, the emphasis is on the unfolding "awareness" from body to mind to spirit. Each increasing circle includes the lower as it moves to the higher level.

In the UR, the "It" space, is the external of the individual. Every state of consciousness has a felt energetic component that is expressed from the wisdom traditions as three recognized bodies: gross, subtle, and causal (Wilber, 2000b, 2005). We can think of these three bodies as the increasing capacities of a person toward higher levels of consciousness. Each level is a specific vehicle that provides the actual support for any state of awareness. The *gross* body is the individual physical, material, sensorimotor body that we experience in our daily activities. The *subtle* body occurs when we are not aware of the gross body of dense matter, but of a shifting to a light, energy, emotional feelings, and fluid and flowing images. Examples might be in our shift during a dream, during different types of bodywork, walks in nature, or other experiences that move us to a profound state of bliss. The causal body is the body of the infinite that is beyond space and time. Causal also includes *nonlocality* where minds of individuals are not separate in space and time (Dossey, 1989). When this is applied to consciousness, separate minds behave as if they are linked regardless of how far apart in space and time they may be. Nonlocal consciousness may underlie phenomena such as remote healing, intercessory prayer, telepathy, premonitions, as well as so-called miracles. Nonlocality also implies that the soul does not die with the death of the physical body—hence, immortality forms some dimension of consciousness. Nonlocality can also be both upper and lower quadrant phenomena.

The LL, the "We" space, is the interior collective dimension of individuals that come together. The concentric circles from the center outward represent increasing levels of complexity of our relational aspect of shared cultural values, as this is where teamwork and the interdisciplinary and transpersonal disciplinary development occur. The inner circle represents the individual labeled as *me*; the second circle represents a larger group labeled *us*; the third circle is labeled as *all of us* to represent the largest group consciousness that expands to all people. These last two circles may include people, but also animals, nature, and nonliving things that are important to individuals.

The LR, the "Its" space, the exterior social system and structures of the collective, is represented with concentric circles. An example within the inner circle might be a *group* of health care professionals in a hospital clinic or department or the complex hospital system and structure. The middle circle expands in increased complexity to include a *nation*; the third concentric circle represents even greater increased complexity to the *global* level where the health of all humanity and the world are considered. It is also helpful to emphasize that these groupings are the physical dynamics such as the working structure of a group of health care professionals versus the relational aspect that is a LL aspect, and the physical and technical structural of a hospital or a clinic.

Integral nurses strive to integrate concepts and practices related to body, mind, and spirit (the all-levels) in self, culture, and nature ("all quadrants" part). The individual interior and exterior—"I" and "It"—as well as the collective interior and exterior—"We" and "Its"—must be developed, valued, and integrated into all aspects of culture and society. The AQAL integral approach suggests that we consciously touch all of these areas and do so in relation to self, to others, and the natural world. Yet to be integrally informed does *not* mean that we have to master all of these areas; we just need to be aware of them and choose to integrate integral awareness and integral practices. Because these areas are already part of our being-in-the-world and cannot be imposed from the outside (they are part of our makeup from the inside), our challenge is to identify specific areas for development and find new ways to deepen our daily integral life practices.

Structure

The structure of the Theory of Integral Nursing is shown in Figure 14-1G. All content components are represented together as an overlay that creates a mandala to symbolize wholeness. Healing is placed at the center, then the metaparadigm of nursing, the patterns of knowing, the four quadrants, and all quadrants and all levels of growth, development, and evolution. [*Note: Although the patterns of knowing are superimposed as they are in the various quadrants, they can also fit into other quadrants.*]

Using the language of Ken Wilber (2000b) and Don Beck (Beck, 2007) and his Spiral Dynamics Integral, individuals move through primitive, infantile consciousness to an integrated language that is considered *first-tier* thinking. As they move up the spiral of growth, development, and evolution and expand their integral worldview and integral consciousness, they move into what is *second-tier* thinking and

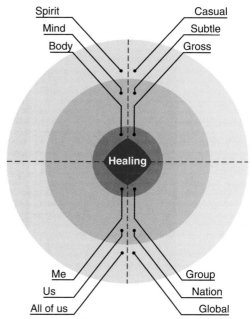

Figure 14 • 1   *G*, Theory of Integral Nursing (healing, metaparadigm, patterns of knowing in nursing, four quadrants, and AQAL).

participation. This is a *radical leap* into holistic, systemic, and integral modes of consciousness. Wilber also expands to a *third-tier* of stages of consciousness that addresses an even deeper level of transpersonal understanding that is beyond the scope of this chapter (Wilber, 2006).

Context

Context in a nursing theory is the environment in which nursing acts occur and the nature of the world of nursing. In an integral nursing environment the nurse strives to be an *integralist*, which means that she or he strives to be integrally informed and is challenged to further develop an integral worldview, integral life practices, and integral capacities, behaviors, and skills. The term *nurse healer* is used to describe that a nurse is an instrument in the healing process and a major part of the external healing environment of a patient or family. An integral nurse values, articulates, and models the integral process and integral worldview and integral life practices and self-care. Nurses assist and facilitate the individual person/s (client/patient, family, and co-workers) to access their own healing process and potentials; they do not do the actual healing. An integral nurse recognizes her/himself as a healing environment interacting with a person, family, or colleague in a *being with* rather than an always *doing to* or *doing for* another person, and enters into a shared experience (or field of consciousness) that promotes healing potentials and an experience of well-being.

Relationship-centered care is valued and integrated as a model of caregiving that is based in a vision of community where three types of relationships are identified: (1) patient–practitioner relationship, (2) community–practitioner relationship, and (3) practitioner–practitioner relationship (Tresoli, 1994). *Relationship-based care* is also valued as it provides the map and highlights the most direct routes to achieve the highest levels of care and serve to patients and families (Koloroutis, 2004).

Process

Process in a nursing theory is the method by which the theory works. An *integral healing process* contains both nurse processes and patient/family and health care workers processes (individual interior and individual exterior), and collective healing processes of individuals and of systems/structures (interior and exterior). This is the understanding of the unitary whole person interacting in mutual process with the environment.

How the Theory of Integral Nursing Guides Nursing Practice

The Theory of Integral Nursing can guide nursing practice and strengthen our 21st-century nursing endeavors. It considers equally important data, meanings, and experiences from the personal interior, the collective interior, the individual exterior, and the collective exterior. Nursing and health care are

fragmented. Collaborative practice has not been realized because only portions of reality are seen as being valid within health care and society.

The nursing profession asks nurses to wrap around "all of life" on so many levels with self and others that we can often feel overwhelmed. So how do we get a handle on "all of life?" The question always arises, How can overworked nurses and student nurses use an integral approach or apply the Theory of Integral Nursing? How do we connect the complexity of so much information that arises in clinical practice? The answer is to start right now. Remember that healing, the core concept in this theory, is the innate natural phenomenon that comes from within a person and reflects the indivisible wholeness, the interconnectedness of all people, all things. This practice situation that follows addresses these questions.

Imagine that you are caring for a very ill patient who needs to be transported to the radiology department for a procedure. The current transportation protocol between the unit and the radiology department lacks continuity. In this moment, shift your feelings and your interior awareness (and believe it!) to: "I am doing the best that I can in this moment," and "I have all the time needed to take a deep breath and relax my tight chest and shoulder muscles." This helps you connect these four perspectives as follows: (1) the interior self (caring for yourself in this moment); (2) the exterior self (using a research-based relaxation and imagery integral practice to change your physiology); (3) the self in relationship to others (shifting your awareness creates another way of being with your patient and the radiology team member); and (4) the relationship to the exterior collective of systems/structures (considering how to work with the radiology team and department to improve a transportation procedure in the hospital).

Professional burnout is high, with many nurses disheartened. Self-care is a low priority; time is not given or valued within practice settings to address basic self-care such as short breaks for personal needs and meals. This is worsened by short staffing and overtime. Also, we do not consistently listen to the pain and suffering that nurses experience within the profession, nor do we consistently listen to the pain and suffering of the patient and family members or our colleagues. Often there is a lack of respect for each other, with verbal abuse occurring on many levels in the workplace.

Nurse retention and a global nursing shortage are at a crisis level throughout the world. As nurses deepen their understanding related to an integral process and integral worldview and use daily integral life practices, we will more consistently be healthy and model health and understand the complexities within healing and society. This enhances nurses' capacities for empowerment, leadership, and acting as change agents for a healthy world.

An integral worldview and approach can help each nurse and student nurse increase her or his self-awareness, as well as the awareness of how self affects others, that is the patient, family, colleagues, and the workplace and community. As the nurse discovers her or his own innate healing from within, he/she is able to model self-care and how to release stress, anxiety, and fear that manifest each day in this human journey. All nursing curricula can be mapped in the integral quadrants so that students learn to think integrally about how these four perspectives create the whole.

Meaning of the Theory of Integral Nursing for Practice

A key concept in the Theory of Integral Nursing is *meaning*, which addresses that which is indicated, referred to, or signified (Dossey, 2003). *Philosophical meaning* is related to one's view of reality and the symbolic connections that can be grasped by reason. *Psychological meaning* is related to one's consciousness, intuition, and insight. *Spiritual meaning* is related to how one deepens personal experience of a connection with the Divine, to feel a sense of oneness, belonging

and feeling of connection in life. In the next section, four integral nursing principles are discussed that provide further insight into how the Theory of Integral Nursing guides nursing practice and meaning in practice. See Figure 14-1F for specifics for each principle.

Integral Nursing Principle 1: Nursing Starts with "I"

Integral Nursing Principle 1 recognizes the interior individual "I" (subjective) space. Each of us must value the importance of exploring one's health and well-being starting with our own personal work on many levels. In this "I" space *integral self-care* is valued, which means that integral reflective practices become part of and can be transformative in our developmental process. This includes how each of us continually addresses our own stress, burnout, suffering, and soul pain. It can assist us to understand the necessity of personal healing and self-care related to nursing as art where we develop qualities of nursing presence and inner reflection.

Nurse presence is also used and is a way of approaching a person in a way that respects and honors the person's essence; it is relating in a way that reflects a quality of "being with" and "in collaboration with." Our own inner work also helps us to hold deeply a conscious awareness of our own roles in creating a healthy world. We recognize the importance of addressing one's own shadow as described by Jung (1981). This is a composite of personal characteristics and potentials that have been denied expression in life and of which a person is unaware; the ego denies the characteristics because they are in conflict and incompatible with a person's chosen conscious attitude.

Mindfulness is the practice of giving attention to what is happening in the present moment such as our thoughts, feelings, emotions, and sensations. To cultivate the capacity of mindfulness practice one may include mindfulness meditation practice, centering prayer, and other reflective practices such as journaling, dream interpretation, art, music, or poetry that leads to an experience of non-separateness and love; it involves developing the qualities of stillness and to be present for one's own suffering that will also allow for full presence when with another.

In our personal process, we recognize *conscious dying* where time and thought is given to contemplate one's own death. Through a reflective practice one rehearses and imagines one's final breath to practice preparing for one's own death. The experience prepares us to not be so attached to material things and spending so much time thinking about the future but living in the moment as often as we can and to live fully until death comes. We are more likely to participate with deeper compassion in the death process and to become more fully engaged in the death process. *Death* is seen as the mirror in which the entire meaning and mystery of life is reflected—the moment of liberation. Within an integral perspective the state of *transparency*, the understanding that there is no separation between our practice and our everyday life is recognized. This is a mature practice that is wise and empty of a separate self.

Integral Nursing Principle 2: Nursing is Built Upon "We"

Integral Nursing Principle 2 recognizes the importance of the "We" (intersubjective) space. In this "We" space nurses come together and are conscious of sharing their worldviews, beliefs, priorities and values related to working together in ways to enhance integral self-care and integral health care. *Deep listening*, the being present and focused with intention to understand what another person is expressing or not expressing is used. *Bearing witness* to others, the state achieved through reflective and mindfulness practices is also valued (Dossey, 2008a,b; Halifax et al., 2007). Through mindfulness one is able to achieve states of *equanimity*, that is, the stability of mind that allows us to be present with a good and impartial heart no matter how beneficial or difficult the conditions; it is being present for the sufferer and suffering just as it is while maintaining a spacious mindfulness in the midst of life's changing conditions. *Compassion*

is where bearing witness and loving kindness manifest in the face of suffering and is part of our integral practice. The realization of the self and another as *not* being separate are experienced; it is the ability to open one's heart and be present for all levels of suffering so that suffering may be transformed for others, as well as for the self. A useful phrase to consider is "I'm doing the best that I can." Compassionate care assists us in living as well as when being with the dying person, the family, and others. We can touch the roots of pain and become aware of new meaning in the midst of pain, chaos, loss, grief, and also in the dying process.

An integral nurse considers *transpersonal* dimensions. This means that interactions with others move from conversations to a deeper dialogue that goes beyond the individual ego; it includes the acknowledgment and appreciation for something greater that may be referred to as spirit, nonlocality, unity, or oneness. Transpersonal dialogues contain an integral worldview and recognize the role of *spirituality* that is the search for the sacred or holy that involves feelings, thoughts, experiences, rituals, meaning, value, direction, and purpose as valid aspects of the universe. It is a unifying force of a person with all that is— the essence of beingness and relatedness that permeates all of life and is manifested in one's knowing, doing, and being; it is usually, though not universally, considered the interconnectedness with self, others, nature, and God/Life Force/Absolute/Transcendent.

Within nursing, health care, and society, there is much suffering (may be physical, mental, emotional, social, spiritual), moral suffering, moral distress, and soul pain. We are often called upon to "be with" these difficult human experiences and to use our nursing presence. Our sense of "We" supports us to recognize the phases of suffering—"mute" suffering, "expressive" suffering, and "new identity" in suffering (Halifax et al., 2007). When we feel alone, as nurses, we experience mute suffering; this is an inability to articulate and communicate with others one's own suffering. Our challenge in nursing is to more skillfully enter into the phase of "expressive" suffering where sufferers seek language to express their frustrations and experiences such as in sharing stories in a group process. Outcomes of this experience often move toward new identity in suffering through new meaning-making wherein one makes new sense of the past, interprets new meaning in suffering, and can envision a new future. A shift in one's consciousness allows for a shift in one's capacity to be able to transform her or his suffering from causing distress to finding some new truth and meaning of it. As we create times for sharing and giving voice to our concerns, new levels of healing may happen.

From an integral perspective, *spiritual care* is an interfaith perspective that takes into account dying as a developmental and natural human process that emphasizes meaningfulness and human and spiritual values. *Religion* is recognized as the codified and ritualized beliefs, behaviors, and rituals that take place in a community of like-minded individuals involved in spirituality. Our challenge is to enter into deep dialogue to more fully understand religions different than our own so that we may be tolerant where there are differences.

Integral action is the actual practice and process that creates the condition of trust wherein a plan of care is co-created with the patient and care can be given and received. Full attention and intention to the whole person, not merely the current presenting symptoms, illness, crisis, or tasks to be accomplished, reinforces the person's meaning and experience of community and unity. Engagement between an integral nurse and a patient and the family or with colleagues is done in a respectful manner; each patient's subjective experience about health, health beliefs, and values are explored. We deeply care for others and recognize our own mortality and that of others.

The integral nurse uses *intention*, the conscious awareness of being in the present moment with self or another person to help facilitate the healing process; it is a volitional act of love. An awareness of the role of *intuition*

is also recognized, which is the perceived knowing of events, insights, and things without a conscious use of logical, analytical processes; it may be informed by the senses to receive information. Integral nurses recognize *love* as the unconditional unity of self with others. This love then generates *loving kindness* and the open, gentle, and caring state of mindfulness that assist one's with nursing presence.

Integral communication is a free flow of verbal and nonverbal interchange between and among people and pets and significant beings such as God/Life Force/Absolute/Transcendent. This type of sharing leads to explorations of meaning and ideas of mutual understanding and growth and loving kindness. *Intuition* is a sudden insight into a feeling, a solution, or problem wherein time and actions and perceptions fit together in a unified experience such as understanding about pain and suffering, or a moment in time with another. This is an aspect that may lead to recognizing and being with the pattern of not knowing.

Integral Nursing Principle 3: "It" Is About Behavior and Skill Development

Integral Nursing Principle 3 recognizes the importance of the individual exterior "It" (objective) space. In this "It" space of the individual exterior each person develops and integrates her or his integral self-care plan. This includes skills, behaviors, and action steps to achieve a fit body and to consider body strength training and stretching, and conscious eating of healthy foods. It also includes modeling integral life skills. For the integral nurse and patient it is also the space where the "doing to" and "doing for" occurs. However, the integral nurse also combines her or his nursing presence with nursing acts to assist the patient to access personal strengths, to release fear and anxiety, and to provide comfort and safety. There is awareness of conscious dying to assist the patient who wishes to have minimal medication and treatment to stay as alert as possible while receiving comfort care until she or he makes their death transition.

Integral nurses, with nursing colleagues and health care team members, compile the data around physiological and pathophysiological assessment, nursing diagnosis, outcomes, plans of care (including medications, technical procedures, monitoring, treatments, traditional and integrative practice protocols), implementation, and evaluation. This is also the space that includes patient education and evaluation. Integral nurses co-create plans of care with patients, when possible combining *caring–healing interventions/modalities* and integral life practices that can interface and enhance the success of traditional medical and surgical technology and treatment. Some common interventions are relaxation, music, imagery, massage, touch therapies, stories, poetry, healing environment, fresh air, sunlight, flowers, soothing and calming pictures, pet therapy, and more.

**Integral Nursing Principle 4:
"Its" Is Systems and Structures**

Integral Nursing Principle 4 recognizes the importance of the exterior collective "Its" (interobjective) space. In this "Its" space integral nurses and the health care team come together to examine their work, their priorities, use of technologies and any aspect of the technological environment, and create exterior healing environments that incorporate nature and the natural world when possible such as with outdoor healing gardens, green materials inside with soothing colors, and sounds of music and nature. Integral nurses identify how they might work together as an interdisciplinary team to deliver more effective patient care and to coordinate care while creating external healing environments.

Application of the Theory of Integral Nursing in Practice, Education, Research, Health Care Policy, Global Nursing

The world is currently anchored in one of the most dramatic social shifts in health care history, and the Theory of Integral Nursing can inform and shape nursing practice, education, research, and policy—local to global—to achieve a healthy world. The Theory of Integral Nursing engages us to think deeply and purposefully about our role as nurses as we face a changing picture of health due to globalization that knows no natural or political boundaries.

Practice

The Theory of Integral Nursing was published in this author's co-authored text in 2008 and is currently being used in many clinical settings. The textbook clearly develops the integral and holistic process and clinical application in traditional settings. It includes guidance about the use of complementary and integrative interventions.

Education

The Theory of Integral Nursing can assist educators to be aware of all quadrants while organizing and designing curriculum, continuing education courses, health education presentations, teaching guides, and protocols. In most nursing curricula there is minimal focus on the individual subjective "I" and the collective intersubjective "We"; the emphasis is on teaching concepts such as physiology and pathophysiology and passing an examination or learning a new skill or procedure. Thus the learner retains only small portions of what is taught. Before teaching any technical skills, the instructor might guide a student or patient in an integral practice such as relaxation and imagery rehearsal of the event to encourage the student to be in the present moment.

At Quinnipiac University, Hamden, Connecticut, Cynthia Barrere, PhD, RN, HNC and Mary Helming, PhD, RN, AHN-BC introduced the Theory of Integral Nursing to their nurse educator colleagues who use the theory in their holistic undergraduate and graduate curricula as they prepare holistic nurses for the future. Darlene Hess, PhD, NP, AHN-BC (Barrere, 2008) has used the Theory of Integral Nursing in her Brown Mountain Visions consulting practice to design an RN to BSN curriculum (Hess, 2008). Hess also uses the integral process in her private practice. Diane Pisanos, RNC, MS, NNP (Pisanos, 2008) integrates integral theory and process to organize her life and health coaching practice. Linda Bark, PhD, RN, MCC (Bark, 2007) uses the integral theory and process in her *As One Integral Coaching* and holistic nursing practice.

The Theory of Integral Nursing principles and the integral model were used in 2006 to organize major concepts in an eight-day intensive integral end-of-life care professional training program at Upaya Zen Center, Santa Fe, New Mexico (Halifax et al., 2007). This training program balances didactic presentations and experiential group process work. For every 90 minutes of didactic, there is a related 90 minutes of experiential integral process practices that reinforce the didactic.

Integral Theory is emerging as a distinct academic discipline. More than 500 scholars representing 50 different disciplines gathered at the First Biennial Integral Theory Conference, *Integral Theory in Action: Serving Self, Others & Kosmos* held August 7–10, 2008, at JFK University in Pleasant Hills, California. At the conference, the Theory of Integral Nursing was featured in a plenary session and panel.

Research

A Theory of Integral Nursing can assist nurses to consider the importance of qualitative and quantitative research (Dossey, 2008a,b; Esbjorn-Hargens, 2006). Our challenges in integral nursing are to consider the findings from both qualitative and quantitative data and always consider triangulation of data when appropriate. We must always value introspective, cultural, and interpretive experiences, and expand our personal and collective capacities of consciousness as evolutionary progression towards achieving our goals. In other words, knowledge does emerge from all four quadrants.

Health Care Policy

A Theory of Integral Nursing can guide us to consider many areas related to health care policy. Compelling evidence in all of the health care professions shows that the origins of health and illness cannot be understood by focusing only on the physical body. Only by expanding the equations of health, exemplified by an integral approach or an AQAL approach to include our entire physical, mental, emotional, social, and spiritual dimensions and interrelationships can we account for a host of health events. Some of these include, for example, the correlations, between poverty, poor health and shortened lifespan; job dissatisfaction and acute myocardial infarction; social shame and severe illness; immune suppression and increased death rates during bereavement; improved health and longevity as spirituality and spiritual awareness is increased.

Global Health Nursing

The Theory of Integral Nursing can assist us as we engage in global health partnerships and projects. Global health is the exploration of the emerging value base and new relationships and agendas that emerge when health becomes an essential component and expression of global citizenship (Gostin, 2007; Karpf, 2009; WHO, 2007). It is an increased awareness that health is a basic human right and a global good that needs to be promoted and protected by the global community. Severe health needs exist in almost every community and nation throughout the world as previously described in the UN Millennium Goals (MDGs). Thus, all nurses must raise their voices and speak about global nursing as their health and healing endeavors assist individuals to become healthier. As Nightingale said... "We must create a public opinion, which must drive the government instead of the government having to drive us.... an enlightened public opinion, wise in principle, wise in detail" (Nightingale, 1892).

Practice Exemplar

A nurse can use the Theory of Integral Nursing in any clinical situation; it assists us to integrate the art and science of nursing simultaneously with all actions/interactions. As discussed previously, healing, the core concept, can occur on many levels (physical, mental, emotional, social, spiritual). Having an integral awareness and creating a space for the possibility that healing can occur allows for a unique field of experience. As nurses engage in their own healing, reflective integral practices, personal development and self-care, they literally embody a very special way of being with others. That is, they "walk their talk" of caring-healing. There is a mutual respect for self and others in each encounter as the nurse is always part of the patient's external environment. (See Process section and Integral Nursing Principles.) Even while giving medications and performing various acute care technical skills, a nurse's healing presence in each encounter can reflect a "being with" and "in collaboration with." Nurses must engage in their own development and also personally experience the various reflective practices (relaxation, imagery, reframing) before engaging the patient in these practices.

Background

J. D. is a lean, extroverted, competitive, 6´4" 64-year-old global energy corporate executive who travels internationally. J. D., an avid jogger, had a recent executive physical with normal stress test and blood work and was declared "a picture of good health." His father and paternal grandfather both died of heart attacks in their 60s. He eats a Mediterranean diet when possible and drinks several glasses of wine with meals. He uses a treadmill or runs daily. J. D. has been a widower for 2 years after a tragic head-on automobile accident in which his wife was hit by a DWI driver. He has four grown children who live in the same city who quarrel over loopholes in their inheritance left by their mother and maternal grandmother. The two sons are both

executives and have problems with alcohol abuse. His two daughters are happily married and each has two preschool children.

One Sunday, J. D. placed second in a city marathon and was very disappointed he didn't win. On finishing a morning shower on Monday morning after a restful night's sleep before a scheduled international trip, J. D. had severe back pain. He tried stretching exercises and the pain went away, so he related it to a back strain from the marathon. He then drove to his office and collapsed onto the steering wheel after he parked his car. A friend saw this and immediately called 911. He was taken to a nearby emergency room, where he was immediately assessed and sent for cardiac catheterization where he received a stent to open the complete occlusion of his right coronary artery. Later that night in the CCU, his cardiologist confirmed from his electrocardiogram that he had a severe inferior myocardial infarction with cardiac irritability; a few days later he developed pericarditis secondary to the infarction.

His cardiac situation was even more complicated. His cardiologist informed him that he also had an 80% blockage at the bifurcation in his left anterior descending coronary artery and circumflex that was in a difficult place for a stent. Because he had excellent collateral circulation, he was placed on cardiac medications and told that he would be monitored over the next few months to determine if he needed further invasive procedures or possibly open heart surgery. He was started on gradual CCU cardiac rehabilitation.

J. D. was very quiet when the nurse entered the room after the cardiologist left. The nurse had a hunch that J. D. might want to talk about what he was experiencing. After a brief exchange, the nurse followed with further exploration of the meaning and negative images that he conveyed. She asked him if he wanted to pursue some new ideas that might help him relax as well as his inner healing resources and strengths. He said that he would. This encounter took 10 minutes.

Nurse: In your recovery now with your heart healing, how do you experience your healing?

J. D.: There is this sac around my heart; every time I take a deep breath, my breath is cut off by the pain [pericarditis]. My heart is like a broken vase. I don't think it is healing.

Nurse: I can understand some of your frustration and concern. However, some important things that are present right now show me that you are better than when you first came to the CCU. Your persistent chest pain is gone and your heartbeats are now regular, which shows that the stent is very effective. If you focus on what is going right, you can help your heart and lift your spirits. Let me share some ideas so that you might be able to shift to some positive thoughts.

J. D.: I don't know if I can.

Nurse: I would like to show you how to breathe more comfortably. Place your right hand on your upper chest, and your left hand on your belly, and begin to breathe with your belly. With your next breath in, through your nose, let the breath fill your belly with air. And as you exhale through your mouth, let your stomach fall back to your spine. As you focus on this way of breathing, notice how still your upper chest feels.

J. D.: (After three complete breaths). This is the easiest breathing I've done today.

Nurse: As you focused on breathing with your belly, you let go of fearing the discomfort with your breathing. Can you tell me more about the image you have of your heart as a broken vase?

J. D.: I saw this crack down the front of my heart right after the doctor told me about my big arteries that have the 80% blockage. This is very scary.

Nurse: (Taking a small plastic bag full of crayons out of her pocket and picking up a piece of paper). Is it possible for you to choose a few crayons and draw your broken heart using those images you just talked about?

J. D.: I can't draw.

Nurse: This has nothing to do with drawing, but something usually happens when you place a few marks to create an image of your words.

J. D.: Do you mean the image of a broken vase?

He began to place an image on the paper. When halfway through with the drawing he said, "I know this sounds crazy, but my father had a heart attack when he was 63. I was visiting my parents. Dad hadn't been feeling well, even complained of his stomach hurting that morning. He was in the living room, and as he fell, he knocked over a large Chinese porcelain vase that broke in two pieces. I can remember so clearly running to his side. I can see that vase now, cracked in a jagged edge down the front. He made it to the hospital, but died 2 days later. You know, I think that might be where that image of a broken heart came from."

Nurse: Your story contains a lot of meaning. Remembering this image and event can be very helpful to you in your healing. What are some of the things that you are most worried about just now?

J. D.: Dying young.

Tears filled his eyes. "I have this funny feeling in my stomach just now. I don't want to die. I'm too young. I have so much to contribute to life. I've been driving myself to excess at work. I need to learn to relax and manage my stress and change my life."

Nurse: J. Each day you are getting stronger. This time over the next few weeks can be a time to reflect on what are the most important things in your life. Whenever you feel discouraged, let images come to you of a beautiful vase that has a healed crack in it. This is exactly what your heart is doing right now. Even as we are talking, the area that has been damaged is healing. As it heals, there will be a solid scar that will be very strong, just in the same way that a vase can be mended and become strong again. New blood supplies also come into the surrounding area of your

Continued

Practice Exemplar cont.

heart to help it heal. Positive images can help you heal, because you send a different message from your mind to your body when you are relaxed and thinking about becoming strong and well. You help your body, mind, and spirit function at their highest level. Is it possible for you to once again draw an image of your heart as a healed vase, and notice any difference in your feelings?

J. D.: Thanks for this talk. With a smile, he picked up several crayons and began to draw a healing image to encourage hope and healing.

When J. D. entered the outpatient cardiac rehabilitation program he was motivated to learn stress management skills and express his emotions. Two weeks into the program, J. D. did not appear to be his usual extroverted self. The cardiac rehabilitation nurse engaged him in conversation, and before long, he had tears in his eyes. He stated that he was very discouraged about having heart disease. He said, "It just has a grip on me." The nurse took him into her office and they continued the dialogue. After listening to his story, she asked J. D. if he would like to explore his feelings further. He nodded yes. This next session took 15 minutes.

To facilitate the healing process, she thought it might be helpful to have J.D. get in touch with his images and their locations in his body. She began by saying, "If it seems right to you, close your eyes and begin to focus on your breathing just now." She guided him in a general exercise of head-to-toe relaxation, accompanied by an audiocassette music selection of sounds in nature. As his breathing patterns became more relaxed and deeper, indicating relaxation, she began to guide him in exploring "the grip" in his imagination.

Nurse: Focus on where you experience the grip. Give it a size, … a shape, … a sound, … a texture, … a width, … and a depth.

J. D.: It's in my chest, but not like chest pain. It's dull, deep, and blocks my knowing

what I need to think or feel about living. I can't believe that I'm using these words. Well, it's bigger than I thought. It's very rough, like heavy jute rope tied in a knot across my chest. It has a sound like a rope that keeps a sailboat tied to a boat dock. I'm now rocking back and forth. I don't know why this is happening.

Nurse: Stay with the feeling, and let it fill you as much as it can. If you need to change the experience, all you have to do is take several deep breaths.

J. D.: It's filling me up. Where are these sounds, feelings, and sensations coming from?

Nurse: They are coming from your wise, inner self, your inner healing resources. Just let yourself stay with the experience. Continue to use as many of your senses as you can to describe and feel these experiences.

J. D.: Nothing is happening. I've gone blank.

Nurse: Focus again on your breath in … and feel the breath as you let it go. … Can you allow an image of your heart to come to you under that tight grip?

J. D.: It is so small I can hardly see it. It's all wrapped up.

Nurse: In your imagination, can you introduce yourself to your heart as if you were introducing yourself to a person for the first time? Ask your heart if it has a name?

J. D.: It said hello, but it was with a gesture of hello, no words.

Nurse: That is fine. Just say, "Nice to meet you," and see what the response might be.

J. D.: My heart seems like an old soul, very wise. This feels very comfortable.

Nurse: Ask your heart a question for which you would like an answer. Stay with this and listen for what comes.

After long pause:

J. D.: The answer is practice patience that I am on the right track, that my heart disease has a message, don't know what it is.

Nurse: Just stay with your calmness and inner quiet. Notice how the grip has changed for you. There are many more answers to come for you. This is your wise self that has much to offer you. Whenever you want, you can get back to this special kind of knowing. All you have to do is take the time. When you set aside time to be quiet with your rich images, you will get more information. You might also find special music to assist you in this process. … Your skills with this way of knowing will increase each time you use this process … now that whatever is right for you in this moment is unfolding, just as it should. In a few moments, I will invite you back into a wakeful state. On five, be ready to come back into the room and feel wide-awake and relaxed. One … two … three … four … eyelids lighter, taking a deep breath … and five, back into the room, awake and alert, ready to go about your day.

J. D.: Where did all that come from? I've never done that before.

Nurse: All of these experiences are your inner healing resources that are always with you to help you recognize quality and purpose in living each day. All you have to do is take the time to remember to use them and direct your self-talk and images towards a desired outcome. If you want, I can teach and share more of these skills.

J. D.: Ever since my wife died I have had a sense of what is the meaning of my life, what is my purpose. Some days I feel like I have lost my soul. I go through my days doing and doing, and yes I do accomplish a lot. But deep down I am not happy. I have been asking myself the question, "What am I doing…or NOT doing…that is feeding the problems I don't want and believing that I can find happiness out there. Today with you in this experience a light switch got turned on in me. My happiness is buried inside me. I have to gain access to it again somehow. I try to fix my kids by giving them more money. I actually don't really sit down with them. Sometimes I feel like I don't really

know anything about them. I have grandkids that I rarely see. I get frustrated with my corporation as I feel we are contributing to environmental pollution. We (the corporation) can do more about changing this. You helped me identify my needs and how I can contribute differently. I feel a new kind of ownership about my life."

Evaluation and Outcomes

Together the patient and the nurse evaluate an encounter and determine whether the relaxation and imagery experience were useful and discuss future outcomes. Such sessions frequently open up profound information and possibilities. To evaluate the session further, the nurse may again explore the subjective effects of the experience with the patient. Relaxation and imagery are integral life practices for connecting with our unlimited capabilities and capacities. The patient can experience more self-awareness, self-acceptance, self-love, and self-worth. These integral life practices can be transferred to daily life as resources for self-care. The best way to develop confidence and skill in using relaxation and imagery in a clinical setting is for the nurse to embody these practices in her or his own life as a part of personal self-care and enrichment.

Learning how to be authentic and fresh in interactions and in each moment can be enhanced as we learn to bear witness by deep listening and "simply noticing" what is going on. It is so easy to get locked into our analytical logic that we block ourselves from reaching into our hearts and moving into our intuitions or emotions. With time and practice, we give space to what might appear. Both good and negative thoughts always contain some wisdom. After such a patient encounter, it is a time to really reflect on what happened: how did you stay focused for the patient and stay in the moment? In this kind of encounter, we can never predict what will happen. As we engage in our work, our challenge is to be

Continued

Practice Exemplar cont.

aware of learning to bear witness and not try to fix anything and just to explore the moment with self and other(s). It seems that when we least expect it, we might experience or access a deeper place on inner wisdom. Reflection is often how the contrast of the light and shadow, the "dark nights of the soul" are resolved.

■ Summary

The Theory of Integral Nursing addresses how we can increase our integral awareness, our wholeness and healing, and strengthen our personal and professional capacities to more fully open to the mysteries of life's journey and the wondrous stages of self-discovery with self and others. There are many opportunities to increase our integral awareness, application, and understanding each day. Reflect on all that you do each day in your work and life—analyzing, communicating, listening, exchanging, surveying, involving, synthesizing, investigating, interviewing, mentoring, developing, creating, researching, teaching, and creating new schemes for what is possible. Before long, you will realize how all these four quadrants and realities fit together. You might find you are completely missing a quadrant, thus an important part of reality. As we address and value the individual interior and exterior, the "I" and "It," as well as the collective interior and exterior, the "We" and "Its" a new level of integral understanding emerges and we may find that there is also more balance and harmony each day.

Our time demands a new paradigm and a new language where we take the best of what we know in the science and art of nursing that includes holistic and human caring theories and modalities. With an integral approach and worldview we are in a better position to share with others the depth of nurses' knowledge, expertise, and critical-thinking capacities and skills for assisting others in creating health and healing. Only an attention to the heart of nursing, for "sacred" and "heart" reflect a common meaning, can we generate the vision, courage, and hope required to unite nursing in healing. This assists us as we engage in health care reform to address the challenges in these troubled times—local to global. It is not an abstract matter of philosophy, but of survival.

See Barbara Dossey's Web site at http://www.dosseydossey.com to download the Theory of Integral Nursing PowerPoint and one-page handout

References

American Holistic Nurses Association and the American Nurses Association. (2007). *American Holistic Nurses Association and the American Nurses Association Holistic Nursing Practice: Scope and Standards.* Silver Spring, MD: Nursesbooks.org.

Averill, J. B., & Clements, P. T. (2007). Patterns of knowing as a foundation for action-sensitive pedagogy. *Qual Health Research, 17*(3), 386-399.

Bark, L. (2007). As one coaching. Retrieved from http://www.asonecoaching.com (Accessed August 1, 2007).

Barnum, B. (2003). *Spirituality in nursing: From traditional to new age* (2nd ed.). New York: Springer.

Barnum, B. S. (2004). *Nursing theory: Analysis, application, evaluation* (6th ed.). Philadelphia: Lippincott Williams & Wilkins.

Barrere, C. C. (2008). Teaching our future holistic nurses: Integrating holism into an Undergraduate Nursing Curriculum. In: B. M. Dossey & L. Keegan (Eds.), *Holistic nursing: A handbook for practice* (5th ed., pp. 709-717). Sudbury, MA: Jones and Bartlett.

Baye, J. Nursing in Canada with the integral framework. Personal communication, June 25, 2007.

Baye, J. Royal Jubilee Hospital pre-acudose deployment integral assessment. Personal communication, June 25, 2007.

Beck, D. (2007). Spiral dynamics integral. Retrieved from http://www.spiraldynamics.net (Accessed July 20, 2007).

Burkhardt, M. A., & Najai-Jacobson, M. G. (2008). Spirituality and healing. In: B. M. Dossey & L. Keegan (Eds.), *Holistic nursing: A handbook for practice* (5th ed.). Sudbury, MA: Jones and Bartlett.

Carper, B. A. (1978). Fundamental patterns of knowing in nursing. *Advances in Nursing Science, 1*(1), 13–23.

Chinn, P. L., & Kramer, M. K. (2004). *Theory and nursing: Integrated knowledge development* (6th ed.). St. Louis, MO: C. V. Mosby.

Clark, C. S. (2006). An integral nursing education: Exploration of the Wilber quadrant model. *International Journal of Human Caring, 10*(3), 22–29.

Cowling, W. R. (2004). Pattern, participation, praxis, and power in unitary appreciative inquiry. *Advances in Nursing Science, 27*(3), 202–214.

Dossey, B. (2010). *Florence Nightingale: Mystic, visionary, healer.* (Commemorative Edition) Philadelphia: F. A. Davis.

Dossey, B. M. (2008a). Integral and holistic nursing. In: B. M. Dossey & L. Keegan (Eds.), *Holistic nursing: A handbook for practice* (5th ed., pp. 1–46). Sudbury, MA: Jones and Bartlett.

Dossey, B. M. (2008b). Theory of Integral Nursing. *Advances in Nursing Science, 31*(1), E52–73.

Dossey, B. M., Beck, D. M., & Rushton, C. H. (2008). Nightingale's vision for collaboration. In: S. Weinstein & A. M. Brooks (Eds.), *Nursing without borders: Values, wisdom and success markers.* Indianapolis, IN: Sigma Theta Tau. .

Dossey, B. M., Selanders, L. C., Beck, D. M., & Attewell, A. (2005). *Florence Nightingale today: Healing, leadership, global action.* Washington, DC: NurseBooks.org.

Dossey, L. (2003). Samueli conference on definitions and standards in healing research: Working definitions and terms. *Alternative Therapies in Health and Medicine, 9*(3), A11.

Dossey, L. (1989). *Recovering the soul: A scientific and spiritual search.* New York: Bantam.

Engebretson, E. (1998). A heterodox model of healing. *Alternative Therapy in Health and Medicine, 4*(2), 37–43.

Esbjorn-Hargens, S. (2006). Integral research: A multi-method approach to investigating phenomena. *Constructivism in the Human Sciences, 11*(1), 79–107.

Fawcett, J., Watson, J., Neuman, B., Walker, P. H., & Fitzpatirck, J. J. (2001). On nursing theories and evidence. *Journal of Nursing Scholarship, 33*(2), 115–119. ff102–105.

Fiandt, K., Forman, J., Megel, M. E., Pakieser, R. A., & Burge, S. (2003). Integral nursing: An emerging framework for engaging the evolution of the profession. *Nursing Outlook, 51*(3), 130–137.

Frisch, N. C. (2008). Nursing theory in holistic nursing practice. In: B. Dossey & L. Keegan (Eds.), *Holistic nursing: A handbook for practice* (5th ed.). Sudbury, MA: Jones and Bartlett.

Gaydos, H. L. (2004). The co-creative aesthetic process: A new model for aesthetics in nursing. *International Journal of Human Caring, 7,* 40–43.

Gaydos, H. L. (2005). The experience of immobility due to trauma. *Holistic Nursing Practice, 19*(1), 40–43.

Gostin, L. O. (2007). Meeting the survival needs of the world's least healthy people. *JAMA, 298*(2), 225–227.

Halifax, J., Dossey, B. M., & Rushton, C. H. (2007). *Being with dying: Compassionate end-of-life care.* Santa Fe, NM: Prajna Mountain Press.

Harvey, A. (2007). Sacred activism. Retrieved from http://www.andrewharvey.net/sacred_activism.html (Accessed July 18, 2007).

Hess, D. R. (2008). *Curriculum for an RN to BSN program using the theory of integral nursing.* In: B. M. Dossey & L. Keegan (Eds.), *Holistic nursing: A handbook for practice* (5th ed., pp. 38–42). Sudbury, MA: Jones and Bartlett.

International Council of Nurses (ICN). (2004). *The global shortage of registered nurses: An overview of issues and action.* Geneva: International Council of Nurses. Retrieved from http://www.icn.ch/global/shortage.pdf (Accessed April 1, 2007).

Jarrín, O. F. (2007). An integral philosophy and definition of nursing. *AQAL: Journal of Integral Theory and Practice, 2*(4), 79–101.

Jung, C. G. (1981). *The archetypes and the collective unconscious* (2nd ed., vol. 9, part I). Princeton, NJ: Bollingen.

Karpf, T., Swift, R., Ferguson, T., & Lazarus, J. (2008). *Restoring hope: Decent care in the midst of HIV/AIDS.* London: Palgrave MacMillan Press and World Health Organization.

Koerner, J. G. (2007). *Nursing presence: The essence of nursing.* New York: Springer.

Koloroutis, M. (Ed.). (2004). *Relationship-based care: A model for transforming practice.* Minneapolis, MN: Creative Health Care Management.

McKivergin, M. (2008). Nurse as an instrument of healing. In: B. M. Dossey & L. Keegan (Eds.), *Holistic nursing: A handbook for practice* (5th ed.). Sudbury, MA: Jones and Bartlett..

Meleis, A. L. (2005). *Theoretical nursing: Development and progress* (3rd. ed. rev.). Philadelphia: Lippincott Williams & Wilkins.

Munhall, P. L. (1993). Unknowing: Toward another pattern of knowing in nursing. *Nursing Outlook, 41*(3), 125–128.

Newman, M. A. (2003). A world of no boundaries. *Advances in Nursing Science, 26*(4), 240–245.

Nightingale, F. Letter to Sir Frederick Verney. 23 November 1892, Add. Mss. 68887.

Nightingale Initiative for Global Health (2007). *Nightingale Declaration.* Retrieved from http://www.nightingaledeclaration.net (Accessed October 12, 2007).

Quinn, J. F., Smith, M., Rittenbaugh, C., Swanson, K., & Watson, J. (2003). Research guidelines for assessing the impact of the healing relationship in clinical nursing. *Alternative Therapies in Health and Medicine, 9*(3), A65–A79.

Tresoli, C. (1994). *Pew-Fetzer Task Force on Advancing Psychosocial Health Education: Health professions education and relationship-centered care.* San Francisco: Commission at the Center for the Health Professions, University of California.

United Nations (2000). *United Nations millennium development goals.* New York: United Nations. Retrieved from http://www.un.org/millenniumgoals/html (Accessed July 20, 2007).

Walker, PhD, RN, FAAN, who coined the terms and concept "nurses as health diplomats," "integral nurse coaches" and "coaching for integral change".

Watson, J. (2005). *Caring science as sacred science.* Philadelphia: F. A. Davis.

White, J. (1995). Patterns of knowing: Review, critique, and update. *Advances in Nursing Science 17*(4), 73–86.

Wilber, K. (1999). *The collected works of Ken Wilber* (vols. 1–4). Boston: Shambhala.

Wilber, K. (2000a). *The collected works of Ken Wilber* (vols. 5–8). Boston: Shambhala.

Wilber, K. (2000b). *Integral psychology.* Boston: Shambhala.

Wilber, K. (2005a). *Integral operating system.* Louisville, CO: Sounds True.

Wilber, K. (2005b). *Integral life practice.* Denver, CO: Integral Institute.

Wilber, K. (2006). *Integral spirituality.* Boston: Shambhala.

World Health Organization (WHO). *Primary care.* Retrieved from http://www.paho.org/English/DD/PIN/ptoday12_nov05.htm (Accessed July 20, 2007).

Zahourek, R. (2008). Holistic nursing research. In: B. Dossey & L. Keegan (Eds.), *Holistic nursing: A handbook for practice* (5th ed.). Sudbury, MA: Jones and Bartlett.

Zahourek, R. (2004). Intentionality forms the matrix of healing: A theory. *Alternative Therapies in Health and Medicine, 10*(6), 40–49.

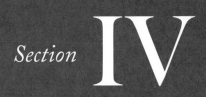

Section IV

Conceptual Models/Grand Theories in the Unitary–Transformative Paradigm

Conceptual Models/Grand Theories in the Unitary–Transformative Paradigm

There are three grand theories clustered in the Unitary–Transformative Paradigm. In this paradigm the human being and environment are conceptualized as irreducible fields, open with the environment. The person and environment are continuously changing and evolving through mutual patterning toward greater complexity. In Chapter 15, Rogers' Science of Unitary Human Beings (SUHB) is explicated by Howard Butcher and Violet Malinski. The SUHB is based on the premise that humans and environments are patterned, pandimensional energy fields in continuous mutual process with each other. Persons participate in their well-being, which is relative and personally defined. Several theories, research traditions, and practice traditions have evolved from this conceptual system. Parse's Humanbecoming School of Thought is featured in Chapter 16, written by the theorist herself. Humanbecoming is defined as a basic human science that has co-created human experiences as its central focus. The School of Thought portends a view that unitary human beings are expert in their own health and lives. For Parse, human beings choose meanings that reflect value priorities co-created in transcending with the possibles. The School of Thought has well-developed research and practice methods that guide the inquiry and practice of nurses embracing humanbecoming. Newman's Theory of Health as Expanding Consciousness (HEC) is explicated in Chapter 17 by Margaret Dexheimer Pharris. According to HEC, health is an evolving unitary pattern of the whole, including patterns of disease. Consciousness, or the informational capacity of the whole, is revealed in the evolving pattern. Pattern identifies the human–environmental process and is characterized by meaning. Concepts important to nursing practice include expanding consciousness, time, presence, resonating with the whole, pattern, meaning, insights as choice points, and the mutuality of the nurse–patient relationship. These concepts are reflected in the praxis method developed to guide practice-research.

Chapter 15

Martha E. Rogers' Science of Unitary Human Beings

HOWARD KARL BUTCHER AND
VIOLET M. MALINSKI

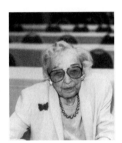

Martha E. Rogers

Introducing the Theorist

Martha E. Rogers, one of nursing's foremost scientists, was a staunch advocate for nursing as a basic science from which the art of practice would emerge. A common refrain throughout her career was the need to differentiate skills, techniques, and ways of using knowledge from the body of knowledge that would guide practice to promote well-being for humankind. "The practice of nursing is not nursing. Rather, it is the use of nursing knowledge for human betterment" (Rogers, 1994a, p. 34). Rogers identified the human–environmental mutual process as nursing's central focus, not health and illness. She repeatedly emphasized the need for nursing science to encompass human beings in space as well as on Earth. Who was this visionary who introduced a new worldview to nursing?

Martha Elizabeth Rogers was born in Dallas, Texas, on May 12, 1914, a birthday she shared with Florence Nightingale. Her parents soon returned home to Knoxville, Tennessee, where Martha and her three siblings grew up. Rogers spent 2 years at the University of Tennessee in Knoxville before entering the nursing program at Knoxville General Hospital. Next, she attended George Peabody College in Nashville, Tennessee, where she earned her Bachelor of Science degree in public health nursing, choosing that field as her professional focus. Rogers spent the next 13 years in rural public health nursing in Michigan, Connecticut, and Arizona, where she established the first visiting nurse service in Phoenix, serving as its executive director (Hektor, 1989/1994). Recognizing the need for advanced education, in 1945 she earned a master's degree in nursing from Teachers College, Columbia University, in the program developed by another nurse theorist, Hildegard Peplau. In 1951 she left public health nursing in Phoenix to return to academia, this time earning a master's of public health and a doctor of science degree from Johns Hopkins University in Baltimore, Maryland.

In 1954, Rogers was appointed head of the Division of Nursing at New York University (NYU), beginning the second phase of her career overseeing baccalaureate, master's, and doctoral programs in nursing and developing the nursing science she knew was integral to the knowledge base nurses needed. She articulated the need for a "valid baccalaureate education" that would serve as the basis for graduate and doctoral studies in nursing. Such a program, she believed, required 5 years of study in theoretical content in nursing, as well as liberal arts and the biological, physical, and social sciences. Under her leadership, NYU established such a program. At the doctoral level, Rogers opposed the federally funded nurse-scientist doctoral programs that prepared nurses in disciplines other than the science of nursing. During the 1960s, she successfully shifted the focus of doctoral research from nurses and their functions to humans in mutual process with the environment. She wrote three books that explicated her ideas: *Educational Revolution in Nursing* (1961), *Reveille in Nursing* (1964), and the landmark *An Introduction to the Theoretical Basis of Nursing* (1970). From 1963 to 1965 she edited *Nursing Science*, a journal that was far ahead of its time; it offered content on theory development, the emerging science of nursing, as well as research and issues in education and practice.

In 1974, Rogers and a number of nursing colleagues established the Society for Advancement in Nursing. Among other issues, this group supported differentiation in education and practice for professional and technical careers in nursing. They drafted legislation to amend the Education Law in New York State, proposing licensure as an independent nurse (IN) for those who had a minimum of a baccalaureate degree. The group also introduced a new exam and licensure as a registered nurse (RN) for those with either a diploma or an associate degree in nursing who passed the traditional boards (Governing Council of the Society for Advancement in Nursing, 1977/1994).

Rogers is best remembered for the paradigm she introduced to nursing that displays her visionary, future-oriented perspective. Early stages of theoretical ideas appeared in her 1961 and 1964 books and were more fully developed in the 1970 book, then revised and refined in a number of articles and book chapters written between 1980 and 1994. She helped create the Society of Rogerian Scholars, Inc., chartered in New York in 1988, as one avenue for furthering the development of her nursing science. Rogers' (1970, 1980, 1988, 1992) Science of Unitary Human Beings is a major conceptual system unique to nursing that offers nurses a radically new way of viewing persons and their universe. It is congruent with the most contemporary emerging scientific theories describing a worldview of wholeness (Bohm, 1980; Briggs & Peat, 1984, 1989; Capra, 1996; Lovelock, 1991; Mitchell, 1996; Sheldrake, 1988; Talbot, 1991; Woodhouse, 1996). Although the Science of Unitary Human Beings was first postulated nearly 40 years ago, scientific support for her postulates of energy fields, pandimensionality, openness, and pattern is increasing every year (Capra, 2002; Gleick, 2000; Green, 1999; Kaku, 2005; Laszlo, 1996; Lorenz, 1994; McTaggert, 2008; Radin, 2006; Randall, 2005; Rosenblum & Kuttner, 2006). Boxes 15-1 and 15-2 provide additional information on hospitals that currently use her work, see Applications of the Conceptual System section on page 261.

Rogers died in 1994, leaving a rich legacy in her writings on nursing science, the space age, research, education, and professional and political issues in nursing.

Overview of Rogers' Science of Unitary Human Beings

The historical evolution of the Science of Unitary Human Beings has been described by Malinski and Barrett (1994). This chapter presents the science in its current form and identifies work in progress to expand it further.

Rogers' Worldview

Rogers (1992) identified the need for and articulated a new worldview in nursing, one that was commensurate with new knowledge emerging across disciplines, which rooted nursing science in "a pandimensional view of people and their world" (p. 28). Rogers (1994a) identified the unique focus of nursing as "the irreducible human being and its environment, both defined as energy fields" (p. 33). "Human" encompasses both *Homo sapiens* and *Homo spatialis*, the evolutionary transcendence of humankind as we voyage into space, and environment encompasses outer space, the cosmos itself.

Beginning in 1968, Rogers described the new worldview underpinning her conceptual system to students and colleagues. It has been available in print with some revisions in language since 1986 (Madrid & Winstead-Fry, 1986; Malinski, 1986a; Rogers, 1990a, 1990b, 1992, 1994a, 1994b). Rogers (1992) described the evolution from older to newer worldviews in such shifting perspectives as cell theory to field theory, entropic to negentropic universe, three-dimensional to pandimensional, person–environment as dichotomous to person–environment as integral, causation and adaptation to mutual process, dynamic equilibrium to innovative growing diversity, homeostasis to homeodynamics, waking as a basic state to waking as an evolutionary emergent, and closed to open systems. She pointed out that in a universe of open systems, energy fields are continuously open, infinite, and integral with one another. A view of change as predictable, or even probabilistic, yields to change as diverse, creative, innovative, and unpredictable.

Rogers was aware that the world looks very different from the vantage point of the newer view as contrasted with the older, traditional worldview. She pointed out that we are already living in a new reality, one that is "a synthesis of rapidly evolving, accelerating ways of using knowledge" (Rogers, 1994a, p. 33), even if people are not always fully aware that these shifts have occurred or are in process. She urged that nurses be visionary, looking forward and not backward, and not allowing themselves to become "stuck" in the present, in the details of how things are now, but envision how they might be in a universe where continuous change is the only given. Rogers (1994b) cautioned that, although traditional modalities of practice and methods of research serve a purpose, they are inadequate for the newer worldview, which urges nurses to use the knowledge base of Rogerian nursing science creatively to develop innovative new modalities and research approaches that would promote the betterment of humankind.

Postulates of Rogerian Nursing Science

Rogers (1992) identified four fundamental postulates that form the basis of the new reality:

- Energy fields
- Openness
- Pattern
- Pandimensionality (formerly called both four-dimensionality and multidimensionality)

Rogers (1990a) defined the energy field as "the fundamental unit of the living and the non-living," noting that it is dynamic, infinite, and continuously moving (p. 7). Although Rogers did not define energy per se, Todaro-Franceschi's (1999) wide-ranging philosophical study of the enigma of energy sheds light on a Rogerian conceptualization of energy. She highlighted the communal, transformative nature of energy, noting that energy is everywhere and is always changing and actualizing potentials. Energy transformation is the basis of all that is, both in living and dying.

Rogers identified two energy fields of concern to nurses, which are distinct but not separate: the human field and the environmental field. The human field can be conceptualized as person, group, family, or community. Parts have no meaning in unitary science. The human and environmental fields are irreducible; they cannot be broken down into component parts or subsystems. For example, the unitary human is not described as a bio–psycho–sociocultural or body–mind–spirit entity. Rogers (1994b) interpreted such designations as representative of current uses of "holistic," meaning a summation of parts to arrive at the whole, wherein a nurse would assess the domains, subsystems, or components identified, then synthesize the accumulated data to arrive at a picture of the total person. Instead, she maintained that each field, human and environmental, is identified by pattern, defined as "the distinguishing characteristic of an energy field perceived as a single wave" (Rogers, 1990a, p. 7). Pattern manifestations and characteristics are specific to the whole.

Because human and environmental fields are integral with each other, they cannot be separated. They are always in mutual process. A concept such as adaptation, a change in one preceding a change in another, loses meaning in this nursing science. Change occurs simultaneously for human and environment.

The fields are pandimensional, defined as "a non-linear domain without spatial or temporal attributes" (Rogers, 1992, p. 29). Pandimensional reality transcends traditional notions of space and time, which can be understood as perceived boundaries only. Examples of pandimensionality include phenomena commonly labeled "paranormal" that are, in Rogerian nursing science, manifestations of the changing diversity of field patterning and examples of pandimensional awareness.

The postulate of openness resonates throughout the preceding discussion. In an open universe, there are no boundaries other than perceptual ones. Therefore, human and environment are not separated by boundaries. The energy of each flows continuously through the other in an unbroken wave. Rogers repeatedly emphasized that person and environment are themselves energy fields; they do not have energy fields, such as auras, surrounding them. In an open universe, there are multiple potentials and possibilities. Nothing is predetermined or foreordained. Causality breaks down, paving the way for a creative, unpredictable future. People experience their world in multiple ways, evidenced by the diverse manifestations of field patterning that continuously emerge.

Rogers (1992, 1994a) described pattern as changing continuously while giving identity to each unique human–environmental field process. Although pattern is an abstraction, not something that can be observed directly, "it reveals itself through its manifestations" (Rogers, 1992, p. 29). Individual characteristics of a particular person are not characteristics of field patterning. Pattern manifestations reflect the human–environmental field mutual process as a unitary, irreducible whole. Person and environment cannot be examined or understood as separate entities. Pattern manifestations reveal innovative diversity flowing in lower and higher frequency rhythms within the human–environmental mutual field process. Rogers identified some of these manifestations as lesser and greater diversity; longer, shorter, and seemingly continuous rhythms; slower, faster, and seemingly continuous motion; time experienced as slower, faster, and timeless; pragmatic, imaginative, and visionary; and longer sleeping, longer waking, and beyond waking. Beyond waking refers to emergent experiences and perceptions such as hyperawareness, unitive experiences attained in meditation, precognition, déjà vu, intuition, tacit knowing, mystical experiences, clairvoyance, and telepathy. She explained "seems continuous" as "a wave frequency so rapid that the observer perceives it as a single, unbroken event" (Rogers, 1990a, p. 10). This view of the ongoing process of change is captured in Rogers' principles of homeodynamics.

Principles of Homeodynamics

Like adaptation, homeostasis—maintaining balance or equilibrium—is an outdated concept in the worldview represented in Rogerian nursing science. Rogers chose "homeodynamics" to convey the dynamic, ever-changing nature of life and the world. Her three principles of homeodynamics—resonancy, helicy, and integrality—describe the nature and process of change in the human–environmental field process. *Resonancy* specifies the nonlinear, continuous flow of lower and higher frequency wave patterning in the human–environmental field process, the way change occurs.

Both lower and higher frequency awareness and experiencing are essential to the wholeness of rhythmical patterning. As Phillips (1994, p. 15) described it, "[W]e may find that growing diversity of pattern is related to a dialectic of low frequency–high frequency, similar to that of order–disorder in chaos theory. When the rhythmicities of lower-higher frequencies work together, they yield innovative, diverse patterns."

Helicy describes the creative and diverse nature of ongoing change in field patterning. *Integrality* specifies the context of change as the integral human–environmental field process where person and environment are inseparable.

Together the principles suggest that the mutual patterning process of human and environmental fields changes continuously, innovatively, and unpredictably, flowing in lower and higher frequencies. Rogers (1990a, p. 9) believed that they serve as guides both to the practice of nursing and to research in the science of nursing.

Theories Derived from the Science of Unitary Human Beings

Rogers clearly stated her belief that multiple theories can be derived from the Science of Unitary Human Beings. They are specific to nursing and reflect not what nurses do, but an understanding of people and our world (Rogers, 1992). Nursing education is identified

by transmission of this theoretical knowledge, and nursing practice is the creative use of this knowledge. "Research is done in relation to the theories" (Rogers, 1994a, p. 34) to illuminate the nature of the human–environmental field change process and its many unpredictable potentials.

Theory of Accelerating Evolution

The Theory of Accelerating Evolution was derived by Rogers, who purported that the only "norm" is accelerating change. Higher frequency field patterns that manifest growing diversity open the door to wider ranges of experiences and behaviors, calling into question the very idea of "norms" as guidelines. Human and environmental field rhythms are accelerating. We experience faster environmental motion now than ever before, in cars and high-speed trains and planes, for example. It is common for people to experience time as rapidly speeding by. People are living longer. Rather than viewing aging as a process of decline or as "running down," as in an entropic worldview, this theory views aging as a creative process whereby field patterns show increasing diversity in such manifestations as sleeping, waking, and dreaming.

Rogers hypothesized that hyperactive children provide a good example of speeded-up rhythms relative to other children. They would be expected to show indications of faster rhythms, increased motion, and other behaviors indicative of this shift. She expected that relative diversity would manifest in different patterns for individuals within any age cohort, concluding that chronological age is not a valid indicator of change in this system: "[I]n fact, as evolutionary diversity continues to accelerate, the range and variety of differences between individuals also increase; the more diverse field patterns evolve more rapidly than the less diverse ones" (Rogers, 1992, p. 30).

The Theory of Accelerating Evolution provides the basis for reconceptualizing the aging process. Rogers (1970, 1980) used the principle of helicy and the Theory of

Accelerating Evolution to put forward the notion that aging is a continuously creative process of growing diversity of field patterning. Therefore, aging is not a process of decline or "running down." Rather, field patterns become increasingly diverse as we age, as older adults need less sleep; are more satisfied with personal relationships; are better able to handle their emotions; are better able to cope with stress; and have increasing crystallized intelligence, wisdom, and improved problem-solving abilities (Whitbourne, 2008). Butcher (2003) expanded on Rogers "negentropic" view of aging in outlining key elements for a "unitary model of aging as emerging brilliance" that includes replacing ageist stereotypes with new positive images of aging; and developing policies, lifestyles, and technologies that enhance successful aging and longevity. Within a unitary view of aging, later life becomes a potential for growth, "a life imbued with splendor, meaning, accomplishment, active involvement, growth, adventure, wisdom, experience, compassion, glory, and brilliance ..." (Butcher, 2003, p. 64).

Theory of Emergence of Paranormal Phenomena

Another theory derived by Rogers is the Emergence of Paranormal Phenomena, in which she suggests that experiences commonly labeled "paranormal" are actually manifestations of changing diversity and innovation of field patterning. They are pandimensional forms of awareness, examples of pandimensional reality that manifest visionary, beyond waking potentials. Meditation, for example, transcends traditionally perceived limitations of time and space, opening the door to new and creative potentials. Therapeutic touch provides another example of such pandimensional awareness. Both participants often share similar experiences during therapeutic touch, such as a visualization of common features that evolves spontaneously for both, a shared experience arising within the mutual process both are experiencing, with neither able to lay claim to it as a personal, private experience.

The idea of a pandimensional or nonlinear domain provides a framework for understanding paranormal phenomena. A nonlinear domain unconstrained by space and time provides an explanation of seemingly inexplicable events and processes. Rogers (1992) even asserted that within the Science of Unitary Human Beings, psychic phenomena become "normal" rather than "paranormal." Dean Radin, director of the Conscious Research Laboratory at the University of Nevada in Las Vegas, suggests that an understanding of nonlocal connections along with the relationship between awareness and quantum effects provides a framework for understanding paranormal phenomena (Radin, 1997). "Deep interconnectedness" demonstrated by Bell's Theorem embraces the interconnectedness of everything unbounded by space and time. In addition, the work of Dossey (1993, 1999), Nadeau and Kafatos (1999), Sheldrake (1988), and Talbot (1991) explicates the role of nonlocality in evolution, physics, cosmology, consciousness, paranormal phenomena, healing, and prayer.

Within a nonlinear–nonlocal context, paranormal events are our experience of the deep nonlocal interconnections that bind the universe together. Existence and knowing are locally and nonlocally linked through deep connections of awareness, intentionality, and interpretation. Pandimensionality embraces the infinite nature of the universe in all its dimensions and includes processes of being more aware of naturally occurring changing energy patterns. Pandimensionality also includes intentionally participating in mutual process with a nonlinear–nonlocal potential of creating new energy patterns. Distance healing, the healing power of prayer, therapeutic touch, out-of-body experiences, phantom pain, precognition, dejá vu, intuition, tacit knowing, mystical experiences, clairvoyance, and telepathic experiences are a few of the energy field manifestations patients and nurses experience that can be better understood as natural events in a pandimensional universe characterized by nonlinear–nonlocal human–environmental field integrality propagated by increased awareness and intentionality.

Todaro-Franceschi (2006) identified the existence of synchronicity experiences in many who were grieving the loss of a spouse, a pioneering effort in delineating a unitary view of death and dying. From the results of her qualitative study she described how such experiences help the bereaved to relate to their deceased loved ones in a new, meaningful way rather than in the traditional view of learning to let go and move on.

Manifestations of Field Patterning

Rogers' third theory, Rhythmical Correlates of Change, was changed to manifestations of field patterning in unitary human beings, discussed earlier. Here Rogers suggested that evolution is an irreducible, nonlinear process characterized by increasing diversity of field patterning. She offered some manifestations of this relative diversity, including the rhythms of motion, time experience, and sleeping–waking, encouraging others to suggest further examples. The next part of this chapter covers Rogerian science–based practice and research in more detail.

In addition to the theories that Rogers derived, a number of others have been developed by Rogerian scholars that are useful in informing Rogerian pattern–based practice including the Theory of Enlightenment (Hills & Hanchett, 2001) and the Theory of Enfolding Health-as-Wholeness-and-Harmony (Carboni, 1995a). Two additional theories are presented in the text that follows.

Theory of Power as Knowing Participation in Change

Barrett's (1989) Theory of Power as knowing participation in change was derived directly from Rogers' postulates and principles, and it interweaves awareness, choices, freedom to act intentionally, and involvement in creating changes. Power is a natural continuous theme in the flow of life experiences and dynamically describes how humans participate with the environment to actualize their potential. Barrett (1983) pointed out that most theories of power are causal and define power as the ability to influence; prevent; or cause change

with dominance, force, and hierarchy. Power, within a Rogerian perspective, is being aware of what one is choosing to do, feeling free to do it, doing it intentionally, and being actively involved in the change process. A person's ability to participate knowingly in change varies in given situations. Thus, the intensity, frequency, and form in which power manifests vary. Power is neither inherently good nor evil; however, the form in which power manifests may be viewed as either constructive or destructive, depending on one's value perspective (Barrett, 1989). Barrett (1989) stated that her theory does not value different forms of power, but instead recognizes differences in power manifestations.

The Power as Knowing Participation in Change Tool (PKPCT) is a measure of one's relative frequency of power. Barrett (1989) suggests that the Power Theory and the PKPCT may be useful in a wide variety of nursing situations. Barrett's Power Theory is useful with clients who are experiencing hopelessness, suicidal ideation, hypertension, obesity, drug and alcohol dependence, grief and loss, self-esteem issues, adolescent turmoil, career conflicts, marital discord, cultural relocation trauma, or the desire to make a lifestyle change. In fact, all health/illness experiences involve issues concerning knowing participation in change. The nurse invites the client to complete the PKPCT as a means to identify the client's power pattern. To prevent biased responses, the nurse should refrain from using the word "power." The power score is determined on each of the four subscales: awareness, choices, freedom to act intentionally, and involvement in creating changes. The scores are documented as part of the client's pattern profile and shared with the client during voluntary mutual patterning. Scores are considered as a tentative and relative measure of the ever-changing nature of one's field pattern in relation to power.

Instead of focusing on issues of control, the nurse helps the client identify the changes and the direction of change the client desires to make. Using open-ended questions, the nurse and the client mutually explore choices and options and identify barriers preventing change, strategies, and resources to overcome barriers; the nurse facilitates the client's active involvement in creating the changes. For example, asking the questions, "What do you want?" "What choices are open to you now?" "How free do you feel to do what you want to do?" and "How will you involve yourself in creating the changes you want?" can enhance the client's awareness, choice-making, freedom to act intentionally, and his or her involvement in creating change (Barrett, 1998).

A wide range of voluntary mutual patterning strategies may be used to enhance knowing participation in change, including meaningful dialogue, dance/movement/motion, sound, light, color, music, rest/activity, imagery, humor, therapeutic touch, bibliotherapy, journaling, drawing, and nutrition (Barrett, 1998). The PKPCT can be used at intervals to evaluate the client's relative changes in power.

Theory of Kaleidoscoping in Life's Turbulence

Butcher's (1993) Theory of Kaleidoscoping in Life's Turbulence was derived from Rogers' Science of Unitary Human Beings, chaos theory (Briggs & Peat, 1989; Peat, 1991), and Csikszentmihalyi's (1990) Theory of Flow. It focuses on facilitating well-being and harmony amid turbulent life events. Turbulence is a dissonant commotion in the human–environmental field characterized by chaotic and unpredictable change. Any crisis may be viewed as a turbulent event in the life process. Nurses often work closely with clients who are in a "crisis." The turbulent life event may be an illness, the uncertainty of a medical diagnosis, marital discord, or loss of a loved one. Turbulent life events are often chaotic in nature, unpredictable, and always transformative.

Kaleidoscoping is a way of engaging in a mutual process with clients who are in the midst of experiencing a turbulent life event by mutually flowing with turbulent manifestations of patterning (Butcher, 1993). Flow is an intense harmonious involvement in the human–environmental mutual field process.

The term "kaleidoscoping" was used because it evolves directly from Rogers' writings and conveys the unpredictable and continuously shifting flow of patterns, sometimes turbulent, that one experiences when looking through a kaleidoscope. Rogers (1970) explained that the "organization of the living system is maintained amidst kaleidoscopic alterations in the patterning of system" (p. 62).

The Theory of Kaleidoscoping with Turbulent Life Events is used in conjunction with the pattern manifestation knowing and appreciation and voluntary mutual patterning processes. In addition to engaging in the processes already described in pattern manifestation knowing and appreciation, the nurse identifies manifestations of patterning and mutually explores the meaning of the turbulent situation with the client. A pattern profile describing the essence of the client's experiences, perceptions, and expressions related to the turbulent life event is constructed and shared with the client.

In the Theory of Kaleidoscoping, voluntary mutual patterning also incorporates the processes of transforming turbulent events by cultivating purpose, forging resolve, and recovering harmony (Butcher, 1993). Cultivating purpose involves assisting clients in identifying goals and developing an action system. The action system comprises patterning strategies designed to promote harmony amid adversity and facilitate the actualization of the potential for well-being.

In moments of turbulence, clients may want to increase their awareness of the complexity of the situation. Creative suspension is a technique that may be used to facilitate comprehension of the situation's complexity (Peat, 1991). Guided imagery is a useful strategy for facilitating creative suspension because it potentially enhances the client's ability to enter a timeless suspension directed toward visualizing the whole situation and facilitating the creation of new strategies and solutions. Forging resolve is assisting the clients in becoming involved and immersed in their action system. Because chaotic and turbulent systems are infinitely sensitive, actions are "gentle" or subtle in nature and are distributed over the entire system involved in the change process. Entering chaotic systems with a "big splash" or trying to force a change in a particular direction will likely lead to increased turbulence (Butcher, 1993).

Forging resolve involves incorporating flow experiences into the change process. Flow experiences promote harmonious human–environmental field patterns. A wide range of flow experiences can be incorporated into daily activities: art, music, exercise, reading, gardening, meditation, dancing, sports, sailing, swimming, carpentry, sewing, yoga, or any activity that is a source of enjoyment, concentration, and deep involvement. The incorporating of flow experiences into daily patterns potentiates the recovery of harmony. Recovering harmony is achieving a sense of courage, balance, calm, and resilience amid turbulent and threatening life events. The art of kaleidoscoping with turbulence is a mutual creative expression of beauty and grace and is a way of enhancing perseverance through difficult times.

Applications of the Conceptual System

New worldviews require new ways of thinking, sciencing, languaging, and practicing. Rogers' nursing science postulates a pandimensional universe of human–environmental energy fields manifesting as continuously innovative, increasingly diverse, creative, and unpredictable unitary field patterns. The principles of homeodynamics provide a way to understand the process of human-environmental change, paving the way for Rogerian theory–based practice. Rogers often reminded us that unitary means whole. Therefore, people are always whole, regardless of what they are experiencing in the moment, and therefore do not need nurses to facilitate their wholeness. Rogers identified noninvasive modalities as the basis for nursing practice now and in the future. She stated that nurses must use "nursing knowledge in non-invasive ways in a direct effort to promote well-being" (Rogers, 1994a, p. 34).

Box 15–1 Nursing Practice Evolves

The relevance of Rogerian nursing science to both human well-being and nursing is precisely the transformative vision of people and the world that it offers. Recognizing this, the nursing department at Bronx Lebanon Hospital Center, Bronx, New York, has made the decision to use Rogerian nursing science as the framework for practice throughout the hospital. People are complex, society is changing, and nursing's image is changing and so is our practice, which is driven by the science of nursing, according to Jeanine M. Frumenti, Vice President, Patient Care Services/Chief Nursing Officer (personal communication, July 21, 2008). Rogerian nursing science was chosen because it is inclusive and reflective of people's ever changing relationship to their environment, whereas many other nursing theories are reflective of the art of nursing. According to Frumenti, nurses need to be open to unfolding pattern and pandimensional experiences; everything is integrated and changing. It is her hope that Rogerian nursing science will assist Bronx Lebanon nurses in actualizing transformative practice for themselves and their clients.

Box 15–2 Providing Leadership in Nursing Education

The Washburn University School of Nursing in Topeka, Kansas, was a pioneer in the use of Rogerian nursing science as a framework for its curriculum. The school's Web site (www.washburn.edu) provides a summary of Rogerian nursing science and contains the statement that "The School of Nursing has become a national model in the use of the Rogerian theoretical framework."

This focus gives nurses a central role in health care rather than medical care. She also noted that health services should be community based, not hospital based. Hospitals are properly used to provide satellite services in specific instances of illness and trauma; they do not provide health services. Rogers urged nurses to develop autonomous, community-based nursing centers.

Larkin, one unitary nurse who has answered the call for noninvasive nursing modalities, has pioneered the use of Ericksonian hypnothera-peutic support groups. In a study comparing individuals diagnosed with chronic physical illnesses in Ericksonian versus traditional sup-port groups, persons in the former experienced pandimensional health and power, contrary to the view within the prevailing biomedical para-digm that such individuals experience dimin-ishing health and powerlessness (Larkin, 2007).

Unfortunately, a number of ideas relevant to nursing practice that Rogers discussed verbally never made it into print, for example, healing, intentionality, and expanded views on therapeutic touch. In three audiotaped and transcribed dialogues among Rogers, Malinski, and Meehan on January 26, 1988, for example, she described healing as a process, everything that happens as persons actualize potentials they identify as enhancing health and wellness for themselves. Todaro-Franceschi (1999) described healing in a similar way, with nurses knowingly participat-ing in the healing process by helping people actualize "their unique potentials—whatever those potentials may be" (p. 104). Cowling (2001) described healing as appreciating wholeness, offering unitary pattern apprecia-tion as the praxis for exploring wholeness within the unitary human–environmental mutual process.

Rogers also reminded us that change is a neutral process, neither good nor bad, one that we cannot direct but in which we par-ticipate. In this vein, in the transcribed dia-logue among Rogers, Malinski, and Meehan on therapeutic touch, Rogers described therapeutic touch as a neutral process, one that facilitates the patterning most com-mensurate with well-being for the person, whatever that is. There is no exchange of energy, no identification of desired out-comes. Rather than intentionality, Rogers suggested knowing participation as most congruent with her thinking, seeing inten-tionality as too closely tied to will and intent. However, she did suggest that a unitary view of intentionality was worthy of study. Zahourek's (2004, 2005) grounded theory study of intentionality differentiates

intentionality from both intent and intention and identifies it as the matrix for healing, a transformative process.

Rogers also questioned the concept of spir-ituality, which she saw as too often confused with religiosity. Smith (1994) and Malinski (1991, 1994) have both explored a Rogerian view of spirituality. For example, Malinski (2004) described it as the experience of wholeness and unity with all living beings and the natural environment, whereby people find meaning and purpose in both living and dying. As such, spirituality is a unitary experience with relevance for healing and well-being. Butcher (2008) reviewed the last 15 years of advances in Rogerian science list-ing additional concepts that have been con-ceptualized within the Science of Unitary Human Beings including hope, compassion, caring, despair, time, awareness, risk-taking, and empowerment.

Rogerian Practice Methods

A hallmark of a maturing scientific practice discipline is the development of specific prac-tice and research methods evolving from the discipline's extant conceptual systems. Rogers (1992) asserted that practice and research methods must be consistent with the Science of Unitary Human Beings in order to study irreducible human beings in mutual process with a pandimensional universe. Therefore, Rogerian practice and research methods must be congruent with Rogers' postulates and principles if they are to be consistent with Rogerian science.

The goal of nursing practice is the pro-motion of well-being and human better-ment. Nursing is a service to people wher-ever they may reside. Nursing practice—the art of nursing—is the creative application of substantive scientific knowledge devel-oped through logical analysis, synthesis, and research. Since the 1960s, the nursing process has been the dominant nursing practice method. The nursing process is an appropriate practice methodology for many nursing theories. However, there has been some confusion in the nursing literature concerning the use of the traditional nursing process within Rogers' nursing science.

In early writings, Rogers (1970) did make reference to nursing process and nursing diagnosis. But in later years she asserted that nursing diagnoses were not consistent with her scientific system. Rogers (quoted in Smith, 1988, p. 83) stated:

Nursing diagnosis is a static term that is quite inappropriate for a dynamic system … it (nursing diagnosis) is an outdated part of an old worldview, and I think by the turn of the century, there are going to be new ways of organizing knowledge.

Furthermore, nursing diagnoses are particularistic and reductionist labels describing cause and effect (i.e., "related to") relationships inconsistent with a "nonlinear domain without spatial or temporal attributes" (Rogers, 1992, p. 29). The nursing process is a stepwise sequential process inconsistent with a nonlinear or pandimensional view of reality. In addition, the term "intervention" is not consistent with Rogerian science. Intervention means to "come, appear, or lie between two things" (*American Heritage Dictionary*, 2000, p. 916). The principle of integrality describes the human and environmental field as integral and in mutual process. Energy fields are open, infinite, dynamic, and constantly changing. The human and environmental fields are inseparable, so one cannot "come between." The nurse and the client are already inseparable and interconnected. Outcomes are also inconsistent with Rogers' principle of helicy: expected outcomes infer predictability. The principle of helicy describes the nature of change as being unpredictable. Within an energy-field perspective, nurses in mutual process assist clients in actualizing their field potentials by enhancing their ability to participate knowingly in change (Butcher, 1997).

Given the inconsistency of the traditional nursing process with Rogers' postulates and principles, the Science of Unitary Human Beings requires the development of new and innovative practice methods derived from and consistent with the conceptual system.

During the last decade, a number of practice methods have been derived from Rogers' postulates and principles.

Barrett's Rogerian Practice Method

Barrett's Rogerian practice methodology for health patterning is the accepted alternative to the nursing process for Rogerian practice and is currently the most widely used Rogerian practice model. Barrett's (1988) practice model was derived from the Science of Unitary Human Beings and consisted of two phases: pattern manifestation appraisal and deliberative mutual patterning. Barrett (1998) expanded and updated the methodology by refining each of the phases, now more appropriately referred to as "processes." Each of the processes has also been renamed for greater clarity and precision. Pattern manifestation knowing is the continuous process of apprehending the human and environmental field (Barrett, 1998). "Appraisal" means to estimate an amount or to judge the value of something, negating the egalitarian position of the nurse, whereas "knowing" means to recognize the nature, achieve an understanding, or become familiar or acquainted with something. Voluntary mutual patterning is the continuous process whereby the nurse assists clients in freely choosing—with awareness—ways to participate in their well-being (Barrett, 1998). The change to the term "voluntary" emphasizes freedom, spontaneity, and choice of action. The nurse does not invest in changing the client in a particular direction, but rather facilitates and mutually explores with the client options and choices and provides information and resources so the client can make informed decisions regarding his or her health and well-being. Thus, clients feel free to choose with awareness how they want to participate in their own change process.

The two processes are continuous and nonlinear; therefore they are not necessarily sequential. Patterning is continuous and occurs simultaneously with knowing. Control and predictability are not consistent with Rogers' postulate of pandimensionality and principles of integrality and helicy. Rather, acausality allows for freedom of choice and means outcomes are unpredictable. The goal of voluntary mutual patterning is the actualization of potentialities for well-being through knowing participation in change.

Cowling's Rogerian Practice Constituents

Cowling (1990) proposed a template comprising 10 constituents for the development of Rogerian practice models. Cowling (1993b, 1997) refined the template and proposed that "pattern appreciation" was a method for unitary knowing in both Rogerian nursing research and practice. Cowling preferred the term "appreciation" rather than "assessment" or "appraisal" because appraisal is associated with evaluation. Appreciation has broader meaning, which includes "being fully aware or sensitive to or realizing; being thankful or grateful for; and enjoying or understanding critically or emotionally" (Cowling, 1997, p. 130). Pattern appreciation has a potential for deeper understanding.

The first constituent for unitary pattern appreciation identifies the human energy field emerging from the human–environmental mutual process as the basic referent. Pattern manifestations emerging from the human–environmental mutual process are the focus of nursing care. Next, the person's experiences, perceptions, and expressions are unitary manifestations of pattern and provide a focus for pattern appreciation. Third, "pattern appreciation requires an inclusive perspective of what counts as pattern information (energetic manifestations)" (Cowling, 1993b, p. 202). Thus, any information gathered from and about the client, family, or community—including sensory information, feelings, thoughts, values, introspective insights, intuitive apprehensions, laboratory values, and physiological measures—are viewed as "energetic manifestations" emerging from the human/environmental mutual field process.

The fourth constituent is that the nurse uses pandimensional modes of awareness when appreciating pattern information. In other words, intuition, tacit knowing, and other forms of awareness beyond the five senses are ways of apprehending manifestations of pattern. Fifth, all pattern information has meaning only when conceptualized and interpreted within a unitary context. Synopsis and synthesis are requisites to unitary knowing. Synopsis is a process of deliberately viewing together all aspects of a human experience (Cowling, 1997). Interpreting pattern information within a unitary perspective means that all phenomena and events are related nonlinearly. Also, phenomena and events are not discrete or separate but rather coevolve together in mutual process. Furthermore, all pattern information is a reflection of the human/environmental mutual field process. The human and environmental fields are inseparable. Thus, any information from the client is also a reflection of his or her environment. Physiological and other reductionistic measures have new meaning when interpreted within a unitary context. For example, a blood pressure measurement interpreted within a unitary context means the blood pressure is a manifestation of a pattern emerging from the entire human/environmental field mutual process rather than being simply a physiological measure. Thus, any expression from the client is unitary and not particular by reflecting the unitary field from which it emanates (Cowling, 1993b).

The sixth constituent in Cowling's practice method describes the format for documenting and presenting pattern information. Rather than stating nursing diagnoses and reporting "assessment data" in a format that is particularistic and reductionistic by dividing the data into categories or parts, the nurse constructs a "pattern profile." Usually the pattern profile is in the form of a narrative summarizing the client's experiences, perceptions, and expression inferred from the pattern appreciation process. The pattern profile tells the story of the client's situation and should be expressed in as many of the client's own words as possible. Relevant particularistic data such as physiological data interpreted within a unitary context may be included in the pattern profile. Cowling (1990, 1993b) also identified additional forms of pattern profiles, including single words or phrases and listing pattern information, diagrams, pictures, photographs, or metaphors that are meaningful in conveying the themes and essence of the pattern information.

Seventh, the primary source for verifying pattern appreciation and profile is the client. Verifying can occur by sharing the pattern profile with the client for revision and confirmation. During verification, the nurse also discusses options, identifies goals with the client, and plans mutual patterning strategies. Sharing the pattern profile with the client enhances participation in the planning of care and facilitates the client's knowing participation in the change process (Cowling, 1997).

The eighth constituent identifies knowing participation in change as the foundation for health patterning. Knowing participation in change is being aware of what one is choosing to do, feeling free to do it, doing it intentionally, and being actively involved in the change process. The purpose of health patterning is to assist clients in knowing participation in change (Barrett, 1988). Ninth, pattern appreciation incorporates the concepts and principles of unitary science; approaches for health patterning are determined by the client. Last, knowledge derived from pattern appreciation reflects the unique patterning of the client (Cowling, 1997).

Unitary Pattern–Based Praxis Method

Butcher (1997, 1999a, 2001) synthesized Cowling's Rogerian practice constituents with Barrett's practice method to develop a more inclusive and comprehensive practice model. In a 2006 publication, Butcher expanded the "praxis" model by illustrating how the Rogerian cosmology, ontology, epistemology, aesthetics, ethics, postulates, principles, and theories all form an "interconnected nexus" informing both Rogerian-based practice and research models (Butcher, 2006a, p. 9). The unitary pattern–based practice (Fig. 15-1) consists of two nonlinear and simultaneous

processes: pattern manifestation appreciation and knowing, and voluntary mutual patterning. The focus of nursing care guided by Rogers' nursing science is on pattern transformation by facilitating pattern recognition during pattern manifestation knowing and appreciation and by facilitating the client's ability to participate knowingly in change, harmonizing person–environment integrality, and promoting healing potentialities and well-being through voluntary mutual patterning.

Pattern Manifestation Knowing and Appreciation

Pattern manifestation knowing and appreciation is the process of identifying manifestations of patterning emerging from the human–environmental field mutual process and involves focusing on the client's experiences, perceptions, and expressions. "Knowing" refers to apprehending pattern manifestations (Barrett, 1988), whereas "appreciation" seeks a perception of the "full force of pattern" (Cowling, 1997). Pattern is the distinguishing feature of the human–environmental field. Everything experienced, perceived, and expressed is a manifestation of patterning. During the process of pattern manifestation knowing and appreciation, the nurse and client are coequal participants. In Rogerian practice, nursing situations are approached and guided by a set of Rogerian-ethical values, a scientific base for practice, and a commitment to enhance the client's desired potentialities for well-being.

Unitary pattern–based practice begins by creating an atmosphere of openness and freedom so clients can freely participate in the process of knowing participation in change. Approaching the nursing situation with an appreciation of the uniqueness of each person and with unconditional love, compassion, and empathy can help create an atmosphere of openness and healing patterning. Rogers (1966/1994) defined nursing as a humanistic science dedicated to compassionate concern for humans. Compassion includes energetic acts of unconditional love and means (1) recognizing the interconnectedness of the nurse and client by being able to fully understand

Unitary pattern-based praxis

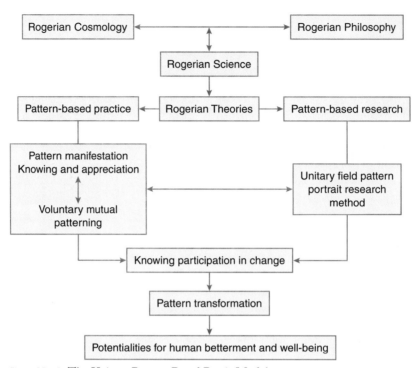

Figure 15 • 1   The Unitary Pattern-Based Praxis Model. *(Model from Butcher, H. K. [2006a]. Unitary pattern-based praxis: A nexus of Rogerian cosmology, philosophy, and science. Visions: The Journal of Rogerian Nursing Science, 14[2], 8–33.)*

and know the suffering of another; (2) creating actions designed to transform injustices; and (3) not only grieving in another's sorrow and pain, but also rejoicing in another's joy (Butcher, 2002).

Pattern manifestation knowing and appreciation involves focusing on the experiences, perceptions, and expressions of a health situation, revealed through a rhythmic flow of communion and dialogue. In most situations, the nurse can initially ask the client to describe his or her health situation and concern. The dialogue is guided toward focusing on uncovering the client's experiences, perceptions, and expressions related to the health situation as a means to reaching a deeper understanding of unitary field pattern. Humans are constantly all-at-once experiencing, perceiving, and expressing (Cowling, 1993a). Experience involves the rawness of living through sensing and being aware as a source of knowledge and includes any item or ingredient the client senses (Cowling, 1997). The client's own observations and description of his or her health situation includes his or her experiences. "Perceiving is the apprehending of experience or the ability to reflect while experiencing" (Cowling, 1993a, p. 202). Perception is making sense of the experience through awareness, apprehension, observation, and interpreting. Asking clients about their concerns, fears, and observations is a way of apprehending their perceptions. Expressions are manifestations of experiences and perceptions that reflect human field patterning. In addition, expressions are any form of information that comes forward in the encounter with the client. All expressions are energetic manifestations of field patterns. Body language, communication patterns, gait, behaviors, laboratory values, and vital signs are examples of energetic manifestations of human–environmental field patterning.

Because all information about the client–environment–health situation is relevant, various health assessment tools, such as the comprehensive holistic assessment tool developed by Dossey, Keegan, and Guzzetta (2004), may also be useful in pattern knowing and appreciation. However, all information must be interpreted within a unitary context. A unitary context refers to conceptualizing all information as energetic/dynamic manifestations of pattern emerging from a pandimensional human–environmental mutual process. All information is interconnected, is inseparable from environmental context, unfolds rhythmically and acausally, and reflects the whole. Data are not divided or understood by dividing information into physical, psychological, social, spiritual, or cultural categories. Rather, a focus on experiences, perceptions, and expressions is a synthesis more than and different from the sum of parts. From a unitary perspective, what may be labeled as abnormal processes, nursing diagnoses, or illness or disease are conceptualized as episodes of discordant rhythms or nonharmonic resonancy (Bultemeier, 2002).

A unitary perspective in nursing practice leads to an appreciation of new kinds of information that may not be considered within other conceptual approaches to nursing practice. The nurse is open to using multiple forms of knowing, including pandimensional modes of awareness (intuition, meditative insights, tacit knowing) throughout the pattern manifestation knowing and appreciation process. Intuition and tacit knowing are artful ways to enable seeing the whole, revealing subtle patterns, and deepening understanding. Pattern information concerning time perception, sense of rhythm or movement, sense of connectedness with the environment, ideas of one's own personal myth, and sense of integrity are relevant indicators of human–environment–health potentialities (Madrid & Winstead-Fry, 1986). A person's hopes and dreams, communication patterns, sleep–rest rhythms, comfort–discomfort, waking–beyond waking experiences, and degree of knowing participation in change provide important information regarding each client's thoughts and feelings concerning a health situation.

The nurse can also use a number of pattern appraisal scales derived from Rogers' postulates and principles to enhance the collecting and understanding of relevant information specific to Rogerian science. For example, nurses can use Barrett's (1989) power as knowing participation in change tool as a way of knowing clients' energy field patterns in relation to their capacity to knowingly participate in the continuous patterning of human and environmental fields as manifest in frequencies of awareness, choice making ability, sense of freedom to act intentionally, and degree of involvement in creating change. Watson's (1993) assessment of dream experience scale can be used to know and appreciate the clients' dream experiences, and Ference's (1979) human field motion tool is an indicator of the wave frequency pattern of the energy field.

Hastings-Tolsma's (1992) diversity of human field pattern scale may be used as a means for knowing and appreciating a clients' perception of the diversity of their energy field pattern, Johnston's (1994) human image metaphor scale can be used as a way of knowing and appreciating the clients' perception of the wholeness of their energy field, and the well-being picture scale of Gueldner et al. (2005) affords a way to measure a person's sense of unitary well-being. Paletta (1990) developed a tool consistent with Rogerian Science that measures the subjective awareness of temporal experience.

The pattern manifestation knowing and appreciation is enhanced through the nurse's ability to grasp meaning, create a meaningful connection, and participate knowingly in the client's change process (Butcher, 1999a). "Grasping meaning entails using sensitivity, active listening, conveying unconditional acceptance, while remaining fully open to the rhythm, movement, intensity, and configuration of pattern manifestations" (Butcher, 1999a, p. 51). Through integrality, nurse and client are always connected in mutual process. However, a meaningful connection with the client is facilitated by creating a rhythm and flow through the intentional expression of unconditional love, compassion, and empathy. Together, in mutual process, the nurse and client explore the meanings, images, symbols, metaphors, thoughts, insights, intuitions, memories, hopes, apprehensions, feelings, and dreams associated with the health situation.

Rogerian ethics are integral to all unitary pattern–based practice situations. Rogerian ethics are pattern manifestations emerging from the human–environmental field mutual process that reflect those ideals concordant with Rogers' most cherished values and are indicators of the quality of knowing participation in change (Butcher, 1999b). Thus, unitary pattern–based practice includes making the Rogerian values of reverence, human betterment, generosity, commitment, diversity, responsibility, compassion, wisdom, justice-creating, openness, courage, optimism, humor, unity, transformation, and celebration intentional in the human–environmental field mutual process (Butcher, 1999b, 2000).

When initial pattern manifestation knowing and appreciation is complete, the nurse synthesizes all the pattern information into a meaningful pattern profile. The pattern profile is an expression of the person–environment–health situation's essence. The nurse weaves together the expressions, perceptions, and experiences in a way that tells the client's story. The pattern profile reveals the hidden meaning embedded in the client's human–environmental mutual field process. Usually the pattern profile is in a narrative form that describes the essence of the properties, features, and qualities of the human–environment–health situation. In addition to a narrative form, the pattern profile may also include diagrams, poems, listings, phrases, and/or metaphors. Interpretations of any measurement tools may also be incorporated into the pattern profile.

Voluntary Mutual Patterning

Voluntary mutual patterning is a process of transforming human–environmental field patterning. The goal of voluntary mutual patterning is to facilitate each client's ability to participate knowingly in change, harmonize person–environment integrality, and promote healing potentialities, lifestyle changes, and well-being in the client's desired direction of change without attachment to predetermined outcomes. The process is mutual in that both the nurse and the client are changed with each encounter, each patterning one another and coevolving together. "Voluntary" signifies freedom of choice or action without external compulsion (Barrett, 1998). The nurse has no investment in changing the client in a particular way.

Whereas patterning is continuous, voluntary mutual patterning may begin by sharing the pattern profile with the client. Sharing the pattern profile with the client is a means of validating the interpretation of pattern information and may spark further dialogue, revealing new and more in-depth information. Sharing the pattern profile with the client facilitates pattern recognition and also may enhance the client's knowing participation in his or her own change process. An increased awareness of one's own pattern may offer new insight and increase one's desire to participate in the change process. In addition, the nurse and client can continue to explore goals, options, choices, and voluntary mutual patterning strategies as a means to facilitate the client's actualization of his or her human–environmental field potentials.

A wide variety of mutual patterning strategies may be used in Rogerian practice, including many "interventions" identified in the Nursing Intervention Classification (Bulechek, Butcher, & Dochterman, 2008). However, "interventions," within a unitary context, are not linked to nursing diagnoses and are reconceptualized as voluntary mutual patterning strategies, and the activities are reconceptualized as patterning activities. Rather than linking voluntary mutual patterning strategies to nursing diagnoses, the strategies emerge in dialogue whenever possible out of the patterns and themes described in the pattern profile. Furthermore, Rogers (1988, 1992,

1994) placed great emphasis on modalities that are traditionally viewed as holistic and noninvasive. In particular, the use of sound, dialogue, affirmations, humor, massage, journaling, exercise, nutrition, reminiscence, aroma, light, color, artwork, meditation, storytelling, literature, poetry, movement, and dance are just a few of the voluntary mutually patterning strategies consistent with a unitary perspective. In addition, patterning modalities have been developed that are conceptualized within the Science of Unitary Human Beings such as Butcher's metaphoric unitary landscape narratives (2006b) and written emotional expression (2004a), therapeutic touch (Malinski, 1993), guided imagery (Butcher & Parker, 1988; Levin, 2006), magnet therapy (Kim, 2001), and music (Horvath, 1994; Johnston, 2001). Sharing of knowledge through health education and providing health education literature and teaching also have the potential to enhance knowing participation in change. These and other noninvasive modalities are well described and documented in both the Rogerian (Barrett, 1990; Madrid, 1997; Madrid & Barrett, 1994) and the holistic nursing practice literature (Dossey, 1997; Dossey, Keegan, & Guzzetta, 2004).

The nurse continuously apprehends changes in patterning emerging from the human–environmental field mutual process throughout the simultaneous pattern manifestation knowing and appreciation and voluntary mutual patterning processes. While the concept of "outcomes" is incompatible with Rogers' notions of unpredictability, outcomes in the Nursing Outcomes Classification (Moorhead, Johnson, Maas, & Swanson, 2008) can be reconceptualized as potentialities of change or "client potentials" (Butcher, 1997, p. 29), and the indicators can be used as a means to evaluate the client's desired direction of pattern change. At various points in the client's care, the nurse can also use the scales derived from Rogers' science (previously discussed) to co-examine changes in pattern. Regardless of which combination of voluntary patterning strategies and evaluation methods is used, the intention is for clients to actualize

their potentials related to their desire for well-being and betterment.

The unitary pattern–based practice method identifies the aspect that is unique to nursing and expands nursing practice beyond the traditional biomedical model dominating much of nursing. Rogerian nursing practice does not necessarily need to replace hospital-based and medically driven nursing interventions and actions for which nurses hold responsibility. Rather, unitary pattern–based practice complements medical practices and places treatments and procedures within an acausal, pandimensional, rhythmical, irreducible, and unitary context. Unitary pattern–based practice provides a new way of thinking and being in nursing that distinguishes nurses from other health care professionals and offers new and innovative ways for clients to reach their desired health potentials.

The Science of Unitary Human Beings reflects Rogers' optimism and hope for the future. She envisioned humankind poised "on the threshold of a fantastic and unimagined future" (Rogers, 1992, p. 33), looking toward space while simultaneously engaging in a transformative Rogerian revolution in health care on Earth. One manifestation will surely be the establishment of autonomous Rogerian nursing centers here on Earth and ultimately in space. Research Applications of the Science of Unitary Human Beings Research is the bedrock of nursing practice. The Science of Unitary Human Beings has a long history of theory-testing research. As new practice theories and health patterning modalities evolve from the Science of Unitary Human Beings, there remains a need to test the viability and usefulness of Rogerian theories and voluntary health patterning strategies. The mass of Rogerian research has been reviewed in a number of publications (Caroselli & Barrett, 1998; Dykeman & Loukissa, 1993; Fawcett, 2005; Fawcett & Alligood, 2003; Kim, 2008; Malinski, 1986a; Phillips, 1989; Watson, Barrett, Hastings-Tolsma, Johnston, & Gueldner, 1997). For additional information, please visit DavisPlus at http://davisplus.fadavis.com.

Practice Exemplar

Elizabeth Ann Manhart Barrett

Barrett continues to refine her theory and practice method, as evidenced at "A Celebration of Barrett's Theory of Power" held June 6, 2008, when she and other researchers, practitioners, and administrators presented papers. Her brochure describes how to live powerfully through Health Patterning, with the therapist and client engaging in "a dialogue of meaning" and various health patterning modalities individualized through a Power Prescription "aimed toward power enhancement, with no attachment to outcomes...Power Prescriptions enrich power-as-freedom and diminish power-as-control, thereby facilitating well-being and healing...." The following is a vignette from her practice.

John, a tall, thin, 37-year-old man, dressed in a business suit, white shirt, and tie, walked into my office for our first session pulling a large backpack on wheels. Before sitting down, he opened the backpack, removed many papers, and began to place several stacks on the floor. "I'm desperate. I need your help with this mess," he said. "Is there anything in your life that feels like a mess you need to sort out?" I asked. At that point, John welled up and a few tears trickled down his cheeks. "I'm afraid I'm going to be fired from my job as a salesman. I haven't kept clear records and now my boss is claiming I haven't billed customers for many orders that have been delivered. These papers are all mixed up and I can't make heads or tails out of them. I counted them last night and there are 569 sheets of paper, some duplicates, some with dates before the time frame my boss is questioning. I want you to read them and help me straighten out this mess. I've been trying for weeks and I just can't think straight anymore."

John's pattern manifestations of flushed face; rapid, pressured speech; and clammy hands during an initial handshake revealed that his discomfort was intense. I suggested a therapeutic touch session, briefly explained the process, and he agreed. Afterward, he told me he felt more relaxed, so I invited him to complete the PKPCT (Power as Knowing Participation in Change Tool) and I scored it immediately. Then I briefly explained the power theory and pointed out that his scores on the four power dimensions on this semantic differential type tool with 12 opposite adjective pairs rated on a 1- to 7-point scale provided a 48-item snapshot of how he viewed his capacity to participate in change in a knowing manner. His scores indicated that for all four power dimensions—awareness, choices, freedom to act intentionally, and involvement in creating change—his power was chaotic rather than orderly, avoiding rather than seeking, and unpleasant rather than pleasant. "That's exactly how I feel about what is going on in my job right now. Of course, it's unpleasant; everything about straightening out this mess seems like constant chaos, and I am the first to admit I have been avoiding it like the plague."

We worked together to come up with a Power Prescription Plan that would allow him to identify from his paperwork what he had billed and what he had neglected to bill and to throw away duplicates and other extraneous material. Being relaxed after the TT experience allowed him to offer the necessary information so that I could help him design the plan. As we talked, I emphasized that carrying out the plan required giving himself the freedom to act on his intention to straighten out his life by beginning with straightening out his papers. He could see that avoidance just prolonged the chaos of confusion and if, he involved himself in creating this change, it would certainly be a pleasant relief.

After some suggestions as to how he could organize his paperwork, he left feeling he had a direction and was relieved to know that the outcome of his job situation was unpredictable and that rather than attaching to an outcome, he would focus on what he was doing to correct the situation. He planned to laminate the Power Prescription that I gave him and carry it with him as a reminder. It goes like this: "I am free to choose with awareness how I participate in changes I intend to create."

John returned the following week carrying only a small briefcase. He opened it and handed me two folders. "I can hardly believe that I have sorted those papers I brought here last week into two small groups. One folder contains invoices that have been paid and the other folder contains information regarding delivered materials that I have neglected to complete the paperwork that would allow for payment. I am showing you copies of what I showed my boss. He said he appreciated my clarification of what had happened and that the necessary procedures would be carried out so that the outstanding funds could be collected. By seeking a solution in an orderly way, I not only did what I had not been able to do in the midst of chaos, but the nightmare turned into a pleasant experience."

John, where do you see yourself in your life right now?" He said the "mess" he came in with the previous week had been cleaned up and he felt like his old self. He came for a specific purpose and the issue was resolved and he felt no need to continue. He asked if I could give him a way to help himself to relax on his own. Short imagery exercises are integral to my Health Patterning practice. So, I briefly instructed him in the use of imagery and gave him an imagery exercise that incorporated color, sound, light, and motion. Rogers believed those four modalities would be used increasingly in the future of nursing practice. I suggested he tape record the exercise and that hearing his own voice could reinforce his confidence to believe that he was taking charge of his life. I gave him a copy of my brochure that describes Health Patterning and the Power as Knowing Participation in Change(sm) Theory. I explained that our work had been about helping him further develop and use his power-as-freedom,

sourced from oneself, and not to be intimidated by power-as-control, where others may attempt to dominate. Then, a therapeutic touch session brought a close to our time together.

As a nurse with a practice based on Rogers' Science of Unitary Human Beings, I see the world and clients, whom I prefer to call healing partners, in a nonlinear, acausal way. The simple approach used with John, based on the Rogerian practice methodology, could serve as a prototype for him to realize he had power and could use it in any situation in his life. Pattern manifestation knowing and appreciation and voluntary mutual patterning flowed in a moment-to-moment changing rhythm. Therapeutic touch and imagery were not used as solutions to a problem defined by a diagnosis; rather, these are Health Patterning modalities. The therapeutic touch sessions based on his pattern manifestations and the specific selection of an imagery exercise for this particular person are what I define as Power Prescriptions. Health patterning modalities are general; Power Prescriptions are specific to the person or group. Rogers' four postulates and three principles describe the way change works in this particular worldview of people and their environments.

Power is the capacity to participate knowingly in change, and my work is intended to teach people how to participate knowingly in creating changes in their lives. Health Patterning is helping people make the changes they want to make. I see power as a phenomenon that just exists in the world and there are two types, power-as-control, based on the causal, material worldview, and power-as-freedom reflecting the acausal, spiritual worldview. Practice, in accord with Rogers' science, helps people actualize their power-as-freedom in accord with the legacy she laid out as a framework for nurses to use in all the many ways of being a nurse.

■ Summary

"Nursing is the study of caring for persons experiencing human–environment–health transitions" (Butcher, 2004b, p. 76). If nursing's content and contribution to the betterment of the health and well-being of a society is not distinguishable from other disciplines and has nothing unique or valuable to offer, then nursing's continued existence may be questioned. Thus, nursing's survival rests on its ability to make a difference in promoting the health and well-being of people. Making a difference refers to nursing's contribution to the client's desired health goals, and offering care is distinguishable from the services of other disciplines.

Every discipline's uniqueness evolves from its philosophical and theoretical perspective. The Science of Unitary Human Beings offers nursing a distinguishable and new way of conceptualizing health events concerning human well-being that is congruent with the most contemporary scientific theories. As with all major theories embedded in a new worldview, new terminology is needed to create clarity and precision of understanding and meaning. Rogers' nursing science leads to a new understanding of the experiences, perceptions, and expressions of health events and leads to innovative ways of practicing nursing. There is an ever-growing body of literature demonstrating the application of Rogerian science to practice and research. Rogers' nursing science is applicable in all nursing situations. Rather than focusing on disease and cellular biological processes, the Science of Unitary Human Beings focuses on humans as irreducible wholes inseparable from their environment.

For 30 years, Rogers advocated that nurses should become the experts and providers of noninvasive modalities that promote health. Now, the growth of "alternative medicine" and noninvasive practices is outpacing the growth of traditional medicine. If nursing continues to be dominated by biomedical frameworks that are indistinguishable from medical care, nursing will lose an opportunity to become expert in holistic health care modalities. The Science of Unitary Human Beings offers nursing a distinguishable and new way of conceptualizing health events concerning human well-being that is congruent with the most contemporary scientific theories.

References

American Heritage Dictionary. (2000). (4th ed.). New York: Houghton Mifflin.

Barrett, E. A. M. (1983). An empirical investigation of Martha E. Rogers' principle of helicy: The relationship of human field motion and power. Unpublished dissertation, New York University, New York.

Barrett, E. A. M. (1988). Using Rogers' science of unitary human beings in nursing practice. *Nursing Science Quarterly, 1,* 50–51.

Barrett, E. A. M. (1989). A nursing theory of power for nursing practice: Derivation from Rogers' paradigm. In: J. Riehl-Sisca, J. (Ed.), *Conceptual models for nursing practice* (3rd ed., pp. 207–217). Norwalk, CT: Appleton & Lange.

Barrett, E. A. M. (1990). Health patterning with clients in a private practice environment. In E. A. M. Barrett (Ed.), *Visions of Rogers' science-based practice* (pp. 105–115). New York: National League for Nursing.

Barrett, E. A. M. (1996). Canonical correlation analysis and its use in Rogerian research. *Nursing Science Quarterly, 9,* 50–52.

Barrett, E. A. M. (1998). A Rogerian practice methodology for health patterning. *Nursing Science Quarterly, 11,* 136–138.

Barrett, E. A. M., & Caroselli, C. (1998). Methodological ponderings related to the power as knowing participation in change tool. *Nursing Science Quarterly, 11,* 17–22.

Barrett, E. A. M., Cowling, W. R., Carboni, J. T., & Butcher, H. K. (1997). Unitary perspectives on methodological practices. In: M. Madrid (Ed.), *Patterns of Rogerian knowing* (pp. 47–62). New York: National League for Nursing.

Bohm, D. (1980). *Wholeness and the implicate order.* London: Ark Paperbacks.

Briggs, J. P., & Peat, F. D. (1984). *Looking glass universe: The emerging science of wholeness.* New York: Simon & Schuster.

Briggs, J., & Peat, F. D. (1989). *Turbulent mirror: An illustrated guide to chaos theory and the science of wholeness*. New York: Harper & Row.

Bulechek, G. M., Butcher, H. K., & Dochteman, J. M. (Eds.). (2008). *Nursing interventions classification (NIC)* (5th ed). St. Louis, MO: Mosby-Elsevier.

Bultemeier, K. (2002). Rogers' Science of Unitary Human Beings in nursing practice. In: M. R. Alligood & A. Marriner-Tomey (Eds.), *Nursing theory: Utilization and application* (pp. 267–288). St. Louis, MO: Mosby.

Butcher, H. K. (1993). Kaleidoscoping in life's turbulence: From Seurat's art to Rogers' nursing science. In: M. E. Parker (Ed.), *Patterns of nursing theories in practice* (pp. 183–198). New York: National League for Nursing.

Butcher, H. K. (1994). The unitary field pattern portrait method: Development of research method within Rogers' science of unitary human beings. In M. Madrid & E. A. M. Barrett (Eds.), *Rogers' scientific art of nursing practice* (pp. 397–425). New York: National League for Nursing.

Butcher, H. K. (1996). A unitary field pattern portrait of dispiritedness in later life. *Visions: The Journal of Rogerian Nursing Science, 4*, 41–58.

Butcher, H. K. (1997). Energy field disturbance. In G. K. McFarland & E. A. McFarlane, (Eds.), *Nursing diagnosis and intervention* (3rd ed., pp. 22–33). St. Louis, MO: Mosby.

Butcher, H. K. (1998). Crystallizing the processes of the unitary field pattern portrait research method. *Visions: The Journal of Rogerian Nursing Science, 6*, 13–26.

Butcher, H. K. (1999a). The artistry of Rogerian practice. *Visions: The Journal of Rogerian Nursing Science, 7*, 49–54.

Butcher, H. K. (1999b). Rogerian-ethics: An ethical inquiry into Rogers' life and science. *Nursing Science Quarterly, 12*, 111–117.

Butcher, H. K. (2000). Critical theory and Rogerian science: Incommensurable or reconcilable. *Visions: The Journal of Rogerian Nursing Science, 8*, 50–57.

Butcher, H. K. (2001). Nursing science in the new millennium: Practice and research within Rogers' science of unitary human beings. In: M. Parker (Ed.), *Nursing theories and nursing practice* (pp. 205–226). Philadelphia: F. A. Davis.

Butcher, H. K. (2002). Living in the heart of helicy: An inquiry into the meaning of compassion and unpredictability in Rogers' nursing science. *Visions: The Journal of Rogerian Nursing Science, 10*, 6–22.

Butcher, H. K. (2003). Aging as emerging brilliance: Advancing Rogers' unitary theory of aging. *Visions: The Journal of Rogerian Nursing Science, 11*, 55–66.

Butcher, H. K. (2004a). Written expression and the potential to enhance knowing participation in change. *Visions: The Journal of Rogerian Nursing Science, 12*, 37–50.

Butcher, H. K. (2004b). Nursing's distinctive knowledge. In L. Haynes, H. Butcher, & T. Boese (Eds.), *Nursing in contemporary society: Issues, trends, and transition to practice* (pp. 71–103). Upper Saddle River, NJ: Prentice-Hall.

Butcher, H. K. (2005). The unitary field pattern portrait research method: Facets, processes and findings. *Nursing Science Quarterly, 18*, 293–297.

Butcher, H. K. (2006a). Unitary pattern-based praxis: A nexus of Rogerian cosmology, philosophy, and science. *Visions: The Journal of Rogerian Nursing Science, 14*(2), 8–33.

Butcher, H. K. (2006b). Using metaphoric unitary landscape narratives to facilitate pattern transformation: Fires in the tallgrass prairie as a wellspring of possibilities. *Visions: The Journal of Rogerian Nursing Science, 13*, 41–58.

Butcher, H. K. (2008). Progress in the explanatory power of the Science of Unitary Human Beings: Frubes in a lull or surfing in the barrel of the wave. *Visions: The Journal of Rogerian Nursing Science, 15*(2), 23–26.

Butcher, H. K., & Parker, N. (1988). Guided imagery within Martha Rogers' science of unitary human beings: An experimental study. *Nursing Science Quarterly, 1*, 103–110.

Capra, F. (1996). *The web of life: A new understanding of living systems*. New York: Anchor Books.

Capra, F. (2002). *The Hidden Connections: Integrating the Biological, Cognitive, and Social Dimensions of Life into a Science of Sustainability*. New York: Random House.

Carboni, J. T. (1992). Instrument development and the measurement of unitary constructs. *Nursing Science Quarterly, 5*, 134–142.

Carboni, J. T. (1995a). Enfolding health-as-wholeness-and-harmony: A theory of Rogerian nursing practice. *Nursing Science Quarterly, 8*, 71–78.

Carboni, J. T. (1995b). A Rogerian process of inquiry. *Nursing Science Quarterly, 8*, 22–37.

Caroselli, C., & Barrett, E. A. M. (1998). A review of the power as knowing participation in change literature. *Nursing Science Quarterly, 11*, 9–16.

Cowling, W. R. (1986). The science of unitary human beings: Theoretical issues, methodological challenges, and research realities. In: V. M. Malinski (Ed.), *Explorations on Martha Rogers' science of unitary human beings* (pp. 65–78). Norwalk, CT: Appleton-Century-Crofts.

Cowling, W. R. (1990). A template for unitary pattern-based nursing practice. In: E. A. Barrett (Ed.), *Visions of Rogers' science-based nursing* (pp. 45–65). New York: National League for Nursing.

Cowling, W. R. (1993a). Unitary knowing in nursing practice. *Nursing Science Quarterly, 6*, 201–207.

Cowling, W. R. (1993b). Unitary practice: Revisionary assumptions. In: M. E. Parker (Ed.), *Patterns of nursing theories in practice* (pp. 199–212). New York: National League for Nursing.

Cowling, W. R. (1997). Pattern appreciation: The unitary science/practice of reaching essence. In: M. Madrid (Ed.), *Patterns of Rogerian knowing* (pp. 129–142). New York: National League for Nursing.

Cowling, W. R. (1998). Unitary case inquiry. *Nursing Science Quarterly, 11,* 139–141.

Cowling, W. R. (2001). Unitary appreciative inquiry. *Advances in Nursing Science, 23*(4), 32–48.

Csikszentmihalyi, M. (1990). *Flow: The psychology of optimal experience.* New York: Harper & Row.

Dossey, B. (1997). *Core curriculum for holistic nursing.* Gaithersburg, MD: Aspen.

Dossey, B., Keegan, L., & Guzzetta, C. (2004). *Holistic nursing: A handbook for practice* (4th ed.). Boston: Jones & Bartlett.

Dossey, L. (1993). *Healing words: The power of prayer and the practice of medicine.* New York: Harper Collins

Dossey, L. (1999). *Reinventing medicine: Beyond mind-body to a new era of healing.* New York: HarperCollins.

Dykeman, M. C., & Loukissa, D. (1993). The science of unitary human beings: An integrative review. *Nursing Science Quarterly, 6,* 179–188.

Fawcett, J. (1996). Issues of (in) compatibility between the worldview and research views of the science of unitary human beings: An invitation to dialogue. *Visions: The Journal of Rogerian Nursing Science, 4,* 5–11.

Fawcett, J. (2005). *Contemporary nursing knowledge: Analysis and evaluation of nursing models and theories.* Philadelphia: F. A. Davis.

Fawcett, J., & Alligood, M. R. (2003). The science of unitary human beings: Analysis of qualitative research approaches. *Visions: The Journal of Rogerian Nursing Science, 11,* 7–20.

Ference, H. (1979). The relationship of time experience, creativity traits, differentiation, and human field motion. Unpublished doctoral dissertation, New York University, New York.

Ference, H. M. (1986). The relationship of time experience, creativity traits, differentiation, and human field motion. In V. M. Malinski (Ed.), *Explorations on Rogers' science of unitary human beings* (pp. 95–105). Norwalk, CT: Appleton-Century-Crofts.

Gleick, J. (2000). *Faster: The Acceleration of Just About Everything.* New York: Knopf.

Governing Council of the Society for the Advancement of Nursing (SAIN). (1977/1994). SAIN Perspective. In: V. M. Malinski & E. A. M. Barrett (Eds.), *Martha E. Rogers: Her life and her work* (pp. 182–191). Philadelphia: F. A. Davis. (Reprinted from SAIN Newsletter, pp. 4–6, 1977, January.)

Green, B. (1999). *The elegant universe: Superstrings, hidden dimensions, and the quest for the ultimate theory.* New York: Norton.

Guba, E. G., & Lincoln, Y. S. (1989). *Fourth generation evaluation.* Newbury Park, CA: Sage.

Gueldner, S. H., Michel, Y., Bramlett, M. H., Liu, C-F., Johnston, L. W., Endo, E., Minegishi, H., & Carlyle, M. S. (2005). The Well-Being Picture Scale: A Revision of the Index of Field Energy. *Nursing Science Quarterly, 18,* 42–50.

Guzzetta, C. E. (Ed.). (1998). *Essential readings in holistic nursing.* Gaithersburg, MD: Aspen.

Hastings-Tolsma, M. T. (1992). The relationship among diversity and human field pattern, risk taking, and time experience: An investigation of Rogers' principles of homeodynamics. Unpublished doctoral dissertation, New York University, New York.

Hektor, L. M. (1989/1994). Martha E. Rogers: A life history. In: V. M. Malinski & E. A. Barrett (Eds.), *Martha E. Rogers: Her life and her work* (pp. 10–27). Philadelphia: F. A. Davis. (Reprinted from Nursing Science Quarterly, 2, 63–73).

Hills, R. G. S., & Hanchett, E. (2001). Human change and individuation in pivotal life situation: Development and testing of the theory of enlightenment. *Visions: The Journal of Rogerian Nursing Science, 9,* 6–19.

Horvath, B. (1994). The science of unitary human beings as a foundation for nursing practice with persons experiencing life patterning difficulties: Transforming theory into motion. In: M. Madrid & E. A. M. Barrett (Eds.), *Rogers' scientific art of nursing practice* (pp. 163–176). New York: National League for Nursing.

Johnston, L. W. (1994). Psychometric analysis of Johnson's Human Field Metaphor Scale. *Visions: The Journal of Rogerian Nursing Science, 2,* 7–11.

Johnston, L. W. (2001). An exploration of individual preferences for audio enhancement of the dying experience. *Visions: The Journal of Rogerian Nursing Science, 9,* 20–26.

Kahku, M. (2005). *Parallel worlds: A journey through creation, higher dimensions, and the future of the cosmos.* New York: Doubleday.

Kim, T. S. (2001). The relation of magnetic field therapy to pain and power over time in persons with chronic primary headache: A pilot study. *Visions: The Journal of Rogerian Nursing Science, 9,* 27–42.

Kim, T. S. (2008). Science of unitary human beings: An update on research. *Nursing Science Quarterly, 21,* 294–299.

Larkin, D. M. (2007). Ericksonian hypnosis in chronic care support groups: A Rogerian exploration of power and self-defined health promoting goals. *Nursing Science Quarterly, 20,* 357–369.

Laszlo, E. (1996). *The systems view of the world: A holistic vision for our time (Advances in systems theory, complexity, and the human sciences).* Cresskill, NJ: Hampton Press.

Levin, J. D. (2006). Unitary transformative nursing: using metaphor and imagery for self-reflection and theory informed practice. *Visions: The Journal of Rogerian Nursing Science, 14,* 27–35.

Lorenz, E. N. (1994). *The essence of chaos.* Seattle: University of Washington Press.

Lovelock, J. E. (1991). *Gaia.* Oxford: Oxford University Press.

Madrid, M. (Ed.). (1997). *Patterns of Rogerian knowing.* New York: National League for Nursing.

Madrid, M., & Barrett, E. A. M. (Eds.). (1994). *Rogers' scientific art of nursing practice.* New York: National League for Nursing.

Madrid, M., & Winstead-Fry, P. (1986). Rogers' conceptual model. In P. Winstead-Fry (Ed.), *Case studies in nursing theory* (pp. 73–102). New York: National League for Nursing.

Malinski, V. M. (Ed.). (1986a). *Explorations on Martha Rogers' Science of Unitary Human Beings.* Norwalk, CT: Appleton-Century-Crofts.

Malinski, V. M. (1986b). Further ideas from Martha Rogers. In: V. M. Malinski (Ed.), *Explorations on Martha Rogers' Science of Unitary Human Beings* (pp. 9–14). Norwalk, CT: Appleton-Century-Crofts.

Malinski, V. M. (1991). Spirituality as integrality: A Rogerian perspective on the path of healing. *Journal of Holistic Nursing, 9,* 54–64.

Malinski, V. (1993). Therapeutic touch: The view from Rogerian nursing science. *Visions: The Journal of Rogerian Nursing Science, 1,* 45–54.

Malinski, V. M. (1994). Spirituality: A pattern manifestation of the human/environmental mutual process. *Visions: The Journal of Rogerian Nursing Science, 2,* 12–18.

Malinski, V. M. (2004). Compassion and lovingkindness: Heartsongs for healing spirit. *Spirituality and Health International, 5,* 89–98.

Malinski, V. M., & Barrett, E. A. M. (Eds.). (1994). *Martha E. Rogers: Her life and her work.* Philadelphia: F. A. Davis.

McTaggert, L. (2008). *The field: The quest for the secret force of the universe.* New York: HarperCollins.

Mitchell, E. (1996). *The way of the explorer.* New York: Putnam.

Moorhead, S., Johnson, M., Maas, M., & Swanson, E. (2008). *Nursing outcomes classification (NOC)* (4th ed.). St. Louis, MO: Mosby-Elsevier.

Nadeau, R., & Kafatos, M. (1999). *The non-local universe: The new physics and matters of the mind.* Oxford: Oxford University Press.

Paletta, J. L. (1990). The relationship of temporal experience to human time. In: E. A. M. Barrett (Ed.), *Visions of Rogers' science-based nursing* (pp. 239–253). New York: National League for Nursing.

Peat, F. D. (1991). *The philosopher's stone: Chaos, synchronicity, and the hidden world of order.* New York: Bantam.

Phillips, J. (1989). Science of unitary human beings: Changing research perspectives. *Nursing Science Quarterly, 2,* 57–60.

Phillips, J. R. (1990). Research and the riddle of change. *Nursing Science Quarterly, 3,* 55–56.

Phillips, J. R. (1994). The open-ended nature of the science of unitary human beings. In M. Madrid & E. A. M. Barrett (Eds.), *Rogers' scientific art of nursing practice* (pp. 11–25). New York: National League for Nursing.

Radin, D. (1997). *The conscious universe: The scientific truth of psychic phenomena.* San Francisco: Harper.

Radin, D. (2006). *Entangled minds: Extrasensory experiences in a quantum reality.* New York: Paraview.

Randall, L. (2005). *Warped passages: Unraveling the mysteries of the universe's hidden dimensions.* New York: HarperCollins.

Rawnsley, M. M. (1994). Multiple field methods in unitary human field science. In: M. Madrid & E. A. M. Barrett (Eds.), *Rogerian scientific art of nursing practice* (pp. 381–395). New York: National League for Nursing.

Reason, P. (1994). Three approaches to participative inquiry. In: N. K. Denzin & Y. S. Lincoln (Eds.), *Handbook of qualitative research* (pp. 324–339). Thousand Oaks, CA: Sage.

Reeder, F. (1986). Basic theoretical research in the conceptual system of unitary human beings. In: V. M. Malinski (Ed.), *Explorations on Martha E. Rogers' science of unitary human beings* (pp. 45–64). Norwalk, CT: Appleton-Century-Crofts.

Rogers, M. F. (1961). *Educational revolution in nursing.* New York: Macmillan.

Rogers, M. F. (1964). *Reveille in nursing.* Philadelphia: F. A. Davis.

Rogers, M. E. (1970). *An introduction to the theoretical basis of nursing.* Philadelphia: F. A. Davis.

Rogers, M. E. (1980). Nursing: A science of unitary man. In: J. P. Riehl & C. Roy (Eds.), *Conceptual models for nursing practice* (2nd ed., pp. 329–337). New York: Appleton-Century-Crofts.

Rogers, M. E. (1966/1994). Epilogue. In: V. M. Malinski & E. A. M. Barrett (Eds.), *Martha E. Rogers and her work* (pp. 337–338). Philadelphia: F. A. Davis. (Reprinted from the Education Violet, the New York University newspaper, 1966.)

Rogers, M. E. (1988). Nursing science and art: A prospective. *Nursing Science Quarterly, 1,* 99 102.

Rogers, M. E. (1989). Response to Questions for Dr. Martha E. Rogers. *Rogerian Nursing Science News, 1*(3), 6.

Rogers, M. E. (1990a). Nursing: Science of unitary, irreducible human beings: Update 1990. In Barrett, E. A. M. (Ed.), *Visions of Rogers' science-based nursing* (pp. 5–11). New York: National League for Nursing.

Rogers, M. E. (1990b). Space-age paradigm for new frontiers in nursing. In: M. E. Parker (Ed.), *Nursing theories in practice* (pp. 105–113). New York: National League for Nursing.

Rogers, M. E. (1992). Nursing and the space age. *Nursing Science Quarterly, 5,* 27–34.

Rogers, M. E. (1994a). The science of unitary human beings: Current perspectives. *Nursing Science Quarterly, 7,* 33–35.

Rogers, M. E. (1994b). Nursing science evolves. In: M. Madrid & E. A. M. Barrett (Eds.), *Rogers' scientific art of nursing practice* (pp. 3–9). New York: National League for Nursing.

Rosenblum, B., & Kuttner, F. (2006). *Quantum enigma: Physics encounters consciousness.* Oxford: Oxford University Press.

Shearer, N. B. C., & Reed, P. (2004). Empowerment: Reformulation of a non-Rogerian concept. *Nursing Science Quarterly*, 253–259.

Sheldrake, R. (1988). *The presence of the past: Morphic resonance and the habits of nature*. New York: Times Books.

Smith, D. W. (1994). Toward developing a theory of spirituality. *Visions: The Journal of Rogerian Nursing Science, 2*, 35–43.

Smith, M. C. (1999). Caring and the science of unitary human beings. *Advances in Nursing Science, 21*(4), 14–28.

Smith, M. C., & Reeder, F. (1996). Clinical outcomes research and Rogerian science: Strange or emergent bedfellows. *Visions: The Journal of Rogerian Nursing Science, 6*, 27–38.

Smith, M. J. (1988). Perspectives on nursing science. *Nursing Science Quarterly, 1*, 80–85.

Talbot, M. (1991). *The holographic universe*. New York: HarperCollins.

Todaro-Franceschi, V. (1999). *The enigma of energy: Where science and religion converge*. New York: Crossroad Publishing.

Todaro-Franceschi, V. (2006). Synchronicity related to dead loved ones: A natural healing modality. *Spirituality and Health International, 7*, 151–161.

Watson, J. (1993). The relationships of sleep-wake rhythm, dream experience, human field motion, and time experience in older women. Unpublished doctoral dissertation, New York University, New York.

Watson, J., Barrett, E. A. M., Hastings-Tolsma, M., Johnston, L., & Gueldner, S. (1997). Measurement in Rogerian Science: A review of selected instruments. In: M. Madrid (Ed.), *Patterns of Rogerian knowing* (pp. 87–99). New York: National League for Nursing.

Whitbourne, S. K. (2008). *Adult development & aging: Biopsychosocial perspectives* (3rd ed.). Hoboken, NJ: John Wiley & Sons.

Woodhouse, M. B. (1996). *Paradigm wars: Worldviews for a new age*. Berkeley, CA: Frog, Ltd.

Zahourek, R. P. (2004). Intentionality forms the matrix of healing: A theory. *Alternative Therapies in Health and Medicine, 10*(6), 40–49.

Zahourek, R. P. (2005). Intentionality: Evolutionary development in healing: A grounded theory study for holistic nursing. *Journal of Holistic Nursing, 23*, 89–109.

16

Rosemarie Rizzo Parse's Humanbecoming School of Thought

ROSEMARIE RIZZO PARSE

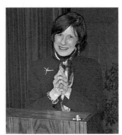

Rosemarie Rizzo Parse

Introducing the Theorist

Rosemarie Rizzo Parse is a Distinguished Professor Emeritus at Loyola University Chicago as well as a Fellow in the American Academy of Nursing, where she initiated and is immediate past chair of the Nursing Theory–Guided Practice Expert Panel. She is founder and editor of *Nursing Science Quarterly*; president of Discovery International, which sponsors international nursing theory conferences; and founder of the Institute of Humanbecoming, where each summer in Pittsburgh she teaches new material on the ontological, epistemological, and methodological aspects of the humanbecoming school of thought. There are also sessions on the Humanbecoming Community Change Model (Parse, 2003a), the Humanbecoming Teaching–Learning Model (Parse, 2004), the Humanbecoming Mentoring Model (Parse, 2008c), the Humanbecoming Leading–Following Model (Parse, 2008b), and the Humanbecoming Family Model (Parse, 2008a). The goal of all sessions is the understanding of the meaning of humanuniverse from a humanbecoming perspective.

Dr. Parse has published more than 100 articles and 9 books. Her books include *Nursing Fundamentals* (Parse, 1974); *Man-Living-Health: A Theory of Nursing* (Parse, 1981); *Nursing Research: Qualitative Methods* (Parse, Coyne, & Smith, 1985); *Nursing Science: Major Paradigms, Theories, and Critiques* (Parse, 1987); *Illuminations: The Human Becoming Theory in Practice and Research* (Parse, 1995); *The Human Becoming School of Thought* (Parse, 1998a); *Hope: An International Human Becoming Perspective* (Parse, 1999a); *Qualitative*

Inquiry: The Path of Sciencing (Parse, 2001), and *Community: A Human Becoming Perspective* (Parse, 2003a). Her books and other publications have been translated into many languages, as her theory is a guide for practice in health care settings and her research methodologies are used by nurse scholars in Australia, Canada, Denmark, Finland, Greece, Italy, Japan, South Korea, Sweden, Switzerland, Taiwan, the United Kingdom, the United States, and many other countries.

Dr. Parse has received two lifetime achievement awards, one from the Midwest Nursing Research Society and one from the Asian Nurses' Association. The Rosemarie Rizzo Parse Scholarship was endowed in her name at the Henderson State University School of Nursing. She is a sought-after speaker and consultant for local, national, and international venues.

Dr. Parse is a graduate of Duquesne University in Pittsburgh and received her master's and doctorate from the University of Pittsburgh. She was a member of the faculty of the University of Pittsburgh, dean of the School of Nursing at Duquesne University, professor and coordinator of the Center for Nursing Research at Hunter College of the City University of New York (1983–1993), and professor and Niehoff Chair in Nursing Research at Loyola University Chicago (1993–2006). Since January 2007, she has been a consultant and visiting scholar at the New York University College of Nursing.

Author's Reflections on the Discipline and Profession of Nursing

At present, nurse leaders in research, administration, education, and practice are focusing attention on expanding the knowledge base of nursing through enhancement of the discipline's frameworks and theories. Nursing is both a discipline and a profession (Parse, 1999b). The goal of the *discipline* is to expand knowledge about human experiences through creative conceptualization and research. The knowledge base of the discipline is the scientific guide to living the art of nursing. The discipline-specific knowledge is born and fostered in academic settings where research

and education advance knowledge to new realms of understanding. The goal of the *profession* is to provide service to humankind through living the art of the science. Members of the nursing profession are responsible for regulating the standards of practice and education based on disciplinary knowledge that reflects safe health service to society in all settings (Parse, 1999b).

The Profession of Nursing

The profession of nursing consists of people educated according to nationally regulated, defined, and monitored standards that are intended to preserve the integrity of health care for members of society. They are specified predominantly in medical terms, according to a tradition largely related to nursing's early subservience to medicine. Recently, nurse leaders in health care systems and in regulating organizations have been developing standards (Mitchell, 1998) and regulations (Damgaard & Bunkers, 1998) consistent with discipline-specific knowledge as articulated in the theories and frameworks of nursing. This is a very significant development that will fortify the identity of nursing as a discipline with its own body of knowledge—one that specifies the service that society can expect from members of the profession. With the rapidly changing health policies and the general dissatisfaction of consumers with health care delivery, clearly stated expectations for services from each of nursing's paradigms are a welcome change (Parse, 1999b).

The Discipline of Nursing

The discipline of nursing encompasses at least two paradigmatic perspectives about human-universe. The totality paradigm posits the human as body–mind–spirit whose health is considered a state of biological, psychological, social, and spiritual well-being. The body–mind–spirit perspective is particulate—focusing on the bio–psycho–social–spiritual parts of the whole human as the human interacts with and adapts to the environment. The ontology leads to research and practice on phenomena related to preventing disease and maintaining and promoting health according to societal norms. The totality paradigm frameworks and theories are more closely aligned with the medical model tradition. Nurses practicing according to this paradigm are concerned with participation of persons in health care decisions, but have specific regimens and goals to bring about change for the people they serve (Parse, 1999b).

In contrast, the simultaneity paradigm views the human as indivisible, unpredictable, everchanging (Parse, 1987, 1998a, 2007b), wherein health is considered personal becoming recognized with changing value priorities. Health is not static but, rather, is everchanging as humans choose ways of living. The ontology leads research and practice scholars to focus on, for example, energy field patterns (Rogers, 1992), lived experiences, and quality of life (Parse, 1981, 1992, 1997a, 1998a). Nurses living the simultaneity paradigm beliefs hold that their primary concern is people's perspectives of their health situations and their desires. Nurses focus on knowing participation (Rogers, 1992) and bearing witness, as persons in the nurse's presence choose ways of changing health patterns (Parse, 1981, 1987, 1992, 1995, 1997a). Because the ontologies of these paradigmatic perspectives are different, they lead to different research and practice modalities, different ethical considerations, and different professional services to humankind. As in other disciplines, various theories constitute each paradigm. Humanbecoming emanates from the simultaneity paradigm and is a basic *human science* that has co-created human experiences as a central focus. It is called a school of thought because it encompasses an ontology, epistemology, and methodologies (Parse, 1997b).

Overview of Parse's Humanbecoming School of Thought

Parse's (1981) original work was titled *Man-Living-Health: A Theory of Nursing*. When the term *mankind* was replaced with *male gender* in the dictionary definition of *man*, the name of the theory was changed to *human becoming* (Parse, 1992). No aspect of the principles changed at that time. With the publication of *The Human Becoming School of Thought* (1998a), Parse expanded the original work to include descriptions of three research methodologies and additional specifics related to the practice methodology (Parse, 1987), thus classifying the science of humanbecoming as a school of thought (Parse, 1997b). The fundamental idea of humanbecoming that humans are indivisible, unpredictable, everchanging, as specified in the ontology, precludes any use of terms such as physiological, biological, psychological, or spiritual to describe the human. These terms are particulate, thus inconsistent with the ontology. Other terms inconsistent with humanbecoming include words often used to describe people, such as noncompliant, dysfunctional, and manipulative.

In 2007, Parse set forth a clarification of the ontology of the school of thought. She specified *humanbecoming* as one word and *humanuniverse* as one word (Parse, 2007b). Joining the words creates one concept and further confirms the idea of indivisibility. She also described postulates to clarify the ontology further (Parse, 2007b). The ontology—that is, the assumptions, postulates, and principles—sets forth beliefs that are clearly different from other nursing frameworks and theories. Discipline-specific knowledge is articulated in unique language specifying a position on the phenomenon of concern for each discipline. The humanbecoming language is unique to nursing. For example, the three humanbecoming principles contain nine concepts written in verbal form with -*ing* endings to make clear the importance of the ongoing process of change as basic to humanuniverse emergence. In addition, each concept is explicated with paradoxes as apparent opposites, further specifying the uniqueness of the humanbecoming language.

The humanbecoming school of thought encompasses the ontology, the epistemology, and the research and practice methodologies.

The Ontology

The assumptions, postulates, and principles of the humanbecoming school of thought comprise the ontology (Parse, 2007b).

Philosophical Assumptions

The assumptions of the humanbecoming school of thought are written at the philosophical level of discourse (Parse, 1998a). There are nine fundamental assumptions, four about the human and five about becoming (Parse, 1998a, 2008b). Three additional assumptions about humanbecoming were synthesized from these nine assumptions (Parse, 1998a, 2008b). The assumptions arose from a synthesis of ideas from the Science of Unitary Human Beings (Rogers, 1992) and from existential phenomenological thought (Parse, 1981, 1992, 1994a, 1995, 1997a, 1998a). In the assumptions, Parse posits humans as indivisible, unpredictable, and everchanging, cocreating a unique becoming. She also posits humans as experts on their own health and quality of life. Humans live an all-at-onceness in freely choosing meanings that arise with illimitable experiences. The chosen meanings are the value priorities co-created in transcending with the possibles (Parse 1998a).

Postulates and Principles

In 2007, Parse (2007b) elaborated certain truths embedded in the conceptualizations of the ontology. In so doing she expanded the idea of co-creating reality as a seamless symphony of becoming (Parse, 1996), a central thought foundational to the ontology, as foregrounded with four postulates of illimitability, paradox, freedom, and mystery [see Parse (2007b) for detailed descriptions of the postulates]. The meanings of the postulates permeate all three of the principles; the words of the postulates are not used in the statements of the principles. Thus, the wording has been clarified to provide semantic consistency without changing the original meaning of the principles. The principles of humanbecoming, often referred to as the theory, describe the central phenomenon of nursing (humanuniverse), and

arise from the three major themes of the assumptions: meaning, rhythmicity, and transcendence. Each principle describes a theme with three concepts. Each of the concepts explicates fundamental paradoxes of humanbecoming (Parse, 1998a, 2007b). The paradoxes are rhythms lived all-at-once as pattern preferences (Parse, 2007b). Paradoxes are not opposites or problems to be solved but rather are ways humans live their chosen meanings. This way of viewing paradox is unique to the humanbecoming school of thought (Mitchell, 1993a; Parse, 1981, 1994b, 2007b).

The new statements of principles are presented in detail in Parse (2007b). With the first principle (see Parse, 1981, 1998a, 2007b), Parse explicates the idea that humans construct personal realities with unique choosings arising with illimitable humanuniverse options. Reality, the meaning given to a situation, is the individual human's everchanging seamless symphony of becoming (Parse, 1996). The seamless symphony is the unique story of the human as mystery emerging with the explicit-tacit knowings of *imaging*. The human lives the confirming–not confirming of *valuing* as cherished beliefs, while *languaging* with speaking–being silent and moving–being still [see Parse (2007b) for details].

The second principle (Parse, 1981, 1998a, 2007b) describes the rhythmical humanuniverse patterns of relating. The paradoxical rhythm "*revealing–concealing* is disclosing–not disclosing all-at-once" (Parse, 1998a, p. 43). Not all is explicitly known or can be told in the unfolding mystery of humanbecoming. "*Enabling–limiting* is living the opportunities–restrictions present in all choosings all-at-once" (Parse, 1998a, p. 44). There are opportunities and restrictions irrespective of the choice; all choosings are potentiating–restricting (see Parse, 2007b for details). "*Connecting–separating* is being with and apart from others, ideas, objects and situations all-at-once" (Parse, 1998a, p. 45). It is coming together and moving apart; there is closeness in the separation and distance in the closeness—a rhythmical attending–distancing [see Parse (2007b) for details].

With the third principle, Parse (1981, 1998a, 2007b) explicated the idea that humans are everchanging, that is, moving on with the possibilities of their intended hopes and dreams. A changing diversity unfolds as humans affirm and do not affirm in the pushing–resisting of *powering*, as creating new ways of living the conformity–nonconformity and certainty–uncertainty of *originating* sheds new light on the familiar–unfamiliar of *transforming*. *Powering* is the pushing–resisting of affirming–not affirming being in light of nonbeing (Parse, 1998a). The being–nonbeing rhythm is all-at-once living the everchanging now moment as it melts with the not-yet. Humans, in *originating*, seek to conform–not conform, that is, to be like others and unique all-at-once, while living the ambiguity of the certainty–uncertainty embedded in all change. The changing diversity arises with *transforming* the familiar–unfamiliar, as illimitable possibles are viewed in a different light.

The three principles, together with the postulates and assumptions, comprise the ontology of the humanbecoming school of thought. The principles are referred to as the humanbecoming theory. The concepts, with the paradoxes, describe humanuniverse. This ontological base gives rise to the epistemology and methodologies of humanbecoming. Epistemology refers to the focus of inquiry. Consistent with the humanbecoming school of thought, the focus of inquiry is on humanly lived experiences.

Humanbecoming Research Methodologies

Sciencing humanbecoming is coming to know; it is an ongoing inquiry to discover and understand the meaning of lived experiences. The humanbecoming research tradition has two basic research methods and one applied research method (Parse, 1998a, 2005). The three methods flow from the ontology of the school of thought. The basic research methods are the Parse Method (Parse, 1987, 1990, 1992, 1995, 1997a, 1998a, 2001) and the Humanbecoming Hermeneutic Method (Cody, 1995; Parse, 1995, 1998a, 2001, 2005).

The Humanbecoming Hermeneutic Method was created in congruence with the assumptions and principles of Parse's theory, drawing from works by Bernstein (1983), Gadamer (1976, 1960/1998), Heidegger (1962), Langer (1976), and Ricoeur (1976, 1981).

The purpose of these two basic research methods is to advance the science of humanbecoming by studying lived experiences from participants' descriptions (Parse Method) and from written texts and art forms (Humanbecoming Hermeneutic Method). The phenomena for study with the Parse Method are universal lived experiences such as joy, sorrow, hope, grieving, and courage, among others. Written texts from any literary source or art form may be the subject of research with the Humanbecoming Hermeneutic Method. The processes of both methods call for a unique dialogue, researcher with participant, or researcher with text or art form. The researcher in the Parse Method is in true presence as the participant moves with an unstructured dialogue about the lived experience under study. The researcher in the Humanbecoming Hermeneutic Method is in true presence with the emerging possibilities in the horizon of meaning arising in dialogue with texts or art forms. True presence is an intense attentiveness to unfolding essences and emergent meanings. The researcher's intent with these research methods is to discover structures (Parse Method) and emergent meanings (Humanbecoming Hermeneutic Method). The contributions of the findings from studies using these two methods include "new knowledge and understanding of humanly lived experiences" (Parse, 1998a, p. 62).

Many nurse scholars worldwide have conducted studies using the Parse Method, some of which have been published (see Doucet & Bournes, 2007). Parse (1999a) was also a principal investigator for a research study on the lived experience of hope using the Parse Method, with participants from Australia, Canada, Finland, Italy, Japan, Sweden, Taiwan, the United Kingdom, and the United States. The findings from these studies and the stories of the participants are published in

Hope: An International Human Becoming Perspective (Parse, 1999a). Collaborative research projects using the Parse Research Method also have been published on feeling very tired (Baumann, 2003; Huch & Bournes, 2003; Parse, 2003b). Four studies have been published in which authors used the Humanbecoming Hermeneutic Method (Cody, 1995, 2001; Ortiz, 2003; Parse, 2007a; see Doucet & Bournes, 2007).

The applied research method is the qualitative descriptive preproject–process–postproject method. It is used when a researcher wishes to evaluate the changes, satisfactions, and effectiveness of health care when humanbecoming guides practice (Parse, 1998a, 2001, 2006). The major purpose of the method is to understand what happens when humanbecoming is lived nurse with person, family, and community. A number of researchers have conducted studies using this method (Bournes & Ferguson-Paré, 2007, 2008; Bournes et al., 2007; Jonas, 1995a; Legault & Ferguson-Paré, 1999; Maillard-Strüby, 2007; Mitchell, 1995; Northrup & Cody, 1998; Santopinto & Smith, 1995), and a synthesis of the findings of these and other such studies was written and published (Bournes, 2002; Doucet & Bournes, 2007).

Humanbecoming: The Art

From the humanbecoming perspective, the discipline's goal is quality of life. The goal of the nurse living the humanbecoming beliefs is true presence in bearing witness and being with others in their changing health patterns. True presence is lived nurse with person, family, and community in illuminating meaning, synchronizing rhythms, and mobilizing transcendence (Parse, 1987, 1992, 1994a, 1995, 1997a, 1998a). The nurse with individuals or groups is in true presence with the unfolding meanings as persons explicate, dwell with, and move on with changing patterns of diversity.

Living true presence is unique to the art of humanbecoming. True presence is not to be confused with terms now prevalent in the literature such as authentic presence, transforming presence, presencing, and others. It is

sometimes misinterpreted as simply asking persons what they want and respecting their desires. Often nurses say it is what they always do (Mitchell, 1993b); this is not true presence. "True presence is an intentional reflective love, an interpersonal art grounded in a strong knowledge base" (Parse, 1998a, p. 71). The knowledge base underpinning true presence is specified in the assumptions, postulates, and principles of humanbecoming (Parse, 1981, 1992, 1995, 1997a, 1998a, 2007b). True presence is a free-flowing attentiveness that arises from the belief that the humanuniverse is indivisible, unpredictable, everchanging. Humans freely choose with situations, structure personal meaning, live paradoxical rhythms, and move beyond with changing diversity (Parse, 1998a, 2007b). Parse (1987, 1998b) states that to know, understand, and live the beliefs of human becoming requires concentrated study of the ontology, epistemology, and methodologies and a commitment to a different way of being with people. The different way that arises from the humanbecoming beliefs is true presence.

True presence is a powerful human universe connection. It is lived in face-to-face discussions, silent immersions, and lingering presence (Parse, 1987, 1998a). Nurses may be with persons, families, and communities in discussions, imaginings, or remembrances through stories, films, drawings, photographs, movies, metaphors, poetry, rhythmical movements, and other expressions (Parse, 1998a).

Many publications explicate the art of true presence and humanbecoming-guided practice (see, e.g., Arndt, 1995; Banonis, 1995; Bournes, 2000, 2003, 2006; Bournes & Flint, 2003; Bournes, Bunkers, & Welch, 2004; Bournes & Naef, 2006; Butler, 1988; Butler & Snodgrass, 1991; Chapman, Mitchell, & Forchuk, 1994; Cody, Mitchell, Jonas-Simpson, & Maillard-Strüby, 2004; Hansen-Ketchum, 2004; Hutchings, 2002; Jonas, 1994, 1995b; Jonas-Simpson & McMahon, 2005; Karnick, 2005, 2007; Lee & Pilkington, 1999; Mattice & Mitchell, 1990; Mitchell, 1988, 1990; Mitchell & Bournes, 2000; Mitchell, Bournes, & Hollett, 2006; Mitchell & Bunkers,

2003; Mitchell & Cody, 1999; Mitchell & Copplestone, 1990; Mitchell & Pilkington, 1990; Naef, 2006; Norris, 2002; Paille & Pilkington, 2002; Quiquero, Knights, & Meo, 1991; Rasmusson, 1995; Rasmusson, Jonas, & Mitchell, 1991; Smith, 2002; Stanley & Meghani, 2001; and others).

The Art of Humanbecoming Lived with Persons and Others

It is important here to clarify some terminology. *Nursing practice* is a generic term that refers to the genre of activities of the profession in general. The term *practice* is not appropriate to use when referring to humanbecoming, because according to various dictionary definitions it means a habit, or to drill, exercise, try repeatedly, or do over and over again. The word *practice* is antithetical to the ontology, as a major focus of humanbecoming is human freedom and dignity. Humanbecoming nurses live the art of the science of humanbecoming. The art of humanbecoming refers to living true presence, which arises directly from a sound understanding of the ontology of the school of thought. True presence flows only from nurses and health professionals who have studied; understand; believe in; and live the humanbecoming assumptions, postulates, and principles. The term living is the proper term to describe what nurses experience when with recipients of health care. Nurses and others who live humanbecoming believe that persons, families, and communities are the experts on their own health care situations.

In nurse with person health care situations, nurses in true presence come to persons with an availability to be with and bear witness, as persons illuminate the meaning of the situation, synchronize rhythms, and mobilize transcendence (Parse, 1981, 1987, 1998a, 2007b). The illuminating of meaning, synchronizing of rhythms, and the mobilizing of transcendence occurs in the true presence of the humanbecoming nurse, as persons explicate their situations, dwell with the moment, and move on all-at-once. In explicating, dwelling with, and moving on, they experience new insights and even surprises, as situations are seen in the new light that arises with the true presence of nurses who bear witness and do not label. Labeling or diagnosing is objectifying, ignoring the importance of persons' dignity and freedom. Humanbecoming nurses believe that persons know their way and live their health situations according to their unique value priorities. When with recipients of health care, the humanbecoming nurse asks what is most important for the moment, and explores meanings, wishes, intents, and desires related to the situation from the perspective of the recipients. Nurses are with persons in ways that honor these wishes and desires. Persons are seamless symphonies of becoming and nurses are only one note in the symphony.

The Art of Humanbecoming Lived with Community

The humanbecoming school of thought is a guide for research, practice, education, and administration in settings throughout the world. Scholars from five continents have embraced the belief system and live humanbecoming in a variety of venues, including health care centers and university nursing programs. The Humanbecoming Community Change Concepts (Parse, 2003a), the Humanbecoming Teaching–Learning Model (Parse, 2004), The Humanbecoming Mentoring Model (Parse, 2008c), and the Humanbecoming Leading–Following Model (Parse, 2008b) are disseminated and utilized in practice settings worldwide. Many health centers throughout the world have humanbecoming as a guide to health care (Bournes, Bunker, & Welch, 2004; Cody, Mitchell, & Jonas, 2004). In several university-affiliated practice settings in Canada, humanbecoming practice has been evaluated, and the theory has provided underpinnings for standards of care (Bournes, 2002; Legault & Ferguson-Paré, 1999; Mitchell, 1998; Mitchell, Closson, Coulis, Flint, & Gray, 2000; Northrup & Cody, 1998) and nursing best practice guidelines (Nelligan et al., 2002). For example, in Toronto, Sunnybrook Health Science Centre and University Health Network have both created multidisciplinary standards of care that arise from the beliefs and values of the humanbecoming school of thought.

In the settings worldwide where humanbecoming has guided nursing practice on a large scale, researchers examined the effects on the nurses and persons who were involved (Bournes & Ferguson Paré, 2007, 2008; Bournes et al., 2007; Jonas, 1995a; Legault & Ferguson-Paré, 1999; Maillard-Strüby, 2007; Mitchell, 1995; Northrup & Cody, 1998; Santopinto & Smith, 1995). The findings of the studies describe what happened when humanbecoming was used as a guide for nursing practice on an orthopedic surgery and rheumatology unit (Bournes & Ferguson-Paré, 2007), on a cardiac surgery unit (Bournes et al., 2007), on a medical oncology unit and a general surgery unit (Bournes & Ferguson-Paré, 2008), in a family practice unit affiliated with a large teaching hospital (Jonas, 1995a), on a 41-bed vascular and general surgery unit (Legault & Ferguson-Paré, 1999), on an acute care medical unit (Mitchell, 1995), on three acute care psychiatry units (Northrup & Cody, 1998), on three units in a 400-bed community teaching hospital (Santopinto & Smith, 1995), and on a medical oncology unit (Maillard-Strüby, 2007). The findings from five of the studies are summarized in Bournes (2002) and are consistent with those of more recent evaluations (Bournes & Ferguson-Paré, 2007, 2008; Bournes et al., 2007; Maillard-Strüby, 2007).

Bournes and Ferguson-Paré (2007, 2008) and Bournes, Plummer, Hollett, and Ferguson-Paré (2008) examined the impact of an innovative academic employment model (the humanbecoming 80/20 model—in which nurses spend 80% of their paid work time in direct patient care guided by humanbecoming and 20% of their paid work time learning about humanbecoming and engaging in related professional development activities). The humanbecoming 80/20 model has been implemented on four units—three in Toronto, Ontario (Bournes & Ferguson-Paré, 2007, 2008) and one in Regina, Saskatchewan

(Bournes et al., 2007). The Regina project was implemented in collaboration with Regina Qu'Appelle Health Region and the Saskatchewan Union of Nurses.

Findings from the research (Bournes & Ferguson-Paré, 2007, 2008; Bournes et al., 2007) to evaluate implementation of the humanbecoming 80/20 model have been extremely positive. For example, interviews with nurses, patients, families, and other health professionals in the Bournes and Ferguson-Paré (2007) study "supported the humanbecoming theory as an effective basis for learning and implementing patient-centered care that benefits both nurses and patients" (p. 251). Patients and families in that study "reported that they appreciated the reverent consideration given to them by nurses who had learned about humanbecoming-guided patient-centered care" (p. 251). They also described "being confident engaging in discussions with nurses who were understanding and attentive experts interested in who they were and what was important to them" (p. 251). Similarly, the nurse participants in Bournes and Ferguson-Paré's (2007) and Bournes and colleagues' (2008) studies reported that after learning about humanbecoming-guided nursing practice "they were more concerned with listening to patients and families, being with them, getting to know what is important to them, and respecting them as the experts about their quality of life. They also reported being more satisfied with their work—a theme noted by nurse leaders and allied health participants who shared that nurses...listened more and focused on patients' perspectives" (Bournes & Ferguson-Paré, 2007, p. 251). Participants in both studies described the benefits of the program, not only in relation to how it changed their relationships with patients, but also in relation to how it changed their view of how to be with their colleagues in more meaningful ways (see Bournes & Ferguson-Paré, 2007; Bournes et al., 2007). In addition, study findings show that the cost of providing education about humanbecoming-guided practice and staffing the 80/20 aspect of the model is offset by higher nurse and patient satisfaction scores and a reduction in sick time and overtime (Bournes & Ferguson-Paré, 2007; Bournes et al., 2007). At a large academic teaching hospital, the humanbecoming 80/20 model is currently being tested as the basis for a mentoring program among experienced critical care nurses and new nurses who want to work in critical care (Bournes et al., 2008). The mentoring program is based on the Humanbecoming Mentoring Model (Parse, 2008c).

In South Dakota, a parish nursing model was built on the Eight Beatitudes and the principles of humanbecoming to guide nursing practice in the health model at the First Presbyterian Church in Sioux Falls (Bunkers, 1998a, 1998b; Bunkers, Michaels, & Ethridge, 1997; Bunkers & Putnam, 1995). Bunkers and Putnam (1995) state, "The nurse, in practicing from the human becoming perspective and emphasizing the teachings of the Beatitudes, believes in the endless possibilities present for persons when there is openness, caring, and honoring of justice and human freedom" (p. 210). Also, the Board of Nursing of South Dakota has adopted a decisioning model based on the humanbecoming school of thought (Damgaard & Bunkers, 1998). Augustana College (in Sioux Falls) has humanbecoming as one theoretical focus of the curricula for the baccalaureate and master's programs. The humanbecoming theory is the basis of Augustana's Health Action Model for Partnership in Community (Bunkers, Nelson, Leuning, Crane, & Josephson, 1999). "The purpose of the model is to respond in a new way to nursing's social mandate to care for the health of society by gaining an understanding of what is wanted from those living these health experiences" (Bunkers et al., 1999, p. 94). The creation of the model was "for persons homeless and low income who are challenged with the lack of economic, social and interpersonal resources" (Bunkers et al., 1999, p. 92).

The humanbecoming school of thought is the theoretical foundation of the baccalaureate and master's curricula at the California Baptist University College of Nursing in Riverside, California. Faculty and students learn and live the art of humanbecoming in the various venues where they practice. The Nursing Center for Health Promotion with the Charlotte Rainbow PRISM Model was established in Charlotte, North Carolina, as a venue for nurses to offer health care delivery to homeless women and children with diverse backgrounds. The PRISM Model, based on humanbecoming, is the guide to practice (Cody, 2003). At the Espace Mediane community nursing center in Geneva, Switzerland (for persons who have concerns about cancer and palliative care), practice and teaching–learning are guided by humanbecoming, meaning that nurses in the center live true presence with visitors. They also link with academic partners to provide an academic service for postgraduate nursing students specializing in oncology and palliative care (Cody et al., 2004). A study to evaluate what happens when the art of humanbecoming is initiated in a palliative care inpatient setting is currently in process in Fribourg, Switzerland (F. Maillard-Strüby, personal communication, August, 7, 2008).

Shifting practice from the traditional medical model mode to living the art of humanbecoming is a challenge for healthcare institutions and requires high-level administrative commitment for resources, including educational opportunities for nurses. The commitment to humanbecoming practice requires a change in value priorities system-wide (Bournes, 2002; Bournes & DasGupta, 1997; Linscott et al., 1999; Mitchell et al., 2000).

Approximately 300 participants worldwide who are interested in living the art of humanbecoming subscribe to Parse-L, an e-mail listserv where Parse scholars share ideas. There is a Parse home page on the Internet that is updated regularly (see www.humanbecoming.org). Every other year, most of the 100 or more members of the International Consortium of Parse Scholars meet in Canada for a weekend immersion in humanbecoming research and practice. The DVD *The Human Becoming School of Thought: Living the Art of Human Becoming*

(International Consortium of Parse Scholars, 2007) (available from the International Consortium of Parse Scholars at www.humanbecoming.org) shows Parse nurses in true presence with persons in different settings and features Rosemarie Rizzo Parse talking about humanbecoming in practice. Parse is also featured on the video in the Portraits of Excellence Series called *Rosemarie Rizzo Parse: Human Becoming* (Fitne, 1997), available from Fitne (www.fitne.net). Another video showing nurse with persons is *The Grief of Miscarriage* (Gerretsen & Pilkington, 1990). There is also a video called *I'm Still Here*, which is a humanbecoming research-based drama on living with dementia (Ivonoffski, Mitchell, Krakauer, & Jonas-Simpson, 2006). It is available from the Murray Alzheimer Research and Education Program at the University of Waterloo.

■ Summary

Through the efforts of Parse scholars, the humanbecoming school of thought will continue to emerge as a major force in the 21st-century evolution of nursing knowledge. Knowledge gained from basic research studies will continue to be synthesized to explicate further the meaning of lived experiences. The findings from applied research projects related to fostering understanding of humanbecoming in practice also will continue to be synthesized. These syntheses will guide decisions for continually creating the vision for sciencing and living the art of the humanbecoming school of thought for the betterment of humankind.

References

Arndt, M. J. (1995). Parse's theory of human becoming in practice with hospitalized adolescents. *Nursing Science Quarterly, 8,* 86–90.

Banonis, B. C. (1995). Metaphors in the practice of the human becoming theory. In: R. R. Parse (Ed.), *Illuminations: The human becoming theory in practice and research* (pp. 87–95). New York: National League for Nursing Press.

Baumann, S. L. (2003). The lived experience of feeling very tired: A study of adolescent girls. *Nursing Science Quarterly, 16,* 326–333.

Bernstein, R. J. (1983). *Beyond objectivism and relativism: Science, hermeneutics, and praxis.* Philadelphia: University of Pennsylvania Press.

Bournes, D. A. (2000). A commitment to honoring people's choices. *Nursing Science Quarterly, 13,* 18–23.

Bournes, D. A. (2002). Research evaluating human becoming in practice. *Nursing Science Quarterly, 15,* 190–195.

Bournes, D. A. (2003). Stories of courage and confidence: Interpretation with the human becoming community change concepts. In: R. R. Parse, *Community: A human becoming perspective* (pp. 131–145). Sudbury, MA: Jones and Bartlett.

Bournes, D. A. (2006). Human becoming–guided practice. *Nursing Science Quarterly, 19,* 329–330.

Bournes, D. A., Bunker, S. S., & Welch, A. J. (2004). The theory of human becoming in action: Scope and challenges. *Nursing Science Quarterly, 17*(3), 227–232.

Bournes, D. A., & DasGupta, D. (1997). Professional practice leader: A transformational role that addresses human diversity. *Nursing Administration Quarterly, 21*(4), 61–68.

Bournes, D. A., & Ferguson-Paré, M. (2007). Human becoming and 80/20: An innovative professional development model for nurses. *Nursing Science Quarterly, 20,* 237–253.

Bournes, D. A., & Ferguson-Paré, M. (2008). The humanbecoming 80/20 study: Second study in Toronto. Unpublished manuscript.

Bournes, D. A., Ferguson-Paré, M., Plummer, C., Kyle, C., Larrivee, D., & LeMoal, L. (2007, November). *Innovations in nurse retention and patient centered care: The 80/20 study in Regina.* Poster panel presentation at Celebrating New Knowledge and Innovation, University Health Network Nursing Research Day, Old Mill Inn and Spa, Toronto, ON.

Bournes, D. A., & Flint, F. (2003). Mis-Takes: Mistakes in the nurse-person process. *Nursing Science Quarterly, 16,* 127–130.

Bournes, D. A., & Naef, R. (2006). Human becoming practice around the globe: Exploring the art of living true presence. *Nursing Science Quarterly, 19,* 109–115.

Bournes, D. A., Plummer, C., Hollett, J., & Ferguson-Paré, M. (2008). *Critical care mentoring study: Testing a humanbecoming mentoring program to enhance retention and recruitment of nurses.* Unpublished manuscript.

Bunkers, S. S. (1998a). A nursing theory–guided model of health ministry: Human becoming in parish nursing. *Nursing Science Quarterly, 11,* 7–8.

Bunkers, S. S. (1998b). Translating nursing conceptual frameworks and theory for nursing practice in the parish community. In: A. Solari-Twadell & M. McDermott (Eds.), *Parish nursing* (pp. 205–214). Thousand Oaks, CA: Sage.

Bunkers, S. S., Michaels, C., & Ethridge, P. (1997). Advanced practice nursing in community: Nursing's opportunity. *Advanced Practice Nursing Quarterly, 2*(4), 79–84.

Bunkers, S. S., Nelson, M. L., Leuning, C. J., Crane, J. K., & Josephson, D. K. (1999). The health action model: Academia's partnership with the community. In: E. L. Cohen & V. DeBack (Eds.), *The outcomes mandate: Case management in health care today* (pp. 92–100). St. Louis, MO: C. V. Mosby.

Bunkers, S. S., & Putnam, V. (1995). A nursing theory–based model of health ministry: Living Parse's theory of human becoming in the parish community. In: *Ninth Annual Westberg Parish Nurse Symposium: Parish nursing: Ministering through the arts.* Northbrook, IL: International Parish Nursing Resource Center–Advocate Health Care.

Butler, M. J. (1988). Family transformation: Parse's theory in practice. *Nursing Science Quarterly, 1,* 68–74.

Butler, M. J., & Snodgrass, F. G. (1991). Beyond abuse: Parse's theory in practice. *Nursing Science Quarterly, 4,* 76–82.

Chapman, J. S., Mitchell, G. J., & Forchuk, C. (1994). A glimpse of nursing theory–based practice in Canada. *Nursing Science Quarterly, 7,* 104–112.

Cody, W. K. (1995). Of life immense in passion, pulse, and power: Dialoguing with Whitman and Parse, a hermeneutic study. In: R. R. Parse (Ed.), *Illuminations: The human becoming theory in practice and research* (pp. 269–307). New York: National League for Nursing Press.

Cody, W. K. (2001). "Mendacity" as the refusal to bear witness: A human becoming hermeneutic study of a theme from Tennessee Williams' "Cat on a Hot Tin Roof." In: R. R. Parse (Ed.), *Qualitative inquiry: The path of sciencing* (pp. 205–220). Sudbury, MA: Jones and Bartlett.

Cody, W. K. (2003). Human becoming community change concepts in an academic nursing practice setting. In: R. R. Parse (Ed.), *Community: A human becoming perspective* (pp. 49–71). Sudbury, MA: Jones and Bartlett.

Cody, W. K., Mitchell, G. J., Jonas-Simpson, C., & Maillard-Strüby, F. V. (2004). Human becoming: Scope and challenges continued. *Nursing Science Quarterly, 17,* 324–329.

Damgaard, G., & Bunkers, S. S. (1998). Nursing science–guided practice and education: A state board of nursing perspective. *Nursing Science Quarterly, 11,* 142–144.

Doucet, T., & Bournes, D. A. (2007). Review of research related to Parse's theory of human becoming. *Nursing Science Quarterly, 20,* 16–32.

Fitne. (1997). Portraits of excellence: Rosemarie Rizzo Parse: Human becoming [CD-ROM]. Athens, OH: Author. (Available from www.fitne.net)

Gadamer, H. -G. (1976). *Philosophical hermeneutics* (D. E. Linge, trans.). Berkeley, CA: University of California.

Gadamer, H. -G. (1998). *Truth and method* (2nd rev. ed.; J. Weinsheimer & D. G. Marshall, Trans.). New York: Continuum. (Original work published 1960)

Gerretsen, P. (Producer), & Pilkington, F. B. (Consultant). (1990). *The grief of miscarriage* [Video]. Toronto, Canada: St. Michael's Hospital.

Hansen-Ketchum, P. (2004). Parse's theory in practice. *Journal of Holistic Nursing, 22,* 57–72.

Heidegger, M. (1962). *Being and time* (J. Macquarrie & E. Robinson, trans.). New York: Harper & Row.

Huch, M. H., & Bournes, D. A. (2003). Community dwellers' perspectives on the experience of feeling very tired. *Nursing Science Quarterly, 16,* 334–339.

Hutchings, D. (2002). Parallels in practice: Palliative nursing practice and Parse's theory of human becoming. *American Journal of Hospice and Palliative Care, 19,* 408–414.

International Consortium of Parse Scholars. (2007). *The human becoming school of thought: Living the art of human becoming* [DVD]. Toronto, Ontario, Canada: Author.

Ivonoffski, V., Mitchell, G. J., Krakauer, R., Jonas-Simpson, C. (Writers), & Dennis, G. (Producer). (2006). *I'm still here* [DVD]. Waterloo, Ontario, Canada: Murray Alzheimer Research and Education Program.

Jonas, C. M. (1994). True presence through music. *Nursing Science Quarterly, 7,* 102–103.

Jonas, C. M. (1995a). Evaluation of the human becoming theory in family practice. In: R. R. Parse (Ed.), *Illuminations: The human becoming theory in practice and research* (pp. 347–366). New York: National League for Nursing Press.

Jonas, C. M. (1995b). True presence through music for persons living their dying. In: R. R. Parse (Ed.), *Illuminations: The human becoming theory in practice and research* (pp. 97–104). New York: National League for Nursing Press.

Jonas-Simpson, C., & McMahon, E. (2005). The language of loss when a baby dies prior to birth: Cocreating human experience. *Nursing Science Quarterly, 18,* 124–130.

Karnick, P. M. (2005). Human becoming theory with children. *Nursing Science Quarterly, 18,* 221–226.

Karnick, P. M. (2007). Nursing practice: Imaging the possibles. *Nursing Science Quarterly, 20,* 44–47.

Langer, S. (1976). *Philosophy in a new key.* Cambridge, MA: Harvard University Press.

Lee, O. J., & Pilkington, F. B. (1999). Practice with persons living their dying: A human becoming perspective. *Nursing Science Quarterly, 12,* 324–328.

Legault, F., & Ferguson-Paré, M. (1999). Advancing nursing practice: An evaluation study of Parse's theory of human becoming. *Canadian Journal of Nursing Leadership, 12*(1), 30–35.

Linscott, J., Spee, R., Flint, F., & Fisher, A. (1999). Creating a culture of patient-focused care through a learner-centred philosophy. *Canadian Journal of Nursing Leadership, 12*(4), 5–10.

Maillard-Strüby, F. (2007, March). *Evaluation of the humanbecoming theory in practice.* Paper presented at the 2nd International Congress of the University of Applied Studies. Freiburg, Switzerland.

Mattice, M., & Mitchell, G. J. (1990). Caring for confused elders. *The Canadian Nurse, 86*(11), 16–18.

Mitchell, G. J. (1988). Man-living-health: The theory in practice. *Nursing Science Quarterly, 1,* 120–127.

Mitchell, G. J. (1990). Struggling in change: From the traditional approach to Parse's theory-based practice. *Nursing Science Quarterly, 3,* 170–176.

Mitchell, G. J. (1993a). Living paradox in Parse's theory. *Nursing Science Quarterly, 6,* 44–51.

Mitchell, G. J. (1993b). The same-thing-yet-different phenomenon: A way of coming to know—or not? *Nursing Science Quarterly, 6,* 61–62.

Mitchell, G. J. (1995). The lived experience of restriction-freedom in later life. In: R. R. Parse (Ed.), *Illuminations: The human becoming theory in practice and research* (pp. 159–195). New York: National League for Nursing Press.

Mitchell, G. J. (1998). Standards of nursing and the winds of change. *Nursing Science Quarterly, 11,* 97–98.

Mitchell, G. J., & Bournes, D. A. (2000). Nurse as patient advocate? In search of straight thinking. *Nursing Science Quarterly, 13,* 204–209.

Mitchell, G. J., Bournes, D. A., & Hollett, J. (2006). Human becoming–guided patient-centered care: A new model transforms nursing practice. *Nursing Science Quarterly, 19,* 218–224.

Mitchell, G. J., & Bunkers, S. S. (2003). Engaging the abyss: A mis-take of opportunity? *Nursing Science Quarterly, 16,* 121–125.

Mitchell, G. J., Closson, T., Coulis, N., Flint, F., & Gray, B. (2000). Patient-focused care and human becoming thought: Connecting the right stuff. *Nursing Science Quarterly, 13,* 216–224.

Mitchell, G. J., & Cody, W. K. (1999). Human becoming theory: A complement to medical science. *Nursing Science Quarterly, 12,* 304–310.

Mitchell, G. J., & Copplestone, C. (1990). Applying Parse's theory to perioperative nursing: A nontraditional approach. *AORN Journal, 51,* 787–798.

Mitchell, G. J., & Pilkington, B. (1990). Theoretical approaches in nursing practice: A comparison of Roy and Parse. *Nursing Science Quarterly, 3,* 81–87.

Naef, R. (2006). Bearing witness: A moral way of engaging in the nurse-person relationship. *Nursing Philosophy, 3,* 146–156.

Nelligan, P., Balfour, J., Connolly, L., Grinspun, D., Jonas-Simpson, C., Lefebre, N., et al. (2002). *Nursing best practice guideline: Client centred care.* Toronto, Ontario, Canada: Registered Nurses Association of Ontario.

Norris, J. R. (2002). One-to-one teleapprenticeship as a means for nurses teaching and learning Parse's theory of human becoming. *Nursing Science Quarterly, 15,* 113–116.

Northrup, D. (2002). Time passing: A Parse research method study. *Nursing Science Quarterly, 15,* 318–326.

Northrup, D., & Cody, W. K. (1998). Evaluation of the human becoming theory in practice in an acute care psychiatric setting. *Nursing Science Quarterly, 11,* 23–30.

Ortiz, M. R. (2003). Lingering presence: A study using the human becoming hermeneutic method. *Nursing Science Quarterly, 16,* 146–154.

Paille, M., & Pilkington, F. B. (2002). The global context of nursing: A human becoming perspective. *Nursing Science Quarterly, 15,* 165–170.

Parse, R. R. (1974). *Nursing fundamentals.* Flushing, NY: Medical Examination.

Parse, R. R. (1981). *Man-living-health: A theory of nursing.* New York: John Wiley & Sons.

Parse, R. R. (1987). *Nursing science: Major paradigms, theories, and critiques.* Philadelphia: W. B. Saunders.

Parse, R. R. (1990). Parse's research methodology with an illustration of the lived experience of hope. *Nursing Science Quarterly, 3,* 9–17.

Parse, R. R. (1992). Human becoming: Parse's theory of nursing. *Nursing Science Quarterly, 5,* 35–42.

Parse, R. R. (1994a). Laughing and health: A study using Parse's research method. *Nursing Science Quarterly, 7,* 55–64.

Parse, R. R. (1994b). Quality of life: Sciencing and living the art of human becoming. *Nursing Science Quarterly, 7,* 16–21.

Parse, R. R. (Ed.). (1995). *Illuminations: The human becoming theory in practice and research.* New York: National League for Nursing Press.

Parse, R. R. (1996). Reality: A seamless symphony of becoming. *Nursing Science Quarterly, 9,* 181–183.

Parse, R. R. (1997a). The human becoming theory: The was, is, and will be. *Nursing Science Quarterly, 10,* 32–38.

Parse, R. R. (1997b). The language of nursing knowledge: Saying what we mean. In: J. Fawcett & I. M. King (Eds.), *The language of theory and metatheory* (pp. 73–77). Indianapolis, IN: Sigma Theta Tau International Center Nursing Press.

Parse, R. R. (1998a). *The human becoming school of thought.* Thousand Oaks, CA: Sage.

Parse, R. R. (1998b). On true presence. *Illuminations, 7*(3), 1.

Parse, R. R. (1999a). *Hope: An international human becoming perspective.* Sudbury, MA: Jones and Bartlett.

Parse, R. R. (1999b). Nursing: The discipline and the profession. *Nursing Science Quarterly, 12,* 275.

Parse, R. R. (2001). *Qualitative inquiry: The path of sciencing.* Sudbury, MA: Jones and Bartlett.

Parse, R. R. (2003a). *Community: A human becoming perspective.* Sudbury, MA: Jones and Bartlett.

Parse, R. R. (2003b). The lived experience of feeling very tired: A study using the Parse research method. *Nursing Science Quarterly, 16,* 319–325.

Parse, R. R. (2004). A human becoming teaching-learning model. *Nursing Science Quarterly, 17,* 33–35.

Parse, R. R. (2005). The human becoming modes of inquiry: Emerging sciencing. *Nursing Science Quarterly, 18,* 297–300.

Parse, R. R. (2006). Research findings evince benefits of nursing theory–guided practice. *Nursing Science Quarterly, 19,* 87.

Parse, R. R. (2007a). Hope in "Rita Hayworth and Shaw-shank Redemption": A human becoming hermeneutic study. *Nursing Science Quarterly, 20,* 148–154.

Parse, R. R. (2007b). The humanbecoming school of thought in 2050. *Nursing Science Quarterly, 20,* 308.

Parse, R. R. (2008a, June). *The humanbecoming family model.* Paper presented at the Institute of Human-becoming, Pittsburgh, PA.

Parse, R. R. (2008b). *The humanbecoming leading-following model. Nursing Science Quarterly, 21*(4), 369–375.

Parse, R. R. (2008c). A humanbecoming mentoring model. *Nursing Science Quarterly, 21,* 195–198.

Parse, R. R., Coyne, B. A., & Smith, M. J. (1985). *Nursing research: Qualitative methods.* Bowie, MD: Brady.

Quiquero, A., Knights, D., & Meo, C. O. (1991). Theory as a guide to practice: Staff nurses choose Parse's theory. *Canadian Journal of Nursing Administration, 4*(1), 14–16.

Rasmusson, D. L. (1995). True presence with homeless persons. In: R. R. Parse (Ed.), *Illuminations: The human becoming theory in practice and research* (pp. 105–113). New York: National League for Nursing Press.

Rasmusson, D. L., Jonas, C. M., & Mitchell, G. J. (1991). The eye of the beholder: Parse's theory with homeless individuals. *Clinical Nurse Specialist, 5*(3), 139–143.

Ricoeur, P. (1976). *Interpretation theory: Discourse and the surplus of meaning.* Fort Worth, TX: Texas Christian University Press.

Ricoeur, P. (1981). *Hermeneutics and human sciences* (J. B. Thompson, trans.). Paris: Cambridge.

Rogers, M. E. (1992). Nursing science and the space age. *Nursing Science Quarterly, 5,* 27–34.

Santopinto, M. D. A., & Smith, M. C. (1995). Evaluation of the human becoming theory in practice with adults and children. In: R. R. Parse (Ed.), *Illuminations: The human becoming theory in practice and research* (pp. 309–346). New York: National League for Nursing Press.

Smith, M. K. (2002). Human becoming and women living with violence. *Nursing Science Quarterly, 15,* 302–307.

Stanley, G. D., & Meghani, S. H. (2001). Reflections on using Parse's theory of human becoming in a palliative care setting in Pakistan. *Canadian Nurse, 97,* 23–25.

Chapter 17

Margaret Newman's Theory of Health as Expanding Consciousness

MARGARET DEXHEIMER PHARRIS

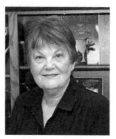

Margaret A. Newman

I don't like controlling, manipulating other people.
I don't like deceiving, withholding, or treating people as subjects or objects.
I don't like acting as an objective non-person.
I do like interacting authentically, listening, understanding, communicating freely.
I do like knowing and expressing myself in mutual relationships.

—MARGARET NEWMAN (1985)

Introducing the Theorist

Nurses who base their practice on Margaret Newman's theory of health as expanding consciousness (HEC) focus on being fully present to meaning and patterns in the lives of their patients. Newman (2005) stated, "[O]ne does not practice nursing *using* the theory, but rather the theory becomes a way of being with the client—a way of offering clients an opportunity to know and be known and to find their way (p. xiv)." Through their relationship with a nurse who understands the theory of HEC and attends to the evolving pattern of what is meaningful in their lives, patients are able to realize a previously undiscovered path for action. Just as patients' health predicaments are situated within the evolving pattern of complex relationships and events in their lives, so too, Newman's theory has evolved within the context of the meaningful relationships and events of her life.

The foundation for Newman's theory was laid long before she entered nursing school (Newman, 1997c). When she was a child, Newman's father, who was an avid reader of philosophical works, would often say to her, "Mind over matter!" Newman learned early on that the way you look at a situation helps you move through it; this was an outlook that carried her through many difficult times and taught her that there are various ways in which to view situations.

As a child growing up in Memphis, Tennessee, Newman had many friends, attended dance school, loved math and the arts, and enjoyed interacting with guests at her parents' tourist home. When it was time to choose a college, Margaret's mother's position as the secretary at the Baptist church strongly influenced Newman's decision to attend college at Baylor University in Texas.

Although Newman did not major in nursing as an undergraduate, two experiences at Baylor sparked her interest in the nursing profession. First, she contemplated entering missionary service but felt she could not attend to people's spiritual well-being without also attending to their physical needs; this realization created a tug toward nursing. The other strong tug occurred during her junior year when Newman's roommate, a nursing student, was called to assist in the aftermath of a tornado. But these influences were not strong enough to persuade her to change college majors at that time.

After graduating from Baylor University Newman returned to Memphis to work and to care for her mother who had been diagnosed a few years earlier with amyotrophic lateral sclerosis (ALS), a degenerative neurological disease that progressively diminishes the movement of all muscles except those of the eyes. The process of caring for her mother over a 5-year period was transformative. Not knowing the trajectory of the disease, Newman learned to live day by day, fully immersed in the present (Newman, 2008b). Newman (2008a) stated she learned that "each day is precious and that the time of one's life is contained in the *present*" (p. 225).

Caring for her mother provided Newman with two additional significant realizations. The first was that simply having a disease does not make a person unhealthy. Although Newman's mother's life was *confined* by the

disease, her life was not *defined* by it. In other words, she could experience health and wholeness in the midst of having a chronic and progressive disease. The second important realization was that time, movement, and space are in some way interrelated with health, which can be manifested by increased connectedness and quality of relationships.

The restrictions of movement that Newman's mother experienced due to the ALS altered her experience of time, space, and consciousness. While caring for her physically immobilized mother, Newman experienced similar alterations in her own movement, space, time, and consciousness (Newman, 1997c). Previously both Margaret Newman and her mother had been very active. They were leaders of organizations and both were involved in several social groups; they were always busy. In the midst of this terminal disease process, with its resultant constrictions on time, space, and movement, both mother and daughter experienced a greater sense of connectedness and increased insight into the meaning of their experience and the meaning of health. Newman came to know her mother in a very deep and significant way (Newman, 2008b). These early seeds of the HEC theory found fertile ground in 1959 when Newman entered nursing school at the University of Tennessee (UT) in Memphis. Her mother died 2 weeks before the beginning of the fall semester for the nursing program at UT. In her first semester of nursing school at UT, Newman realized that nursing would require everything she had—all of her intelligence and all of her humanness (2008b). One of her professors, Marie Buckley, stressed the importance of graduate school for nurses and encouraged the nursing students to consider how to construct an independent nursing practice; this was an idea that intrigued Newman and that she continued to promote in various ways throughout her career.

Another professor, Dorothy Hocker, who held high expectations for students during their clinical rotations, also had a strong impact on Newman's view of the nature of nursing practice. As a student, Newman was frustrated with nursing texts and lectures with lengthy discussions on diseases and their medical treatments but had only a few sentences about the nursing care for people diagnosed with the disease. At that time, most of the knowledge in nursing texts was medical, with only a sprinkling of nursing knowledge added at the very end. Newman wanted to acquire more knowledge specific to the profession of nursing. On one clinical rotation day, she had a very challenging teenage patient with type 1 diabetes. The teen had been hospitalized many times for diabetic comas. Newman watched in horror as a resident physician berated the patient, telling her she was going to die if she didn't shape up. Newman had studied everything there was to know about type 1 diabetes, yet felt at a loss as to how to reach the patient. She did not know what she as a nurse should do. She consulted Dorothy Hocker, who went into the room and asked one or two questions and immediately connected with the patient in a significant and caring manner, which allowed the teenager to open up and talk about her situation. In this interaction, Newman witnessed the power of nursing presence.

A 1961 article by Dorothy Johnson on the significance of nursing care provided the theoretical basis for what Newman had witnessed in the interaction between Dorothy Hocker and the young patient with diabetes. Johnson's writings influenced Newman's desire to explore more thoroughly the nature of nursing practice. Johnson differentiated nursing knowledge from medical knowledge and proposed that nurses provide a dynamic equilibrium for patients as they experience crises.

After graduating from UT's baccalaureate nursing program, Newman stayed on at UT as a clinical instructor. The next year she went to the University of California, San Francisco to obtain her master's degree in medical–surgical nursing. While there, she conducted two studies of nursing practice. One study explored the usefulness of nurse-directed abdominal exercises for preventing constipation in medical–surgical patients on bed rest. The other was influenced by the nursing shortage and looked at nursing interactions during short spans of time (Newman, 1966).

When she graduated from UCSF in 1964, Newman was recruited back to Memphis to become the director of the Clinical Research Center. In this position, Newman went against the conventional grain of the day; she educated the medical director on the nature of nursing functions so that the nursing staff would not be asked to do things physicians could do for themselves or which staff from other departments could do. Newman encouraged the scholarly development of the nursing staff and created time for nurses to go to the library to enrich their knowledge base. Further studies and reflection helped Newman articulate that nurses who can be fully present with patients while doing tasks are able to comprehend in a holistic sense what patients need to achieve a greater sense of health. Seeing and honoring the whole of patients' lives as the important context in which the task at hand is being performed requires a paradigm shift, a shift in point of view. Newman felt that nurse theorist Martha Rogers at New York University (NYU) was articulating a new paradigm of health that expanded the nature of nursing practice. Rogers' Science of Unitary Human Beings theory resonated with Newman's evolving conceptualizations of nursing and health; it enhanced Newman's ability to see the whole by entering into the part (Newman, 1997b).

After directing the Clinical Research Center for 2½ years, Newman decided to pursue doctoral studies in nursing at NYU where she would be able to study with Martha Rogers. She was also excited about living in New York City. Newman received 4 years of funding for her doctoral studies. In her doctoral work at NYU, Newman began studying movement, time, and space as parameters of health; however, she did so out of a logical positivist scientific paradigm. She designed an experimental study that manipulated participants' movements, then measured their perception of time (Newman, 1982). Her results showed a changing perception of time across the life span, with subjective time (as compared to objective time) increasing with age (Newman, 1987). Although her results seemed to support what she later would term "health as expanding consciousness," at the time Newman felt they did little to inform or shape nursing practice, which was what most interested her (Newman, 1997a).

After receiving her PhD in 1971, Newman joined the NYU faculty. While there, Newman published a seminal article in *Nursing Outlook* on nursing's theoretical evolution (Newman, 1972), and with colleague Florence Downs coauthored two editions of a book on research in nursing (Downs & Newman, 1977). She also conducted postdoctoral workshops at NYU on nursing theory development and spent the summer of 1976 consulting with nurses in Brazil. Newman's early career in academia was centered on articulating the knowledge of the discipline and how it is developed.

In 1977, Newman joined the faculty at Penn State as the professor-in-charge of graduate studies. At that time, she was invited to speak at a theory conference to be held in New York in 1978. It was in that address that she first clearly articulated her theory of health. The transcript of her talk was published as a chapter in a book she wrote about theory development in nursing (Newman, 1979), which was one of the first books published on the subject. Newman also organized a Nursing Theory Think Tank, which was limited to 15 PhD prepared nurse scholars who were involved in nursing theory development. Newman remained actively involved with this group until its tenth year. She was also a member of a group of nurse theorists facilitated by Sister Callista Roy to discern how to organize nursing diagnoses so that they would be rooted in the knowledge of the discipline of nursing. This group presented papers in 1978 and 1980 to the North American Nursing Diagnosis Association (NANDA). In 1982, they presented an organizing framework they had developed for nursing diagnoses called *Patterns of Unitary Man (Humans)*.

In 1984, Newman took a position as nurse theorist at the University of Minnesota. As part of her theory development work, she conducted a pilot study of pattern identifcation. She invited Richard Cowling from Case Western and Jim Vail from the Army Nurse Corps to collaborate with her. Newman was at that time also a consultant to the Army Nurse Corps. The study participants were nurses at Walter Reed Hospital. Newman interviewed a nurse while Vail and Cowling watched from another room. She asked the woman to describe meaningful events in her life and diagrammed the unfolding trajectory of her life. When she returned to the woman the next day to reflect the sequential patterns Newman had identified, the woman was able to see that experiences she had previously viewed as being extremely negative (e.g., a divorce), actually were stepping stones to expanded possibilities; she was suddenly able to view her life in a new way. The nurse researchers and participants were excited about the insights they gained. Newman went on to develop a pattern recognition nursing praxis (theory, practice, and research as one) process.

Newman's pattern recognition process served as the basis for the work of several graduate students at the University of Minnesota, most notably Susan Moch (1990), Merian Litchfield (1993, 1999), Helga Jonsdottir (1998), Frank Lamendola (1998), Emiko Endo (1998), Patricia Tommet (2003), and Norma Kiser-Larson (2002). This group met regularly with Newman to dialogue about the evolution of the theory of HEC as they experienced it in their work. The graduate students' studies and the group dialogue, which focused on the meaning of the studies, elaborated and expanded the theory.

While at the University of Minnesota, Newman published two editions of her book, *Health as Expanding Consciousness* (Newman, 1986, 1994a), which attracted international attention. She conducted a series of lectures and dialogues in New Zealand in 1985 and in Finland in 1987 on health as expanding consciousness and nursing knowledge development.

Together with colleagues in Tucson, Arizona, Newman conducted a study of nurses working with a nurse case management project; she found that as nurses reflected on their pattern over time, they gained insights for improved practice and increased general well-being (Newman, Lamb, & Michaels, 1991). This work substantiated the theory of health as expanding consciousness.

Shortly after retiring from her position at the University of Minnesota, Margaret Newman returned to Memphis, Tennessee, where she continues to work on nursing knowledge development through her writing and by dialoguing with students and scholars from around the world. Most recently she published a book titled *Transforming Presence: The Difference that Nursing Makes* (Newman, 2008b). Another book edited by Carol Picard and Dorothy Jones (2005), *Giving Voice to What we Know: Margaret Newman's Theory of Health as Expanding Consciousness in Nursing Practice, Research, and Education,* provides examples of how the theory of HEC has been applied to shape nursing practice, administration, and education.

The honors awarded to Dr. Newman include being named a Fellow of the American Academy of Nursing and a New York University Distinguished Scholar in Nursing. She has received Sigma Theta Tau International's Founders Award for Excellence in Nursing Research and the E. Louise Grant Award for Nursing Excellence from the University of Minnesota. She has been honored as an outstanding alumnus by both the University of Tennessee and New York University. In 2008 Dr. Newman was named a Living Legend by the American Academy of Nursing.

Overview of the Theory

As previously described, the seeds for the theory of health as expanding consciousness (HEC) were planted in Margaret Newman's childhood and experience of caring for her mother as a young adult. Newman's undergraduate studies at the University of Tennessee, master's studies at the University of California, San Francisco, and doctoral studies at New York University also greatly influenced her quest for exploring and articulating the knowledge of the discipline of nursing. Reading and reflecting on the philosophical work of scholars from various disciplines—mainly Bentov (1978), Bohm (1980), Johnson (1961), Prigogene (1976), Rogers (1970), and Young (1976)—stretched Newman's view of the possibilities of nursing, and thus enriched the theory of HEC. Work and dialogue with colleagues and students further explicated the theory.

Academic and Philosophical Influences on the Theory

During her time at the University of California, San Francisco, Newman explored how nurses could respond to patients in a meaningful way during short time spans. Newman's interest in attending to what is meaningful to the patient was influenced by Ida Jean Orlando's deliberative nursing approach. Inspired by Orlando's theoretical work, Newman began making deliberative observations about patients and reflecting what she observed back to the patient. The specific attention stimulated patients to respond by talking about what was meaningful in their unique circumstances.

In a publication of the results of her exploration of this approach to nursing during short time spans, Newman (1966) recounted walking into the room of a patient who had been in the hospital for some time. The patient was reading the newspaper and Newman noticed that the woman was reading the want ads. Newman simply stated, "Reading the want ads, huh?" and waited for a response. The woman, who had been diagnosed with a chronic lung problem, worked in a factory that exuded toxic fumes and she would no longer be able to work there. She was deeply concerned about her future. What ensued through their dialogue was a breakthrough for the patient, whose health care predicament was couched in the larger context of her potential loss of income. Newman asked the woman if she had discussed this with her physician, and the woman responded that she had not discussed it with anyone. When Newman asked why not, the woman replied that no one had asked her about it. Once the meaning of her illness was understood within the context of her entire life, not just her physical state, a path toward health became apparent for the patient. This process of focusing on meaning in patients' lives to understand where the current health predicament fits in the whole of people's lives has endured as central to HEC.

Newman's theoretical insights evolved as she delved into the works of Martha Rogers and Itzhak Bentov, while at the same time reflecting back on her own experience (Newman, 1997b). Several of Martha Rogers' assumptions became central in enriching Margaret Newman's theoretical perspective (Newman, 1997b). First and foremost, Rogers saw health and illness not as two separate realities, but rather as a unitary process. This was congruent with Margaret Newman's earlier experience with her mother and with her patients. On a very deep level, Newman knew that people can experience health even when they are physically or mentally ill. Health is not the opposite of illness, but rather health and illness are both manifestations of a greater whole. One can be very healthy in the midst of a terminal illness.

Second, Rogers argued that all of reality is a unitary whole and that each human being exhibits a unique pattern. Rogers (1970) saw energy fields to be the fundamental unit of all that is living and nonliving, and she posited that there is interpenetration between the fields of person, family, and environment. Person, family, and environment are not separate entities, but rather are an interconnected, unitary whole (Rogers, 1990). Finally, Rogers saw the life process as showing increasing complexity. These assumptions from Rogers' theory, along with the work of Itzhak Bentov (1978), helped to enrich Margaret Newman's (1997b) conceptualization of health and eventually the articulation of her theory. Bentov viewed life as a process of expanding consciousness, which he defined as the informational capacity of the system and the quality of interactions with the environment.

Basic Assumptions of the Theory of Health as Expanding Consciousness

Reflecting on these theoretical works helped Newman prepare for her *Toward a Theory of Health* presentation at the 1978 nursing theory conference in New York City. It was at that conference that the theory of health as expanding consciousness was first formally explicated. In her address (Newman, 1978) and in a written overview of the address (Newman, 1979), Newman outlined the basic assumptions that were integral to her theory at that time. Drawing on the work of Martha Rogers and Itzhak Bentov and on her own experience and insight, she proposed that:

- Health encompasses conditions known as disease or pathology, as well as states where disease is not present.
- Disease/pathology can be considered a manifestation of the underlying pattern of the person.
- The pattern of the person manifesting itself as disease was present before the structural and functional changes of disease.
- Removal of the disease/pathology will not change the pattern of the individual.
- If becoming "ill" is the only way a person's pattern can be manifested, then that is health for the person.
- Health is the expansion of consciousness (Newman, 1979).

Newman's presentation drew thunderous applause as she ended with, "[t]he responsibility of the nurse is not to make people well, or to prevent their getting sick, but to assist people to recognize the power that is within them to move to higher levels of consciousness" (Newman, 1978).

Although Margaret Newman never set out to become a nursing theorist, in that 1978 presentation in New York City she articulated a theory that resonated with what was meaningful in the practice of nurses in many countries throughout the world. Nurses wanted to go beyond combating diseases; they wanted to accompany their patients in the process of discovering meaning and wholeness in their lives. Margaret Newman's proposed theory served as a guide for them to do so; it offered a new way of looking at the essence of nursing practice.

Developing the Theory of HEC

After identifying the basic assumptions of the theory of HEC, the next step was to focus on how to test the theory with nursing research and how the theory could inform nursing practice. Newman began to concentrate on:

- The mutuality of the nurse–client interaction in the process of pattern recognition
- The uniqueness and wholeness of the pattern in each client situation
- The sequential configurations of pattern evolving over time
- Insights occurring as choice points of action potential
- The movement of the life process toward expanded consciousness (Newman, 1997a).

To test the theory of HEC, which embraces reality as an undivided whole, Newman found that Western scientific research methodologies, which isolate particulate variables and analyze the relationships between them, were insufficient.

Newman saw a need to articulate that her work fell within a new paradigm of nursing. Like Martha Rogers (1970, 1990), Newman sees human beings as unitary and inseparable from the larger unitary field that combines person, family, and community all at once. Seeing change as unpredictable and transformative, she named the paradigm within which her work and the work of Martha Rogers are situated the unitary-transformative paradigm (Newman, Sime, and Corcoran-Perry, 1991). A nurse practicing within the unitary–transformative paradigm does not think of mind, body, spirit, and emotion as separate entities, but rather sees them as manifestations of an undivided whole.

Newman's theory (1979, 1990, 1994a, 1997a, 1997b, 2008b) proposes that we cannot isolate, manipulate, and control variables in order to understand the whole of a phenomenon. The nurse and client form a mutual partnership to attend to the pattern of meaningful relationships and experiences in the client's life. In this way, a patient who has had a heart attack can understand the experience of the heart attack in the context of all that is meaningful in his or her life, and through the insight gained with pattern recognition, experience expanding consciousness. Newman's (1994a, 1997a, 1997b) methodology does not divide people's lives into fragmented variables, but rather attends to the nature and meaning of the whole, which becomes apparent in the nurse–patient dialogue.

A nurse practicing within the HEC theoretical perspective possesses multifaceted levels of awareness and is able to sense how physical signs, emotional conveyances, spiritual insights, physical appearances, and mental insights are all meaningful manifestations of a person's underlying pattern. These manifestations also provide insight into the nature of the person's interactions with his or her environment. It takes disciplined study and reflection on practical experience applying the theory for nurses to be able to see pattern as insight into the whole. Newman (2008b) states that practicing within a unitary paradigm requires a completely new way of seeing reality—it is like moving to Copernicus's view of the solar system after always seeing the world as flat—reality is seen from a whole new perspective and there is no going back to the old way of viewing the world.

Newman (1997a) asserted that knowledge emanating from the unitary–transformative paradigm is the knowledge of the discipline and that the focus, philosophy, and theory of the discipline must be consistent with each other and therefore cannot flow out of different paradigms. Newman (1997a) stated:

> The paradigm of the discipline is becoming clear. We are moving from attention on the other as object to attention to the we in relationship, from fixing things to attending to the meaning of the whole, from hierarchical one-way intervention

to mutual process partnering. It is time to break with a paradigm of health that focuses on power, manipulation, and control and move to one of reflective, compassionate consciousness. The paradigm of nursing embraces wholeness and pattern. It reveals a world that is moving, evolving, transforming—a process. (p. 37)

Newman points the way for nurses to practice and conduct research within a unitary–transformative paradigm. The unitary–transformative paradigm sees the process of the nurse–patient partnership as integral to the evolving definition of health for the patient (Litchfield, 1993, 1999; Newman, 1997a), and is synchronous with participatory philosophical thought (Skolimowski, 1994) and research methodology (Heron & Reason, 1997).

When nurses view the world from a unitary perspective, they begin to see the nature of relationships and their meaning in an entirely new light. The work of Frank Lamendola and Margaret Newman (1994) with people with HIV/AIDS illustrates this. In a study they conducted, they found that the experience of HIV/AIDS opened participants to suffering and physical deterioration and at the same time introduced greater sensitivity and openness to themselves and others. Drawing on the work of cultural historian William Irwin Thompson, systems theorist Will McWhinney, and musician David Dunn, Lamendola and Newman, stated:

They [Thompson, McWhinney, and Dunn] see the loss of membranal integrity as a signal of the loss of autopoetic unity analogous to the breaking down of boundaries at a global level between countries, ideologies, and disparate groups. Thompson views HIV/AIDS not simply as a chance infection but part of a larger cultural phenomenon and sees the pathogen not as an object but as heralding the need for living together characterized by a symbiotic relationship. (Lamendola & Newman, 1994, p. 14)

These authors pointed out that the AIDS epidemic has necessitated greater interconnectedness on the interpersonal, community, and global level. It has also called for a re-conceptualization of the nature of the self

and of treatment—inviting a new sense of harmonic integration within the immune system. Lamendola and Newman quoted Thompson (1989), who stated that we need to "learn to tolerate aliens by seeing the self as a cloud in a clouded sky and not as a lord in a walled-in fortress." This change in perspective helps nurses and patients move away from military metaphors in relationship to patients' bodies (i.e., *combating* disease, *waging battles* against *invading* cells, etc.) to focus instead on harmony and balance. Nursing care within a unitary perspective unveils meaning and opens the possibility for a new way of living for people with chronic conditions.

Applications of the Theory

Essential Aspects of Nursing Practice within the HEC Perspective

Newman (2008b) synthesizes the basic assumptions of HEC in the following way:

- Health is an evolving *unitary pattern* of the whole, including patterns of disease.
- Consciousness is the *informational capacity* of the whole and is revealed in the evolving pattern.
- Pattern identifies the human–environmental process and is characterized by *meaning*. (p. 6)

Concepts important to nursing practice grounded in the theory of HEC include expanding consciousness, time, presence, resonating with the whole, pattern, meaning, insights as choice points, and the mutuality of the nurse–patient relationship.

Expanding Consciousness

Ultimate consciousness has been equated with love, which embraces all experience equally and unconditionally: pain as well as pleasure, failure as well as success, ugliness as well as beauty, disease as well as nondisease.

—M. A. NEWMAN (2003, P. 241)

Consciousness within the theory of HEC is not limited to cognitive thought. Margaret Newman (1994a) defined consciousness as the information of the system: The capacity of the system to interact with the environment. In the human system the informational capacity includes not only all the things we normally associate with consciousness, such as thinking and feeling, but also all the information embedded in the nervous system, the immune system, the genetic code, and so on. The information of these and other systems reveals the complexity of the human system and how the information of the system interacts with the information of the environmental system (p. 33).

To illustrate consciousness as the interactional capacity of the person–environment, Newman (1994a) drew on the work of Bentov (1978), who presents consciousness on a continuum ranging from rocks on one end of the spectrum (which have little known interaction with their environment), to plants (which draw nutrients and provide carbon dioxide), to animals (which can move about and interact freely), to humans (who can reflect and make in-depth plans regarding how they want to interact with their environment), and ultimately to spiritual beings on the spectrum's other end. Newman sees death as a transformation point, with a person's consciousness continuing to develop beyond the physical life, becoming a part of a universal consciousness (Newman, 1994a).

The *process* of expanding consciousness is characterized by the evolving pattern of the person–environment interaction (Newman, 1994a). The process of expanding consciousness is defined by Newman (2008b) as "a process of becoming more of oneself, of finding greater meaning in life, and of reaching new heights of connectedness with other people and the world" (p. 6). Nurses and their clients know that there has been an expansion of consciousness when there is a richer, more meaningful quality to their relationships. Relationships that are more open, loving, caring, connected, and peaceful are a manifestation of expanding consciousness. These deeper, more meaningful relationships, may be interpersonal, or they may be relationships with the wider community or biosphere. Expanding consciousness is evident when

people transcend their own egos, dedicate their energy to something greater than the individual self, and learn to build order against the trend of disorder. The process of expanding consciousness may look differently with changes in cognitive function; nurses must carefully discern patterns of meaning when this is the case. For example, when being present to people with dementia or to very young children, nurses realize that there is no past or future—there is only the present and they must be fully present in the present on a deeper level than cognitive and verbal processes can take them (Newman, 2008b). People are best able to experience expanding consciousness when they are not chained to linear time.

Time and Presence

The time experienced
In a moment
Expands or diminishes
With consciousness.
If I am fully present
There is
No time.
Only consciousness.

—MARGARET NEWMAN (2008A, P. 225)

Newman's earliest published work points to the ability of nurses to quickly and effectively, in a short time span, attend to what is most important to patients and by engaging patients in a dialogue about what is of utmost importance to them, to discern the patient's unique path toward health (Newman, 1966). Newman's latest work asserts that it is only when nurses move away from a sense of linear time to a more universal frequency of synchronization that they can be truly present to patients in a meaningful and whole manner (Newman, 2008a). Newman stated:

There is a need to get back to the natural cycles of the universe. The time of civilization (clock time and the Gregorian calendar) is not the same as the time of the rest of the biosphere, our living planet earth. Natural time is radial in nature, projecting from the center, and continuously moving in the direction of greater consciousness (2008a, p. 227).

Newman asserted that the artificial time frame of clinic schedules and hospital shift work places nurses at odds with the natural rhythm of nurse–patient relationships, serves the needs of health systems administrations more than those of patients, and disrupts a meaningful nursing practice. She pointed out that the discipline of nursing has followed a trajectory from adherence to artificial linear time to the synchronization of time in interpersonal relationships, and now must move to the "instantaneous flow of information in each center of consciousness" and that "it is time to opt for practice that reflects this dimension" (Newman, 2008a, p. 227). When nurses must move out of a Western sense of time, they can be more fully present to patients.

Newman (2008b) asserted that it is only in relationship that people can fully come to know themselves. She drew on the work of Smith (2001), who suggested that "when the nurse considers the patient a *mystery to be engaged in* rather than a *problem to be solved*, the relationship is characterized by presence" (Newman, 2008b, p. 53). Newman further stated that "presence is enhanced by the nurse's openness and sensitivity to the other" and involves the nurse letting go of judgments of "good" or "bad" in relationship to patients' health behaviors.

When nurses are truly present to patients they concentrate more on intuitive knowing than on the gathering of facts and health-related data. They enter into a relaxed alertness and realize that transforming presence involves a keen awareness of their oneness with the patient (Newman, 2008b; Newman, Smith, Pharris, & Jones, 2008). Understanding the concept of resonance enables a transforming presence.

Resonating with the Whole

Newman (2008b) described resonance as the mechanism for acquiring essential information to guide nursing actions and to understand meaning in patients' lives. She stated, "This is an important distinction in the explication of nursing knowledge. Knowledge at the unitary, transformative level includes and transcends energy transfer at the sensorial level. It is *nonenergetic, nonlocal, and present everywhere*" (p. 35). She differentiated this information transfer from the transfer of sensory information (like heat and touch, which involve physical energy transfer) and suggests nurses continually rely on this information transfer when intuitive insights arise during the care of patients. Newman cautioned that "intellectualization breaks the field of resonance. If we analyze or evaluate an experience before we have resonated with it, the field is broken—the resonance is damped" (p. 37). "For instance, sometimes when we see familiar symptoms of a disease, we jump into a diagnostic conclusion and preclude receptivity to other data that would present a more complete picture. It assumes we are all the same" (p. 45). Resonance enables nurses to sense the unique situation and concerns of patients.

To resonate with patients and form open relationships, nurses must let go of personal judgments about patients and transcend cultural beliefs and values. In other words, the nurse needs to free him- or herself of all "should" and "ought to" attitudes and all personal preoccupations that might prevent total presence. Newman states there is no prescriptive way to sense the whole through resonance. She recommended that nurses pay attention to the client at the simplest level, begin with whatever presents itself, and assume that it is purposeful (Newman, 2008b). Learning to resonate with patients involves relational engagement and reflection.

Most conventional education programs teach analytic processes attending to what is "logical." This leads students away from understanding the whole. Methods that involve empirical investigation assume that the whole comes after the parts; these methods tend to blind investigators to their relationship with the whole. Newman (2008b) drew on the work of Bohm (1980) to stress that "wholeness is what is real, with fragmentation as our response to fragmentary thought. The whole is irreducible and omnipresent" (p. 40). Newman (2008b) differentiated between the general and the universal. "Seeing comprehensively is concrete and holistic, whereas generalization is abstract and analytical; these ways of seeing go in opposite directions" (p. 47). Resonance is a way to sense into the whole through attention to one aspect or part of it, always with an eye on comprehending the whole. Resonance enables nurses to tap into the pattern of the whole.

Attention to Pattern and Meaning

Essential to Margaret Newman's theory is the belief that each person exhibits a distinct pattern, which is constantly unfolding and evolving as the person interacts with the environment. Pattern is information that depicts the whole of a person's relationship with the environment and gives an understanding of the meaning of the relationships all at once (Endo, 1998; Newman, 1994a). Pattern is characterized by meaning (Newman, 2008b) and is a manifestation of consciousness.

To describe the nature of pattern, Newman draws on the work of David Bohm (1980), who said that anything *explicate* (that which we can hear, see, taste, smell, touch) is a manifestation of the *implicate* (the unseen underlying pattern) (Newman, 1997b). In other words, there is information about the underlying pattern of each person in all that we sense about them, such as their movements, tone of voice, interactions with others, activity level, genetic pattern, vital signs. People can be identified from a distance by someone who knows them, just from the way in which they move. There is also information about their underlying pattern in all that they tell us about their experiences and perceptions, including stories about their life, recounted dreams, and portrayed meanings.

The HEC perspective sees disease, disorder, disconnection, and violence as an explication of the underlying implicate pattern of the person, family, and community. Reflecting on the meaning of these conditions can be part of the process of expanding consciousness (Newman, 1994a, 1997a, 1997b).

Pharris (1999) offered the example of a 16-year-old young man placed in an adult correctional facility after a murder conviction. This young man was constantly getting into fights and generally feeling lost. As he and the nurse researcher met over several weeks to gain insight into patterns of meaningful people and events in his life, the process seemed to be blocked, with no pattern emerging and little insight gained. He spoke of how he felt he had lost himself several years back when he went from being a straight-A student from a stable family to stealing cars, drinking, getting into fights, and eventually murdering someone. One week he walked into the room where the nurse was waiting and his movements seemed more controlled and labored; he sat with his arms tightly cradling his bloated abdomen, and his chest was expanded as though he were about to explode. His palms were glistening with sweat. His face was erupting with acne. He talked as usual in a very detached manner, but his words came out in bursts. The nurse chose to give him feedback about what she was seeing and sensing from his body. She reflected that he seemed to be exerting a great deal of energy holding back something that was erupting within him. With this insight, he was quiet for a few minutes and tears began rolling down his cheeks. Suddenly he began talking about a very painful family history of sexual abuse that had been kept secret for many years. It became obvious that the experience of covering up the abuse had been so all-encompassing that it was suppressing his pattern.

This young man had reached a point at which he realized his old ways of interacting with others were no longer serving him, and he chose to interact with his environment in a different way. By the next meeting, his movements had become smooth and sure, his complexion had cleared up, he was now able to reflect on his insights, and he no longer was involved in the chaos and fighting in his cell-block. He was able to let go of his need to control everything and was able to connect with the emotions of his childhood experiences; he was also able to cry for the first time in years.

In their subsequent work together, this young man and the nurse were able to distinguish between his implicate pattern, which had now become clear through their dialogue, and the impact that keeping the abusive experience a secret had had on him and on other members of his family. He was able to free himself of the shame he was carrying, which did not belong to him. Since that time, the young man has been able to transcend previous limitations and has become involved in several efforts to help others, both in and out of the prison environment. He has entered into several warm and loving relationships with family members and friends and has achieved academic success. This was evidence of expanding consciousness for the young man. He reflected that he wished he had had a nurse to talk with prior to "catching his case" (being arrested for murder). He had been seen by a nurse in the juvenile detention center, who performed a physical examination and gave him aspirin for a headache. A few days before the murder, he saw a nurse practitioner in a clinic who wrote a prescription for antibiotics and talked with him about safe sex. These interactions are explications of the pattern of the U.S. health care system and the increasingly task-oriented role that nursing is being pressured to take (Jonsdottir, Litchfield, & Pharris, 2003, 2004).

The focus of nursing is on pattern and meaning. That which is underlying makes itself known in the physical realm. Nurses grounded in the theory of HEC are able to be in relationships with patients, families, and communities in such a way that insights arising in their pattern recognition dialogue shed light on an expanded horizon of potential actions (Newman, 1997a; Litchfield, 1999).

Insights Occurring as Choice Points of Action Potential

The disruption of disease and other traumatic life events may be critical points in the expansion of consciousness. To explain this phenomenon, Newman (1994a, 1997b) drew on the work of Ilya Prigogine (1976), whose theory of dissipative structures asserts that a

system fluctuates in an orderly manner until some disruption occurs, and the system moves in a seemingly random, chaotic, disorderly way until at some point it chooses to move into a higher level of organization (Newman, 1997b). Nurses see this all the time—the patient who is lost to his work and has no time for his family or himself, and then suddenly has a heart attack, which leaves him open to reflecting on how he has been using his energy. Insights gained through this reflection give rise to transformation and decisions about where energy will be spent; and his life becomes more creative, relational, and meaningful. Nurses also see this in people diagnosed with a terminal illness that causes them to reevaluate what is really important, attend to it, and then to state that for the first time they feel as though they are really living. The expansion of consciousness is an innate tendency of humans; however, some experiences and processes precipitate more rapid transformations. Nurse researchers working within the theory of HEC have clearly demonstrated how nurses can create a mutual partnership with their patients to reflect on their evolving pattern and the points of transformation. Through this process, expanding consciousness is realized (Barron, 2005; Endo, 1998; Endo, Minegishi, & Kubo, 2005; Endo et al., 2000; Flanagan, 2005; Jonsdottir, 1998; Jonsdottir et al., 2003, 2004; Kiser-Larson, 2002; Lamendola, 1998; Lamendola & Newman, 1994; Litchfield, 1993, 1999, 2005; Moch, 1990; Neill, 2002a, 2002b; Newman, 1995; Newman & Moch, 1991; Noveletsky-Rosenthal, 1996; Pharris, 2002, 2005; Pharris & Endo, 2007; Picard, 2000, 2005; Ruka, 2005; Tommet, 2003).

Newman (1999) pointed out that nurse–client relationships often begin during periods of disruption, uncertainty, and unpredictability in patients' lives. When patients are in a state of chaos because of disease, trauma, loss, etc., they often cannot see their past or future clearly. In the context of the nurse–patient partnership, which centers on the meaning the patient gives to the health predicament, insight for action arises and it becomes clear to the patient how to get on with life (Jonsdottir et al., 2003, 2004; Litchfield, 1999; Newman, 1999). Litchfield (1993, 1999) sees this as experiencing an expanding present that connects to the past and creates an extended horizon of action potential for the future.

Endo (1998), in her work in Japan with women with cancer; Noveletsky-Rosenthal (1996), in her work in the United States with people with chronic obstructive pulmonary disease; and Pharris (2002), in her work with U.S. adolescents convicted of murder, found that it is when patients' lives are in the greatest states of chaos, disorganization, and uncertainty that the HEC nursing partnership and pattern recognition process is perceived as most beneficial to patients (Fig. 17-1).

Many nurses who encounter patients in times of chaos strive for stability; they feel they have to *fix* the situation, not realizing that this disorganized time in the patient's life presents an opportunity for growth. Newman (1999) states:

The "brokenness" of the situation . . . is only a point in the process leading to a higher order. We need to join in partnership with clients and dance their dance, even though it appears arrhythmic, until order begins to emerge out of chaos. We know, and we can help clients know, that there is a basic, underlying pattern evolving even though it might not be apparent at the time. The pattern will be revealed at a higher level of organization. (p. 228)

The disruption brought about by the presence of disease, illness, and traumatic or stressful events creates an opportunity for transformation to an expanded level of consciousness (Newman, 1997b, 1999) and represents a time when patients most need nurses who are attentive to that which is most meaningful. Newman (1999, p. 228) stated, "Nurses have a responsibility to stay in partnership with clients as their patterns are disturbed by illness or other disruptive events." This disrupted state presents a *choice point* for the person to either continue going on as before, even

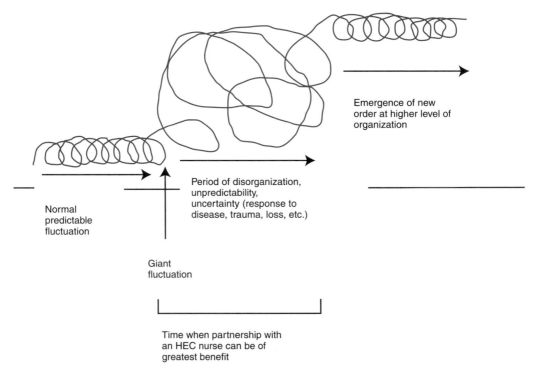

Emergence of new
order at higher level of
organization

Period of disorganization,
unpredictability,
uncertainty (response to
disease, trauma, loss, etc.)

Normal
predictable
fluctuation

Giant
fluctuation

Time when partnership with
an HEC nurse can be of
greatest benefit

Figure 17 • 1 Prigogine's theory of dissipative structures applied to health as expanding consciousness (HEC) nursing.

though the old rules are not working, or to shift into a new way of being. To explain the concept of a *choice point* more clearly, Newman drew on Arthur Young's (1976) theory of the evolution of consciousness.

Young suggested that there are seven stages of binding and unbinding, which begin with total freedom and unrestricted choice, followed by a series of losses of freedom. After these losses comes a choice point and a reversal of the losses of freedom, ending with total freedom and unrestricted choice. These stages can be conceptualized as seven equidistant points on a V shape (Fig. 17-2). Beginning at the uppermost point on the left is the first stage, *potential freedom.* The next stage is *binding.* In this stage, the individual is sacrificed for the sake of the collective, with no need for initiative because everything is being regulated for the individual. The third stage, *centering,* involves the development of an individual identity, self-consciousness, and self-determination. "Individualism emerges in the self's break with authority" (Newman, 1994b). The fourth stage, *choice,* is situated at the base of the V. In this stage, the individual learns that the old ways of being are no longer working. It is a stage of self-awareness, inner growth, and transformation. A new way of being becomes necessary. Newman (1994b) described the fifth stage, *decentering,* as being characterized by a shift from the development of self (individuation) to dedication to something greater than the individual self. The person experiences outstanding competence; his or her works have a life of their own beyond the creator. The task is transcendence of the ego. Form is transcended, and the energy becomes the dominant feature—in terms of animation, vitality, a quality that is somehow infinite. In this stage, the person experiences the power of unlimited growth and has learned how to build order against the trend of disorder (pp. 45–46).

Newman (1994b) stated that few experience the sixth stage, *unbinding,* or the seventh stage, *real freedom,* unless they have had these experiences of transcendence characterized by the fifth stage. It is in the moving through the

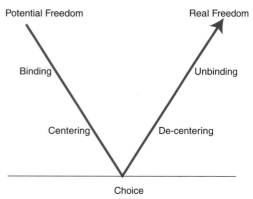

Figure 17 • 2 Young's spectrum of the evolution of consciousness.

choice point and the stages of decentering and unbinding that a person moves on to higher levels of consciousness (Newman, 1999). Newman proposed a corollary between her theory of health as expanding consciousness and Young's theory of the evolution of consciousness in that we "come into being from a state of potential consciousness, are bound in time, find our identity in space, and through movement we learn 'the law' of the way things work and make choices that ultimately take us beyond space and time to a state of absolute consciousness" (Newman, 1994b, p. 46).

The Mutuality of the Nurse–Client Interaction in the Process of Pattern Recognition

We come to the meaning of the whole not by viewing the pattern from the outside, but by entering into the evolving pattern as it unfolds.

—M. A. NEWMAN

Nursing within the HEC perspective involves being fully present to the patient without judgments, goals, or intervention strategies. It involves *being with* rather than *doing for.* It is caring in its deepest, most respectful sense with a focus on what is important to the patient. The nurse–patient interaction becomes like a pure reflection pool through which both the nurse and the patient achieve a clear picture of their pattern and come away transformed by the insights gained.

To illustrate the mutually transforming effect of the nurse–patient interaction, Newman (1994a) offers the image of a smooth lake into which two stones are thrown. As the stones hit the water, concentric waves circle out until the two patterns reach one another and interpenetrate. The new pattern of their interaction ripples back and transforms the two original circling patterns. Nurses are changed by their interactions with their patients, just as patients are changed by their interactions with nurses. This mutual transformation extends to the surrounding environment and relationships of the nurse and patient.

In the process of doing this work, it is important that the nurse sense his or her own pattern. Newman states: "We have come to see nursing as a process of relationship that co-evolves as a function of the interpenetration of the evolving fields of the nurse, client, and the environment in a self-organizing, unpredictable way. We recognize the need for process wisdom, the ability to come from the center of our truth and act in the immediate moment" (Newman, 1994b, p. 155). Sensing one's own pattern is an essential starting point for the nurse. In her book *Health as Expanding Consciousness,* Newman (1994a, pp. 107–109) outlines a process of focusing to assist nurses as they begin working in the HEC perspective. It is important that the nurse be able to practice from the center of his or her own truth and be fully present to the patient. The nurse's consciousness, or pattern, becomes like the vibrations of a tuning fork that resonate at a centering frequency, and the client has the opportunity to resonate and tune to that clear frequency during their interactions (Newman, 1994a; Quinn, 1992). The nurse–patient relationship ideally continues until the patient finds his or her own rhythmic vibrations without the need of the stabilizing force of the nurse–patient dialogue. Newman (1999) points out that the partnership demands that nurses develop tolerance for uncertainty, disorganization, and dissonance, even though it

may be uncomfortable. It is in the state of disequilibrium that the potential for growth exists. She states, "The rhythmic relating of nurse with client at this critical boundary is a window of opportunity for transformation in the health experience" (Newman, 1999, p. 229).

Relevance of HEC Across Cultures

Margaret Newman's theory of health as expanding consciousness is being used throughout the world, but it has been more quickly embraced and understood by nurses from indigenous and Eastern cultures, who are less bound by linear, three-dimensional thought and physical concepts of health and who are more immersed in the metaphysical, mystical aspect of human existence. Increasingly, however, HEC is being enthusiastically embraced by nurses in industrialized nations who are finding it difficult to nurse in the modern technologically driven and intervention-oriented health care system, which is dependent on diagnosing and treating diseases (Jonsdottir et al., 2003, 2004). Practicing from an HEC perspective involves a holistic approach, which places what is meaningful to patients back into the center of the nurses' focus and what is meaningful to students back into the center of the focus of nurse educators. This person-centered approach has wide appeal across cultures.

Focusing on the Process of Health Patterning and the Nurse–Patient Partnership

Merian Litchfield (1993), from New Zealand, was the first researcher to apply the theory of health as expanding consciousness to a nursing partnership with families. Litchfield (1993, 1999, 2005) has led the way in focusing on the process of the nursing partnership with patients and families. In her first study, Litchfield (1993) described health patterning as "a process of nursing practice whereby, through dialogue, families with researcher as practitioner, recognize pattern in the life process providing opportunity for insight as the potential for action; a process by which there may be increased self-determination as a feature of health" (p. 10). Litchfield (1993) describes her research as a "shared process of inquiry through which participants are empowered to act to change their circumstances" (p. 20). Through her research over several years with families with complex health predicaments requiring repeated hospitalizations, Litchfield (1993, 1999, 2005) found that she could not stand outside of the process of recognizing pattern to observe a fixed health pattern of the family. She sees the pattern as continuously evolving dialectically in the dialogue within the nursing partnership. The findings are literally created in the participatory process of the partnership (Litchfield, 1999). For this reason, Litchfield did not use diagrams to reflect pattern, as she thought they would imply that the pattern is static rather than continually evolving. As the family reflects on the pattern of their interactions with each other and the environment, insight into action may involve a transformative process, with the same events being seen in a new light. Family health is seen as a function of the nurse–family relationship. Many of the families in partnership with Litchfield gained insight into their own predicaments in such a way that they required less interaction and service from traditional health care services and thus a cost saving in health care services was realized (1999, 2005).

Exploring Pattern Recognition as a Nursing Intervention

Emiko Endo (1998) explored HEC pattern recognition as a nursing intervention in Japan with women living with ovarian cancer. She asked, "When a person with cancer has an opportunity to share meaning in the life process within the nurse–client relationship, what changes may occur in the evolving pattern?" Attending to the flow of meaningful thoughts for each participant and building on the previous work of Litchfield (1993), Endo found four common phases of the process of expanding consciousness for all participants: client–nurse mutual concern, pattern recognition,

vision and action potential, and transformation. Participants differed in the pace of evolving movement toward a turning point and in the characteristics of personal growth at the turning point. The characteristics of growth ranged from assertion of self, to emancipation of self, to transcendence of self. Reflecting on her experience, Endo (1998) put forth that pattern recognition is "not intended to fix clients' problems from a medical diagnostic standpoint, but to provide individuals with an opportunity to know themselves, to find meaning in their current situation and life, and to gain insight for the future" (p. 60).

Endo et al. (2000) conducted a similar study with Japanese families in which the wife-mother was hospitalized because of a cancer diagnosis. Families found meaning in their patterns and reported increased understanding of their present situation. In the pattern recognition process, most families reconfigured from being a collection of separated individuals to trustful, caring relationships as a family unit, showing more openness and connectedness. The researchers concluded that pattern recognition as a nursing intervention was a "meaning-making transforming process in the family–nurse partnership" (p. 604).

Early research emanating from Margaret Newman's HEC theoretical perspective added to understanding the interrelatedness of time, movement, space, and consciousness as manifestations of health. These studies pointed to the need to look at health as expanding consciousness using a research methodology that acknowledges, understands, and honors the undivided wholeness of the human health experience. They pointed to a need to *step inside* to view the whole from within—which is simply a metaphorical process since the researcher has been integrally within the whole all along. These studies cleared away the murky waters surrounding what previously appeared to be separate islands, but are now clearly visible as mountaintops on one undivided piece of land, newly emerged but always there as a whole. As a result, a new generation of qualitative HEC research emerged, and a deeper understanding of health from a holistic perspective has surfaced. This new understanding inspires practice.

HEC-Inspired Practice

Patricia Tommet (2003) used the HEC hermeneutic dialectic methodology to explore the pattern of nurse–parent interaction in families faced with choosing an elementary school for their medically fragile children. She found a pattern of *living in uncertainty* in the families during the intense period of disruption and disorganization after the birth of their medically fragile child through the first few years. After 2 to 3 years, the families exhibited a pattern of *order in chaos* where they learned how to live in the present, letting go of the way they lived in the past. Tommet found that "families changed from being passive recipients to active participants in the care of their children" (p. 90) and that the "experience of their children's birth and life transformed these families and through them, transformed systems of care" (p. 86). Tommet demonstrated insights gained in family pattern recognition and concluded that a nurse–parent partnership could have a more profound impact on these families, and hence the services they use, during the first 3 years of their children's lives.

Working with colleagues in New Zealand, Litchfield undertook a pilot project that included 19 families in a predicament of strife (Litchfield & Laws, 1999). The goal of the pilot project, which built on Litchfield's previous work (1993, 1999), was to explore a model of nurse case management incorporating the use of a family nurse who understands the theory of health as expanding consciousness. In the context of a family–family nurse partnership, the unfolding pattern of family living was attended to. Family nurses shared their stories of the families with the research group, who reflected together on the families' changing predicaments and the whole picture of family living in terms of how each family moved in time and place. Subsequent visits with the families focused on recognition of pattern and potential for action. The family nurse mobilized relief services if necessary and orchestrated services as needs emerged in the process of pattern recognition. The research group found that families became more open and spontaneous through the process of pattern recognition, and their interactions evidenced more focus, purposefulness, and cooperation. In analyzing costs of medical care for one participating family, it was estimated that a 3 to 13 percent savings could be seen by employing the model of family nursing, with greater savings being possible when family nurses are available immediately after a family disruption takes place (Litchfield & Laws, 1999). Based on Litchfield's work with families with complex health predicaments, the government funded a large demonstration project to support family nurses who would be able to nurse from unitary-transformative perspective and partner with families without having predetermined goals and outcomes that the families and nurses must achieve. These nurses are free to focus on family health as defined and experienced by the families themselves.

Endo and colleagues (Endo, Minegishi, & Kubo, 2005; Endo, Miyahara, Suzuki, & Ohmasa, 2005) in Japan have expanded their work to incorporate the pattern recognition process at the hospital nursing unit level. After engaging the professional nursing staff in reading and dialogue about the theory of HEC, nurses are encouraged to incorporate the exploration of meaningful events and people into their practice with their patients. Nurses keep journals and come together to reflect on the experience of expanding consciousness in their patients and in themselves. Endo, Miyahara, Suzuki, and Ohmasa (2005) conclude: Retrospectively it was found through dialogue in the research/project meetings that in the usual nurse-client relationships, nurses were bound by their responsibilities within the medical model to help clients get well, but in letting go of the *old rules*, they encountered an amazing experience with clients' transformations. The nurses' transformation occurred concomitantly, and they were free to follow the clients' paths and incorporate all realms of nursing interventions in everyday practice into the unitary perspective. (p. 145)

Jane Flanagan (2005) transformed the practice of presurgical nursing by developing the pre-admission nursing practice model, which is based on HEC. The nursing practice model shifted from a disease focus to a process focus, with attention being given to the nurses knowing their patients and that which is meaningful to them so that the surgery experience could be put in proper context and appropriate care provided. Nursing presurgical visits were emphasized. Flanagan reported that the nursing staff was exuberant to be free to be a nurse once again, and patients frequently stopped by to comment on their preoperative experience and evolving life changes.

Similarly, Susan Ruka (2005) made HEC pattern recognition the foundation of care at a long-term-care nursing facility, transforming the nursing practice and the sense of connectedness among staff, families, and residents: each became more peaceful, relaxed, and loving.

Application of HEC at the Community Level

Pharris (2002, 2005) attempted to understand a community pattern of rising youth homicide rates by conducting a study with incarcerated teens convicted of murder. The youth in the study reported the pattern recognition process to be transformative, and expanding consciousness was visible in changed behaviors, increased connectedness, and more loving attention to meaningful relationships. The experience of the young men demonstrated that alterations in movement, time, and space inherent in the prison system can intensify the process of expanding consciousness. When the experiences of meaningful events and relationships were compared across participants, the pattern of disconnection with the community became evident. People from various aspects of the community (youth workers, juvenile detention staff, emergency hospital staff, pediatric nurses and physicians, social workers, educators, etc.) were engaged in dialogues reflecting on the youths' stories and the community pattern. Insights transformed community responses to youths at risk for violent perpetration. System change ensued.

Pharris (2005) and colleagues extended the community pattern recognition process through partnerships within a multiethnic community interested in understanding and transforming patterns of racism and health disparities. They engaged women and girls from all walks of life in the community in dialogue about their experiences of health, well-being, and racism. Findings were woven into a spoken word narrative that was presented in various forms (performances at meetings and gatherings, through community television and radio, and showing of DVD recordings) to members of the community so that meaningful dialogue could ensue. The process of reflecting on the community pattern generated insight into the nature of the community and what actions could be taken to dismantle racism and enhance health and well-being.

In a related study comparing the evolving patterns of Hmong women living in the United States with diabetes, Yang, Xiong, Vang, and Pharris (2009) found that the women's blood sugars rose and fell with their experiences of trauma, loss, separation, and isolation. Dialogue on these findings, which were presented as a play at a community dinner for Hmong women living with diabetes, shed light on needed individual, family, and community actions so that Hmong women living with diabetes could lead happy and healthy lives.

Sharon Falkenstern (2003, 2009) found the community pattern to emerge as significant when she studied the process of HEC nursing with families with a child with special health care needs. She reports that the nursing partnership is very important to families as they struggle to make sense of their experiences and try to discern how to get on with their lives. The evolving pattern of the families in Falkenstern's study illuminated the social and political forces on families from the educational, disabilities support, and health care systems, as well as community patterns of caring, prejudice, and racism. Falkenstern summarized her experience of using HEC with families with children with special health care needs in the following way:

My experience with this study has rekindled my passion for nursing. I felt affirmed that in the world of managed health care and educational cutbacks, a movement is growing to recapture the essence and value of nursing. While there is still much to be done for nursing within the political realm of health care, each nurse can control where and how they choose to practice. Especially, I realized that a nurse can experience joy and renewed energy by choosing to practice nursing within health as expanding consciousness. (2003, p. 232)

The pattern of the community is visible in the stories of individuals and families. Nurses can play an important role in engaging communities in dialogue as these stories are shared and reflected upon. More work needs to be done on methods of engaging communities in dialogue about patterns of health and their meanings. For example, if an HEC nurse were to take on the task of engaging nurses at the national level in a dialogue about what is meaningful in their practice, expanding consciousness would be manifest as the profession reorganizes at a higher level of functioning, promoting health care systems change. In the process, the population would no doubt experience a fuller, more equitable, and deeper sense of health and meaning.

Practice Exemplar

Sandra is an adult nurse practitioner working in a community clinic in an urban area of the United States; she is about to enter the room of Gloria, a new patient with diabetes and hypertension. Gloria was referred by Anna, a physician colleague who felt that Gloria was "noncompliant," as evidenced by her uncontrolled hypertension and hemoglobin A1c levels that consistently hovered around 10. Anna felt that Gloria needed more care than she could provide for her.

Sandra's graduate program in nursing was based on the theory of health as expanding consciousness; the faculty paid attention to knowing her and what was meaningful to her in her educational and vocational journey. She experienced a relationship-based education process where the teacher is seen as "a catalyst to help students become who they will become rather than be 'trained'" and the learning process is a "dance between content and resonance" (Newman, 2008b, p. 75). Sandra felt known and loved by the faculty. She had ample experience performing problem-solving approaches through the medical paradigm that leads to diagnoses yet, she realized that her nursing actions were best guided by a dialogue focused on understanding Gloria's physical health within the context of her life situation. She knew that the focus of her care for Gloria would arise out of their dialogue; she could not prescribe or predetermine the best care for Gloria.

Before entering the room where Gloria is waiting, Sandra consciously attends to freeing herself of any personal preoccupations or expectations of what might happen. She wants to fully attend to Gloria and sense what is of greatest importance to her right now, knowing that this will guide Sandra's nursing actions so that they can be of most benefit to Gloria. Sandra is confident that she will get a sense of this not only by asking questions and listening deeply, but also through intuitive hunches that will arise through her resonant presence with Gloria.

On entering the room, Sandra warmly greets Gloria and concentrates on what she is sensing from Gloria's presence. She sits down next to Gloria in a relaxing and open manner. What most strongly called Sandra's attention is that Gloria is wringing her hands, which are sweaty; and her muscles seem very tense.

After pausing for a moment, Sandra chooses to reflect back to Gloria what she sees. "Your muscles seem tense, like you might be anxious about something. How has life been going for you?" Gloria looks at Sandra, curious that

Sandra is interested in her life. She responds, "Well things have been hard." Sandra responds, "Hmm, tell me about that." Gloria explains that it has been difficult to take care of the two children she provides day care for. She says she doesn't have the energy, but needs the money to pay her rent, which leaves her very little money to buy food and she cannot afford her medications.

Sandra assures Gloria that the clinic has a plan that will provide her with her medications and that she will see that this is taken care of today—that she will go home with adequate medications. She tells Gloria that she would like to learn a little more about what has been meaningful in her life and asks her to describe meaningful events. Sandra uses the exam table paper to draw a diagram of what Gloria tells her. In very little time Sandra has sketched a diagram of the flow of important events in Gloria's life. She learns that when immigrating to the United States from Africa. Gloria suffered intense abuse and was separated from her family and friends. She has children in the United States who constantly call her to babysit their children and to help them out. Gloria has also experienced intimate partner violence and her current economic stress and depression have flowed from this experience. Gloria lives in a small apartment in a neighborhood where she would need to walk 2 miles to get to a store that sells fresh fruits and vegetables. She tells Sandra she is hesitant to leave her apartment.

Sandra reflects back to Gloria that she sees all of Gloria's energy going out to others and none coming back to her. She has gone from being very active to only moving around within her apartment. Tears run down Gloria's cheeks as she listens to Sandra's reflection. "That is so true!" They talk about sources of support, nurturance, and energy. Gloria identifies a woman in her building whose company she enjoys. They talk about the possibility of the two women walking to the supermarket together and simply getting together to talk. They identify a neighborhood women's walking group, which might be a source of support. They also talk about a women's group at the local library, but Gloria seems hesitant.

During the course of their conversation, Sandra has tried to clear herself of her own concerns, yet, as they talk, she keeps thinking about an experience of racism she witnessed at that library. She decides that it is important information and shares the story with Gloria. This provokes an outpouring of emotion from Gloria as she recounts her experiences of racism. They discuss how distorting these experiences are and how to move through them. They talk about how blood sugar and pressure respond to these situations and ways in which Gloria can best cope.

Sandra does all of the things for Gloria that her medical colleagues would do. She also discusses the services of the social worker, dietician, and psychologist at the clinic so that Gloria can choose what might be most helpful to her at this time. Gloria hugs Sandra as she leaves, saying that she feels so much better, and adding, "You are a very good nurse!" Gloria leaves with a greater understanding of herself, of what is meaningful to her, and what actions she might take. Sandra is left with the same enhanced understanding of herself and her practice.

Sandra tucks the diagram they have drawn into a folder so that it can be elaborated upon at subsequent visits. Sandra knows that Gloria's experience of health and well being will evolve and that she can serve as a catalyst, witnessing and engaging in dialogue about the meaning of the pattern of Gloria's evolving health. Sandra will continue to focus on what she senses as meaningful to Gloria and engage in a relationship centered on Gloria's unfolding pattern of health. Hemoglobin A1c levels and blood pressure readings are only one aspect of that pattern.

As Sandra engages with more and more patients with similar predicaments, she gets a sense of the community pattern of health. She brings her insight to the clinic staff

Continued

Practice Exemplar cont.

meetings where a rich dialogue about community health ensues. Sandra joins the CEO for a dialogue with the clinic's community board of directors to offer their insights. Through the subsequent dialogue, the board of directors and CEO commit themselves to ensuring that health care providers have sufficient time to attend to patients in a holistic manner, sponsoring community forums on racism and how to deal with it, embedding a mental health practitioner in the medical clinic, partnering with a community recreational facility so that patients have a safe place to exercise, encouraging community microeconomic enterprises for women, working with a community coop to provide an affordable source of nutritious food in the immediate neighborhood, and lobbying for health care financing reform.

The circle of dialogue continues for Sandra. Her attention is on pattern and meaning in the evolving health of her patients and the community. She trusts that health is inherently present in her patients and the community; and that reflection on what is meaningful is a catalyst for its evolving pattern. With this realization, Sandra is able to return home where she can be fully present to her family.

◼ Summary

Margaret Newman's theory of health as expanding consciousness (HEC) calls nurses to focus on that which is meaningful in their practice and in the lives of their patients. It attends to the evolving pattern of interactions with the environment for individuals, families, and communities. It is a theory that is relevant across practice settings and cultures. It informs and guides nursing practice, health care administration, and education. The theory of HEC presents a philosophy of *being with* rather than simply *doing for*. It involves a different way of knowing—of resonating with patients, students, and health care colleagues.

The HEC nurse brings to the patient encounter all that she or he has learned in school and in practice yet, begins with a sense of nonknowing so that she or he can take in and begin with what is most meaningful to the patient. The nurse attends to the patient's definition of health and sees it in the context of the patient's expression of meaningful relationships and events. The focus is not on predetermined outcomes mandated by the health system or on *fixing* the patient, but rather on partnering with the patient in his or her experience of health. Rather than simply using technological tools and following prescribed clinical pathways, nurses offer their own transforming presence, knowing that the direction of their interaction with patients will arise out of the relationshp's focus on the patient's evolving experience of health. Insights gained inform population level dialogue for health policy transformation.

Newman (2008b) stated, "This theory asserts that every person in every situation, no matter how disordered and hopeless it may seem, is part of a process of expanding consciousness—a process of becoming more of oneself, of finding greater meaning in life, and of reaching new heights of connectedness with other people and the world" (p. 6). HEC nurses attend to that process.

Acknowledgments

The author thanks St. Catherine University for sabbatical support and scholarly research funding to review the Margaret A. Newman archives housed at the University of Tennessee and to interview Dr. Newman. That work has informed this chapter.

More information about Margaret Newman's theory of health as expanding consciousness can be found on the Internet at www.healthasexpandingconsciousness.org

References

Barron, A. M. (2005). Suffering, growth, and possibility: Health as expanding consciousness in end-of-life care. In C. Picard & D. Jones (Eds.), *Giving voice to what we know: Margaret Newman's theory of health as expanding consciousness in research, theory, and practice* (pp. 43–52). Boston: Jones and Bartlett.

Bentov, I. (1978). *Stalking the wild pendulum.* New York: E. P. Dutton.

Bohm, D. (1980). *Wholeness and the implicate order.* London: Routledge & Kegan Paul.

Connor, M. (1998). Expanding the dialogue on praxis in nursing research and practice. *Nursing Science Quarterly, 11*(2), 51–55.

Downs, F. S., & Newman, M. A. (1977). *A source book on nursing research* (2nd ed.). Philadelphia: F. A. Davis.

Endo, E. (1998). Pattern recognition as a nursing intervention with Japanese women with ovarian cancer. *Advances in Nursing Science, 20*(4), 49–61.

Endo, E., Minegishi, H., & Kubo, S. (2005). Creating action research teams: A praxis model of care. In: C. Picard & D. Jones (Eds.), *Giving voice to what we know: Margaret Newman's theory of health as expanding consciousness in research, theory, and practice* (pp. 143–152). Boston: Jones and Bartlett.

Endo, E., Miyahara, T., Suzuki, S., & Ohmasa, T. (2005). Partnering of researcher and practicing nurses for transformative nursing. *Nursing Science Quarterly, 18*(2), 138–145.

Endo, E., Nitta, E., Inayoshi, M., Saito, R., Takemura, K., Minegishi, H., et al. (2000). Pattern recognition as a caring partnership in families with cancer. *Journal of Advanced Nursing, 32*(3), 603–610.

Falkenstern, S. K. (2003). *Nursing facilitation of expanding consciousness in families who have a child with special health care needs.* Unpublished doctoral thesis. The Pennsylvania State University, University Park, PA.

Falkenstern, S. K., Gueldner, S. H., & Newman, M. A. (2009). Health as expanding consciousness with families with a child with special healthcare needs. *Nursing Science Quarterly, 22*(3), 267–279.

Flanagan, J. (2005). Creating a healing environment for staff and patients in a pre-surgery clinic. In: C. Picard & D. Jones (Eds.), *Giving voice to what we know: Margaret Newman's theory of health as expanding consciousness in research, theory, and practice* (pp. 53–64). Boston: Jones and Bartlett.

Guba, E. G., & Lincoln, Y. S. (1989). *Fourth generation evaluation.* Newbury Park, CA: Sage.

Heron, J., & Reason, P. (1997). A participatory inquiry paradigm. *Qualitative Inquiry, 3*(3), 274–294.

Johnson, D. E. (1961). The significance of nursing care. *American Journal of Nursing, 61*(11), 63–66.

Jonsdottir, H. (1998). Life patterns of people with chronic obstructive pulmonary disease: Isolation and being closed in. *Nursing Science Quarterly, 11*(4), 160–166.

Jonsdottir, H., Litchfield, M., & Pharris, M. D. (2003). Partnership in practice. *Research and Theory for Nursing Practice, 17*(3), 51–63.

Jonsdottir, H., Litchfield, M., & Pharris, M. D. (2004). The relational core of nursing practice. *Journal of Advanced Nursing, 47*(3), 241–250.

Jonsdottir, H., Litchfield, M., Pharris, M. D., & Picard, C. L. (2001). *Partnership as a nursing intervention?* Symposium presentation at the International Council of Nurses 22nd Quadrennial Congress, Copenhagen, Denmark. June 11, 2001.

Kiser-Larson, N. (2002). Life pattern of native women experiencing breast cancer. *International Journal for Human Caring, 6*(2), 61–68.

Lamendola, F. (1998). *Patterns of the caregiver experiences of selected nurses in hospice and HIV/AIDS care.* Unpublished doctoral thesis, University of Minnesota, Minneapolis.

Lamendola, F., & Newman, M. A. (1994). The paradox of HIV/AIDS as expanding consciousness. *Advances in Nursing Science, 16*(3), 13–21.

Litchfield, M. C. (1993). *The process of health patterning in families with young children who have been repeatedly hospitalized.* Unpublished master's thesis, University of Minnesota, Minneapolis.

Litchfield, M. (1999). Practice wisdom. *Advances in Nursing Science, 22*(2), 62–73.

Litchfield, M. C. (2005). The nursing praxis of family health. In: C. Picard & D. Jones (Eds.), *Giving voice to what we know: Margaret Newman's theory of health as expanding consciousness in research, theory, and practice* (pp. 73–83). Boston: Jones and Bartlett.

Litchfield, M., & Laws, M. (1999). Achieving family health and cost-containment outcomes. In: E. L. Cohen & V. De Back (Eds.), *The outcomes mandate: Case management in health care today* (pp. 306–314). St. Louis, MO: C. V. Mosby.

Moch, S. D. (1990). Health within the experience of breast cancer. *Journal of Advanced Nursing, 15,* 1426–1435.

Moss, R. (1991). *The I that is we.* Millbrae, CA: Celestial Arts.

Neill, J. (2002a). Transcendence and transformation in the life patterns of women living with rheumatoid arthritis. *Advances in Nursing Science, 24*(4), 27–47.

Neill, J. (2002b). From practice to caring praxis through Newman's theory of health as expanding consciousness: A personal journey. *International Journal for Human Caring, 6*(2), 48–54.

Newman, M. A. (1966). Identifying and meeting patients' needs in short-span nurse-patient relationships. *Nursing Forum, 5*(1), 76–86.

Newman, M. A. (1972). Nursing's theoretical evolution. *Nursing Outlook, 20*(7), 449–453.

Newman, M. A. (1976). Movement tempo and the experience of time. *Nursing Research, 25,* 173–179.

Newman, M. A. (1978). *Nursing theory*. (Audiotape of an address to the 2nd National Nurse Educator Conference in New York.) Chicago: Teach'em, Inc.

Newman, M. A. (1979). *Theory development in nursing*. Philadelphia: F. A. Davis.

Newman, M. A. (1982). Time as an index of expanding consciousness with age. *Nursing Research, 31,* 290–293.

Newman, M. A. (1986). *Health as expanding consciousness*. St. Louis, MO: C. V. Mosby.

Newman, M. A. (1987). Aging as increasing complexity. *Journal of Gerontological Nursing, 12,* 16–18.

Newman, M. A. (1990). Newman's theory of health as praxis. *Nursing Science Quarterly, 3,* 37–41.

Newman, M. A. (1994a). *Health as expanding consciousness* (2nd ed.). Boston: Jones and Bartlett (NLN Press).

Newman, M. A. (1994b). Theory for nursing practice. *Nursing Science Quarterly, 7*(4), 153–157.

Newman, M. A. (1995). *A developing discipline*. Boston: Jones and Bartlett (formerly, New York: National League for Nursing Press).

Newman, M. A. (1997a). Experiencing the whole. *Advances in Nursing Science, 20*(1), 34–39.

Newman, M. A. (1997b). Evolution of the theory of health as expanding consciousness. *Nursing Science Quarterly, 10*(1), 22–25.

Newman, M. A. (1997c). Margaret Newman: Health as expanding consciousness. In: Fuld Institute for Technology in Nursing Education, *The nurse theorists: Portraits of excellence* [CD-ROM]. Athens, OH: FITNE, Inc.

Newman, M. A. (1999). The rhythm of relating in a paradigm of wholeness. *Image: Journal of Nursing Scholarship, 31*(3), 227–230.

Newman, M. A. (2002). The pattern that connects. *Advances in Nursing Science, 24*(3), 1–7.

Newman, M. A. (2003). A world with no boundaries. *Advances in Nursing Science, 26*(4), 240–245.

Newman, M. A. (2005). Preface. In C. Picard & D. Jones (Eds.), *Giving voice to what we know: Margaret Newman's theory of health as expanding consciousness in research, theory, and practice* (pp. xxiii–xxvi). Sudbury, MA: Jones and Bartlett.

Newman, M. A. (2008a). It's about time. *Nursing Science Quarterly, 21*(3), 225–227.

Newman, M. A. (2008b). *Transforming presence: The difference that nursing makes*. Philadelphia: F. A. Davis.

Newman, M. A., Lamb, G. S., & Michaels, C. (1991). Nurse case management: The coming together of theory and practice. *Nursing & Health Care, 12*(8), 404–408.

Newman, M. A., & Moch, S. D. (1991). Life patterns of persons with coronary heart disease. *Nursing Science Quarterly, 4,* 161–167.

Newman, M. A., Sime, A. M., & Corcoran-Perry, S. A. (1991). The focus of the discipline of nursing. *Advances in Nursing Science, 14*(1), 1–6.

Newman, M. A., Smith, M. C., Pharris, M. D., & Jones, D. (2008). The focus of the discipline revisited. *Advances in Nursing Science, 31*(1), E16–E27.

Noveletsky-Rosenthal, H. T. (1996). *Pattern recognition in older adults living with chronic illness*. Unpublished doctoral thesis, Boston College.

Pharris, M. D. (1999). *Pattern recognition as a nursing intervention with adolescents convicted of murder*. Unpublished doctoral thesis, University of Minnesota, Minneapolis.

Pharris, M. D. (2002). Coming to know ourselves as community through a nursing partnership with adolescents convicted of murder. *Advances in Nursing Science, 24*(3), 21–42.

Pharris, M. D. (2005). Engaging with communities in a pattern recognition process. In: C. Picard & D. Jones (Eds.), *Giving voice to what we know: Margaret Newman's theory of health as expanding consciousness in research, theory, and practice* (pp. 83–94). Boston: Jones and Bartlett.

Pharris, M. D., & Endo, E. (2007). Flying free: The evolving nature of nursing practice guided by the theory of health as expanding consciousness. *Nursing Science Quarterly, 20*(2), 136–140.

Picard, C. (2000). Pattern of expanding consciousness in mid-life women: Creative movement and the narrative as modes of expression. *Nursing Science Quarterly, 13*(2), 150–158.

Picard, C. (2005). Parents of persons with bipolar disorder and pattern recognition. In: C. Picard & D. Jones (Eds.), *Giving voice to what we know: Margaret Newman's theory of health as expanding consciousness in research, theory, and practice* (pp. 133–141). Boston: Jones and Bartlett.

Picard, C., & Jones, D. (Eds.). (2005). *Giving voice to what we know: Margaret Newman's theory of health as expanding consciousness in research, theory, and practice*. Boston: Jones and Bartlett.

Prigogine, I. (1976). Order through fluctuation: Self-organization and social system. In: Jantsch, E., & Waddington, C. H. (Eds.), *Evolution and consciousness* (pp. 93–133). Reading, MA: Addison-Wesley.

Quinn, J. F. (1992). Holding sacred space. The nurse as healing environment. *Holistic Nursing Practice, 6*(4), 26–36.

Rogers, M. E. (1970). *An introduction to the theoretical basis of nursing*. Philadelphia: F. A. Davis.

Rogers, M. E. (1990). Nursing science and the space age. *Nursing Science Quarterly, 5*(1), 27–34.

Ruka, S. (2005). Creating balance, rhythm and patterns in people with dementia living in a nursing home. In: C. Picard & D. Jones (Eds.), *Giving voice to what we know: Margaret Newman's theory of health as expanding consciousness in research, theory, and practice* (pp. 59–104). Boston: Jones and Bartlett.

Skolimowski, H. (1994). *The participatory mind*. London: Arkana.

Smith, T. D. (2001). The concept of nursing presence: State of the science. *Scholarly Inquiry for Nursing Practice: An International Journal, 15*(4), 299–322.

Thompson, W. I. (1989). *Imaginary landscape: Making worlds of myth and science.* New York: St. Martin's Press.

Tommet, P. (2003). Nurse-parent dialogue: Illuminating the evolving pattern of families with children who are medically fragile. *Nursing Science Quarterly, 16*(3), 239–246.

Yamashita, M. (1998). Newman's theory of health as expanding consciousness: Research of family caregiving in mental illness in Japan. *Nursing Science Quarterly, 11*(3), 110–115.

Yamashita, M. (1999). Newman's theory of health as expanding consciousness: Research of family caregiving in mental illness in Japan. *Nursing Science Quarterly, 12*(1), 73–79.

Yang, A., Xiong, D., Vange, E., & Pharris, M.D. (2009). *Hmong American women living with diabetes. Journal of Nursing Scholarship, 41*(2), 139–148.

Young, A. M. (1976). *The reflexive universe: Evolution of consciousness.* San Francisco, CA: Robert Briggs Associates.

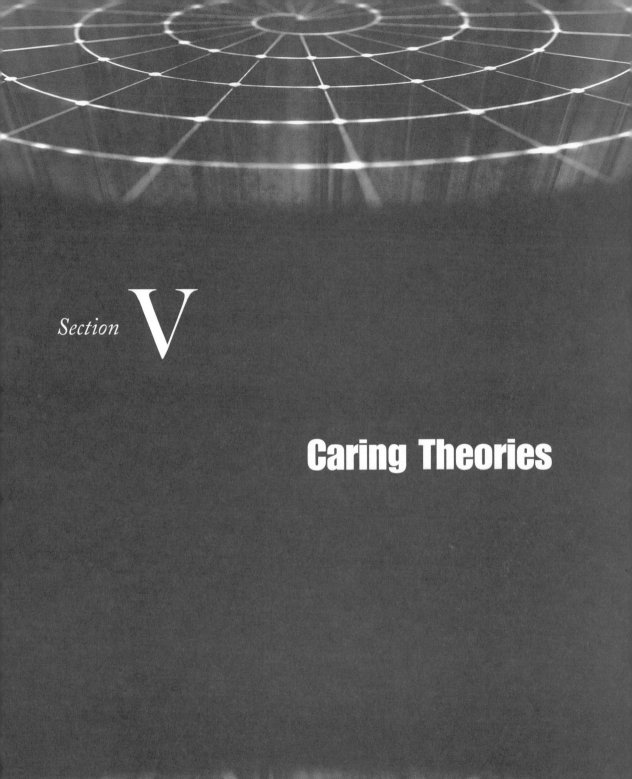

Section V

Caring Theories

Caring Theories

Four of the grand theories in this book focus on the phenomenon of care or caring. Three of these authors describe care or caring as the defining concept of the discipline of nursing. Rather than place these in either the interactive–integrative or unitary–transformative paradigm we situated them in a category of their own. Leininger's Theory of Cultural Care Diversity and Universality is covered in Chapter 18. Leininger describes the theory, while Marilyn McFarland addresses the practice applications related to the theory. This chapter was not updated from the 2nd edition of the book. Leininger was the first to define care as the essence of nursing; she asserts that care or nurturance can be understood only within cultural contexts. In Chapter 19, Paterson and Zderad's Humanistic Nursing Theory is presented by Susan Kleiman. While the theory does not explicitly identify caring as its focus, it serves as a foundation and shares concepts with other theories in this classification. For example, nursing is described as responding to a call from a person, family, community, or humanity toward the purpose of nurturing well-being and more-being. This idea of call and response toward facilitating becoming is foundational to Boykin and Schoenhofer's theory of Nursing as Caring and is related to Watson's Theory of Human Caring, which are presented in Chapters 20 and 21. Watson's theory is composed of the ten caritas processes, the transpersonal caring relationship, the caring occasion, and caring–healing modalities. Watson's theory draws from a spiritual dimension affirming that transpersonal caring is connecting and embracing the spirit or soul of another. She shares examples of how her theory is being advanced and applied as a model for practice through the Watson Caring Science Institute and the International Caritas Consortium. Boykin and Schoenhofer co-authored Chapter 21, on their theory of Nursing as Caring. The focus of nursing is the person living and growing in caring. The theory focuses on coming to know the other as caring, hearing, and answering calls for caring and nurturing the growth of the other as caring. This theory has, and is currently, transforming care in a variety of settings.

Chapter # 18

Madeleine Leininger's Theory of Culture Care Diversity and Universality

MADELEINE M. LEININGER AND
MARILYN R. MCFARLAND

Part One The Theory of Culture Care Diversity and Universality

Part Two Implications for Nursing Practice

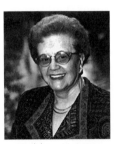

Madeleine M. Leininger

Part One

Introducing the Theorist

Madeleine M. Leininger, founder of the worldwide Transcultural Nursing Society, is the founder and leader of the field of transcultural nursing, focusing on comparative human care theory and research. Dr. Leininger obtained her initial nursing education at St. Anthony School of Nursing in Denver, Colorado. She earned her undergraduate degree from Mt. St. Scholastic College in Atchison, Kansas and her master's degree from the Catholic University of America in Washington, DC. She completed her PhD in social and cultural anthropology at the University of Washington. Dr. Leininger served as dean and professor of nursing at the Universities of Washington and Utah, where she helped initiate and direct the first doctoral programs in nursing. She facilitated the development of master's degree programs in nursing at American and overseas institutions. A fellow and Living Legend of the American Academy of Nursing, she is a professor emeritus in the College of Nursing at Wayne State University and adjunct professor at the University of Nebraska, College of Nursing.

Dr. Leininger has written or edited 30 books, published more than 250 articles, and given more than 1,200 public lectures throughout the United States and abroad. Some of her well known books include *Basic Psychiatric Concepts in Nursing* (Leininger &

Hofling, 1960); *Caring: An Essential Human Need* (1981); *Care: The Essence of Nursing and Health* (1984); *Care: Discovery and Uses in Clinical and Community Nursing* (1988); *Ethical and Moral Dimensions of Care* (1990d); and *Culture Care Diversity and Universality: A Theory of Nursing* (1991a). Some of her books were the first in their areas of nursing to be published. *Nursing and Anthropology: Two Worlds to Blend* (1970) was the first book to bring together nursing and anthropology. The first book on transcultural nursing was *Transcultural Nursing: Concepts, Theories, and Practices* (1978). *Qualitative Research Methods in Nursing* (1985) was the first qualitative research methods book in nursing.

Her published books and articles cover five decades of cumulative transcultural nursing and human care within many cultures throughout the world. In 1989, Dr. Leininger founded the *Journal of Transcultural Nursing*, the first transcultural nursing journal in the world. Dr. Leininger conducted the first field study of the Gadsup of the Eastern Highlands of New Guinea in the early 1960s, and since then has studied approximately 25 Western and non-Western cultures. She developed the first nursing research method called *ethnonursing* and led nurses to use her qualitative ethnonursing research methods. She also outlined new ways to provide culturally competent health care, coining the phrase "culturally congruent care" in the 1960s. In 1987, she initiated the idea of worldwide certification of nurses prepared in transcultural nursing to protect and respect the cultural needs and lifeways of people of diverse cultures.

As a pioneering nurse educator, leader, theorist, and administrator, Dr. Leininger has been a risk taker and innovator. She has never been afraid to bring forth new directions and practical issues in education and service. Her persistent leadership has made transcultural methods and human care central to nursing and respected as formal areas of study and practice. Colleagues and students have called her "the Margaret Mead of the health field" and the "new Nightingale." Her genuine enthusiasm for whatever she pursues is contagious, inspiring, and challenging.

Overview of the Theory

One of Dr. Leininger's most significant and unique contributions was the development of her Culture Care Diversity and Universality Theory, which she introduced in the early 1960s to provide culturally congruent and competent care (Leininger, 1991b, 1995). She believed that transcultural nursing care could provide meaningful, therapeutic health and healing outcomes. As she developed the theory, she identified transcultural nursing concepts, principles, theories, and research-based knowledge to guide, challenge, and explain nursing practices. This was a significant innovation in nursing and has helped open the door to new scientific and humanistic dimensions of caring for people of diverse and similar cultures.

The Theory of Culture Care Diversity and Universality was developed to establish a substantive knowledge base to guide nurses in discovery and use of transcultural nursing practices. At this time, during the post–World War II period, Dr. Leininger realized nurses would need transcultural knowledge and practices to function with people of diverse cultures worldwide (Leininger, 1970, 1978). Many new immigrants and refugees were coming to America, and the world was becoming more multicultural.

Leininger held that caring for people of many different cultures was a critical and essential need, yet nurses and other health professionals were not prepared to meet this global challenge. Instead, nursing and medicine were focused on using new medical technologies and treatment regimens. They concentrated on biomedical study of diseases and symptoms. Shifting to a transcultural perspective was a major but critically needed change.

This part of the chapter presents an overview of the Theory of Culture Care Diversity and Universality, along with its purpose, goals, assumptions, theoretical tenets, predicted hunches, and related general features. The next part of the chapter discusses applications of the knowledge in clinical and community settings. For a more in-depth discussion of the theorist's perspectives, please consult the primary literature on the theory (Leininger, 1970, 1981, 1989a, 1989b, 1990a, 1990b, 1991a, 1995, 1997a, 1998, 2002, 2006).

Factors Leading to the Theory

A frequent question often posed to Dr. Leininger is, "What led you to develop your theory?" Her major motivation was the desire to discover unknown or little known knowledge about cultures and their core values, beliefs, and needs. The idea for the Culture Care Theory came to her while she was a clinical child nurse specialist in a child guidance home in a large Midwestern city (Leininger, 1970, 1991a, 1995). From her focused observations and daily nursing experiences with the children in the home, she became aware that they were from many different cultures, differing in their behaviors, needs, responses, and care expectations. In the home were youngsters who were Anglo-Caucasian, African American, Jewish American, Appalachian, and many other cultures. Their parents responded to them differently, and their expectations of care and treatment modes were different. The reality was a shock to Leininger, as she was not prepared to care for children of diverse cultures. Likewise, nurses, physicians, social workers, and health professionals in the guidance home were also not prepared to respond to such cultural differences.

It soon became evident that she needed cultural knowledge to be helpful to the children. Her psychiatric and general nursing care knowledge and experiences were woefully inadequate. She decided to pursue doctoral study in anthropology. While in the anthropology program, she discovered a wealth of potentially valuable knowledge that would be helpful from a nursing perspective. To care for children of diverse cultures and link such knowledge into nursing thought and actions was a major challenge. It was essential to incorporate into nursing new cultural knowledge that went beyond the traditional physical and emotional needs

of clients. Leininger was concerned about whether such learning would be possible, given nursing's traditional norms and orientation toward medical knowledge.

At that time, she had questioned what made nursing a distinct and legitimate profession. She declared in the mid-1950s that care is (or should be) the essence and central domain of nursing. However, many nurses resisted this idea, because they thought care was unimportant, too feminine, too soft, and too vague, and that it would never explain nursing and be accepted by medicine (Leininger, 1970, 1977, 1981, 1984). Nonetheless, Leininger firmly held to the claim and began to teach, study, and write about care as the essence of nursing, its unique and dominant attribute (Leininger, 1970, 1981, 1988, 1991a). From both anthropological and nursing perspectives, she held that care and caring were basic and essential human needs for human growth, development, and survival (Leininger, 1977, 1981). She argued that what humans need is human caring to survive from birth to old age, when ill or well. Nevertheless, care needed to be specific and appropriate to cultures.

Her next step in the theory was to conceptualize selected cultural perspectives and transcultural nursing concepts derived from anthropology. She developed assumptions of culture care to establish a new knowledge base for the new field of transcultural nursing. Synthesizing or interfacing culture care into nursing was a real challenge. The new Theory of Culture Care Diversity and Universality had to be soundly and logically developed (Leininger, 1976, 1978, 1990a, 1990b, 1991a). Formulating such cultural care knowledge was needed to support the new discipline of transcultural nursing. Findings from the theory could be the knowledge to care for people of different cultures. The idea of providing care was largely taken for granted or assumed to be understood by nurses, clients, and the public (Leininger, 1981, 1984). Yet the meaning of "care" from the perspective of different cultures was unknown to nurses and not in the literature before establishing the nursing theory in the early 1960s. Care knowledge had to be discovered with cultures.

Before her work, there were no theories explicitly focused on care and culture in nursing environments, let alone research studies to explicate care meanings and phenomena in nursing (Leininger, 1981, 1988, 1990a, 1991a, 1995). Theoretical and practice meanings of care in relation to specific cultures had not been studied, especially from a comparative cultural perspective. Leininger saw the urgent need to develop a whole new body of culturally based care knowledge to support transcultural nursing care. Shifting nurses' thinking and attitudes from medical symptoms, diseases, and treatments to that of knowing cultures and caring values and patterns was a major task. But nursing needed an appropriate theory to discover care, and Leininger held that her theory could open many new knowledge doorways.

Rationale for Transcultural Nursing: Signs and Need

The rationale and need for change in nursing in America and elsewhere (Leininger, 1970, 1978, 1984, 1989a, 1990a, 1995) was as follows:

1. There were increased numbers of global migrations of people from virtually every place in the world due to modern electronics, transportation, and communication. These people needed sensitive and appropriate care.
2. There were signs of cultural stresses and cultural conflicts as nurses tried to care for strangers from many Western and non-Western cultures.
3. There were cultural indications of consumer fears and resistance to health personnel as they used new technologies and treatment modes that did not fit their values and lifeways.
4. There were signs that some clients from different cultures were angry, frustrated, and misunderstood by health personnel owing to ignorance of the clients' cultural beliefs, values, and expectations.
5. There were signs of misdiagnosis and mistreatment of clients from unknown cultures because health personnel did not understand the culture of the client.

6. There were signs that nurses, physicians, and other professional health personnel were becoming quite frustrated in caring for cultural strangers. Culture care factors of clients were largely misunderstood or neglected.
7. There were signs that consumers of different cultures, whether in the home, hospital, or clinic, were being treated in ways that did not satisfy them and this influenced their recovery.
8. There were many signs of intercultural conflicts and cultural pain among staff that led to tensions.
9. There were very few health personnel of different cultures caring for clients.
10. Nurses were beginning to work in foreign countries in the military or as missionaries, and they were having great difficulty understanding and providing appropriate caring for clients of diverse cultures. They complained that they did not understand the peoples' needs, values, and lifeways.

For these reasons and many others, it was clearly evident in the 1960s that people of different cultures were not receiving care congruent with their cultural beliefs and values (Leininger, 1978, 1995). Nurses and other health professionals urgently needed transcultural knowledge and skills to work efficiently with people of diverse cultures.

While anthropologists were clearly experts about cultures, many did not know what to do with patients, nor were they interested in nurses' work, in nursing as a profession, or in the study of human care phenomena in the early 1950s. Most anthropologists in those early days were far more interested in medical diseases, archaeological findings, and in physical and psychological problems of culture. Leininger therefore took a leadership role in the new field she called *transcultural nursing*. She needed to develop educational programs to provide culturally safe and congruent care practices that could be beneficial to cultures, to teach nurses about cultures, and to fit the knowledge in with care practices.

She initiated a number of transcultural nursing undergraduate and graduate courses and programs by the mid-1970s and early 1980s. These offerings were gradually accepted by nurses, helping them to care for diverse cultures and enjoy the work with clients (Leininger, 1989a, 1995).

Nurses were the largest and most direct group of health care providers, so excellent opportunities existed for them to change health care to incorporate culturally congruent care practices, the ultimate goal of transcultural nursing. Nurses and those in other health care disciplines urgently needed to become prepared to meet a growing multicultural world. Inadequate culturally based services were leading to client dissatisfaction and new sets of problems. In fact, some clients declined to use health services because the staff were not culturally sensitive to their needs and care.

As more courses and programs became available to educate nurses about transcultural nursing, the interest of nurses in the topic began to grow. As more nurses began to study and use the Theory of Culture Care Diversity and Universality, the concept of transcultural nursing became meaningful. Leininger had defined transcultural nursing as an area of study and practice focused on cultural care (caring) values, beliefs, and practices of particular cultures. The goal was to provide culture-specific and congruent care to people of diverse cultures (Leininger, 1978, 1984, 1995).

The central purpose of transcultural nursing was to use research-based knowledge to help nurses discover care values and practices and use this knowledge in safe, responsible, and meaningful ways to care for people of different cultures. Today the Culture Care Theory has led to a wealth of research-based knowledge to guide nurses in the care of clients, families, and communities of different cultures or subcultures.

Major Theoretical Tenets

In developing the Theory of Culture Care Diversity and Universality, Leininger identified several predictive tenets or premises as essential for nurses and others to use.

Commonalities

A major principal tenet was that cultural care diversities and similarities (or commonalities) would be found within cultures. This tenet challenges nurses to discover this knowledge so that nurses could use cultural data to provide therapeutic outcomes. It was predicted there would be a gold mine of knowledge if nurses were patient and persistent to discover care values and patterns within cultures, a dimension that had been missing from traditional nursing. Leininger has stated that human beings are born, they live, and they die with their specific cultural values and beliefs, as well as with their historical and environmental context, and that care has been important for their survival and well-being. Leininger predicted that discovering which elements of care were culturally universal and which were different would drastically revolutionize nursing and ultimately transform health care systems and practices (Leininger, 1978, 1990a, 1990b, 1991a).

Worldview and Social Structure Factors

Another major tenet of the theory was that worldview and social structure factors—such as religion (and spirituality), political and economic considerations, kinship (family ties), education, technology, language expressions, the environmental context, and cultural history—were important influences on health care outcomes (Leininger, 1995). This broad and multifaceted view provided a holistic perspective for understanding people and grasping their world and environment within a historical context. Data from this holistic research-based knowledge was predicted to guide nurses for the health and well-being of the individual or to help disabled or dying clients from different cultures. These social structural factors influencing care of people from different cultures would provide new insights to provide culturally congruent care. Systematic study by nurse researchers rather than superficial knowledge of culture would be required to provide this level of care. These factors, together with the history of cultures and knowledge of their environmental factors, had to be discovered to create the theory and to bring new insights and new knowledge. Also, these data would disclose ways that clients could stay well and prevent illnesses. Indeed, in order to meet the theory's goal of making decisions that would provide culturally congruent care, holistic cultural knowledge would have to be discovered (Leininger, 1991a).

Discovering cultural care knowledge would require entering the cultural world to observe, listen, and validate ideas. Transcultural nursing is an immersion experience, not a "dip in and dip out" experience. No longer could nurses rely only on fragments of medical and psychological knowledge. Nurses needed to become aware of the social structure, cultural history, language use, and the environment in which people lived in order to understand cultural and care expressions. Thus, nurses had to be taught the philosophy of transcultural nursing, the culture care theory, and how to discover culture knowledge. Transcultural nursing courses and programs would provide the necessary instruction and mentoring.

Professional and Generic Care

Another major and predicted tenet of the theory was that differences and similarities existed between the practices of two kinds of care: professional and generic (traditional, indigenous, or "folk"; Leininger, 1991a). These differences were also predicted to influence the health and well-being of clients. Elucidating these differences would identify gaps in care, inappropriate care, and also beneficial care. Such findings would influence the recovery (healing), health, and well-being of clients of different cultures. Marked differences between generic and professional care ideas and actions could lead to serious client–nurse conflicts, potential illnesses, and even death (Leininger, 1978, 1995). Such differences needed to be identified and resolved.

Three Modalities

Leininger also identified three new creative ways to attain and maintain culturally congruent care (Leininger, 1991a). The three modalities postulated were: (1) culture care preservation or maintenance, (2) culture care accommodation or negotiation, and (3) culture care restructuring or repatterning (Leininger, 1991a, 1995). These three modes were very different from traditional nursing practices, routines, or interventions. They were focused on ways to use theory data creatively to facilitate congruent care to fit clients' particular cultural needs. To arrive at culturally appropriate care, the nurse had to draw on fresh culture care research and discovered knowledge from the people along with theory data findings. The care had to be tailored to client needs. Leininger believed that routine interventions would not always be appropriate and could lead to cultural imposition, tensions, and conflicts. Thus, nurses had to shift from relying on routine interventions and from focusing on symptoms to care practices derived from the clients' culture and from the theory. They had to use holistic care knowledge from the theory and not medical data. Most importantly, they had to use both generic and professional care data. This was a new challenge but a rewarding one for the nurse and the client if thoughtfully done. Examples of the use of the three modalities containing theory findings can be found in several published sources (Leininger, 1995, 1999, 2002) and are presented in the next part of this chapter.

Use of Leininger's theory has led to the discovery of new kinds of transcultural nursing knowledge. Culturally based care has been found to prevent illness and to maintain wellness. Methods for helping people throughout the life cycle from birth to death have been discovered. Cultural patterns of caring and health maintenance also have been appreciated, along with environmental and historical factors. Most importantly, use of Leininger's theory has helped uncover significant cultural differences and similarities.

Theoretical Assumptions: Purpose, Goal, and Definitions of the Theory

This section discusses some of the major assumptions, definitions, and purposes of the theory. The theory's overriding purpose was to discover, document, analyze, and identify the cultural and care factors influencing humans in health, sickness, and dying and to thereby advance and improve nursing practices.

The theory's goal was to use research-based knowledge to provide culturally congruent, safe, beneficial, and satisfying care to people of diverse or similar cultures for their health and well-being or for meaningful dying. Thus, the ultimate and primary goal of the theory was to provide culturally congruent care that was tailor-made for the lifeways and values of people (Leininger, 1991a, 1995).

Theory Assumptions

Leininger postulated several assumptions or basic beliefs (Leininger, 1970, 1977, 1981, 1984, 1991a, 1997b):

1. Care is essential for human growth, development, and survival and for facing death or dying.
2. Care is essential to curing and healing; there can be no curing without caring.
3. **The forms, expressions, patterns, and processes of human care vary among all cultures of the world.**
4. Every culture has generic (lay, folk, or naturalistic) care, and most also have professional care practices.
5. Culture care values and beliefs are embedded in religious, kinship, social, political, cultural, economic, and historical dimensions of the social structure and in language and environmental contexts.
6. Therapeutic nursing care can occur only when culture care values, expressions, and/ or practices are known and used explicitly to provide human care.
7. Differences between caregiver and care receiver expectations need to be understood in order to provide beneficial, satisfying, and congruent care.
8. Culturally congruent, specific, or universal care modes are essential to the health or well-being of people of all cultures.
9. Nursing is essentially a transcultural care profession and discipline.

Orientational Theory Definitions

1. *Culture care diversity:* Variability and/or differences in meanings, patterns, values, lifeways, or symbols of care within or

between cultures that demonstrate assistive, supportive, or enabling human care expressions (Leininger, 1991a, p. 47).
2. *Culture care universality:* Common, similar, or dominant uniform care meanings, patterns, values, lifeways, or symbols that are manifest with cultures and reflect assistive, supportive, facilitative, or enabling ways to help people (Leininger, 1991a, p. 47).
3. *Care:* Abstract and concrete phenomena related to assisting, supporting, or enabling experiences toward or for others with evident or anticipated care needs to ameliorate or improve a human condition or lifeway. "Caring" refers generally to care actions and activities (Leininger, 1991a, p. 46).
4. *Culture:* The learned, shared, and transmitted values, beliefs, norms, and lifeways of a particular group that guides their thinking, decisions, and actions in patterned ways (Leininger, 1991a, p. 47).
5. *Culture care:* Subjectively and objectively learned and transmitted values, beliefs, and patterned lifeways that assist, support, facilitate, or enable another individual or group to maintain well-being and health, to improve their human condition and lifeway, or to deal with illness, handicaps, or death (Leininger, 1991a, p. 47).
6. *Professional care:* Formally taught, learned, and transmitted professional care, health, illness, wellness, and related knowledge and skills that are found in professional institutions and held to be beneficial to clients (they are usually etic or outsiders' views) (Leininger, 1991a, 1995, p. 106).
7. *Generic (folk and lay) care:* Culturally learned and transmitted indigenous (or traditional, folk, lay, and home-based) knowledge or skills used to provide assistive, supportive, enabling, or facilitative acts toward or for another individual or group (they are largely emic or insiders' views) (Leininger, 1995, p. 106).
8. *Health:* A state of well-being that is culturally defined, valued, and practiced and reflects the ability of individuals (or groups) to perform their daily role activities in culturally expressed, beneficial, and patterned ways (Leininger, 1991a, 1995, p. 106).

9. *Culture care preservation or maintenance*: Assistive, supporting, facilitative, or enabling professional actions and decisions that help people of a particular culture to retain and/or preserve relevant care values so that they can maintain their well-being, recover from illness, or face handicaps and/or death (Leininger, 1991a, p. 48).

10. *Culture care accommodation or negotiation:* Assistive, supporting, facilitative, or enabling creative professional actions and decisions that help people of a designated culture to adapt to or negotiate with others for beneficial or satisfying health outcomes (Leininger, 1991a, p. 48).

11. *Culture care repatterning or restructuring:* Assistive, supporting, facilitative, or enabling professional actions and decisions that help clients reorder, change, or greatly modify their own lifeways for new, different, and beneficial health-care patterns while respecting the client(s)' cultural values and beliefs to provide beneficial and healthy lifeways (Leininger, 1991a, p. 49). (These patterns are mutually established between care givers and receivers.)

12. *Ethnohistory:* Past facts, events, instances, and experiences of individuals, groups, cultures, and institutions that have been primarily experienced or known in the past and that describe, explain, and interpret human lifeways within a particular culture over time (Leininger, 1991a, p. 48).

13. *Environmental context:* The totality of an event, situation, or particular experience that gives meaning to human expressions, interpretations, and social actions in particular physical, ecological, sociopolitical, and/or cultural settings (Leininger, 1991a, p. 48).

14. *Worldview:* The way in which people look out on the world or their universe to form a picture or value stance about their life or the world around them (Leininger, 1991a, p. 47).

15. *Kinship and social factors:* Family intergenerational linkages and social interactions based on cultural beliefs, values, and recurrent lifeways over time.

16. *Religion and spiritual factors:* Supernatural and natural beliefs and practices that guide individual and group thoughts and actions toward the good or desired ways to improve one's lifeways.

17. *Political factors:* Authority and power over others that regulates or influences another's actions, decisions, or behavior.

18. *Technological factors:* The use of electrical, mechanical, or physical (nonhuman) objects in the service of humans.

19. *Education factors:* Formal and informal modes of learning.

20. *Economic factors:* Production, distribution, and use of negotiable material or consumable goods held valuable to or needed by humans.

21. *Environmental factors:* The totality of influences within one's geographic or ecological living area.

22. *Culturally congruent care:* Culturally based care knowledge and action modes used with individuals or groups in beneficial and meaningful ways to improve one's health and well-being or to face illness, disability, or death (Leininger, 2002).

The above definitions are called *orientational* rather than *operational*, in order to let the researcher discern previously unknown phenomena or ideas. Orientational terms allow discovery and are usually congruent with the client lifeways. They are important in using the qualitative ethnonursing discovery method, which is focused on how people understand and experience their world using cultural knowledge and lifeways (Leininger, 1985, 1991a, 1997b, 1997c, 2002, 2006).

The Sunrise Enabler: A Conceptual Guide to Knowledge Discovery

Leininger developed the sunrise enabler (Fig. 18-1) to provide a holistic and comprehensive conceptual picture of the major

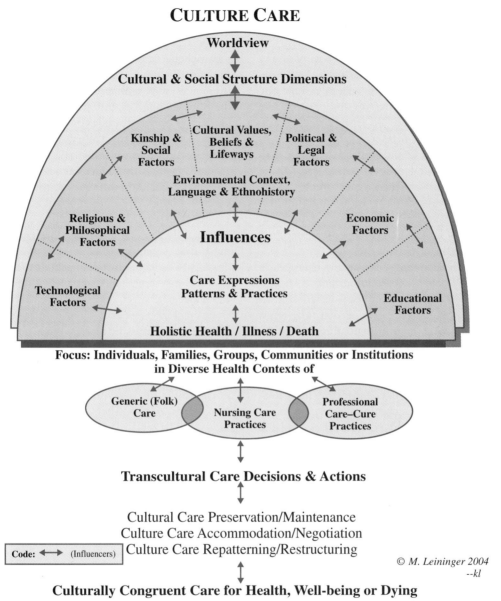

Figure 18 · 1 Leininger's sunrise enabler to discover culture care. (©*M. Leininger 2004.*)

factors influencing Culture Care Diversity and Universality (Leininger, 1995, 1997b; Leininger & McFarland, 2002). The model can be a valuable visual guide to elucidating multiple factors that influence human care and cultural lifeways of different cultures. The enabler serves as a cognitive guide for the researcher to reflect on different predicted influences on culturally based care.

The sunrise enabler can also be used as a valuable aid in cultural and health care assessment of clients. As the researcher uses the model, the different factors alert him or her to find culture care phenomena. Gender, sexual orientation, race, class, and biomedical condition are studied as part of the theory. These determinants tend to be embedded in the worldview and social structure and take time to recognize. Care values and beliefs are usually lodged into environment, religion, kinship, and daily life patterns.

The nurse can begin the discovery at any place in the enabler and follow the informants' ideas and experiences about care. If one starts in the upper part of the enabler, one needs to reflect on all aspects depicted to obtain holistic or total care data. Some nurses start with generic and professional care, then look at how religion, economics, and other influences affect these care modes. One always moves with the informants' interest and story rather than the researcher's interest. Flexibility in using the enabler will lead to a total or holistic view of care.

The three modes of action and decision (in the lower part) are very important to keep in mind. Nursing actions or decisions are studied until one realizes the care needed. The nurse discovers with the informant the appropriate actions, decisions, or plans for care. Throughout this discovery process, the nurse holds his or her own etic biases in abeyance, so that the informants' ideas will come forth, rather than the researcher's. Transcultural nurses are mentored in ways to withhold their biases or wishes and to enter the client's worldview.

The nurse begins the study by making explicit a specific domain of inquiry. For example, the researcher may focus on a *domain of inquiry* (DOI) such as "culture care of Mexican American mothers caring for their children in their home." Every word in the domain statement is important and is studied with the sunrise enabler and the theory tenets. The nurse may have hunches about the domain and care, but until all data have been studied with the theory tenets, she or he cannot prove them. Informants' viewpoints, experiences, and actions are fully documented. Generally, informants select what they like to talk about first, and the nurse accommodates their interest or stories about care. During in-depth study of the domain of inquiry, all areas of the sunrise enabler are identified and confirmed with the informants. The informants become active participants throughout the discovery process in such a way as to feel comfortable and willing to share their ideas.

The real challenge is to focus care meanings, beliefs, values, and practices related to informants' cultures, so subtle and obvious differences and similarities about care are identified among key and general informants. The differences and similarities are important to document with the theory. They may be with historical, environmental, and social structure factors (differences about care with religion, family, and economic, political, legal, or other factors). If informants ask about the researcher's views, the latter must be carefully and sparsely shared. The researcher keeps in mind that some informants may want to please the researcher by talking about the professional medicines and treatments. Professional ideas, however, often cloud or mask the client's real interests and views. If this occurs, the researcher must be alert to such tendencies and keep the focus on the informants' ideas and on the domain of inquiry studied. The informants' knowledge is always kept central to the discovery process about culture care, health, and well-being. If the researcher finds some factors unfamiliar, such as kinship, economics, and political and other considerations depicted in the model, the researcher should listen attentively to the informant's ideas. Obtaining insight into the informant's emic (insider's) views, beliefs, and practices is central to studying the theory (Leininger, 1985, 1991a, 1995, 1997b; Leininger & McFarland, 2002).

Throughout the study and use of the theory, the meanings, expressions, and patterns of culturally based care are important. The nurse listens attentively to informants' accounts about care, and then documents the ideas. What informants know and practice about care or caring in their culture is significant. Documenting ideas from the informant's emic viewpoint is essential to arrive at accurate culturally based care. Unknown care meanings, such as the concepts of protection, respect, love, and many other care concepts, need to be teased out and explored in depth, as they are the key words and ideas in understanding care. Such care meanings and expressions are not always readily known; informants ponder care meanings and are often surprised that nurses are focused on care instead of medical symptoms. Sometimes informants may be reluctant to share social structure and factors such as religion and economical or political ideas, as they fear they may not be accepted or understood by health personnel. Generic (folk or indigenous) knowledge often has rich care data and needs to be explored. Generic care ideas need to be appropriately integrated into the three modes of action and decision for congruent care outcomes. Generic and professional care are integrated so the clients benefit from both types of care.

The sunrise enabler was developed with the idea to "let the sun enter the researcher's mind" and discover largely unknown care factors of cultures. Letting the sun "rise and shine" is important and offers fresh insights about care practices. Generally, a wealth of unexpected nursing care knowledge is discovered that has never been known and used in present-day nursing and medical services.

Current Status of the Theory

Currently, the theory of culture care diversity and universality is being studied and used in many schools of nursing within the United States and other countries (Leininger & McFarland, 2002). The theory has grown in recognition and value for several reasons. First, it is the only nursing theory that focuses explicitly and in depth on discovering the meaning, uses, and patterns of culture care within and between specific cultures. Second, the theory provides a comparison of culture care between and within cultures. Thus, it has greatly expanded nurses' knowledge about care so essential for them to know and use in practices. Third, the theory has a built-in and tailor-made ethnonursing nursing research method that helps to realize the theory tenets. It is different from ethnography and other research methods. The ethnonursing method

is a qualitative method and is valuable in discovering largely covert, complex care knowledge in cultures or subcultures. The fact that it was the first specific research method designed so that the theory and method fit together has brought forth a wealth of new data. Quantitative data methods were not helpful to find hidden care data.

Fourth, the theory of culture care is the only theory that searches for comprehensive care data relying on social structure, worldview, and multiple factors in a culture to construct a holistic knowledge base about care. The theory predicts the health and well-being of people and focuses on the totality of lifeways of individuals, families, groups, communities, and/ or institutions related to culture and care phenomena. It gives a comprehensive picture of care knowledge, often in a historical and environmental context. Some nurse researchers have studied care with limited variables or in regard to medical symptoms and diseases—an approach that is too limited and fails to identify care beliefs and values from the informants' views. Discovering the totality of living with a caring ethos in a culture has provided a wealth of new knowledge about clients' lifeworld and care.

Fifth, the theory has both abstract and practical dimensions. This characteristic helps nurse researchers to discover what has the potential to be known and used for human caring and health practices. What exists and does not exist is important to discover, as is the potential for future discoveries. Some theories deal only with abstract phenomena, but this theory has both abstract and practical realities.

Sixth, the theory of culture care is a synthesized concept; integrated with the ethnonursing method, it has already provided a wealth of many new insights (5 books and 250 articles), showing different ways to care for people of diverse cultures. These transcultural nursing research findings are the new knowledge holdings that support the young discipline of transcultural nursing. They are the "gold nuggets" to transform health care to realize therapeutic outcomes for different cultures. Several transcultural nursing studies reported in the *Journal of Transcultural Nursing* and other transcultural nursing books and journals since 1980 substantiate the theory (Leininger, 1991a, 1995, 1997b, 1997c).

Seventh, the theory and its research findings are stimulating nursing faculty and clinicians to use safe, appropriate, culture-specific care in clinical and community settings. Nursing administrators in service and academia must be active change leaders to use transcultural nursing findings. Nursing faculty members should promote and teach ways to be effective with different cultures (Leininger, 1998). Nurse consultants are using the theory findings for effective consultation services with members of various cultures. The theory is frequently used to conduct culturally congruent health care assessments. Today, transcultural nursing concepts, policies, and standards of care are being developed and used from findings (Leininger, 1991a). Interdisciplinary health personnel are becoming aware of transcultural nursing concepts which help them in their work.

Eighth, informants are often very pleased to have their culture understood and to have care made to fit their values and beliefs, a most rewarding benefit of the theory. Consumers also like the ethnonursing method as they can "tell their story" and guide health researchers to discover truths about their culture. Informants speak of being more comfortable with researchers. They dislike narrowly focused studies on numbers, variables, and short instant responses.

Ninth, users of the theory are thinking reflectively and valuing it. The theory encourages the researcher or clinician to discover culture from the people and to let them be in control of their ideas and their accounts.

Tenth, nurse researchers who have been prepared in transcultural nursing and have used the theory and method commonly say things like, "I love the theory. It is the only theory that makes sense to help cultures. We grow in ideas and enjoy discovering new knowledge of the lifeways of people and their meanings."

Eleventh, nurses who have used the theory and findings over time often speak of how much they have learned about themselves, new cultures, and, caring values and practices. Nurses discover their ethnocentric tendencies as well as racial biases. Their findings are helpful to reduce cultural biases and prejudices that influence quality of care to people of different cultures. Ethnocentrism and racial biases are being reduced with transcultural research. Many nurses also are interested in discovering the differences and similarities among cultures, as it expands their worldviews and deepens their appreciation of humans from diverse cultures. Learning to become immersed in a culture has been a major benefit. Most of all, nurses who thought such research would not yield benefits are overwhelmed to discover care meaning and values from informants. Finally, the strength of the theory is that it can be used in any culture and at any time and within most disciplines. Other disciplines may have to modify the theory slightly to fit their goals. Several disciplines including dentistry, medicine, social work, and pharmacy have reported using the culturally congruent care theory or teaching it in their programs. Most encouraging is the fact that the concept of "culturally congruent care" (a term coined in the early 1960s) has now become a major goal for the U.S. federal government and several of its state governments. The concept is growing in use and will become a global force.

The theory of culture care is of global interest and significance as we continue to understand cultures and their care needs and practices worldwide. Transcultural nursing concepts, principles, theory, and findings must become fully incorporated into professional areas of teaching, practice, consultation, and research. When this occurs, one can anticipate true transcultural health practices and concomitant benefits. Unquestionably, the theory will continue to grow in relevance and use as our world becomes more intensely multicultural. Nurses and all health professionals will be expected in the near future to function competently with diverse cultures. The theory, along with many transcultural nursing concepts, principles, and research findings, will prove indispensable.

The purpose of this part of the chapter is to present the implications for nursing practice of the culture care theory and related ethnonursing research findings. Many nursing theories are rather abstract and do not focus on how practicing nurses might use the research findings related to a theory. However, with the Culture Care Theory, along with the ethnonursing method, there is a built-in means for discovering and confirming data with informants in order to make nursing actions and decisions meaningful and culturally congruent (Leininger, 2002). The Ethnonursing Research Method is provided at http://davisplus.fadavis.com.

Applications of the Theory

Over the past five decades, the culture care theory, along with the ethnonursing method, has been used by nurse researchers to discover knowledge that can be and has been used in nursing practice. Nurses can use such knowledge to care for individual clients and to focus on care practices that are beneficial for families, groups, communities, cultures, and institutions. Our multicultural world has made it imperative that nurses understand different cultures to work and care for people who have diverse and similar values, beliefs, and ideas about nursing, health, caring, wellness, illness, death, and disabilities (Leininger, 1991b, 1995). As stated by Dr. Leininger in the first part of this chapter, the goal of the Theory of Culture Care Diversity and Universality is to improve or maintain health and well-being by providing culturally congruent care to people that is beneficial and fits with the lifeways of the client, family, or cultural group. The sunrise enabler serves as a cognitive map depicting the seven culture and social structure dimensions that influence care, which in turn influence the health and/or illness of clients. The culture care theory and the sunrise enabler include what is similar (universal) and different (diverse) between generic or folk care and professional care, and provides a

focus on both types of care for the provision of culturally congruent care for clients in diverse nursing practice settings. Leininger (1991b) predicted that culturally congruent care would prevent cultural clashes, cultural illnesses, and other unfavorable human conditions under human control. These general ideas are kept in mind as one uses findings related to the theory in clinical practice.

The Three Care Modes and the Sunrise Enabler

To provide a different focus from traditional nursing, Leininger developed the unique three modes of care to incorporate theory findings (refer to sunrise enabler, Fig. 18-1): culture care preservation or maintenance; culture care accommodation or negotiation; and culture care repatterning or restructuring. The theorist has predicted that the researcher can use ethnoresearch findings to guide nursing judgments, decisions, and actions related to providing culturally congruent care (Leininger, 2002).

Leininger prefers not to use the phrase "nursing intervention," because this term often implies to clients from different cultures that the nurse is imposing his or her (etic) views, which may not be helpful. Instead, the term "nursing actions and decisions" is used, but always with the clients helping to arrive at whatever actions or decisions are planned and implemented. The modes fit with the clients' or peoples' lifeways and yet are therapeutic and satisfying for them. The nurse can draw upon scientific nursing, medical, and other knowledge with each mode.

Data collected from the upper and lower parts of the sunrise enabler provide culture care knowledge for nurse researchers to discover and establish useful ways to provide quality care practices. Active participatory involvement with clients is essential to arrive at culturally congruent care with one or all of the three action modes to meet clients' care needs in their particular environmental contexts. The use of these modes in nursing care is one of the most creative and rewarding features of transcultural and general nursing practice with clients of diverse cultures.

It is most important (and a shift in nursing) to carefully focus on the holistic dimensions, as depicted in the sunrise enabler, to arrive at therapeutic culture care practices. All the factors in the sunrise enabler must be considered to arrive at culturally congruent care. These include worldview; technological, religious, kinship, political–legal, economic, and educational factors; cultural values and lifeways; environmental context, language, and ethnohistory; and generic (folk) and professional care practices (Leininger, 2002). Care generated from the culture care theory will become safe, congruent, meaningful, and beneficial to clients only when the nurse in clinical practice becomes fully aware of and explicitly uses knowledge generated from the theory and ethnonursing method, whether in a community, home, or institutional context. The culture care theory, along with the ethnonursing method, are powerful means for new directions and practices in nursing. Incorporating culture-specific care into client care is essential to the practice of professional care and to licensure as registered nurses. Culture-specific care is the safe means to ensure culturally based holistic care that fits the client's culture—a major challenge for nurses who practice and provide services in all health care settings.

The Use of Culture Care Research Findings

Over the past five decades, Dr. Leininger and other research colleagues have used the culture care theory and the ethnonursing method to focus on the care meanings and experiences of 100 cultures (Leininger, 2002). They discovered 187 care constructs in Western and non-Western cultures (Leininger, 1998), as reported in the *Journal of Transcultural Nursing* (1989–1999). Leininger has listed the 11 most dominant constructs of care in priority ranking, with the most universal or frequently discovered first: respect for/about, concern for/about; attention to (details)/in anticipation of; helping–assisting or facilitative acts; active helping; presence (being physically there); understanding (beliefs, values, lifeways,

and environmental); connectedness; protection (gender related); touching; and comfort measures (McFarland, 2002). These care constructs are the most critical and important universal or common findings to consider in nursing practice, but care diversities will also be found and must be considered. The ways in which culture care is applied and used in specific cultures will reflect both similarities and differences among (and sometimes within) different cultures.

Next, three ethnonursing studies are reviewed with focus on the findings, which have implications for nursing practice.

Culture Care of Lebanese Muslims in the United States

In the late 1980s, Luna (1989) conducted an ethnonursing study of the culture care of Arab Muslim cultural groups in a large urban community in the Midwestern United States. In 1989, she published the findings relevant to the culture care of Lebanese Muslim Americans, using Leininger's three modes of nursing decisions and actions to provide culturally congruent and responsible care. The study focused on the care for Lebanese Muslims in the hospital, clinic, and home-community contexts. She stated: "[An] understanding [of] the cultural context in which Lebanese Muslims attempt to adapt, survive, and practice their faith in America necessitates a look into the community into which they migrate" (Luna, 1994, p. 15). Luna's research findings and the nursing practice implications related to the home and community context in the late 1980s remain important as health care shifts from hospital care services to home or community settings. Luna discovered that attending a clinic in a Midwestern United States urban context was often a new and different approach to health care for Lebanese Muslim women, especially during pregnancy and childbirth. Luna's study revealed that many women relied on the traditional midwife in Lebanon for home deliveries. The routine of monthly and weekly visits to the prenatal clinic was incongruent with what these clients had experienced in their home country. In the United States, prenatal care in the clinic context involved long waiting periods with the husband missing work to take his wife to each appointment. Examination by a male physician was culturally incongruent for the women, so *culture care negotiation and repatterning* was essential for culturally congruent care. Luna described the clinic as *culturally decontextualized* for clients and their families because the prenatal care and the environmental clinic context in which the care was provided were not congruent with the clients' cultural values, beliefs, and practices (Luna, 1989). Luna discovered some dominant and universal care constructs for Lebanese Muslim men, which included surveillance, protection, and maintenance of the family. For Lebanese women, the dominant and universal care constructs included emphasizing the positive attributes of educating the children and maintaining a family caring environment according to the precepts of Islam. A number of generic or folk care practices were discovered relating to these care constructs that should be recognized, preserved, and maintained by nurses to enhance the health and well-being of clients. For instance, the female network in the Lebanese Muslim culture is very important at the time of birth; Lebanese women come together to care for one another and offer practical and emotional assistance for new immigrants who are struggling to survive in a new cultural context such as the United States. By recognizing the benefits of this network and by allowing women flexibility in their visiting and presence in the hospital and clinic contexts, the nurse would use culture care preservation to maintain these generic care practices for the health and well-being of clients.

Luna found that female modesty was an important cultural care value for Lebanese women; this was reflected in requests by female clients to have only female nurses, physicians, and other caregivers. Culture care accommodation of this generic care practice was accomplished by nurses negotiating for these women to have female caregivers whenever possible, which would promote health, well-being, and client satisfaction with care.

By including Lebanese Muslim men in health teaching and discharge planning, Luna discovered a way to use culture care preservation that recognized the family as a unit, rather than focusing on the individual. Luna recognized that the patriarchal organization of the family should be preserved as a social structure feature, which acknowledges men for their roles in family care continuity rather than being narrowly interpreted as men always being in control. Negative stereotypes held by nurses about the Arab males' reluctance to participate in the birth process were also discovered, often presenting a barrier to giving nursing care. To counter this, Luna suggested the nurses use culture care preservation to maintain and support the generic culture care practices of men, which included surveillance, protection, and maintenance of the family.

Still another finding from Luna's study was the discovery of the importance of religious rituals to many Muslim clients as an essential component of providing care within their cultural context (Luna, 1989, 1994). Luna found that some Muslims pray three to five times a day, and others do not pray at all. During the assessment of client culture (in the hospital context), Luna suggested the nurse should ask about the client's wishes regarding prayer. Culture care accommodation could be practiced by negotiating for an agreeable time and a private place for clients to pray, which for many Muslims is an important cultural expression for their health and well-being. She also suggested that nurses practice culture care accommodation for clients by negotiating with a social service organization that served Arab clients in order to gather written and video materials in the Arabic language related to health for use in the hospital and clinic settings. Luna (1989) identified approaches for culture care repatterning to improve attendance at the prenatal clinic for Lebanese Muslim women. Nurses should avoid direct confrontation and spend considerable time during the first clinic visit educating women about the benefits of regular prenatal care, including emphasis on the health and well-being of both the mother and the baby.

In 1999, Wehbeh-Alamah conducted a 2-year ethnonursing study using the culture care theory and studied the generic health care beliefs, practices, and expressions of Lebanese American Muslim immigrants in two Midwestern U.S. cities. Her findings, which confirmed many of Luna's from 1989, included the discovery of specific generic folk care beliefs on practices that required culture care accommodation/negotiation in the home as well as in the hospital. These included providing for prayer while facing east five times a day; having large numbers of visitors when in the hospital or at home; and eating only halal meat. Many gender care findings were similar to those from Luna's study, revealing a persistence of many related care patterns over time as predicted in the culture care theory. However, the women in Wehbeh-Alamah's study believed the absence of extended family members in the United States had influenced male family members' thinking about the appropriateness of men caring for family members. The researcher reported that acculturation had changed men's view about providing care from the more traditional belief that the hands-on caring for the children, elderly, and sick belonged to women, to the more contemporary belief in cooperation and participation in direct caregiving by Muslim men (Wehbeh-Alamah, 2006). Wehbeh-Alamah conducted an ethnonursing study of the culture care of Syrian American Muslims living in a Midwestern U.S. city. In addition to discovering the culture care meanings, beliefs, and practices of this group, she will compare this study with her previous studies to arrive at universal and diverse care findings among Muslim immigrants from different cultures living in the United States.

Culture Care of Elderly Anglo and African Americans

In the mid-1990s, the theory of culture care was used to guide a study of the culture care of Anglo and African American elders in a long-term care institution (McFarland, 1997). This study revealed care implications for nurses who practice in retirement homes, nursing homes, apartments for the aged, and other long-term care settings. Many residents from both cultural groups participated in the care of their fellow residents. Residents assisted other residents to the dining room, checked on others who did not appear for meals in the dining room (care as surveillance of others), and assisted in ambulation of those who were not able to walk independently. This focus on *other care* versus only *self-care* was a form of culturally congruent care that residents desired in order to maintain healthy and beneficial lifeways in an institutional setting. Culture care preservation was practiced by nursing staff as these generic care practices were integrated into professional nursing care.

Within the retirement home, both Anglo and African American residents desired spiritual or religious care and had some diverse aspects of such care rooted in their respective cultures. The findings of both universality and diversity within the pattern of religious or spiritual care supported Leininger's theory, which states that "culture care concepts, meanings, expressions, patterns, processes, and structural forms of care are different (diversity) and similar (toward universality) among all cultures of the world" (Leininger, 1991b, p. 45). African American residents received care from church friends who ran errands, did banking and laundry, paid bills, visited, and brought communion to them. Anglo American residents received a more formal type of care from their churches, such as a minister coming to the retirement home to do a worship service or a church choir traveling to the retirement home to entertain the residents. The nurses at the retirement home practiced culture care preservation by maintaining the involvement of churches in the daily lives of both cultural groups to help residents face living in a retirement home with increasing disabilities related to aging and handicaps, and even dealing with the prospect of death. With an increase in the numbers of elderly from both the Anglo and African American cultural groups being admitted to long-term care institutions, the knowledge of culture-specific care for both Anglo and

African American elders is important for nurses who practice in these settings.

The generic care pattern of families helping their elderly relatives enhanced the health and lifeways of both Anglo and African American elders in the retirement home setting. Anglo American residents received help from their spouses and/or adult children. In contrast with the Anglo American findings, African American spouses, children, extended family members, and nonkin who were considered family reflected the care pattern of families helping elderly residents. Grandchildren, great grandchildren, nieces, nephews, grandnieces, and grandnephews, as well as church members or friends who were considered family and were referred to as brothers, sisters, or daughters, were involved in caring for African American elders. The nursing staff recognized the importance of family involvement in the care of residents and practiced culture care preservation to maintain culture-specific family care practices for residents from each cultural group.

The care pattern of protection was important to African American residents but not to Anglo American residents. Most African American residents had left homes that were in unsafe neighborhoods and had moved into the facility partly for that reason. African American nursing staff recognized the importance of protective care and often accompanied African American residents when they wanted to go outside. The nursing staff made efforts to practice culture care accommodation by negotiating to take the residents outside to sit on the small grass strip around the perimeter of the parking lot of the home.

McFarland (1997) also discovered that the nursing care and the lifeways of elderly residents in the nursing home setting were less satisfying than in the apartment setting within the retirement home context. Professional nurses need to be more actively involved in culture care repatterning as *coparticipants with elders* to restructure lifeway practices, care routines, and the environmental context of nursing homes (including room designs and privacy considerations).

Culture care restructuring of these care-related concerns can be accomplished only when nurses assume an advocacy role for the elderly residents and work with governmental and private agencies that provide the funding and make the rules and regulations that affect long-term care. The culture care theory, with the ethnonursing method, assisted the researcher in this study in the discovery of action and decision modes that were culturally specific for Anglo and African American elders residing in a long-term care institution.

Culture Care of German Americans

In 2000, McFarland and Zehnder (2006) conducted a 2-year ethnonursing study of the culture care of German American elders living in a nursing home in a small Midwestern city in the United States. Their findings, which confirmed many of McFarland's (1997) earlier findings, included many care beliefs and practices that required culture care preservation. German American elder care practices included caring for fellow residents by assisting confused residents to find their assigned seat in the dining room or making items for the annual bazaar to raise money to buy flowers for the nursing home courtyard garden, thereby benefitting all of the residents. The finding of the important care of doing for others versus an emphasis on self-care was previously discovered in McFarland's earlier study in 1997 with Anglo American and African American elders and was confirmed in this German American study.

German American elders received spiritual care from the local German American church and pastor. The pastor conducted a worship service and a Bible class in German each week. Spiritual religious care, provided by connections with the Lutheran Church, was essential to German American elders in maintaining their traditional lifeways and health in the nursing home setting. This finding had also been discovered with Anglo American elders in McFarland's (1997) previous study and was confirmed with German American elders.

McFarland is currently comparatively synthesizing culture care findings from ethnonursing studies of elder care conducted by transcultural nurses with diverse cultures worldwide. This will hopefully lead to the discovery of universal and diverse care meanings, beliefs, and practices to meet the needs of the increasing numbers of elders worldwide who value generic culture-specific care to reaffirm their cultural identities in the latter phase of their lives.

Summary

The purpose of the culture care theory (along with the ethnonursing method) has been to discover culture care with the goal of using the knowledge to combine generic and professional care. The goal is to provide culturally congruent nursing care using the three modes of nursing actions and decisions that are meaningful, safe, and beneficial to people of similar and diverse cultures worldwide (Leininger, 1991b, 1995). The clinical use of the three major care modes (culture care preservation or maintenance; culture care accommodation or negotiation; and culture care repatterning or restructuring) by nurses to guide nursing judgments, decisions, and actions is essential in order to provide culturally congruent care that is beneficial, satisfying, and meaningful to the people nurses serve. The studies of the four cultures just reviewed (Lebanese Muslim, Anglo American, African American, and German Americans) substantiate that the three modes are care-centered and are based on the use of generic care (emic) knowledge along with professional care (etic) knowledge obtained from research using the culture care theory along with the ethnonursing method. This chapter has reviewed only a small selection of the culture care findings from ethnonursing research studies conducted over the past four decades. There is a wealth of additional findings of interest to practicing nurses who care for clients of all ages from diverse and similar cultural groups in many different institutional and community contexts around the world. More in-depth culture care findings, along with the use of the three modes, can be found in the *Journal of Transcultural Nursing* (1989–2004)

and in the numerous books and articles by Dr. Madeleine Leininger. Nurses in clinical practice are advised to consult a list of research studies and doctoral dissertations conceptualized within the culture care theory for additional detailed nursing implications for clients from diverse cultures (Leininger & McFarland, 2002).

The Theory of Culture Care Diversity and Universality is one of the most comprehensive yet practical theories to advance transcultural and general nursing knowledge with concomitant ways for practicing nurses to establish or improve care to people. Nursing students and practicing nurses have remained the strongest advocates of the culture care theory (Leininger, 2002). The theory focuses on a long-neglected area in nursing practice—culture care—that is most relevant to our multicultural world.

The Theory of Culture Care Diversity and Universality is depicted in the sunrise enabler as a rising sun. This visual metaphor is particularly apt. The future of the culture care theory shines brightly indeed, because it is holistic, comprehensive, and facilitates discovering care related to diverse and similar cultures, contexts, and ages of people in familiar and naturalistic ways. The theory is useful to nurses and to nursing and to professionals in other disciplines such as physical, occupational, and speech therapy, medicine, social work, and pharmacy. Health care practitioners in other disciplines are beginning to use this theory, because they also need to become knowledgeable about and sensitive and responsible to people of diverse cultures who need care (Leininger, 2002).

References

Berry, A. (1996). Culture care expression, meanings, and experiences of pregnant Mexican American women within Leininger's culture care theory. (UMI No. 9628875). Ann Arbor, MI: UMI Microfilm.

Berry, A. (1999). Mexican American women's expressions of the meaning of culturally congruent prenatal care. *Journal of Transcultural Nursing, 103,* 203–212.

Leininger, M. (1970). *Nursing and anthropology: Two worlds to blend.* New York: John Wiley & Sons.

Leininger, M. (1976). Transcultural nursing presents an exciting challenge. *The American Nurse, 5*(5), 6–9.

Leininger, M. (1977). Caring: The essence and central focus of nursing. *Nursing Research Foundation Report, 12*(1), 2–14.

Leininger, M. (1978). *Transcultural nursing: Concepts, theories, and practices.* New York: John Wiley & Sons.

Leininger, M. (1981). *Caring: An essential human need.* Thorofare, NJ: Slack.

Leininger, M. (1984). *Care: The essence of nursing and health.* Thorofare, NJ: Slack.

Leininger, M. (1985). *Qualitative research methods in nursing* (pp. 33–73). Orlando, FL: Grune & Stratton.

Leininger, M. (1988). *Care: Discovery and uses in clinical and community nursing.* Detroit: Wayne State University Press.

Leininger, M. (1989a). Transcultural nursing: Quo vadis (where goeth the field)? *Journal of Transcultural Nursing, 1*(1), 33–45.

Leininger, M. (1989b). Transcultural nurse specialists and generalists: New practitioners in nursing. *Journal of Transcultural Nursing, 1*(1), 4–16.

Leininger, M. (1990a). Transcultural nursing: A worldwide necessity to advance nursing knowledge and practices. In: J. McCloskey & H. Grace, (Eds.), *Current issues in nursing.* St. Louis, MO: C. V. Mosby.

Leininger, M. (1990b). Culture: The conspicuous missing link to understand ethical and moral dimensions of human care. In: M. Leininger (Ed.), *Ethical and moral dimensions of care.* Detroit: Wayne State University Press.

Leininger, M. (1990c). Ethnomethods: The philosophic and epistemic basis to explicate transcultural nursing knowledge. *Journal of Transcultural Nursing, 1*(2), 40–51.

Leininger, M. (1990d). *Ethical and moral dimensions of care.* Detroit: Wayne State University Press.

Leininger, M. (1991a). *Culture care diversity and universality: A theory of nursing.* New York: National League for Nursing Press.

Leininger, M. (1991b). The theory of culture care diversity and universality. In: M. Leininger (Ed.), *Culture care diversity and universality: A theory of nursing* (pp. 5–68). New York: National League for Nursing Press.

Leininger, M. (1991c). Ethnonursing: A research method with enablers to study the theory of culture care. In: M. Leininger (Ed.), *Culture care diversity and universality: A theory of nursing* (pp. 73–118). New York: National League for Nursing Press.

Leininger, M. (1995). *Transcultural nursing: Concepts, theories, research, and practice.* Columbus, OH: McGraw Hill College Custom Series.

Leininger, M. (1997a). Overview and reflection of the theory of culture care and the ethnonursing research method. *Journal of Transcultural Nursing, 8*(2), 32–51.

Leininger, M. (1997b). Overview of the theory of culture care with the ethnonursing research method. *Journal of Transcultural Nursing, 8*(2), 32–53.

Leininger, M. (1997c). Transcultural nursing research to transform nursing education and practice: 40 years. *Image: Journal of Nursing Scholarship, 29*(4), 341–347.

Leininger, M. (1998). Special research report: Dominant culture care (emic) meanings and practice findings from Leininger's theory. *Journal of Transcultural Nursing, 9*(2), 44–47.

Leininger, M. M. (2002). Part I: The theory of culture care and the ethnonursing research method. In: M. M. Leininger & M. R. McFarland (Eds.), *Transcultural nursing: concepts, theories, and practice* (3rd ed., pp. 71–98). Sudbury, MA: Jones and Bartlett.

Leininger, M., & Hofling, C. (1960). *Basic psychiatric concepts in nursing.* Philadelphia: Lippincott.

Leininger, M. M., & McFarland, M. R. (Eds.) (2002). *Transcultural nursing: Concepts, theories, and practice* (3rd ed.). New York: McGraw-Hill.

Leininger, M. M., & McFarland, M. R. (Eds.) (2006). *Culture diversity & universality: A worldwide nursing theory* (2nd ed.). Sudbury, MA: Jones and Bartlett.

Luna, L. (1989). *Care and cultural context of Lebanese Muslims in an urban U.S. community: An ethnographic and ethnonursing study conceptualized within Leininger's theory.* (UMI No. 9022423). Ann Arbor, MI: UMI Microfilm.

Luna, L. (1994). Care and cultural context of Lebanese Muslim immigrants with Leininger's theory. *Journal of Transcultural Nursing, 5*(2), 12–20.

McFarland, M. R. (1995). *Cultural care of Anglo and African American elderly residents within the environmental context of a long-term care institution.* (UMI No. 9530568). Ann Arbor, MI: UMI Microfilm.

McFarland, M. R. (1997). Use of culture care theory with Anglo and African American elders in a long term care setting. *Nursing Science Quarterly, 10*(4), 186–192.

McFarland, M. R. (2002). Part II: Selected research findings from the culture care theory. In: M. M. Leininger & M. R. McFarland (Eds.), *Transcultural nursing: Concepts, theories, and practice* (3rd ed., pp. 99–116). New York: McGraw-Hill.

McFarland, M. R., & Zehnder, N. (2006). The culture care of German American elders within a nursing home context. In: M. M. Leininger & M. R. McFarland (Eds.), *Culture care universality and diversity: A worldwide theory of nursing* (2nd ed.). Sudbury, MA: Jones and Bartlett.

Qualitative Solutions and Research. (1997). *QSR NUD*IST 4.* Thousand Oaks, CA: Sage.

Wehbeh-Alamah, H. (2006). Generic care of Lebanese Muslim women in the Midwestern USA. In: M. M. Leininger & M. R. McFarland (Eds.), *Culture care universality and diversity: A worldwide theory of nursing* (2nd ed.). Sudbury, MA: Jones and Bartlett.

Zoucha, R. (1998). The experiences of Mexican Americans receiving professional nursing care: An ethnonursing study. *Journal of Transcultural Nursing, 9*(2), 33–43.

Chapter **19**

Josephine Paterson and Loretta Zderad's Humanistic Nursing Theory

SUSAN KLEIMAN

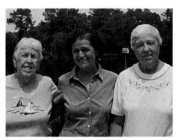

Josephine Paterson
Susan Kleiman
Loretta Zderad

Introducing the Theorists

Dr. Josephine Paterson is originally from the East Coast, where she attended a diploma school of nursing in New York City. She subsequently earned her bachelor's degree in nursing education from St. John's University. In her graduate work at Johns Hopkins University, she focused on public health nursing and then earned her doctor of nursing science degree from Boston University. Her doctoral dissertation focused on patient comfort.

Dr. Loretta Zderad is from the Midwest, where she attended a diploma school of nursing. She later earned her bachelor's degree in nursing education from Loyola University of Chicago and pursued graduate work in psychiatric nursing at the Catholic University of America. She subsequently earned her PhD from Georgetown University. Her dissertation research focused on empathy.

Josephine Paterson and Loretta Zderad met in the mid-1950s while working at Catholic University. As a joint project they created a new program that synthesized the community health and mental health components of the graduate program. This project launched a collaboration and friendship that has lasted for more than 50 years. They shared ideas and developed concepts, approaches, and experiences related to existential phenomenology, which evolved into their Theory of Humanistic Nursing.

In 1971, after their work in academia, Drs. Paterson and Zderad were hired by the Veterans Administration (VA) hospital in

Northport, NY. They accepted positions as "nursologists" created by a forward-thinking administrator who recognized the need for staff support during a period of change in the VA system. The position of nursologist involved a three-pronged approach to the improvement of patient care through clinical practice, education, and research. As part of this project they implemented workshops for the nurses at Northport from 1971 until 1978. In 1978, there was a change in hospital administration that resulted in a reorganization of services.

Dr. Paterson was assigned to the Mental Hygiene Clinic to work as a psychotherapist while Dr. Zderad became the associate chief of nursing service for education. These were the positions they held when I encountered them as a graduate student in psychiatric mental-health nursing. Dr. Paterson agreed to work with me as my clinical supervisor.

The following 2 years brought me a world of enrichment. For Drs. Paterson and Zderad, those years culminated in their retirement and relocation to the South, while I continued the work that they started as fellow theorist, colleague, and friend. They have inspired me to carry on their work, using it in my nursing situations in clinical, administrative, and educational roles, and to share what I have come to know with others.

For more details about the historical and personal backgrounds of Josephine Paterson and Loretta Zderad, told in their own words, refer to the chapter on "Dialogues with Paterson and Zderad" in *Human-Centered Nursing: The Foundation of Quality Care* (Kleiman, 2008).

Overview of the Theory

The Humanistic Nursing Theory emerged from Paterson's and Zderad's search for a way to make things better for nurses and their patients as they engaged in the daily activities of nursing practice; in existential terms, "being in the world of nursing." They wanted to offer a way of responding to the call of human needs. This call, a foundational concept of humanistic

nursing, can be heard where nursing is offered, coming to our attention as a subtle murmur of pain, sorrow, anxiety, desperation, joy, laughter, even silence, that expresses the state-of-being of the protagonists in the drama of health-care delivery, our patients and ourselves.

Unlike the sounds that signal the arrival of equipment or activity, these subtle sounds are always present and can be sensed, even when they fall outside the range of human hearing. It is as if they are awaiting amplification, ready to be transmitted by some mystical force to those who would or would not hear them. When they come into current awareness, they overwhelm the surrounding sounds of the environment, directing our immediate attention to a call for the human touch of a nurse.

Consider, for example, the calls of a mother for her newborn baby:

Where is my baby?
What happened to my baby?
What's wrong with my baby?
Where is my baby?

These calls intensify and bring into the foreground of a nurse's awareness his or her own inner calling to offer that human touch.

When a nurse responds to a call of a health-related concern, she enters the world of another, offering to, metaphorically speaking, go through life with that person. An occasion of humanistic nursing thereby comes into "being." From these moments, nurses can help patients or their loved ones be as much as they can be in the situations in which they find themselves: birth, death, sickness, disability, or health. Helping others to be as much as they can be regardless of their personal situation is the fundamental outcome of humanistic nursing (Kleiman, 2008).

Humanistic Nursing Theory offers nurses a way to illuminate the values and meanings central to their lived experiences so that they may share them with other nurses and integrate them into their nursing practice. Bringing into presence the values and meanings central to these lived experiences helps nurses to realize their self-actualizing potential.

Paterson and Zderad called this process of bringing into presence the essential values and meanings of one's life world "phenomenological reflection on experiences." The process emphasizes synthesis and wholeness rather than reduction and logical analysis. Challenging the notion that the reductionistic approach is the touchstone of explanatory power, they postulated an "all-at-once" character of existence in nurses' experiences of being in the world. They led the way for many of the contemporary nursing theories that emphasize these existential, phenomenologic, and caring aspects of nursing (Benner, 1984; Parse, 1981; Watson, 1988).

Highlights of the Theory

Humanistic Nursing Theory is multidimensional. It speaks to the essences of nursing and embraces the dynamics of being, becoming, and change. It is an interactive nursing theory that provides a methodology for reflection and articulation of nursing essences. It also provides a methodological bridge between theory and practice by providing a broad guide for nursing "dialogue" in a myriad of settings.

Nursing, as seen through Humanistic Nursing Theory, is the ability to struggle with another through "peak experiences related to health and suffering in which the participants are and become in accordance with their human potential" (Paterson & Zderad, 1976, p. 7). The struggle evolves within a dialogue between the participants, illuminating the possibility for each to "become" in concert with the other. According to Paterson and Zderad (1976), in nursing, the purpose of this dialogue, or intersubjective relating, is, "nurturing the well-being and more-being of persons in need" (p. 4).

Humanistic Nursing Theory is grounded in existentialism and emphasizes the lived experience of nursing. One of the existential themes that it builds on is the affirmation of being and becoming of both the patient and the nurse, who are actualized through the choices they make and the intersubjective relationships in which they engage.

The new adventurer in Humanistic Nursing Theory may at first find some of these terms and phrases awkward. When I spoke to a colleague of the "moreness" and of "relating all-at-once," she remarked, "Uh-oh, you're beginning to sound just like them" (Paterson & Zderad). But this vocabulary reflects a grasp of nursing as an ever-changing process. Just as nursing in actual practice is never inert, so Humanistic Nursing Theory is dynamic. Consider the description of humanistic nursing: "Our 'here and now' stage of Humanistic Nursing Theory development at times is experienced as an all-at-once octopus at a discotheque, stimulation personified, gyrating in many colors" (Paterson & Zderad, 1976, p. 4).

If asked to conceptualize Humanistic Nursing Theory succinctly, I would say, "call and response." These three words encapsulate the core themes of this elegant and very profound theory. Through this dialogic movement Paterson and Zderad have presented a vision of nursing that is amenable to variation in practice settings and to the changing patterns of nursing over time.

According to Humanistic Nursing Theory, there is a call from a person, a family, a community, or from humanity for help with some health-related issue. A nurse, a group of nurses, or the community of nurses hearing and recognizing that call respond in a manner that is intended to help the caller with the health-related need. What happens during this dialogue, the "and" in the "call and response," the "between," is nursing.

There is a call from a person, a family, a community, or from humanity for help with some health-related issue. A nurse, a group of nurses, or the community of nurses hearing and recognizing that call respond in a manner that is intended to help the caller with the health-related need. What happens during this dialogue, the "and" in the "call and response," the "between," is nursing.

In their book, *Humanistic Nursing* (1976), Drs. Paterson and Zderad share with other nurses their method for exploring the "between," again emphasizing that it is the "between" that they conceive of as nursing. The method is phenomenological inquiry

(Paterson & Zderad, 1976). Engaging in the phenomenological process sensitizes the inquiring nurse to the excitement, anticipation, and uncertainty of approaching the nursing situation openly. Through a spirit of receptivity, a readiness for surprise, and the courage to experience the unknown, there is an opportunity for authentic relating and intersubjectivity. "The process leads one naturally to repeated experiences of and reflective immersion in the lived phenomena" (Zderad, 1978, p. 8).

This immersion into the intersubjective experience and the phenomenological process helps to guide the nurse in the responsive interchange. During this interchange, the nurse calls forth all that she or he is (education, skills, life experiences, intuition, etc.) and integrates it into her or his response. A common misconception that students of Humanistic Nursing Theory may have is that it asserts that the nurse must provide what it is that the patient is calling for. Remember the response of the nurse is guided by all that she or he is. This includes his or her professional role, ethics, and competencies. A particular nurse may not actually be able or willing to provide what is being called for, but the process of being heard, according to this theory, is in itself a humanizing experience.

The conceptual framework of Humanistic Nursing Theory in Figure 19-1 may illuminate and illustrate some of its basic concepts

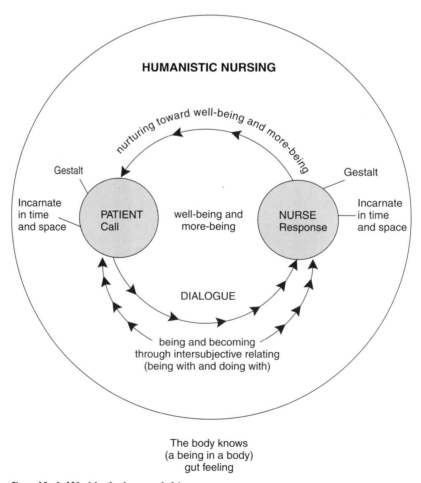

Figure 19 · 1 World of others and things.

and assumptions. Humanistic nursing is a dynamic process that occurs in the living context of human beings, human beings who interface and interact with others and other things in the world. In the world of Humanistic Nursing Theory, when we speak of human beings, we mean patients (e.g., individuals, members of families, members of communities, or members of the human race) and nurses (Fig. 19-2). A person becomes a patient when he or she sends a call for help with some health-related problem. The person hearing and recognizing the call is a nurse. A nurse, by intentionally choosing to become a nurse, has made a commitment to help others with health-related needs.

It is important to emphasize that in Humanistic Nursing Theory, each nurse and each patient is taken to be a unique human being with his or her own particular gestalt (Fig. 19-3). Gestalt, representing all that the particular human being is, includes all past experiences, all current being, and all hopes, dreams, and fears of the future that are experienced in one's own space–time dimension. As illustrated, this gestalt includes past and current social relationships, as well as gender, race, religion, education, work, and all of the individualized patterns for coping that a person has developed. It also includes past experiences with persons in the health care system and a patient's images and expectations of those persons.

Our gestalt is the unique expression of our individuality as incarnate human beings who exist in this particular space at this particular time, with circumscribed resources and in a physical body that senses, filters, and processes our experiences to which we assign subjective meanings. Accordingly, a nurse and a patient perceive and respond to each other as a gestalt, not just as the presentation of a sum of attributes. In humanistic nursing we say that each person is perceived as existing "all-at-once." In the process of interacting with patients, nurses interweave professional identity, education, intuition, and experience with all their other life experiences, creating

Nursing Is Transactional

Figure 19 · 2 Shared human experience.

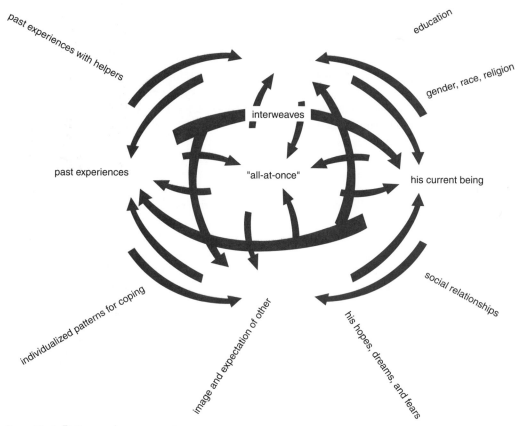

Figure 19 · 3 Patient and nurse gestalts.

their own tapestry, which unfolds during their responses.

One has only to observe nurses going about their nursing to see this process of interrelating as subjective human beings. Consider for example, performing the task of suctioning a patient. This task can be done with tenderness, dignity, and with masterful technical skills that make the procedure almost unnoticeable. I once watched as a nurse performed the task of positioning and suctioning a patient; she made sure she also repositioned the small basket of flowers placed by the patient's bedside. The repositioning of the flowers was not needed to perform the technique of suctioning. However, it showed that the nurse recognized the patient as a unique human being, and she did something special to make the experience less stressful and as comfortable as possible for the patient. Comfort in this instance refers to the idea that through the relationship engendered and nurtured in intersubjective dialogue, there arises the possibility for persons to become all that they can be in particular lived situations.

Philosophical and Methodological Background

The phenomenological movement of the 19th century was a response to what its proponents called the dehumanization and objectification of the world by the logical positivists. Phenomenologists proposed that human beings, the world, and their experiences of their world are inseparable. One can easily see that a nursing theory based in the human context lends itself to phenomenological inquiry rather than reductionism, which attempts to remove subjective humanness and strives to achieve detached objectivity. The early phenomenologists saw their goal as the examination and description of all things, including the human experience of those things, in the particular way they reveal themselves.

Phenomenology is not only a philosophy, but also a method—a method that can be integrated into a general approach or way of viewing the world. Nurses who can relate to this method are inclined to cultivate it and make it a part of their everyday approach to nursing. This method is no less rigorous in its application than methods used in experimental research to build theories. The phenomenological approach is based on description, intuition, analysis, and synthesis. Training and conscientious self-criticism on the part of the unbiased inquirer are essential as he or she investigates the phenomenon as it reveals itself. In phenomenology, a statement's validity is based on whether or not it describes the phenomenon accurately. The truth of all the statements resulting from the critical analysis of each phenomenon described can be verified by examining the phenomenon itself.

Drs. Paterson and Zderad describe five phases to their phenomenological study of nursing. Phenomenology underpins the practice of nursing and study of nursing phenomena. These phases are presented sequentially but are actually interwoven because, as with all of Humanistic Nursing Theory, there is a constant flow between, in all directions, and all-at-once emanating toward a center that is nursing. The phases of humanistic nursing inquiry are:

• Preparation of the nurse knower for coming to know
• Nurse knowing the other intuitively
• Nurse knowing the other scientifically
• Nurse complementarily synthesizing known others
• Succession within the nurse from the many to the paradoxical one

Enfolded in these five phases are three concepts that are very basic to Humanistic Nursing Theory: bracketing, angular view, and noetic loci. These will be taken up as we discuss the phases of inquiry.

Preparation of the Nurse Knower for Coming to Know

In the first phase, the inquirer tries to open him- or herself up to the unknown and to the possibly different. The nurse consciously and conscientiously struggles with understanding and identifying her or his own "angular view." Angular view involves the gestalt of the unique person mentioned earlier. It includes the conceptual and experiential framework that we bring into any situation, a framework that is usually unexamined and casually accepted as we negotiate our everyday world. Later in the process angular view is called upon to help make sense of and give meaning to the phenomena being studied.

By intentionally bringing into consciousness and acknowledging our angular view we are then able to bracket it purposefully so that we do not superimpose it on the lived experience of the other. When we bracket, we hold our own thoughts, experiences, and beliefs in abeyance. This "holding in abeyance" does not deny our unique selves but suspends them temporarily.

A personal experience that helped me grasp the concept of bracketing and the desired state it aims to achieve occurred when I was traveling in Europe. As I entered each new country, I experienced the excitement of the unknown. I realized at the same time how alert, open, and other-directed I was in this uncharted world as compared to my own daily routine at home. In my familiar surroundings, I would often fill in the blanks left by my inattentiveness to a routine experience, sometimes anticipating and answering questions even before they were asked.

Bracketing prepares the inquirer to enter the uncharted world of the other without expectations and preconceived ideas. It helps one to be open to the authentic, to the true experience of the other. Even temporarily letting go of that which shapes our own identity, however, causes anxiety, fear, and uncertainty. Labeling, diagnosing, and routine add a necessary and very valuable predictability, sense of security, and means of conserving energy to our everyday existence and practice. However, as a consequence we may become less open to the new and different in a situation. Being open to the new and different is a necessary stance in being able to know the other intuitively.

Nurse Knowing the Other Intuitively

Knowing the other intuitively is described by Paterson and Zderad (1976) as "moving back and forth between the impressions the nurse becomes aware of in herself and the recollected real experience of the other" (pp. 88–89), which was obtained through the unbiased being with the other. Bracketing and intuiting are not contradictory processes. Both are necessary and interwoven parts of the phenomenological process. The rigor and validity of phenomenology are based on the continually referring back to the phenomenon itself. It is conceptualized as dialectic between the impression and the real. This shifting back and forth allows for sudden insights on the nurse's part, a new overall grasp, which manifests itself in a clearer, or perhaps a new, "understanding." These understandings generate further development of the process. At this time, the nurse's general impressions are in a dialogue with her or his unbracketed view (Fig. 19–4).

Nurse Knowing the Other Scientifically

In the next phase, objectivity is needed as the nurse comes to know the other scientifically. Standing outside the phenomenon, the nurse examines the other through analysis. She or he comes to know the other through parts or elements that are symbolic and known. This phase incorporates the nurse's ability to be conscious of her- or himself and that which she or he has taken in, merged with, and made part of her- or himself. "This is the time when the nurse mulls over, analyzes, sorts out, compares, contrasts, relates, interprets, gives a name to,

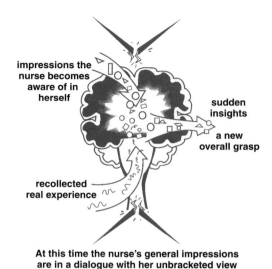

At this time the nurse's general impressions are in a dialogue with her unbracketed view

Figure 19 · 4 Nurse knowing the other intuitively. *(Adapted from Briggs, J., & Peat, D. [1989]. Turbulent Mirror [p. 176]. New York: Harper & Row.)*

and categorizes" (Paterson & Zderad, 1976, p. 79). Patterns and themes are reflective of and rigorously validated by the authentic experience (Fig. 19-5).

Nurse Complementarily Synthesizing Known Others

At this point, the nurse personifies what has been described by Paterson and Zderad as a "noetic locus," a "knowing place" (1976, p. 43). According to this concept, the greatest gift a human being can have is the ability to relate to others, to wonder, search, and imagine about experience, and to create out of what has become known. Seeing themselves as "knowing places" inspires nurses to continue to develop and expand their community of world thinkers through their educative and practical experiences, which then becomes a part of their angular view. This self-expansion, through the internalization of what others have come to know, dynamically interrelates with the nurse's human capacity to be conscious of her own lived experiences. Through this interrelationship, the subjective and objective world of nursing can be reflected upon by each nurse, who is aware of and values herself as a "knowing place" (Fig. 19-6).

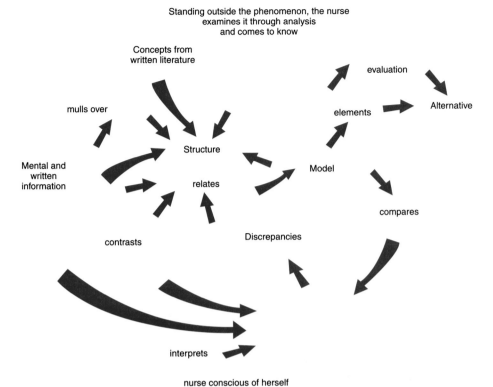

Figure 19 · 5 Nurses knowing the other scientifically. *(Adapted from illustration in Briggs, J., & Peat, D. [1989]. Turbulent Mirror [p. 176]. New York: Harper & Row.)*

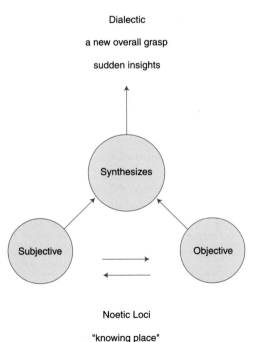

Figure 19 · 6 Nurses complementarily synthesizing knowing others.

Succession Within the Nurse from the Many to the Paradoxical One

This is the birth of the new from the existing patterns, themes, and categories. It is in this phase that the nurse "comes up with a conception or abstraction that is inclusive of and beyond the multiplicities and contradictions" (Paterson & Zderad, 1976, p. 81) in a process that augments and expands her or his own angular view. This is the pattern of the dialectic process, which is reflected throughout Humanistic Nursing Theory. In the dialectic process there is a repetitive pattern of organizing the dissimilar into a higher level (Barnum, 1990, p. 44). At this higher level, differences are assimilated to create the new. This repetitive dialectic process of humanistic nursing is an approach that feels comfortable and natural for those who think inductively. The pervasive theme of dialectic assimilation speaks to universal interrelatedness from the simplest to the most complex level. Humans, by virtue of their ability to self-observe, have the unique capacity to transcend themselves and reflect on their relationship to the universe.

This dialectic process has a pattern similar to that of the call-and-response dialogic movement of Humanistic Nursing Theory. The movement speaks to the interactive dialogue between two different humans from which a unique yet universal instance of nursing emerges. The nursing interaction is limited in time and space, but the internalization of that experience adds something new to each person's angular view. Neither is the same as before. Each is more because of that coming together. The coming together of the nurse and the patient, the between in the lived world, is nursing. Just as in the double helix of the DNA molecule whose interweaving pattern gives structure to the individual, in the fabric of Humanistic Nursing Theory this intentional interweaving between patient and nurse is what gives nursing its structure, form, and meaning.

The Concept of Community

The definition of community presented by Paterson and Zderad (1976) is: "Two or more persons struggling together toward a center" (1976, p. 131). In any community there is the individual and the collective. Plato points to the microcosm and the macrocosm and proposes that the one is reflective of the many. Humanistic Nursing Theory similarly proposes that the interaction of one nurse is a reflection of the recurrent pattern of nursing, and is therefore worth reflecting upon and valuing. According to Humanistic Nursing Theory, there is an inherent obligation of nurses to one another and to the community of nurses. That which enhances one of us, enhances all of us. Through openness, sharing, and caring, we each will expand our angular views, each becoming more than before. Subsequently, we take back into our nursing community these expanded selves, which in turn will touch our patients, other colleagues, and the world of health care.

Applications of the Theory

These descriptive explorations illuminate the concepts of empathy, comfort, and presence innate in applying Humanistic Nursing theory to a clinical setting. Paterson (1977) shared a personal experience in a nursing situation with a person terminally ill with cancer:

> For a while I really beat on myself. I felt nothing, just a kind of indifference and numbness, as Dominic expressed his miseries, fears, and anger. I pride myself on my empathic ability. I felt so inadequate. I could not believe I could not feel with him what he was experiencing. Intellectually I knew his words, his expressions were pain-filled. My feelings of inadequacy, helplessness, and inability to control myself, came through strong. [As] I mulled reflectively about this, suddenly a light dawned amidst my puzzlement. I was experiencing what Dominic was expressing. At this time I was feeling his inadequacy, helplessness, and inability to control his cancer. (p. 13)

This insight brought a greater understanding between Dr. Paterson and this patient, an understanding that brought them closer so that she could endure with him in his fear-filled knowing and unknowing of dying. As his condition deteriorated, she continued to visit at his bedside.

> Often after greeting me and saying what he needed he would fall asleep. First, I thought, 'It doesn't matter whether I come or not.' Then I noticed and validated that when I moved his eyes flew open. I reevaluated his sleeping during my visit. I discussed this with him. He felt safe when I sat with him. He was exhausted, staying awake, watching himself to be sure he did not die. When I was there I watched him, and he could sleep. I no longer made any move to leave before my time with him was up. I told him of this intention so that he could relax more deeply. To alleviate aloneness; this is a most expensive gift. To give this gift of time and presence in the patient's space, a person has to value the outcomes of relating. (p. 13)
>
> This gift of presence is poetically described by Dr. Zderad (1978)

Death lifts his scythe
to swipe down the young man
misdressed in hospital gown
displaced in hospital bed.
The cruel cold blade slashes
the hard mask of his nurse
silently standing there
bleeding forth her presence. (p. 48)

At an interdisciplinary conference on love, intimacy, and connectedness that I attended, one of the opening speakers described the following experience that had been related to him by a dear friend.

His friend had just been diagnosed with a serious form of cancer. The speaker described his friend telling him, "In the early evening the family was all around. We talked, but there was the awkwardness of not knowing what to say or what to expect. Later that night, I was in my room all alone. No longer having to be concerned about my family and what they were struggling with, I began to experience some of my own feelings. I felt so alone. Then the evening nurse who had been working with me over the last two days of testing came in. We looked at each other—neither of us said a word and she just gently touched my hand. I cried. She stayed there for … I don't know how long, until I placed my other hand on top of hers and gently gave it a pat. She left and I was able to go to sleep. This was one of the most intimate moments in my life. This nurse offered to be with me in the known, and unknown; somehow she also conveyed a reassurance that I did not have to go through what was coming, whatever that was, alone."

This ability to be with and endure with a patient in the process of living and dying is frequently taken for granted by us, yet it is what many times differentiates us from other professionals.

Practice Exemplar

The humanistic nursing approach is useful in clinical supervision. In the process of supervision I try to understand the "call" of the nurse when she brings up a clinical issue. This usually is connected to the "call" of the patient to him or her, and some issue that has arisen around the nurse's not being able to hear or respond to that call.

Consider this example. Ms. L. was working with a patient who had recently been told that her HIV test was positive. Although she did not have AIDS, she had been exposed to the AIDS virus, probably through her current boyfriend, who was purportedly an IV drug abuser. The nurse was concerned that the doctor on the interdisciplinary team, who was also the patient's therapist, was not giving the patient the support that the nurse felt the patient was calling out for. The nurse and I explored her perception that the patient did in fact seem to be reaching out. We ask ourselves about the meaning of "reaching out" in terms of what the patient was reaching for. The patient had received clear explanations that she did not have AIDS, but at some point, she might acquire the disease. The patient was told that there were treatments to retard the disease process, but that there were no cures yet. Given this, the doctor, whose primary function was to treat and cure, was feeling ill-prepared to deal with this patient. Perhaps this sense of inadequacy fostered avoidant behavior on his part. But as the nurse and I dialogued together, we came to realize that, in fact, the patient was not calling for doctoring; she was calling for nursing. She was calling for someone to help her get through and grow through this experience in her life. With this clarified, the nurse and I began to explore the nurse's experience of hearing this call. The nurse spoke of the pain of knowing that this young woman might die prematurely. She spoke of how a friend, who reminded her of this

Continued

patient, had also died, and that when she associated the two, she felt sad.

As we explored the nurse's angular view, we were able to identify areas that were unknown. The nurse had difficulty understanding the need or the role of the patient's relationship with her current boyfriend. We worked on helping the nurse to bracket her own thoughts and judgments, so that she could be more open to the patient's experience of this relationship. Subsequently, the nurse was able to understand the patient's intense fear of being alone. As the nurse began to understand that choices are humanizing, she began to explore the need for support systems. To expand her own capability of being a "knowing place" and expanding her angular view, she sought out the help of the nurse practitioner in our gynecology clinic. They worked well together with this patient, who eventually was able to leave the hospital, get a part-time job, and be all that she could in her current life situation.

The nurse in the hospital grew from her experience of working with this patient. Although she is usually quite reserved and shies away from public forums, with encouragement she was able to share the experience with this patient in a large public forum. She not only shared with other professionals the role that she as a nurse played in the care of this patient, but also acknowledged herself in a group of professionals as a "knowing place."

The process enfolded in Humanistic Nursing Theory is beneficial to supervisors and self-reflective practitioners in all areas of nursing. Patients call to us both verbally and nonverbally, with all sorts of health-related needs. It is important to hear the calls and know the process that lets us understand them. In hearing the calls and searching our own experiences of who we are, our personal angular view, we may progress as humanistic nurses.

Policy: Developing a Community of Nurses

Another group experience in which Humanistic Nursing Theory was utilized was the formation of a community of nurses who were mutually struggling with changes in their nursing roles. In Humanistic Nursing Theory, sharing within the community of nurses allows each nurse and the community to become more. I became aware of a common call issued forth by nurses from my own experiences as a nurse manager.

In the report of the secretary of Health and Human Services' Commission on Nursing (December, 1988) we were told that "the perspective and expertise of nurses are a necessary adjunct to that of other health-care professionals in the policy-making, and regulatory, and standard setting process" (p. 31). This mandate is still echoed in today's nursing literature (Wick, 2003), confirming the belief that nurses are challenged to help bring about needed change in the health care system. I

called to the community of nurses where I work, and we joined together to struggle with this challenge. While the importance of organized nursing power cannot be overemphasized, it is the individual nurse in her or his day-to-day practice who can actualize or undermine the power of the profession. As a group, we strove to acknowledge and support one another as individuals of worth so that we in turn could maximize our influence as a profession.

In settings such as hospitals, the time pressure, the unending tasks, the emotional strain, and the conflicts do not allow nurses to relate, reflect, and support one another in their struggle toward a center that is nursing. This isolation and alienation does not allow for the development of either a personal or professional voice. Within our community of nurses, it became clear that developing individual voices was our first task. Talking and listening to one another about our nursing worlds allowed us to become more articulate and clear about function and value as nurses. The theme of developing an articulate voice has pervaded and continues to pervade this group. There is an ever-increasing awareness of both manner and language as we interact with one another and those outside the group. The resolve for an articulate voice is even more firm as members of the group experience and share the empowering effect it can have on both personal and professional life. It has been said that "those that express themselves unfold in health, beauty, and human potential. They become unblocked channels through which creativity can flow" (Hills & Stone, 1976, p. 71).

Group members offered alternative approaches to various situations that were utilized and subsequently brought back to the group. In this way, each member shared in the experience. That experience therefore became available to all members as they individually formulated their own knowledge base and expanded their angular view. As Paterson and Zderad (1976) proposed, "each person might be viewed as a community of the beings with whom she has meaningfully related" (p. 45)

and has a potential resource for expanding herself as a "knowing place."

Through openness and sharing we were able to differentiate our strengths. Once the members could truly appreciate the unique competencies of one another, they were able to reflect that appreciation back. Through this reflection, members began to internalize and then project a competent image of themselves. They learned that this positive mirroring did not have to come from outsiders. They can reflect back to one another the image of competence and power. They, as a community of nurses, can empower one another. This reciprocity is a self-enhancing process, for "the degree to which I can create relationships which facilitate the growth of others as separate persons is a measure of the growth I have achieved in myself" (Rogers, 1976, p. 79). And so by sharing in our community of nurses we can empower one another through mutual confirmation as we help one another move toward a center that is nursing. We strive to do this with our patients. We must also strive to do this for one another and the profession of nursing.

Summary

Today I perceive another call. This call is resounded in and exemplified by the following description of examining a pregnant woman: "Instead of having to approach the woman . . . to feel her breathing, you could now read the information [on her and her fetus] from across the room, from down the hall" (Rothman, 1987, p. 28).

The call I hear is for nursing. It is the call from humanity to maintain the humanness in the health care system, which is becoming increasingly sophisticated in technology, increasingly concerned with cost containment, and increasingly less aware of and concerned with the patient as a human being. The context of Humanistic Nursing Theory is humans. The basic question it

asks of nursing practice is: Is this particular intersubjective–transactional nursing event humanizing or dehumanizing? Nurses as clinicians, teachers, researchers, and administrators can use the concepts and process of Humanistic Nursing Theory to gain a better understanding of the "calls" we are hearing. Through this understanding we are given direction for expanding ourselves as "knowing places" so that we can fulfill our reason for being, which, according to Humanistic Nursing Theory, is nurturing the well-being and more-being of persons in need.

For more information on the subject of Humanistic Nursing see *Human-Centered Nursing: The Foundation of Quality Care* by Susan Kleiman.

References

Barnum, B. J. S. (1990). *Nursing theory: Analysis, application, evaluation.* Glenview, IL: Scott, Foresman.

Benner, P. (1984). *From novice to expert.* Menlo Park, CA: Addison-Wesley.

Buber, M. (1965). *The knowledge of man.* New York: Harper & Row.

Heidegger, M. (1977). *The question concerning technology.* New York: Harper & Row.

Hills, C., & Stone, R. B. (1976). *Conduct your own awareness sessions: 100 ways to enhance self-concept in the classroom.* Englewood Cliffs, NJ: Prentice-Hall.

Husserl, L. (1970). *The idea of phenomenology.* The Hague, Netherlands: Martinus Nijhoff.

Kleiman, S. (2008). *Human Centered Nursing: The foundation of quality care.* Philadelphia: F. A. Davis.

May, R. (1995). *The courage to create.* New York: W. W. Norton.

Oliveira, N. (2003). Lived dialogue between nurse and mothers of children with cancer. 107f. Dissertation (master's degree)—Centro de Ciências da Saúde/Universidade Federal da Paraíba, João Pessoa.

Parse, R. (1981). *Man-living-health: A theory of nursing.* New York: John Wiley & Sons.

Paterson, J. G. (1977). Living until death, my perspective. Paper presented at the Syracuse Veteran's Administration Hospital, New York.

Paterson, J. G., & Zderad, L. T. (1976). *Humanistic nursing.* New York: John Wiley & Sons.

Rogers, C. R. (1976). *Perceiving, behaving, and becoming: 100 ways to enhance self-concept in the classroom.* Englewood Cliffs, NJ: Prentice-Hall.

Rothman, B. (1987). *The tentative pregnancy: Prenatal diagnosis and the future of motherhood.* New York: Penguin.

U.S. Public Health Services. (1988, December). Secretary's commission on nursing, final report. Washington, DC: Department of Health & Human Services.

Watson, J. (1988). *Nursing: Human science and human care.* New York: National League for Nursing.

Wick, G. (2003). A place where the spirit can grow: An answer to recruitment and retention? *Nephrology Nursing Journal, 30*(1), 15.

Zderad, L. T. (1978). From here-and-now theory: Reflections on "how." In: *Theory development: What? Why? How?* Publication no. 15-1708. New York: National League for Nursing.

Chapter 20

Jean Watson's Theory of Human Caring

JEAN WATSON
AND TERRI KAYE WOODWARD

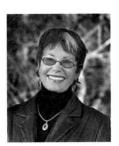

Jean Watson

Introducing the Theorist

Dr. Jean Watson is a distinguished professor of nursing who holds an endowed Chair in Caring Science at the University of Colorado Denver, College of Nursing where she formerly served as dean. She founded the original Center for Human Caring at the University of Colorado Health Sciences Center School of Nursing. She is also a member of the American Academy of Nursing and has served as president of the National League for Nursing. Dr. Watson founded and serves as director of the nonprofit Watson Caring Science Institute, dedicated to furthering the work of caring, science, and heart-centered *Caritas* Nursing, restoring caring and love for nurses' and health care clinicians' healing practices for self and others.

Dr. Watson earned undergraduate and graduate degrees in nursing and psychiatric–mental health nursing and holds a doctorate in educational psychology and counseling from the University of Colorado at Boulder. She is a widely published author and is the recipient of several awards and honors, including an international Kellogg Fellowship in Australia; a Fulbright Research Award in Sweden; and six honorary doctoral degrees, including three international honorary doctorates in Sweden, the United Kingdom, and Canada.

Dr. Watson's published works on the philosophy and theory of human caring and the art and science of nursing are used by clinical nurses and academic programs throughout the world. Her caring philosophy is used to guide new models of caring and healing practices in diverse settings and in several different countries. More recent clinical–research initiatives have been under-way in clinical agencies interested in transforming nursing practice from the inside out, implementing transformative caring-healing practices and models of caring, guided by Watson's theory and philosophy.

Dr. Watson's original book on caring was published in 1979, 6 years after she earned her PhD and joined the faculty at the University of Colorado. Her second book, *Nursing: Human Science and Human Care*, was written while on sabbatical in Australia and reflects the metaphysical, spiritual evolution of her thinking. The third book, *Postmodern Nursing and Beyond*, moves beyond theory to reflect the ontological foundation of nursing as an overarching framework for transforming caring and healing practices in education and clinical care (Watson, 1999).

Additional empirical and clinical caring research foci developments include the first and second editions of the book on caring instruments, *Assessing and Measuring Caring in Nursing and Health Sciences* (2002, 2008). These works offer a critique and collation of more than 20 instruments for assessing and measuring caring. The measurement publications seek to bridge modern and postmodern views of caring and healing in relation to outcomes research and the need for clinical evidence of caring.

Her *Caring Science as Sacred Science* (Watson, 2004/5 *American Journal of Nursing* book of the Year) makes a case for a deep moral–ethical, spirit-filled foundation for caring science and healing that is based on infinite love and an expanding cosmology. This view in turn elicits the finest of nursing as the art, science, and spiritual practice it is meant to be because it reflects the highest ethical ideal form of compassionate service to society and humanity.

The latest 2008 theoretical work, *Nursing: The Philosophy and Science of Caring. Revised New Edition*, University Press of Colorado, revisits and reworks her first book, *Nursing: The Philosophy and Science of Caring* (1979, reprinted 1985), bringing the original publication up to date to include all the changes made during the past 30 years. This latest update introduces Caritas Nursing as the culmination of a Caring Science foundation for professional nursing. The Watson Caring Science Institute and its Faculty Associates are developing educational, clinical, and administrative–leadership and research models that seek to sustain and deepen authentic caring–healing practices for self and other, transforming practitioners and patients alike. The Caring Science model is integrating *Caritas* with the Science of the Heart (www.heartMath.com) as a liberating model to deepen the intelligent heart-centered caring for all.

Overview of the Theory

The Theory of Human Caring was developed between 1975 and 1979 while I was teaching at the University of Colorado. It emerged from my own views of nursing, combined and informed by my doctoral studies in educational, clinical, and social psychology. It was my initial attempt to bring meaning and focus to nursing as an emerging discipline and distinct health profession that had its own unique values, knowledge, and practices, and its own ethic and mission to society. The work was also influenced by my involvement with an integrated academic nursing curriculum and efforts to find common meaning and order to nursing that transcended settings, populations, specialty, and subspecialty areas.

From my emerging perspective, I tried to make explicit that nursing's values, knowledge, and practices of human caring were geared toward subjective inner healing processes and the life world of the experiencing person. This required unique caring–healing arts and a framework called "carative factors," which complemented conventional medicine but stood in stark contrast to "curative factors." At the same time, this emerging philosophy and theory of human caring sought to balance the cure orientation of medicine, giving nursing its unique disciplinary, scientific, and professional standing with itself and its public.

Major Conceptual Elements

The major conceptual elements of the original (and emergent) theory are:

- Ten carative factors (evolving toward "clinical caritas processes")
- Transpersonal caring relationship
- Caring moment/caring occasion
- Caring–healing modalities

Other dynamic aspects of the theory that have emerged or are emerging as more explicit components include:

- Expanded views of self and person (transpersonal mind–body–spirit unity of being, embodied spirit)
- Caring–healing consciousness and intentionality to care and promote healing–caring consciousness as energy within the human–environmental field of a caring moment
- Phenomenal field/unitary consciousness: unbroken wholeness and connectedness of all
- Advanced caring–healing modalities/nursing arts as a future model for advanced practice of nursing qua nursing (consciously guided by one's nursing ethical–theoretical–philosophical orientation).

Caring Science

The emergence of the work is a more explicit development of Caring Science as a deep moral–ethical context of infinite and cosmic love. As soon as one is more explicit about placing the human and caring within their science model, it automatically forces a relational unitary worldview and makes explicit caring as a moral ideal to sustain humanity across time and space, one of the gifts and raison d'etre of nursing in the world, but yet to be recognized within and without. Nevertheless a Caring Science orientation is necessary for the survival of nursing as well as humanity at this crossroads in human evolution.

This view takes nursing and healing work beyond conventional thinking. The latest orientation is located within the ageless wisdom traditions and perennial ingredients of the discipline of nursing, while transcending nursing.

Caring Science as a model for nursing allows nursing's caring–healing core to become both discipline-specific and trans-disciplinary. Thus, nursing's timeless, ancient, enduring, and most noble contributions come of age through a Caring Science orientation—scientifically, aesthetically, and ethically.

Ten Carative Factors

The original (1979) work was organized around 10 carative factors as a framework for providing a format and focus for nursing phenomena. Although "carative factors" is still the current terminology for the "core" of nursing, providing a structure for the initial work, the term "factor" is too stagnant for my sensibilities today. I offer another concept that is more in keeping with my own evolution and future directions for the "theory," the concept of "clinical caritas" and "caritas processes" as consistent with a more fluid and contemporary movement with these ideas and my expanding directions.

Caritas comes from the Latin word meaning "to cherish and appreciate, giving special attention to, or loving." It connotes something that is very fine; indeed, it is precious. The word "caritas" is also closely related to the original word "carative" from my 1979 book. At this time, I now make new connections between carative and caritas and without hesitation compare them to invoke love, which caritas conveys. This allows love and caring to come together for a new form of deep transpersonal caring. This relationship between love and caring connotes inner healing for self and others, extending to nature and the larger universe, unfolding and evolving within a cosmology that is both metaphysical and transcendent with the coevolving human in the universe. This emerging model of transpersonal caring moves from carative to *caritas*. This integrative expanded perspective is postmodern, in that it transcends conventional industrial, static models of nursing while simultaneously evoking both the past and the future. For example, the future of nursing is tied to Nightingale's sense of "calling," guided by a deep sense of commitment and a covenantal ethic of human service, cherishing our phenomena, our subject matter, and those we serve.

It is when we include caring and love in our work and in our life that we discover and affirm that nursing, like teaching, is more than just a job; it is also a life-giving and life-receiving career for a lifetime of growth and learning. Such maturity and integration of past with present and future now require transforming self and those we serve, including our institutions and the profession itself. As we more publicly and professionally assert these positions for our theories, our ethics, and our practices—even for our science—we also locate ourselves and our profession and discipline within a new, emerging cosmology. Such thinking calls for a sense of reverence and sacredness with regard to life and all living things. It incorporates both art and science, as they are also being redefined, acknowledging a convergence among art, science, and spirituality. As we enter into the transpersonal caring theory and philosophy, we simultaneously are challenged to relocate ourselves in these emerging ideas and to question for ourselves how the theory speaks to us. This invites us into a new relationship with ourselves and our ideas about life, nursing, and theory.

Original Carative Factors

The original carative factors served as a guide to what was referred to as the "core of nursing," in contrast to nursing's "trim." *Core* pointed to those aspects of nursing that potentiate therapeutic healing processes and relationships—they affect the one caring and the one being cared for. Further, the basic core was grounded in what I referred to as the philosophy, science, and even art of caring. Carative is that deeper and larger dimension of nursing that goes beyond the "trim" of changing times, setting, procedures, functional tasks, specialized focus around disease, and treatment and technology. Although the "trim" is important and not expendable, the point is that nursing cannot be defined around its trim and what it does in a given setting and at a given point in time. Nor can nursing's trim define and clarify its larger

professional ethic and mission to society—its raison d'être for the public. That is where nursing theory comes into play, and transpersonal caring theory offers another way that both differs from and complements that which has come to be known as "modern" nursing and conventional medical–nursing frameworks.

The 10 carative factors included in the original work are the following:

1. Formation of a humanistic–altruistic system of values.
2. Instillation of faith–hope.
3. Cultivation of sensitivity to one's self and to others.
4. Development of a helping–trusting, human caring relationship.
5. Promotion and acceptance of the expression of positive and negative feelings.
6. Systematic use of a creative problem-solving caring process.
7. Promotion of transpersonal teaching–learning.
8. Provision for a supportive, protective, and/or corrective mental, physical, societal, and spiritual environment.
9. Assistance with gratification of human needs.
10. Allowance for existential–phenomenological–spiritual forces. (Watson, 1979/1985)

Although some of the basic tenets of the original carative factors still hold, and indeed are used as the basis for some theory-guided practice models and research, what I am proposing here, as part of my evolution and the evolution of these ideas and the theory itself, is to transpose the carative factors into "clinical caritas processes." For example, consider the following within the context of clinical caritas and emerging transpersonal caring theory.

From Carative Factor to Clinical Caritas Processes

As carative factors evolve within an expanding perspective, and as my ideas and values evolve, I now offer the following translation of the original carative factors into clinical caritas processes, suggesting more open ways in which they can be considered. For example:

1. Formation of a humanistic–altruistic system of values becomes the practice of loving kindness and equanimity within the context of caring consciousness.
2. Instillation of faith–hope becomes being authentically present and enabling and sustaining the deep belief system and subjective life world of self and one being cared for.
3. Cultivation of sensitivity to one's self and to others becomes cultivation of one's own spiritual practices and transpersonal self, going beyond ego self, opening to others with sensitivity and compassion.
4. Development of a helping–trusting, human caring relationship becomes developing and sustaining a helping–trusting, authentic caring relationship.
5. Promotion and acceptance of the expression of positive and negative feelings becomes being present to, and supportive of, the expression of positive and negative feelings as a connection with deeper spirit of self and the one being cared for.
6. Systematic use of a creative problem-solving caring process becomes creative use of self and all ways of knowing as part of the caring process; to engage in artistry of caring-healing practices.
7. Promotion of transpersonal teaching-learning becomes engaging in genuine teaching-learning experience that attends to unity of being and meaning, attempting to stay within others' frames of reference.
8. Provision for a supportive, protective, and/or corrective mental, physical, societal, and spiritual environment becomes creating a healing environment at all levels (a physical and nonphysical, subtle environment of energy and consciousness, whereby wholeness, beauty, comfort, dignity, and peace are potentiated).
9. Assistance with gratification of human needs becomes assisting with basic needs, with an intentional caring consciousness, administering "human care essentials,"

which potentiate alignment of mind-body-spirit, wholeness, and unity of being in all aspects of care, tending to both embodied spirit and evolving spiritual emergence.

10. Allowance for existential-phenomenological-spiritual forces becomes opening and attending to spiritual-mysterious and existential dimensions of one's own life-death; soul care for self and the one being cared for.

What differs in the clinical caritas framework is that a decidedly spiritual dimension and an overt evocation of love and caring are merged for a new paradigm for this millennium. Such a perspective ironically places nursing within its most mature framework and is consistent with the Nightingale model of nursing—yet to be actualized but awaiting its evolution. This direction, while embedded in theory, goes beyond theory and becomes a converging paradigm for nursing's future.

Thus, I consider my work more a philosophical, ethical, intellectual blueprint for nursing's evolving disciplinary/professional matrix, rather than a specific theory per se. Nevertheless, others interact with the original work at levels of concreteness or abstractness. The caring theory has been, and is still being used as a guide for educational curricula, clinical practice models, methods for research and inquiry, and administrative directions for nursing and health-care delivery.

Reading the Theory

The "theory" can be "read" as a philosophy, an ethic, a paradigm, an expanded science model or a theory. If read as a theory, it can be 'read' as grand theory within the unitary–transformative paradigm when understood at the transpersonal energetic field level of Caritas-Universal Love, and evolving consciousness.

It can be "read" as middle range theory when read at the "Carative factors/Caritas process, which provides the structure and language of the theory, as both middle range and specific. When used in clinical settings nurses are framing their experiences around the caritas processes to sustain the caring science focus, as well as developing language systems including computerized documentation systems to document and study caring within a designated language system" (Rosenberg, 2006, p. 55). The middle range focus also is congruent with clinical caring research projects, utilizing caring language of carative/caritas. Indeed, many of the more formalized caring assessment tools are based on the language of this structure. Several multisite research projects are now underway using consistent caring assessment tools. For example, Dr. Joanne Duffy's: Caring Assessment Tool and the John Nelson, Jean Watson, Inova Health Instrument: Caring Factor Survey (Persky, Nelson, Watson, & Bent, 2008; www.nursing.ucdenver.edu/caring). For more complete access to all the Caring Assessment tools see *Assessing and Measuring Caring in Nursing and Health Sciences,* 2nd ed. (Watson, 2008b).

Heart-Centered Transpersonal Caring Moment: Caritas Field

Whether the "theory" is read at different levels, used as a language system for documentation, used as a guide for professional nursing practice models, or the focus of multisite or individual clinical caring research studies, the essence of the lived theory is in the Caring Moment. The Caring Moment can be located within any caring occasion, as a concept within middle-range or even prescriptive or practice level theory.

However, the Caring Moment is most evident within the transpersonal Caritas energetic field model, in that one's consciousness, intentionality, energetic heart-centered presence is radiating a field beyond the two people or the situation, affecting the larger field. Thus nurses can become more aware, more awake, more conscious of manifesting/radiating a Caritas field of love and healing for self and others, helping to transform self and system. For more comprehensive understanding of this work, see *Nursing: The Philosophy and Science of Caring,* revised 2nd ed. (Watson, 2008a). Indeed, the

latest research based upon the Science of the Heart has demonstrated that the loving heart-centered person is radiating love that can be measured eight to ten feet beyond themselves, affecting the subtle environment of all. Moreover, this research affirms that the heart is actually sending messages to the brain, rather than the other way around. For more information, please visit www.heartMath.com; www.heartMath.org

This work posits a value's explicit moral foundation and takes a specific position with respect to the centrality of human caring, "caritas," and love as an ethic and ontology. It is also a critical starting point for nursing's existence, broad societal mission, and the basis for further advancement for caring–healing practices. Nevertheless, its use and evolution are dependent on "critical, reflective practices that must be continuously questioned and critiqued in order to remain dynamic, flexible, and endlessly self-revising and emergent" (Watson, 1996, p. 143).

Transpersonal Caring Relationship

The terms transpersonal and a transpersonal caring relationship are foundational to the work. Transpersonal conveys a concern for the inner life world and subjective meaning of another who is fully embodied. But transpersonal also energetically goes beyond the ego self and beyond the given moment, reaching to the deeper connections to spirit and with the broader universe. Thus, a transpersonal caring relationship moves beyond ego self and radiates to spiritual, even cosmic, concerns and connections that tap into healing possibilities and potentials.

Transpersonal caring seeks to connect with and embrace the spirit or soul of the other through the processes of caring and healing and being in authentic relation, in the moment. Such a transpersonal relationship is influenced by the caring consciousness and intentionality, and energetic presence of the nurse as she or he enters into the life space or phenomenal field of another person and is able to detect the other person's condition of being (at the soul or spirit level). It implies a focus on the uniqueness of self and other and the uniqueness of the moment, wherein the coming together is mutual and reciprocal, each fully embodied in the moment, while paradoxically capable of transcending the moment, open to new possibilities.

The transpersonal Caritas consciousness nurse seeks to "see" who is that spirit-filled person behind the patient/behind the colleague/behind the disease, diagnosis, the behavior or personality one may not like and connect with the spirit filled individual behind the illusion. This is heart-centered Caritas practice guided by the very first Caritas process: cultivation of loving kindness and equanimity with self and other, allowing for development of more caring, love, compassion, and authentic caring moments.

Transpersonal caring calls for an authenticity of being and becoming, an ability to be present to self and others in a reflective frame. The transpersonal nurse has the ability to center consciousness and intentionality on caring, healing, and wholeness, rather than on disease, illness, and pathology.

Transpersonal caring competencies are related to ontological development of the nurse's human caring literacy and ways of being and becoming. Thus, "ontological caring competencies" become as critical in this model as "technological curing competencies" to the conventional modern, Western nursing-medicine model, which is now coming to an end.

Within the model of transpersonal caring, clinical caritas consciousness is engaged at a foundational ethical level for entry into this framework. The nurse attempts to enter into and stay within the other's frame of reference for connecting with the inner life world of meaning and spirit of the other. Together, they join in a mutual search for meaning and wholeness of being and becoming, to potentiate comfort measures, pain control, a sense of well-being, wholeness, or even a spiritual transcendence of suffering. The person is viewed as whole and complete, regardless of illness or disease (Watson, 1996, p. 153).

Assumptions of the Transpersonal Caring Relationship

The nurse's moral commitment, intentionality, and caritas consciousness exists to protect, enhance, promote, and potentiate human dignity, wholeness, and healing, wherein a person creates or co-creates his or her own meaning for existence, healing, wholeness, and living and dying.

The nurse's will and consciousness affirm the subjective-spiritual significance of the person while seeking to sustain caring in the midst of threat and despair—biological, institutional, or otherwise. This honors the I–Thou relationship versus an I–It relationship.

The nurse seeks to recognize, accurately detect, and connect with the inner condition of spirit of another through genuine presencing and being centered in the caring moment. Actions, words, behaviors, cognition, body language, feelings, intuition, thought, senses, the energy field, and so on all contribute to transpersonal caring connection. The nurse's ability to connect with another at this transpersonal spirit-to-spirit level is translated via movements, gestures, facial expressions, procedures, information, touch, sound, verbal expressions, and other scientific, technical, aesthetic, and human means of communication, into nursing human art/acts or intentional caring-healing modalities.

The caring–healing modalities within the context of transpersonal caring/caritas consciousness potentiate harmony, wholeness, and unity of being by releasing some of the disharmony, the blocked energy that interferes with the natural healing processes. As a result, the nurse helps another through this process to access the healer within, in the fullest sense of Nightingale's view of nursing.

Ongoing personal–professional development and spiritual growth and personal spiritual practice assist the nurse in entering into this deeper level of professional healing practice, allowing the nurse to awaken to the transpersonal condition of the world and to actualize more fully "ontological competencies" necessary for this level of advanced practice of nursing. Valuable teachers for this work include the nurse's own life history and previous experiences, which provide opportunities for focused studies, as the nurse has lived through or experienced various human conditions and has imagined others' feelings in various circumstances. To some degree, the necessary knowledge and consciousness can be gained through work with other cultures and the study of the humanities (art, drama, literature, personal story, narratives of illness journeys), along with an exploration of one's own values, deep beliefs, relationship with self and others, and one's world. Other facilitators include personal-growth experiences such as psychotherapy, transpersonal psychology, meditation, bioenergetics work, and other models for spiritual awakening. Continuous growth is ongoing for developing and maturing within a transpersonal caring model. The notion of health professionals as wounded healers is acknowledged as part of the necessary growth and compassion called forth within this theory/philosophy.

Caring Moment/Caring Occasion

A caring occasion occurs whenever the nurse and another come together with their unique life histories and phenomenal fields in a human-to-human transaction. The coming together in a given moment becomes a focal point in space and time. It becomes transcendent, whereby experience and perception take place, but the actual caring occasion has a greater field of its own, in a given moment. The process goes beyond itself yet arises from aspects of itself that become part of the life history of each person, as well as part of a larger, more complex pattern of life (Watson, 1985, p. 59; 1996, p. 157).

A caring moment involves an action and choice by both the nurse and other. The moment of coming together presents the two with the opportunity to decide how to be in the moment, in the relationship—what to do with and in the moment. If the caring moment is transpersonal, each feels a connection with the other at the spirit level; thus, the moment transcends time and space, opening up new possibilities for healing and human

connection at a deeper level than that of physical interaction. For example:

[W]e learn from one another how to be human by identifying ourselves with others, finding their dilemmas in ourselves. What we all learn from it is self-knowledge. The self we learn about ... is every self. IT is universal—the human self. We learn to recognize ourselves in others ... [it] keeps alive our common humanity and avoids reducing self or other to the moral status of object. (Watson, 1985, pp. 59–60)

Caring (Healing) Consciousness

The dynamic of transpersonal caring (healing) within a caring moment is manifest in a field of consciousness. The transpersonal dimensions of a caring moment are affected by the nurse's consciousness in the caring moment, which in turn affects the field of the whole. The role of consciousness with respect to a holographic view of science has been discussed in earlier writings (Watson, 1992, p. 148) and includes the following points:

- The whole caring–healing–loving consciousness is contained within a single caring moment.
- The one caring and the one being cared for are interconnected; the caring-healing process is connected with the other human(s) and with the higher energy of the universe.
- The caring–healing–loving consciousness of the nurse is communicated to the one being cared for.
- Caring–healing–loving consciousness exists through and transcends time and space and can be dominant over physical dimensions.

Within this context, it is acknowledged that the process is relational and connected. It transcends time, space, and physicality. The process is intersubjective with transcendent possibilities that go beyond the given caring moment.

Implications of the Caring Model

The Caring Model or Theory can be considered a philosophical and moral/ethical foundation for professional nursing and is part of the central focus for nursing at the disciplinary level. A model of caring includes a call for both art and science. It offers a framework that embraces and intersects with art, science, humanities, spirituality, and new dimensions of mind–body–spirit medicine and nursing evolving openly as central to human phenomena of nursing practice.

I emphasize that it is possible to read, study, learn about, and even teach and research the caring theory. However, to truly "get it," one has to experience it personally. The model is both an invitation and an opportunity to interact with the ideas, experiment with and grow within the philosophy, and to live it out in one's personal/professional life.

Applications of the Theory

The ideas as originally developed, as well as in the current evolving phase (Watson, 1979, 1985, 1999, 2003, 2005, 2008), provide us with a chance to assess, critique, and see where or how, or even if, we may locate ourselves within a framework of Caring Science/Caritas as a basis for the emerging ideas in relation to our own theories and philosophies of professional nursing and/or caring practice. If one chooses to use the caring-science perspective as theory, model, philosophy, ethic, or ethos for transforming self and practice, or self and system, the following questions may help (Watson, 1996, p. 161):

- Is there congruence between the values and major concepts and beliefs in the model and the given nurse, group, system, organization, curriculum, population needs, clinical administrative setting, or other entity that is considering interacting with the caring model to transform and/or improve practice?
- What is one's view of "human"? And what does it mean to be human, caring, healing, becoming, growing, transforming, and so on? For example, in the words of Teilhard de Chardin: "Are we humans having a spiritual experience, or are we spiritual beings having a human experience?" Such thinking in regard to this philosophical question can guide one's worldview and help to clarify where one may locate self within the caring framework.
- Are those interacting and engaging in the model interested in their own personal evolution: Are they committed to seeking authentic connections and caring–healing relationships with self and others?
- Are those involved "conscious" of their caring *caritas* or noncaring consciousness and intentionally in a given moment, at individual and system level? Are they interested and committed to expanding their caring consciousness and actions to self, other, environment, nature, and wider universe?
- Are those working within the model interested in shifting their focus from a modern medical science–technocure orientation to a true heart-centered authentic caring–healing–loving model?

This work, in both its original and evolving forms, seeks to develop caring as an ontological–epistemological foundation for a theoretical–philosophical–ethical framework for the profession and discipline of nursing and to clarify its mature relationship and distinct intersection with other health sciences. Nursing caring theory–based activities as guides to practice, education, and research have developed throughout the United States and other parts of the world. The Caring/Caritas model is consistently one of the nursing caring theories used as a guide in Magnet Hospitals in the United States, as found to be culturally consistent with nursing in many other cultures, nations, and countries. Nurses' reflective-critical practice models are increasingly adhering to a caring ethic and ethos as moral and scientific foundation for a profession that is coming of age for a new global era in human history.

Latest Developments

The Watson Caring Science Institute was established in 2007 as a nonprofit foundation. The following statements define and describe the goals, missions, and purposes of the International Caritas Consortium and the WCSI as two interrelated entities.

The general goals and objectives of the Watson Caring Science Institute (WCSI) are to steward and serve the ICC its activities, and more specifically to:

• Transform the dominant model of medical science to a model of caring science by reintroducing the ethic of caring and love, necessary for healing.
• Deepen the authentic caring–healing relationships between practitioner and patient to restore love and heart-centered human compassion as the ethical foundation of healthcare.
• Translate the model of Caring–Healing/ Caritas into more systematic programs and services to help transform health care one nurse, one practitioner, one educator, and one system at a time.
• Ensure caring and healing for the public, reduce nurse turnover, and decrease costs to the system.

International Caritas Consortium Charter

The main purposes of the unfolding and emerging International Caritas Consortium (Watson, 2008a, pp. 278–280) are:

1. To explore diverse ways to bring the caring theory to life in academic and clinical practice settings by supporting and learning from each other
2. To share knowledge and experiences so that we might help guide self and others in the journey to live the caring philosophy and theory in our personal and professional lives

The Consortium gatherings, sponsored by systems implementing Caring Theory in practice:

• Provide an intimate forum to renew, restore, and deepen each person's, and each system's, commitment and authentic practices of human caring in their personal/ professional life and work.
• Learn from each other through shared work of original scholarship, diverse forms of caring inquiry, and model caring–healing practices.
• Mentor self and others in using, extending the Theory of Human Caring to transform education and clinical practices.
• Develop and disseminate Caring Science models of clinical scholarship and professional excellence in the various settings in the world.

Activities for Caritas Consortium Gatherings

• Provide a safe forum to explore, create, renew self and system through reflective time out.
• Share ideas, inspire each other, and learn together.
• Participate in use of Appreciative Inquiry whereby each member is facilitative of each others work, each learning from others.
• Create opportunities for original scholarship and new models of caring science–based clinical and educational practices.
• Generate and share multi-site projects in caring theory/caring science scholarship.
• Network for educational and professional models of advancing caring–healing practices and transformative models of nursing.
• Share unique experiences for authentic self-growth within the Caring Science context.
• Educate, implement, and disseminate exemplary experiences and findings to broader professional audiences through scholarly publications, research and formal presentations.
• Envision new possibilities for transforming nursing and health care.

Because of the many national and international developments and sincere desire for authentic change, new projects using Caring Science; Caritas Theory and Philosophy of Human Caring are now underway in many systems. The Watson Caring Science Institute and the International Caritas Consortium are examples of individuals and representatives of systems convening (in these cases, twice a year) to deepen and sustain what is referred to as *Caritas* Nursing—that is, bringing caring and love and heart-centered human to human practices back into our personal life and work world (Watson, 2008a).

Caring Indicators and Programs

While these above-named systems are identified as sponsors of the growing International Caritas Consortium, examples of how these systems are implementing the theory are captured through identified acts and processes depicting such transformative changes.

Caring theory-in-action reflects transformative processes that are representative of actions taking place in many of the systems in the Caritas Consortium and other systems guided by Caring Science and caring theory as a guide. The following are examples of such caring-in-action indicators:

• Making human caring integral to the organizational vision and culture through new language and documentation of caring, such as posters
• Introducing and naming new professional caring practice models, leading to new patterns of delivery of caring/care, for example, Attending Caring Nursing Project, Patient Care Facilitator Role, the 12-Bed Hospital
• Conscious intentional meaningful rituals. For example, hand washing is for infection control, but also may be a meaningful ritual of self-caring-energetically cleansing, blessing, and releasing last situation or encounter, and being open to the next situation.
• Selected use of caring–healing modalities for self and patients, for example, massage, therapeutic touch, reflexology, aromatherapy, calmative oil of essences; sound, music, arts, variety of energetic modalities
• Dimming the unit lights and having designated "quiet time" for patients/families/staff alike, to soften, slow down, and calm the environment.
• Creating healing spaces for nurses; sanctuaries for their own time out; may include meditation or relaxation rooms for quiet time

• Cultivation of own spiritual heart-centered practices of loving kindness and equanimity to self and others
• Intentionally pausing and breathing, preparing self to be present before entering patient's room
• Centering exercises and mindfulness practices, individually and collectively
• Placing magnets on patient's door with positive affirmations, and reminders of caring practices
• Exploring documentation of caring language and integration in computerized documentation systems
• Participation in multisite research assessing caring among staff and patients.
• Creating healing environments—attending to the subtle environment or Caritas field
• Displaying healing objects, stones, blessing basket
• Creating Caritas Circles to share caring moments
• Caring Rounds at bedside with patients
• Interviewing and selecting staff on basis of "caring" orientation. Asking candidates to describe "Caring Moment"
• Development of "caring competencies"— caritas literacy as guide to assess and promote staff development and assure caring

These and other practices are occurring in a variety of hospitals across the United States, often in Magnet hospitals or those seeking Magnet recognition, where Caring Theory and models of human caring are used to transform nursing and health care for staff and patients alike.

The names of other health care national and international clinical and educational systems incorporating Caring Theory into professional nursing practice models (many hospitals are Magnet hospitals or preparing to become Magnet hospitals) can be found on the following Web sites: www.watsoncaringscience.org; www.nursing.ucdenver.edu/caring

These identified system examples are exemplars of the changing momentum today, and are guided by a shift toward an evolved consciousness. They rely on moral, ethical, philosophical, and theoretical foundations to restore human caring and healing and health in a system that has gone astray – educationally, economically, clinically, and socially. This shift is in a hopeful direction, and is based on a grass roots transformation of nursing, one that is from the inside out. The dedicated leaders who are ushering in these changes serve as an inspiration for sustaining nursing and human caring for practitioners and patients alike.

Conclusion

Consistent with the wisdom and vision of Florence Nightingale, nursing is a lifetime journey of caring and healing, seeking to understand and preserve the wholeness of human existence across time and space and national/geographic boundaries, to offer heart-centered compassionate, informed knowledgeable human caring to society and humankind. This timeless view of nursing transcends conventional minds and mindsets of illness, pathology, and disease that are located in the body physical with curing as end, often at all costs. In nursing's timeless model, caring, kindness, love, and heart-centered compassionate service to humankind are restored. The unifying focus and process is on connectedness with self, other, nature, and God/the Life Force/the Absolute. This vision and wisdom is being reignited today through a blend of old and new values, ethics, and theories and practices of human caring and healing. These Caritas Consciousness practices preserve humanity and human dignity and wholeness, and are the very foundation of transformed thinking and actions.

Such a value's guided relational ontology and expanded epistemology and ethic is embodied in Caring Science as the disciplinary ground for nursing, now and the future. The advancement of nursing theory, which includes both ideals and practical guidance, is increasingly evident as nursing makes its major contribution to health care and matures as a distinct caring–healing profession—one that balances and complements conventional, medical–institutional practices and processes. Nevertheless, much work remains to be done. New transformative, human-spirit–inspired approaches are required to reverse institutional and system lethargy and darkness. To create the necessary cultural change, the human spirit has to be invited back into our health care systems. Professional and personal models are required that open the hearts of nurses and other practitioners. New horizons of possibilities have to be explored to create space whereby compassionate, intentional, heart-centered human caring can be practiced. Such authentic personal/professional practice models of Caring Science are capable of leading us, locally and globally, toward a moral community of caring. This community will restore healing and health at a level that honors and sustains the dignity and humanity of practitioners and patients alike.

The Watson Caring Science Institute is dedicated to create, conduct, and sponsor Caring Science/Caritas education, training, and support to serve the current and future generations of health care professionals globally (www.watsoncaringscience.org

WCSI, 4405 Arapahoe Avenue, Suite 100, Boulder, CO 80303).

Practice Exemplar

Transpersonal Caring Theory and the caring model "can be read, taught, learned about, studied, researched and even practiced: however, to truly 'get it,' one has to personally experience it—interact and grow within the philosophy and intention of the model" (Watson, 1996, p. 160). This is an exemplar of the Transpersonal Caring Theory in action.

October 2002 presented the opportunity for 17 interdisciplinary health-care professionals at The Children's Hospital in Denver, Colorado, to participate in a pilot study designed to: (1) explore the effect of integrating Caring Theory into comprehensive pediatric pain management and (2) examine the Attending Nurse Caring Model® (ANCM) as a care delivery model for hospitalized children in pain. A 3-day retreat launched the pilot study. Participants were invited to explore Transpersonal Human Caring Theory (Caring Theory), as taught and modeled by Dr. Jean Watson, through experiential interactions with caring–healing modalities. The end of the retreat opened opportunities for participants to merge Caring Theory and pain theory into an emerging caring-healing praxis.

Returning from the retreat to the preexisting schedules, customs, and habits of hospital routine was both daunting and exciting. We had lived Caring Theory, and not as a remote and abstract philosophical ideal; rather, we had experienced caring as the very core of our true selves, and it was the call that led us into the health care professions. Invigorated by the retreat, we returned to our 37-bed acute care inpatient pediatric unit, eager to apply Caring Theory to improve pediatric pain management. Our experiences throughout the retreat had accentuated caring as our core value. Caring Theory could not be restricted to a single area of practice.

Wheeler and Chinn (1991) define praxis as "values made visible through deliberate action" (p. 2). This definition unites the ontology or the essence of nursing to nursing actions, to what nurses do. Nursing within acute care inpatient hospital settings is practiced dependently, collaboratively, and independently (Bernardo, 1998). Bernardo describes dependent practice as energy directed by and requiring physician orders, collaborative practice as interdependent energy directed toward activities with other health care professionals, and independent practice as "where the meaningful role and impact of nursing may evolve" (p. 43). Our vision of nursing practice was based in the caring paradigm of deep respect for humanity and all life, of wonder and awe of life's mystery, and the interconnectedness from mind–body–spirit unity into cosmic oneness (Watson, 1996). Gadow (1995) describes nursing as a lived world of interdependency and shared knowledge, rather than as a service provided. Caring praxis within this lived world is a praxis that offers "a combination of action and reflection . . . praxis is about a relationship with self, and a relationship with the wider community" (Penny & Warelow, 1999, p. 260). Caring praxis, therefore, is collaborative praxis.

Collaboration and co-creation are key elements in our endeavors to translate Caring Theory into practice. They reveal the nonlinear process and relational aspect of caring praxis. Both require openness to unknown possibilities, honor the unique contributions of self and other(s), and acknowledge growth and transformation as inherent to life experience. These key elements support the evolution of praxis away from predetermined goals and set outcomes toward authentic caring–healing expressions. Through collaboration and co-creation, we can build on existing foundations to nurture evolution from what is to what can be.

Our mission, to translate Caring Theory into praxis, has strong foundational support. Building on this supportive base, we have committed our intentions and energies toward creating a caring culture. The following is not intended as an algorithm to guide one through varied steps until caring is achieved but is rather a description of our ongoing processes and growth toward an ever-evolving caring praxis. These processes are co-creations that emerged from collaboration with other ANCM participants, fellow health professionals, patients and families, our environment, and our caring intentions.

First Steps

One of our first challenges was to make the ANCM visible. Six tangible exhibits have been displayed on the unit as evidence of our commitment to caring values. First, a large, colorful poster titled "CARING" is positioned at the entrance to our unit. Depicting pictures of diverse families at the center, the

Continued

poster states our three initial goals for theory-guided practice: (1) create caring–healing environments, (2) optimize pain management through pharmacological and caring–healing measures, and (3) prepare children and families for procedures and interventions. Watson's clinical caritas processes are listed, as well as an abbreviated version of her guidelines for cultivating caring–healing throughout the day (Watson, 2002). This poster, written in Caring Theory language, expresses our intention to all and reminds us that caring is the core of our praxis.

Second, a shallow bowl of smooth, rounded river stones is located in a prominent position at each nursing desk. A sign posted by the stones identify them as "Caring–Healing Touch Stones" inviting one to select a stone as "every human being has the ability to share their incredible gift of loving–healing. These stones serve as a reminder of our capacity to love and heal. Pick up a stone, feel its smooth cool surface, let its weight remind you of your own gifts of love and healing. Share in the love and healing of all who have touched this stone before you and pass on your love and healing to all who will hold this stone after you."

Third, latched wicker blessing baskets have been placed adjacent to the caring–healing touch stones. Written instructions invite families, visitors, and staff to offer names for a blessing by writing the person's initials on a slip of paper and placing the paper in the basket. Every Monday through Friday, the unit chaplain, holistic clinical nurse specialist (CNS), and interested staff devote thirty minutes of meditative silence within a healing space to ask for peace and hope for all names contained within the baskets.

Fourth, signs picturing a snoozing cartoon-styled tiger have been posted on each patient's door announcing "Quiet Time." Quiet time is a midday, half-hour pause from hospital hustle-bustle. Lights in the hall are dimmed, voices are hushed, and steps are softened to allow a pause for reflection. Staff tries not to enter patient rooms unless summoned.

Fifth, a booklet has been written and published to welcome families and patients to our unit, to introduce health team members, unit routines, available activities, and define frequently used medical terms. This book emphasizes that patients, parents, and families are members of the health team. A description of our caring attending team is also included.

Sixth and most recently, the unit chaplain, child-life specialist, and social worker have organized a weekly support session called "Goodies and Gathering," offered every Thursday morning. It is held in our healing room—a conference room painted to resemble a cozy room with a beautiful outdoor view and redecorated with comfortable armchairs, soft lighting, and plants. Goodies and Gathering extends a safe retreat within the hospital setting. Offering one hour to parents and another to staff, these professionals provide snacks to feed the body, a sacred space to nourish emotions, and their caring presence to nurture the spirit.

Attending Caring Team (ACT)

To honor the collaborative partnership of our ANCM participants, to include patients and families as equal partners in the health care team, and open participations to all, we have adopted the name Attending Caring Team (ACT). The acronym ACT reinforces that our actions are opportunities to make caring visible. Care as the core of praxis differs from the centrality of cure in the medical model. To describe our intentions to others we compiled the following "elevator" description of ACT, a terse, thirty-second summary that renders the meaning of ACT in the time frame of a shared elevator ride:

The core of the Attending Caring Team (ACT) is caring-healing for patients, families and ourselves. ACT co-creates relationships and collaborative practices between patients, families and health care providers. ACT practice enables health care providers to redefine themselves as caregivers rather than taskmasters. We provide Health Care not Health Tasks.

Large signs have been professionally produced and are hung at various locations on our unit. These signs serve a dual purpose. The largest, posted conspicuously at our threshold, identifies our unit as the home of the Attending Caring Team. Smaller signs, posted at each nurse's station, spell out the above ACT definition, inviting everyone entering our unit to participate in the collaborative co-creation of caring–healing.

Giving ourselves a name and making our caring intentions visible contribute to establishing an identity, yet may be perceived as peripheral activities. For these expressions to be deliberate actions of praxis, the centrality of caring as our core value was clearly articulated. Caring Theory is the flexible framework guiding our unit goals and unit education and has been integrated into our implementation of an institutional customer service initiative.

Unit goals are written yearly. Reflective of the broader institutional mission statement, each unit is encouraged to develop a mission statement and outline goals designed to achieve that mission. In 2003, our mission statement was rewritten to focus on provision of quality *family-centered care,* defined as "an environment of caring-healing recognizing families as equal partners in collaboration with all health care providers." One of the goals to achieve this mission literally spells out caring. We promote a caring-healing environment for patients, families, and staff through:

- Compassion, competence, commitment
- Advocacy
- Respect, research
- Individuality
- Nurturing
- Generosity

Education

Unit educational offerings have also been revised to reflect Caring Theory. Phase classes, a 2-year curriculum of serial seminars designed to support new hires in their clinical, educational, and professional growth, now include a unit on self-care to promote personal healing and support self-growth. The unit on pain management has been expanded to include use of caring–healing modalities. A new interactive session on the caritas processes has been added that asks participants to reflect on how these processes are already evident in their praxis and to explore ways they can deepen caring praxis both individually and collectively as a unit. The tracking tool used to assess a new employee's progress through orientation now includes an area for reflection on growing in caring competencies. In addition to changes in phase classes, informal "clock hours" are offered monthly. Clock hours are designed to respond to the immediate needs of the unit and encompass a diverse range of topics, from conflict resolution, debriefing after specific events, and professional development, to health treatment plans, physiology of medical diagnosis, and in-services on new technologies and pharmacological interventions. Offered on the unit at varying hours to accommodate all work shifts, clock hours provide a way for staff members to fulfill continuing educational requirements during work days.

Customer Service

Caring Theory has provided depth to an institutional initiative to use FISH philosophy to enhance customer service (Lundin, Paul, & Christensen, 2000). Imported from Pike's Fish Market in Seattle, FISH advocates four premises to improve employee and customer satisfaction: presence, make their day, play, and choose your attitude. Briefly summarized, FISH advocates that when employees bring their full awareness through presence, focus on customers to make their day, invoke fun into the day through appropriate play, and through conscious awareness choose their attitude, work environments improve for all. When the four FISH premises are viewed from the perspective of transpersonal caring, they become opportunities for authentic human-to-human connectedness through I–Thou relationships. The merger of Caring Theory with FISH philosophy has inspired

Continued

the following activities. A parade composed of patients, their families, nurses, and volunteers—complete with marching music, hats, streamers, flags, and noise makers—is celebrated two to three times a week just before the playroom closes for lunch. This flamboyant display lasts less than five minutes but invigorates participants and bystanders alike. In addition to being vital for children and especially appropriate in a pediatric setting, play unites us all in the life and joy of each moment. When our parade marches, visitors, rounding doctors, all present on the unit pause to watch, wave, and cheer us on. A weekly bedtime story is read in our healing room. Patients are invited to bring their pillows and favorite stuffed animal or doll and come dressed in pajamas. Night- and day-shift staff have honored one another with surprise beginning-of-the-shift meals, staying late to care for patients and families, and refusing to give off-going report until their oncoming co-workers had eaten. Colorful caring stickers are awarded when one staff member catches another in the ACT of caring, being present, making another's day, playing, and choosing a positive attitude.

ACT Guidelines

Placing Caring Theory at the core of our praxis supports practicing caring–healing arts to promote wholeness, comfort, harmony, and inner healing. The intentional conscious presence of our authentic being to provide a caring–healing environment is the most essential of these arts. Presence as the foundation for co-creating caring relationships has led to writing ACT guidelines. Written in the doctor order section of the chart, ACT guidelines provide a formal way to honor unique families' values and beliefs. Preferred ways of having dressing changes performed, most helpful comfort measures, home schedules, and special needs or requests are examples of what these guidelines might address. ACT members purposefully use the word "guideline" as opposed to "order" as more congruent with co-creative collaborate praxis and to encourage critical thinking and flexibility.

Building practice on caring relationships has led to an increase in both the type and volume of care conferences held on our unit. Previously, care conferences were called as a way to disseminate information to families when complicated issues arose or when communication between multiple teams faltered and families were receiving conflicting reports, plans, and instructions. Now, these conferences are offered proactively as a way to coordinate team efforts and to ensure we are working toward the families' goals. Transitional conferences provide an opportunity to coordinate continuity of care, share insight into the unique personality and preferences of the child, coordinate team effort, meet families, provide them with tours of our unit, and collaborate with families. Other caring–healing arts offered on our unit are therapeutic touch, guided imagery, relaxation, visualization, aromatherapy, and massage. As ACT participants, our challenge is to express our caring values through every activity and interaction. Caring Theory guides us and manifests in innumerable ways. Our interview process, meeting format, and Clinical Nurse Specialist (CNS) role have been transfigured through Caring Theory. Our interview process has transformed from an interrogative three-step procedure into more of a sharing dialogue. We are adopting another meeting style that expresses caring values.

Our unit director had the foresight to budget a position for a CNS to support the co-creation of caring praxis. The traditional CNS roles—researcher, clinical expert, collaborator, educator, and change agent—have allowed the integration of Caring Theory development into all aspects of our unit program. The CNS role advocates self-care and facilitates staff members to incorporate caring-healing arts into their practice through modeling and hands-on support. In addition to providing assistance, searching for resources, acting as liaison with other health care teams, and promoting staff in their efforts, the very presence of the CNS on the unit reinforces our commitment to caring praxis.

Summary

Caring–healing co-creation is fluid, not static. More than 100 years ago, Florence Nightingale wrote, "I entirely repudiate the distinction usually drawn between the man of thought and the man of action" (Vivinus & Nergaard, 1990, p. 310). Nightingale rejected the separation of the ideal (theory) from action (practice). For Nightingale, nursing is not a profession or a job one performs, but rather is a calling. Dedicating her life toward achieving the ideal, she challenged others to "let the Ideal go if you are not trying to incorporate it in your daily life" (Vivinus & Nergaard, 1990, p. 310). We continue to work toward incorporating caring ideals in every action. Currently, we are modifying our competency-based guidelines to emphasize caring competency within tasks and skills. Building relationships for supportive collaborative practice is the most exciting and most challenging endeavor we are now facing as old roles are reevaluated in light of co-creating caring-healing relationships. Watson and Foster (2003) describe the potential of such collaboration: "The new caring-healing practice environment is increasingly dependent on partnerships, negotiation, coordination, new forms of communication pattern and authentic relationships. The new emphasis is on a change of consciousness, a focused intentionality towards caring and healing relationships and modalities, a shift towards a spiritualization of health vs. a limited medicalized view" (p. 361). Our ACT commitment is to authentic relationships and the creation of caring–healing environments.

Summary

Nursing's future and nursing in the future will depend on nursing maturing as the distinct health, healing, and caring profession that it has always represented across time but has yet to fully actualize. Nursing thus ironically is now challenged to stand and mature within its own Caring Science paradigm, while simultaneously having to transcend it and share with others. The future already reveals that all health care practitioners will need to work within a shared framework of caring–healing relationships and human–environmental energetic field modalities. Practitioners of the future pay attention to consciousness, intentionality, energetic human presence, transformed mind–body–spirit medicine, and will need to embrace healing arts and caring practices and processes and the spiritual dimensions of care much more completely.

Thus, nursing is at its own crossroad of possibilities, between worldviews and paradigms. Nursing has entered a new era; it is invited and required to build upon its heritage and latest evolution in science and technology but must transcend itself for a postmodern future yet to be known. However, nursing's future holds promises of caring and healing mysteries and models yet to unfold, as opportunities for offering compassionate caritas services at individual, system, societal, national, and global levels for self, for profession, and for the broader world community. Nursing has a critical role to play in sustaining caring in humanity and making new connections between caring, love, healing, and peace in the world.

References

Bernardo, A. (1998). Technology and true presence in nursing. *Holistic Nursing Practice, 12*(4), 40–49.

Gadow, S. (1995). Narrative and exploration: Toward a poetics of knowledge in nursing. *Nursing Inquiry, 2,* 211–214.

Lundin, S. C., Paul, H., & Christensen, J. (2000). *Fish! A remarkable way to boost morale and improve results.* New York: Hyperion.

Penny, W., & Warelow, P. J. (1999). Understanding the prattle of praxis. *Nursing Inquiry, 6*(4), 259–268.

Persky, G., Nelson, J.W., Watson, J., & Bent, K. (2008). Profile of a nurse effective in caring. *Nursing Administration Quarterly, 32*(1), 15–20.

Rosenberg, S. (2006). Utilizing the language of Jean Watson's Caring Theory within a computerized documentation system. *CIN: Computers, Informatics, Nursing, 24*(1), 53–56.

Swanson, K. M. (1991). Empirical development of a middle range nursing theory. *Nursing Research, 40*(3), 161–166.

Vivinus, M., & Nergaard, B. (1990). *Ever yours, Florence Nightingale.* Cambridge, MA: Harvard University Press.

Watson, J. (1979). Nursing. *The philosophy and science of caring.* Boston: Little Brown. Reprinted. (1985) Boulder, CO: University Press of Colorado.

Watson, J. (1985). *Nursing: Human science and human care.* Norwalk, CT: Appleton Century. Reprinted (1988, 1999, 2008) New York: National League for Nursing Press; Sudbury, MA: Jones and Bartlett.

Watson, J. (1996). Watson's theory of transpersonal caring. In: P. H. Walker & B. Newman (Eds.), *Blueprint for use of nursing models: Education, research, practice and administration.* New York: National League for Nursing Press.

Watson, J. (1999). *Postmodern nursing and beyond.* New York: Churchill Livingstone.

Watson, J. (2001). Post-hospital nursing: Shortage, shifts and scripts. *Nursing Administration Quarterly, 25*(3), 77–82.

Watson, J. (2002). Intentionality and caring-healing consciousness: A practice of transpersonal nursing. *Holistic Nursing Practice, 16*(4), 12–19.

Watson, J. (2003). *Assessing and measuring caring in nursing and health sciences.* New York: Springer.

Watson, J. (2005*). Caring science as sacred science.* Philadelphia: F. A. Davis.

Watson, J. (2008a). *Nursing: The philosophy and science of caring* (rev. 2nd ed. with Caritas Meditation CD). Boulder, CO: University Press of Colorado; www.upcolorado.com

Watson, J. (2008b). *Assessing and measuring caring in nursing and health sciences* (2nd ed.). New York: Springer.

Watson, J., & Foster, R. (2003). The Attending Nurse Caring Model®: Integrating theory, evidence and advanced caring-healing therapeutics for transforming professional practice. *Journal of Clinical Nursing, 12,* 360–365.

Wheeler, C. E., & Chinn, P. L. (1991). *Peace and power: A handbook of feminist process* (3rd ed.). New York: National League for Nursing Press.

Bibliography

For complete listing of all Watson publications, go to: www.nursing.ucdenver.edu/caring and/or www.watsoncaringscience.org

Publications/Audiovisuals

Bevis, E. O., & Watson, J. (1989). *Toward a caring curriculum. A new pedagogy for nursing* (reprinted 2000). Sudbury, MA: Jones and Bartlett.

Chinn, P., & Watson, J. (Eds.). (1994). *Art and aesthetics of nursing.* New York: National League for Nursing Press.

Leininger, M., & Watson, J. (Eds.). (1990). *The caring imperative in education.* New York: National League for Nursing Press.

Taylor, R., & Watson, J. (Eds.). (1989). *They shall not hurt: Human suffering and human caring.* Boulder, CO: Colorado Associated University Press.

Watson, J. (1979). *Nursing: The philosophy and science of caring.* Boston: Little, Brown (2nd printing, 1985. Boulder, CO: University Press of Colorado.) Translated into French and Korean.

Watson, J. (1985). *Nursing: Human science and human care.* East Norwalk, CT: Appleton-Century-Crofts (2nd printing, 1988; 3rd printing, 1999). New York: National League for Nursing Press (Sudbury, MA: Jones and Bartlett) Translated into Japanese, Swedish, Chinese, Korean, German, Norwegian, and Danish.

Watson, J. (Ed.). (1994). *Applying the art and science of human caring.* New York: National League for Nursing Press.

Watson, J. (1999). *Postmodern nursing and beyond* (Japanese translation), Translated into Portuguese. Edinburgh: Churchill Livingstone/W. B. Saunders/Elsevier.

Watson, J. (2002). *Instruments for assessing and measuring caring in nursing and health sciences.* New York: Springer. (*American Journal of Nursing* Book of the Year Award, 2002. Japanese translation 2003.) Revised 2nd edition. 2008.

Watson, J. (2004). *Caring science as sacred science.* Philadelphia: F. A. Davis. (*American Journal of Nursing* Book of the Year award).

Watson, J., & Ray, M. (Eds.). (1988). *The ethics of care and the ethics of cure: Synthesis in chronicity.* New York: National League for Nursing Press.

Journal Articles

Fawcett, J. (2002). The nurse theorists: 21st century updates—Jean Watson. *Nursing Science Quarterly, 15*(3), 214–219.

Fawcett, J., Watson, J., Neuman, B., & Hinton-Walker, P. (2001). On theories and evidence. *Journal of Nursing Scholarship, 33*(2), 121–128.

Quinn, J., Smith, M., Swanson, K., Ritenbaugh, C., & Watson, J. (2003). The healing relationship in clinical nursing: Guidelines for research. *Journal of Alternative Therapies, 9*(3), A65–79.

Watson, J. (1988). Human caring as moral context for nursing education. *Nursing and Health Care, 9*(8), 422–425.

Watson, J. (1988). New dimensions of human caring theory. *Nursing Science Quarterly, 1*(4), 175–181.

Watson, J. (1990). The moral failure of the patriarchy. *Nursing Outlook, 28*(2), 62–66.

Watson, J. (1998). Nightingale and the enduring legacy of transpersonal human caring. *Journal of Holistic Nursing, 16*(2), 18–21.

Watson, J. (2000). Leading via caring–healing: The fourfold way toward transformative leadership. *Nursing Administration Quarterly* (25th Anniversary Edition), *25*(1), 1–6.

Watson, J. (2000). Reconsidering caring in the home. *Journal of Geriatric Nursing, 21*(6), 330–331.

Watson, J. (2000). Via negativa: Considering caring by way of non-caring. *Australian Journal of Holistic Nursing, 7*(1), 4–8.

Watson, J. (2001). Post-hospital nursing: Shortages, shifts, and scripts. *Nursing Administrative Quarterly, 25*(3), 77–82. Available online at http://www.dartmouth.edu/~ahechome/workforce.html, then click "The Nursing Shortage."

Watson, J. (2002). Guest editorial: Nursing: Seeking its source and survival. *ICU NURS WEB J 9,* 1–7. www.nursing.gr/J.W.editorial.pdf

Watson, J. (2002). Holistic nursing and caring: A values based approach. *Journal of Japan Academy of Nursing Science, 22*(2), 69–74.

Watson, J. (2002). Intentionality and caring-healing consciousness: A theory of transpersonal nursing. *Holistic Nursing Journal, 16*(4), 12–19.

Watson, J. (2002). Metaphysics of virtual caring communities. *International Journal of Human Caring, 6*(1), 41–45.

Watson, J. (2003). Love and caring: Ethics of face and hand. *Nursing Administrative Quarterly, 27*(3), 197–202.

Watson, J., & Foster, R. (2003). The attending nurse caring model: Integrating theory, evidence and advanced caring-healing therapeutics for transforming professional practice. *Journal of Clinical Nursing, 12,* 360–365.

Watson, J., & Smith, M. C. (2002). Caring science and the science of unitary human beings: A trans-theoretical discourse for nursing knowledge development. *Journal of Advanced Nursing, 37*(5), 452–461.

Watson, J. (1994). A frog, a rock, a ritual: An eco-caring cosmology. In: E. Schuster & C. Brown (Eds.), *Caring and environmental connection.* New York: National League for Nursing Press.

Watson, J. (1996). Artistry and caring: Heart and soul of nursing. In: D. Marks-Maran & M. Rose (Eds.), *Reconstructing nursing: Beyond art & science* (pp. 54–63). London: Bailliére Tindall.

Watson, J. (1996). Poeticizing as truth on nursing inquiry. In: J. Kikuchi, H. Simmons, & D. Romyn (Eds.), *Truth in nursing inquiry* (pp. 125–139). Thousand Oaks, CA: Sage.

Watson, J. (1996). Watson's theory of transpersonal caring. In: P. H. Walker & B. Neuman (Eds.), *Blueprint for use of nursing models: Education, research, practice, & administration* (pp. 141–184). New York: National League for Nursing Press.

Watson, J. (1999). Alternative therapies and nursing practice. In: J. Watson (Ed.), *Nurse's handbook of alternative and complementary therapies.* Springhouse, PA: Springhouse.

Watson, J., & Chinn, P. L. (1994). Art and aesthetics as passage between centuries. In P. L. Chinn & J. Watson (Eds.), *Art and aesthetics in nursing* (pp. xiii–xviii). New York: National League for Nursing Press.

Audiovisual or Media Productions

CD: Track: Jean Watson A Caring Moment. Care for the Journey CD. www.nursing.ucdenver.edu/caring

CD: Caritas Meditation. Jean Watson. 4 meditations with music by Gary Malkin. In J. Watson (2008). *Nursing: The philosophy and science of caring* (rev. ed.). Boulder, CO: University Press of Colorado. www.upcolorado.com

FITNE. (1997). *The nurse theorists portraits of excellence. Jean Watson: A theory of caring* [video and CD]. To obtain go to: www.fitne.net.

Watson, J. (1988). *The Denver nursing project in human caring* [videotape]. University of Colorado Health Science Center, School of Nursing, Denver, CO. Contact: ellen.janasko@uchsc.edu.

Watson, J. (1988). *The power of caring: The power to make a difference* [videotape]. Center for Human Caring Video, University of Colorado Health Sciences Center, School of Nursing, Denver, CO. Contact: ellen.janasko@uchsc.edu.

Watson, J. (1989). *Theories at work* [videotape]. New York: National League for Nursing. In conjunction with University of Colorado HSC/SoN Chair in Caring Science. Contact ellen.janasko@uchsc.edu.

Watson, J. (1994). *Applying the art and science of human caring,* Parts I and II [videotape]. New York: National League for Nursing. In conjunction with the University of Colorado HSC/SoN, Chair in Caring Science. Contact: ellen.janasko@uchsc.edu.

Watson, J. (1999). *A meta-reflection on nursing's present* [audiotape]. American Holistic Nurses Association. Boulder, CO: SoundsTrue Production.

Watson, J. (1999). *Private psalms. A mantra and meditation for healing* [CD]. Music by Dallas Smith and Susan Mazer. To obtain: e-mail University of Colorado Health Sciences Center Bookstore at traci.mathis@uchsc.edu. (All proceeds from bookstore CDs sales go to support activities of the Murchinson-Scoville Endowed Chair in Caring Science.)

Watson, J. (2001). *Creating a culture of caring* [audiotape]. At the Creative Healthcare Management 9th Annual CHCM, Minneapolis, MN.

Watson, J. (2000). *Importance of story and health care.* Second National Gathering on Relationship-Centered Caring. Fetzer Institute Conference, Miami, Florida.

Watson, J. (2001). *Reconnecting with spirit: Caring and healing our living and dying.* International Parish Nursing Conference. Westberg Symposium. September, 2001. Allenspark, CO.

Chapter **21**

Anne Boykin and Savina O. Schoenhofer's Nursing as Caring Theory

ANNE BOYKIN, SAVINA O. SCHOENHOFER,
AND DANIELLE LINDEN

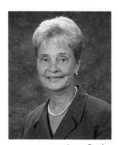

Anne Boykin

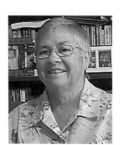

Savina O. Schoenhofer

Introducing the Theorists

Anne Boykin serves as professor and dean of the College of Nursing at Florida Atlantic University where she has demonstrated a long-standing commitment to the International Association for Human Caring, holding the following positions: president-elect (1990–1993), president (1993–1996), and member of the nominating committee (1997–1999). As immediate past president, she served as coeditor of the *International Journal for Human Caring* from 1996 to 1999.

Her scholarly work centers on caring as the grounding for nursing as evidenced in *Nursing as Caring: A Model for Transforming Practice* (coauthored with S. O. Schoenhofer, 1993), and *Living a Caring-based Program* (1994). The latter book illustrates how caring grounds all aspects of a nursing education program. Dr. Boykin has also authored numerous book chapters and articles. She serves as a local, regional, national, and international consultant on the topic of caring.

Dr. Boykin is a graduate of Alverno College in Milwaukee, Wisconsin. She received her master's degree from Emory University in Atlanta, Georgia and her doctorate from Vanderbilt University in Nashville, Tennessee.

Savina Schoenhofer initially studied nursing at Wichita State University, where she earned undergraduate and graduate degrees in nursing, psychology, and counseling. She completed a PhD in educational foundations and administration at Kansas State University in 1983. In 1990, Dr. Schoenhofer cofounded *Nightingale Songs,* an early venue for communicating the beauty of nursing in poetry and prose. In addition to her work on caring, including coauthorship of *Nursing As Caring: A Model for Transforming Practice*, she has written on nursing values, primary care, nursing education, support, touch, personnel management in nursing homes, and mentoring. Her career in nursing has been significantly influenced by three colleagues: Lt. Col. Ann Ashjian (Ret.), whose community nursing practice in Brazil presented an inspiring model of nursing; Marilyn E. Parker, RN, PhD, a faculty colleague who mentored her in the idea of nursing as a discipline, the academic role in higher education, and the world of nursing theories and theorists; and Anne Boykin, PhD, who introduced her to caring as a substantive field of nursing study. Schoenhofer created and manages the website and discussion forum on the theory of nursing as caring (www.nursingascaring.com).

Overview of the Theory

This chapter provides an overview of the Theory of Nursing as Caring, a general theory, framework, or disciplinary view of nursing. The Theory of Nursing as Caring offers a view that permits a broad, encompassing understanding of any and all situations of nursing practice (Boykin & Schoenhofer, 1993). It serves as an organizing framework for nursing scholars in the various roles of practitioner, researcher, administrator, teacher, and developer.

We first present the theory in its most abstract form, addressing assumptions and key themes. We then discuss the meaning of the theory in relation to practice and other nursing roles. In the second part of this chapter, Danielle Linden further describes the theory by illustrating its use as a guide to practice.

Nursing as Caring: Historical Perspective and Current Development

The Theory of Nursing as Caring is an outgrowth of the curriculum development work in the College of Nursing at Florida Atlantic University, where both authors were among the faculty group revising the caring-based curriculum. When the revised curriculum was in place, each of us recognized the potential and even the necessity of continuing to develop and structure ideas and themes toward a comprehensive expression of the meaning and purpose of nursing as a discipline and a profession. The point of departure was the acceptance that caring is the end, rather than the means, of nursing, and that caring is the intention of nursing rather than merely its instrument. This work led to the statement of focus of nursing as "nurturing persons living caring and growing in caring." Further work to identify foundational assumptions about nursing clarified the idea of the nursing situation, a shared lived experience in which the caring between enhances personhood, with personhood understood as living grounded in caring. The clarified focus and the idea of the nursing situation are the key themes that draw forth the meaning of the assumptions underlying the theory and permit the practical understanding of nursing as both a discipline and a profession. As critique of the theory and study of nursing situations progressed, the notion of nursing being primarily concerned with health was seen as limiting, and we now understand nursing to be concerned with human living.

Three bodies of work significantly influenced the initial development of nursing as caring. Roach's (1987/2002) basic thesis that caring is the human mode of being was incorporated into the most basic assumption of the theory. We view Paterson and Zderad's (1988) existential phenomenological theory of humanistic nursing as the historical antecedent of nursing as caring. Seminal ideas such as "the between," "call for nursing," "nursing response," and "personhood" served as substantive and structural bases for our conceptualization of nursing as caring. Mayeroff's (1971) work, *On Caring*, provided a language that facilitated the recognition and description of the practical meaning of caring in nursing situations. In addition to the work of these thinkers, both authors are long-standing members of the community of nursing scholars whose study focuses on caring and who are supported and undoubtedly influenced in many subtle ways by the members of this community and their work.

Fledgling forms of the Theory of Nursing as Caring were first published in 1990 and 1991, with the first complete exposition of the theory presented at a conference in 1992 (Boykin & Schoenhofer, 1990, 1991; Schoenhofer & Boykin, 1993), followed by the publication of *Nursing as Caring: A Model for Transforming Practice* in 1993 (Boykin & Schoenhofer, 1993), which was re-released with an epilogue in 2001 (Boykin & Schoenhofer, 2001a).

Research and development efforts at the time of this writing are concentrated on expanding the language of caring by uncovering personal ways of living caring in everyday life (Schoenhofer, Bingham, & Hutchins, 1998); reconceptualizing nursing outcomes as "value experienced in nursing situations" (Boykin & Schoenhofer, 1997; Schoenhofer & Boykin, 1998a, 1998b); and in consultation with graduate students, nursing faculties, and health-care agencies who are using aspects of the theory to ground research, teaching, and practice.

Assumptions and Key Themes

Certain fundamental beliefs about what it means to be human underlie the Theory of Nursing as Caring. These assumptions, which are illustrated later, reflect a particular set of values and key themes that provide a basis for understanding and explicating the meaning of nursing, listed as follows and detailed here:

- Persons are caring by virtue of their humanness.
- Persons are whole and complete in the moment.
- Persons live caring from moment to moment.
- Personhood is a way of living grounded in caring.
- Personhood is enhanced through participation in nurturing relationships with caring others.
- Nursing is both a discipline and a profession.

Caring

Caring is an altruistic, active expression of love and is the intentional and embodied recognition of value and connectedness. Caring is not the unique province of nursing; however, as a discipline and a profession, nursing uniquely focuses on caring as its central value, its primary interest, and the direct intention of its practice. The full meaning of caring cannot be restricted to a definition but is illuminated in the experience of caring and in the reflection on that experience.

Focus and Intention of Nursing

Disciplines as identifiable entities or "branches of knowledge" grow from the holistic "tree of knowledge" as need and purpose develop. A discipline is a community of scholars (King & Brownell, 1976) with a particular perspective on the world and what it means to be in the world. The disciplinary community represents a value system that is expressed in its unique focus on knowledge and practice.

The focus of nursing, from the perspective of the Theory of Nursing as Caring, is person as living in caring and growing in caring. The general intention of nursing as a practiced discipline is nurturing persons living caring and growing in caring.

Nursing Situation

The practice of nursing, and thus the practical knowledge of nursing, lives in the context of person-with-person caring. The nursing situation involves particular values, intentions, and actions of two or more persons choosing to live a nursing relationship. The nursing situation is understood to mean the shared lived experience in which caring between nurse and nursed enhances personhood. Nursing is created in the caring between. All knowledge of nursing is created and understood within the nursing situation. Any single nursing situation has the potential to illuminate the depth and complexity of nursing knowledge. Nursing situations are best communicated through aesthetic media to preserve the lived meaning of the situation and the openness of the situation as text. Storytelling, poetry, graphic arts, and dance are examples of effective modes of representing the lived experience and allowing for reflection and creativity in advancing understanding.

Personhood

Personhood is understood to mean living grounded in caring. From the perspective of the Theory of Nursing as Caring, personhood is the universal human call. A profound understanding of personhood communicates the paradox of person-as-person and person-in-communion all at once.

Call for Nursing

"A call for nursing is a call for acknowledgment and affirmation of the person living caring in specific ways in the immediate situation" (Boykin & Schoenhofer, 1993, p. 24). Calls for nursing are calls for nurturance through personal expressions of caring. These calls originate within persons as they live out caring uniquely, expressing personally meaningful dreams and aspirations for growing in caring. Calls for nursing are individually relevant ways of saying, "Know me as a caring person in the moment and be with me as I try to live fully who I truly am." Intentionality (Schoenhofer, 2002a) and authentic presence open the nurse to hearing calls for nursing. Because calls for nursing are unique situated personal expressions, they cannot be predicted, as in a "diagnosis." Nurses develop sensitivity and expertise in hearing calls through intention, experience, study, and reflection in a broad range of human situations.

Nursing Response

As an expression of nursing, "caring is the intentional and authentic presence of the nurse with another who is recognized as living caring and growing in caring" (Boykin & Schoenhofer, 1993, p. 25). The nurse enters the nursing situation with the commitment of knowing the other as a caring person, and in that knowing, acknowledging, affirming, and celebrating the person as caring. The nursing response is a specific expression of caring nurturance to sustain and enhance the "other" as he or she lives caring and grows in caring in the situation of concern. Nursing responses to calls for caring evolve as nurses clarify their understandings of calls through presence and dialogue. Nursing responses are uniquely created for the moment and cannot be predicted or applied as preplanned protocols (Boykin & Schoenhofer, 1997). Sensitivity and skill in creating unique and effective ways of communicating caring are developed through intention, experience, study, and reflection in a broad range of human situations.

The "Caring Between"

The caring between is the source and ground of nursing. It is the loving relation into which nurse and nursed enter and co-create by living the intention to care. Without the loving relation of the caring between, unidirectional activity or reciprocal exchange can occur, but nursing in its fullest sense does not occur. It is in the context of the caring between that personhood is enhanced, each expressing self and recognizing the other as a caring person.

Lived Meaning of Nursing as Caring

Abstract presentations of assumptions and themes lay the groundwork and provide an orienting point. However, the lived meaning of nursing as caring can best be understood by the study of a nursing situation. The following poem is one nurse's expression of the meaning of nursing, situated in one particular experience of nursing and linked to a general conception of nursing.

I Care for Him
My hands are moist,
My heart is quick,
My nerves are taut,
He's in the next room,
I care for him.

The room is tense,
It's anger-filled,
The air seems thick,
I'm with him now,
I care for him.

Time goes slowly by,
As our fears subside,
I can sense his calm,
He softens now,
I care for him.

His eyes meet mine,
Unable to speak,
I feel his trust,
I open my heart,
I care for him.

It's time to leave.
Our bond is made,
Unspoken thoughts,
But understood,
I care for him!
—J. M. COLLINS (1993)

Each encounter—each nursing experience—brings with it the unknown. In Collins's reflections, he shares a story of practice that illuminates the opportunity to live and grow in caring.

In the nursing situation that inspired this poem, the nurse and nursed live caring uniquely. Initially, the nurse experiences the familiar human dilemma, aware of separateness while choosing connectedness as he responds to a yet-unknown call for nursing: "My hands are moist/my heart is quick/my nerves are taut . . . I care for him." As he enters the situation and encounters the patient as person, he is able to "let go" of his presumptive knowing of the patient as "angry." The nurse enters with the guiding perspective that all persons are caring. This allows him to see past the "anger-filled" room and to be "with him" (second stanza). As they connect through their humanness, the beauty and wholeness of other is uncovered and nurtured. By living caring moment to moment, hope emerges and fear subsides. Through this experience, both nurse and

nursed live and grow in their understanding and expressions of caring.

In the first stanza, the nurse prepares to enter the nursing relationship with the formed intention of offering caring in authentic presence. Perhaps he has heard a report that the person he is about to encounter is a "difficult patient," and this is a part of his awareness; however, his nursing intention to care reminds him that he and his patient are, above all, caring persons. In the second stanza, the nurse enters the room, experiences the challenge that his intention to nurse has presented, and responds to the call for authentic presence and caring: "I'm with him now/I care for him." Patterns of knowing are called into play as the nurse brings together intuitive, personal knowing, empirical knowing, and the ethical knowing that it is right to offer care, creating the integrated understanding of aesthetic knowing that enables him to act on his nursing intention (Boykin, Parker, & Schoenhofer, 1994; Carper, 1978). Mayeroff's (1971) caring ingredients of courage, trust, and alternating rhythm are clearly evident.

Clarity of the call for nursing emerges as the nurse begins to understand that this particular man in this particular moment is calling to be known as a uniquely caring person, a person of value, worthy of respect and regard. The nurse listens intently and recognizes the unadorned honesty that sounds angry and demanding but is a personal expression of a heartfelt desire to be truly known and worthy of care. The nurse responds with steadfast presence and caring, communicated in his way of being and of doing. The caring ingredient of hope is drawn forth as the man softens and the nurse takes notice.

In the fourth stanza, the "caring between" develops, and personhood is enhanced as dreams and aspirations for growing in caring are realized: "His eyes meet mine ... I open my heart." In the last stanza, the nursing situation is completed in linear time. But each one, nurse and nursed, goes forward, newly affirmed and celebrated as caring persons, and the nursing situation continues to be a source of inspiration for living caring and growing in caring.

Assumptions in the Context of the Nursing Situation

In Collins's poem, the power of the basic assumption that all persons are caring by virtue of their humanness enabled the nurse to find the courage to live his intentions. The idea that persons are whole and complete in the moment permits the nurse to accept conflicting feelings and to be open to the nursed as a person, not merely as an entity with a diagnosis and superficially or normatively understood behavior. The nurse demonstrated an understanding of the assumption that persons live caring from moment to moment, striving to know self and other as caring in the moment with a growing repertoire of ways of expressing caring. Personhood, a way of living grounded in caring that can be enhanced in relationship with caring others, comes through; the nurse is successfully living his commitment to caring in the face of difficulty and in the mutuality and connectedness that emerged in the situation. The assumption that nursing is both a discipline and a profession is affirmed as the nurse draws on a set of values and a developed knowledge of nursing as caring to actively offer his presence in service to the nursed.

Applications of the Theory

The commitment of the nurse practicing nursing as caring is to nurture persons living caring and growing in caring. This implies that the nurse comes to know the other as a caring person in the moment. "Difficult to care" situations are those that demonstrate the extent of knowledge and commitment needed to nurse effectively. An everyday understanding of the meaning of caring is obviously challenged when the nurse is presented with someone for whom it is difficult to care. In these extreme (though not unusual) situations, a task-oriented, nondiscipline-based concept of nursing may be adequate to assure the completion of certain treatment and

surveillance techniques. Still, in our eyes, that is an insufficient response—it certainly is not the nursing we advocate. The theory of nursing as caring calls upon the nurse to reach deep within a well-developed knowledge base that has been structured using all available patterns of knowing, grounded in the obligations and intentionality inherent in the commitment to know persons as caring. These patterns of knowing may develop knowledge as intuition; scientifically quantifiable data emerging from research; and related knowledge from a variety of disciplines, ethical beliefs, and many other types of knowing. All knowledge held by the nurse that may be relevant to understanding the situation at hand is drawn forward and integrated as understanding that guides practice in particular nursing situations (aesthetic knowing). Although the degree of challenge presented from situation to situation varies, the commitment to know self and other as caring persons is steadfast.

The nursing as caring theory, grounded in the assumption that all persons are caring, has as its focus a general call to nurture persons in their unique ways of living caring and growing as caring persons. The challenge for nursing, then, is not to discover what is missing, weakened, or needed in another, but to come to know the other as a caring person and to nurture that person in situation-specific, creative ways and to acknowledge, support, and celebrate the caring that is. We no longer understand nursing as a "process" in the sense of a complex sequence of predictable acts resulting in some predetermined desirable end product. Nursing, we believe, is inherently processual, in the sense that it is always unfolding and is guided by intentionality and the commitment to care.

The nurse practicing within the caring context described here will most often be interfacing with the health care system in two ways: first, communicating nursing so that it can be understood with clarity and richness; and second, articulating nursing service as a unique contribution within the system in such a way that the system itself grows to support nursing.

Nursing as Caring in Nursing Administration

From the viewpoint of nursing as caring, the nurse administrator makes decisions through a lens in which the focus of nursing is on nurturing persons as they live caring and grow in caring. All activities in the practice of nursing administration are grounded in a concern for creating, maintaining, and supporting an environment in which calls for nursing are heard and nurturing responses are given (Boykin & Schoenhofer, 2001b). From this point of view, the expectation arises that nursing administrators participate in shaping a culture that evolves from the values articulated within nursing as caring.

Although often perceived to be "removed" from the direct care of the nursed, the nursing administrator is intimately involved in multiple nursing situations simultaneously, hearing calls for nursing and participating in responses to these calls. As calls for nursing are known, one of the unique responses of the nursing administrator is to enter the world of the nursed either directly or indirectly, to understand special calls when they occur, and to assist in securing the resources needed by each nurse to nurture persons as they live and grow in caring (Boykin & Schoenhofer, 1993). All administrative activities should be approached with this goal in mind. Here, the nurse administrator reflects on the obligations inherent in the role in relation to the nursed. The presiding moral basis for determining right action is the belief that all persons are caring. Frequently, the nurse administrator may enter the world of the nursed through the stories of colleagues who are assuming another role, such as that of nurse manager. The nursing administrator assists others within the organization to understand the focus of nursing and to secure the resources necessary to achieve the goals of nursing.

The nurse administrator is subject to challenges similar to those of the practitioner and often walks a very precarious tightrope between direct caregivers and corporate executives. The nurse administrator, whether at the executive or managerial level of the organizational chart, is held accountable for "customer satisfaction" as well as for "the bottom line." Nurses who "move up the executive ladder" may, on the one hand, be suspected of disassociating from their nursing colleagues, and, on the other hand, of not being sufficiently cognizant of the harsh realities of fiscal constraint. Administrative practice guided by the assumptions and themes of nursing as caring can enhance eloquence in articulating the connection between caregiver and institutional mission: the person seeking care.

Nursing practice leaders who recognize their care role, indirect as it may be, are in an excellent position to act on their committed intention to promote caring environments. Participating in rigorous negotiations for fiscal, material, and human resources and for improvements in nursing practice calls for special skill on the part of the nurse administrator—skill in recognizing, acknowledging, and celebrating the other (e.g., CEO, CFO, nurse manager, or staff nurse) as a caring person. The nurse administrator who understands the caring ingredients (Mayeroff, 1971) recognizes that caring is neither soft nor fixed in its expression. A developed understanding of the caring ingredients helps the nurse administrator mobilize the courage to be honest with self and other, to trust patience, and to value alternating rhythm with true humility while living a hope-filled commitment to knowing self and other as caring persons.

Nursing as Caring in Nursing Education

From the perspective of nursing as caring, all structures and activities should reflect the fundamental assumption that persons are caring by virtue of their humanness. Other assumptions and values reflected in the education program include knowing the person as whole and complete in the moment and living caring uniquely; understanding that person-hood is a way of living grounded in caring and is enhanced through participation in nurturing relationships with caring others; and affirming nursing as a discipline and profession.

The curriculum, the foundation of the education program, asserts the focus and domain of nursing as nurturing persons living caring and growing in caring:

The model for organizational design of nursing education is analogous to the dancing circle. ... Members of the circle include administrators, faculty, colleagues, students, staff, community, and the nursed. What this circle represents is the commitment of each dancer to understand and support the study of the discipline of nursing. The role of education administrators in the circle, represented by deans and department chairpersons is more clearly understood when the origin of the word is reflected upon. The term "administrator" derives from the Latin *ad ministrare,* to serve (according to Webster's, cited in Guralnik, 1976). This definition connotes the idea of rendering service. Administrators within the circle are by nature of [their] role obligated to ministering, to securing, and to providing resources needed by faculty, students, and staff to meet program objectives. Faculty, students, and administrators dance together in the study of nursing. Faculty support an environment that values the uniqueness of each person and sustains each person's unique way of living and growing in caring. This process requires trust, hope, courage, and patience. Because the purpose of nursing education is to study the discipline and practice of nursing, the nursed must be in the circle, and the focus of study must be the nursing situation, the shared lived experience of caring between nurse and nursed and all those who participate in the dance of caring persons. The community created is that of persons living caring in the moment and growing in personhood, each person valued as special and unique. (Boykin & Schoenhofer, 1993, pp. 73–74)

In teaching nursing as caring, faculty assist students to come to know, appreciate, and celebrate both self and other as caring persons. Students, as well as faculty, are in a continual search to discover greater meaning of caring as uniquely expressed in nursing. Examples of a nursing education program based on values similar to those of nursing as caring are illustrated in the book *Living a Caring-based Program* (Boykin, 1994).

Mentoring students as co-learners and creating caring learning environments while concomitantly accepting responsibility for summative evaluation calls for the integrated foundation provided by the guiding intention to know and nurture persons as caring. This intention helps the nurse transcend limiting historical practices while creatively inventing ways to inspire. The humility of unknowing, joined with courage and hope, helps the nurse educator guide the study of nursing as a commitment to knowing and nurturing persons as caring. Many nurse educators are struck with the incongruity of instilling a commitment to nursing as an opportunity to care through means that seem to view the student as an object and view the discipline as a preexisting set of operating rules. Nursing education practiced from the perspective of nursing as caring opens the way for faculty to truly value the discipline and the student.

Questions Nurses Ask About the Theory of Nursing as Caring

The following presents several common questions—and responses—that nurses ask about nursing as caring.

How Does the Nurse Come to Know Self and Other as Caring Persons?

Nursing practice guided by the Theory of Nursing as Caring entails living the commitment to know self and other as living caring in the moment and growing in caring. Living this commitment requires intention, formal study, and reflection on experience. Mayeroff's (1971) caring ingredients offer a useful starting point for the nurse committed to knowing self and other as caring persons. These ingredients include knowing, alternating rhythm, honesty, courage, trust, patience, humility, and hope. Roach's (1987/2002) five C's—commitment, confidence, conscience, competence, and compassion—offer another conceptual framework that is helpful in providing a language of caring. Coming to know self as caring is facilitated by:

- Trusting in self, freeing self up to become what one can truly become, and valuing self.
- Learning to let go, to transcend—to let go of problems, difficulties, in order to remember the interconnectedness that enables us to know self and other as living caring, even in suffering and in seeking relief from suffering.
- Being open and humble enough to experience and know self, to be at home with one's feelings.
- Continuously calling to consciousness that each person is living caring in the moment and that we are each developing uniquely in our personhood.
- Taking time to experience our humanness fully; one can only truly understand in another what one can understand in self.
- Finding hope in the moment. (Schoenhofer & Boykin, 1993, pp. 85–86)

Must I Like My Patients to Nurse Them?

The simple answer to this question is yes. To know the other as caring, the nurse must find some basis for respectful human connection with the person. Does this mean that the nurse must like everything about the person, including personal life choices? Perhaps not; however, the nurse as nurse is not called upon to judge the other, only to care for the other. A concern with judging or censuring another's actions is a distraction from the real purpose for nursing—that is, coming to know the other as caring person, as one with dreams and aspirations of growing in caring, and responding to calls for caring in ways that nurture personhood.

What About Nursing a Person for Whom It Is Difficult to Care?

Related to the previous dilemma, this question presents the crucible within which one's commitment to the assumptions and themes of nursing as caring is tested to the limit. The underlying question is, "Does the person to be nursed deserve or merit my care?" Again, as before, the simple answer is yes. All persons are caring, even when not all chosen actions of the person live up to the ideal to which we are all called by virtue of our humanness. In discussions of hypothetical situations involving child molesters, serial killers, and even political figures who have attempted mass destruction and racial annihilation, certain ethical systems permit and even call for making judgments. However, when such a person presents to the nurse for care, the nursing ethic of caring supersedes all other values. The Theory of Nursing as Caring asserts that it is *only* through recognizing and responding to the other as a caring person that nursing is created and personhood enhanced in that nursing situation. This question and the previous one make it clear that caring is much more than "sweetness and light"; caring effectively in "difficult to care" situations is the most challenging prospect a nurse can face. It is only with sustained intentionality, commitment, study, and reflection that the nurse is able to offer nursing in these situations. Falling short in one's commitment does not necessitate self-deprecation nor does it warrant condemnation by others, rather, it presents an opportunity to care for self and other and to grow in personhood. Making real the potential of such an opportunity calls for seeing with clarity, reaffirming commitment, and engaging in study and reflection, individually and in concert with caring others.

Is It Impossible to Nurse Someone Who Is in an Unconscious or Altered State of Awareness?

The key point here is the "caring between" that *is* the nursing creation: When nursing a person who is unconscious, the nurse lives the commitment to know the other as caring person. How is that commitment lived? It requires that all ways of knowing be brought into action. The nurse must make self as caring person available to the one nursed. The fullness of the nurse as caring person is called forth. This requires use of Mayeroff's caring ingredients: the alternating rhythm of knowing about the other and knowing the other directly through authentic presence and attunement; the hope and courage to risk opening self to one who cannot communicate verbally; patiently trusting in self to understand the other's mode of living caring in the moment; honest humility as one brings all that one knows and remains open to learning from the other. The nurse attuned to the other as person might, for example, experience the vulnerability of the person who lies unconscious from surgical anesthetic or traumatic injury. In that vulnerability, the nurse recognizes that the one nursed is living caring in humility, hope, and trust. Instead of responding to the vulnerability, merely "taking care of" the other, the nurse practicing nursing as caring might respond by honoring the other's humility, by participating in the other's hopefulness, and by steadfast trustworthiness. Creating caring in the moment in this situation might come from the nurse resonating with past and present experiences of vulnerability. Connected to this form of personal knowing might be an ethical knowing that power as a reciprocal of vulnerability has the potential to develop undesirable status differential in the nurse–patient role relationship. As the nurse sifts through a myriad of empirical data, the most significant information emerges—this is a *person* with whom I am called to care. Ethical knowing again merges with other pathways as the nurse forms the decision to go beyond vulnerability and engage the other as caring person, rather than as helpless object of another's concern. Aesthetic knowing comes in the praxis of caring, in living chosen ways of honoring humility, joining in hope, and demonstrating trustworthiness in the moment (Schoenhofer & Boykin, 1993, pp. 86–87).

How Does the Nursing Process Fit with this Theory?

Process, as it is understood in the term "nursing process," connotes a systematic and sequential series of steps resulting in a predetermined, specifiable product. Nursing process, as introduced into nursing by Orlando (1961), is a linear stepwise decision-making tool based on rational analysis of empirical data (known in other disciplines as the problem-solving process) and is a key structural theme of many nursing theories developed in past decades. Proponents of the theory of nursing as caring view nursing not as a process with an endpoint, but as an ongoing process, that is, as dynamic and unfolding, guided by intentionality, although not directed by a pre-envisioned outcome or product. Nursing responses of care arise in aesthetic knowing, in the creative and evolving patterns of appreciation and understanding, and in the context of a shared lived experience of caring. Instead of preselected and quantifiable outcomes, the value of nursing to the nursed and to others is that which is experienced as valuable arising in and evolving through the "caring between" of the nursing situation. Much of that value is neither measurable nor empirically verifiable. That which is measurable and empirically verifiable is relevant in the situation, however, and may be called upon at any time to contribute to and through the nurse's empirical knowing. Information that the nurse has available becomes knowledge within the nursing situation. Knowing the person directly is what guides the selection and patterning of relevant points of factual information in a nursing situation. That is, any fact or set of facts from nursing research or related bodies of information can be considered for relevance and drawn into the supporting knowledge base. This knowledge base remains open and evolving as the nurse employs an alternating rhythm of scanning and considering facts for relevance while remaining grounded in the nursing situation (Schoenhofer & Boykin, 1993, pp. 89–90).

In addition to empirical knowing, knowing for nursing purposes also requires personal knowing, including intuition and ethical knowing, all converging in aesthetic knowing within each unique nursing situation.

How Practical Is This Theory in the Real World of Nursing?

Nurses are frequently heard to say they have no time for caring, given the demands of the role. All nursing roles are lived out in the context of a contemporary environment. At the beginning of the twenty-first century, the environment for practice, administration, education, and research is fraught with many challenges, such as

• Technological advancement and proliferation that can promote routinization and depersonalization on the part of the caregiver as well as the one seeking care
• Demands for immediate and measurable outcomes that favor a focus on the simplistic and the superficial
• Organizational and occupational configurations that tend to promote fragmentation and alienation
• Economic focus and profit motive ("time is money") as the apparent prime institutional value

Nurses express frustration when evaluating their own caring efforts against an idealized, rule-driven conception of caring. Practice guided by the theory of nursing as caring reflects the assumption that caring is created from moment to moment and does not demand idealized patterns of caring. Caring in the moment (and moment to moment) occurs when the nurse is living a committed intention to know and nurture the other as caring person (Boykin & Schoenhofer, 2000). No predetermined ideal amount of time or form of dialogue is prescribed. A simple example of living this intention to care is the nurse who goes to the IV or the monitor *through* the person, rather than going directly to the technology and failing to acknowledge the person. When the nurse goes *through* the person, it becomes clear that the use of technology is one way the nurse expresses caring *for the person* (Schoenhofer, 2001). In

proposing his model of machine technologies and caring in nursing, Locsin (1995, 2001) distinguishes between mere technological competence and technological competence as an intentional expression of caring in nursing. Simply avowing an intention to care is not sufficient. The committed intention to care is supported by serious study of caring and ongoing reflection. As Locsin (1995, p. 203) so aptly states:

[A]s people seriously involved in giving care know, there are various ways of expressing caring. Professional nurses will continue to find meaning in their technological caring competencies, expressed intentionally and authentically, to know another as a whole person. Through the harmonious coexistence of machine technology and caring technology the practice of nursing is transformed into an experience of caring.

The practicality of the theory of nursing as caring has been tested in various nursing practice settings. Nursing practice models have been developed in acute and long-term care settings. Research studies focused on designing, implementing, and evaluating a theory-based practice model using nursing as caring on a telemetry unit of a for-profit hospital and in the emergency department of a community hospital demonstrated that when nursing practice is intentionally focused on coming to know a person as caring and on nurturing and supporting those nursed as they live their caring, transformation of care occurs. Within this new model, those nursed could articulate the "experience of being cared for"; patient and nurse satisfaction increased dramatically; retention increased; and the environment for care became grounded in the values of and respect for person (Boykin, Schoenhofer, Smith, St. Jean, & Aleman, 2003; Boykin, Bulfin, Baldwin, & Southern, 2004; Boykin, Schoenhofer, Bulfin, Baldwin, & McCarthy, 2005).

Current research is focused on transforming an entire for-profit health care organization by intentionally grounding it in Nursing as Caring. Caring from the heart—a model for interdisciplinary practice in a long-term care facility and based on the theory of nursing as caring—was designed through collaboration between project personnel and all stakeholders. Foundational values of respect and coming to know grounded the model, which revolves around the major themes of responding to that which matters; caring as a way of expressing spiritual commitment; devotion inspired by love for others; commitment to creating a home environment; and coming to know and respect person as person (Touhy, Strews, & Brown, 2003). The major building blocks of the nursing models for an acute care hospital and for a long-term care facility each reflect central themes of nursing as caring, but those themes are drawn out in ways unique to the setting and to the persons involved in each setting. The differences and similarities in these two practice models demonstrate the power of nursing as caring to transform practice in a way that reflects unity without conformity, uniqueness within oneness.

Practice Exemplar

The application of nursing as caring in my practice has been fulfilling both professionally and personally. I have been invited to share this experience.

Nursing as caring requires the nurse to use many different ways of knowing to come to know "other" in the fullness of one's existence. Each domain contains a vast amount of knowledge. The nurse must be knowledgeable of each and artfully apply this knowledge in an effort to transcend the physical boundaries of the human body to come to know other's complex existence. Personally, this effort is rewarded by enhancing who I am as a person.

As an advanced registered nurse practitioner (ARNP) in family practice, I see patients in a primary care setting. Grounded in nursing as caring, I borrow knowledge from other disciplines such as pathophysiology, microbiology, pharmacology, and philosophy and use this knowledge to come to know other in each moment of our visit. Some patients have immediate acute needs. Others have chronic problems that require maintenance therapy. All of them need to be recognized as holistic and complex humans with a unique existence in this world, living in caring and growing in caring. I am a facilitator of this process and risk entering into another's world with the intent of living caring in that nursing situation.

In practice, I emphasize wellness and prevention. Nursing as caring guides the nursing situation, serving as a framework in my patient encounters. I walk in the room with the intent of coming to know other as a holistic being with a body, mind, and spirit. The call for nursing then begins to unfold and reveals itself to me. My presence with other is authentic, and there exists a genuine responsiveness to come to know other. Authentic presence allows one to know that which is not spoken. A person can speak one's mind. A physical assessment can reveal an ailment. The spirit, however, must be attended to as well. Everything is revealed in one's spirit. When you are in authentic presence with other, the call for nursing unfolds before you. These are the profound encounters that never leave you.

Then there are the more frequent encounters where reflection becomes a useful tool to uncover the deeper meaning behind these chance nursing situations. Sometimes the patient's call for nursing is physical. I recognize it and treat accordingly. Reflection allows me to answer these questions: Was I nursing? What did I do differently from another health-care provider? My answer is the perspective from which I practice. I walked into the room with the willingness to come to know other, whatever may have been revealed in that moment. It was the way I touched the patient, my tone of voice, my unhurried pace, and my smile—all the tools I use to convey to other that I am there and that I care. The

Continued

Practice Exemplar cont.

goal is to enhance other as he or she lives and grows in caring.

I take time regularly to reflect upon the profound and not-so-profound nursing situations in my life. Reflection uncovers those hidden meanings that are not readily apparent in the moment. It is also a time for self-growth and validation—a process of coming to know self and others as caring persons.

Another form of reflection is the sharing of nursing situations with others. There are many different ways one can present a nursing situation, such as case presentations, poems, projects, and various other art forms. When one shares a nursing situation with others, new possibilities for knowing other unfold exponentially. Each practitioner brings the wealth of his or her education and experiences. New revelations come to life.

I share with you here a nursing situation I encountered. First, I will present it in the traditional medical model, and then I will present the same story in a nursing perspective grounded in the nursing as caring theory. Through comparison, the lived experience of both of these models will make clearer the difference between practice perspectives.

Medical Model Perspective

E. S. was a 76-year-old white woman who came to the office with the complaint of a lump in her abdomen. She remarked that she did not like going to the doctor and had neglected to have any checkups in quite a few years. A comprehensive history and physical exam was unremarkable with the exception of her abdomen, which revealed a small, palpable, nontender mass in the right lower quadrant. I ordered blood tests, all of which were unremarkable with the exception of the Ca125, which was 625, well above normal parameters. My suspicion for ovarian cancer was confirmed.

Three days after our initial visit, I asked her to return to the office so we could discuss the results. She did so, and brought a gift. She said I had done so much for her in our visit, she

wanted to share with me a precious gift the Lord had given her—her voice. There, in the office, I sat with her labs in my lap as she serenaded me with a song. I don't remember the name of the song, but the verse told me Jesus was calling her home and she was not afraid.

When she was done, we discussed the findings. I advised her that although the blood test was not diagnostic, the possibility of cancer did exist and she needed to see an oncological gynecologist. She cried and we hugged.

After a month of invasive testing at the family's prompting, exploratory surgery and biopsies confirmed the diagnosis of ovarian cancer with extensive metastasis. The patient underwent a total abdominal hysterectomy and bilateral salpingo-oophorectomy with debulking, and she died shortly thereafter.

There is much one can learn from a case presentation such as this one, but it does not reflect the essence of what occurred between the nurse and the one nursed. The reader is left wondering what the nurse did that prompted such a special present in return.

Nursing as Caring Perspective

As the morning rolled along, I began to dream. I dreamed I was a tree. My roots entwined deep within the foundation upon which I stood. I took from the Earth what I needed to nourish and strengthen me. My roots drank from the spring of knowledge beneath me. I felt strong. I grew tall. My arms outstretched, reached for the sun, found the sky, and in it, a gentle breeze that surrounded and calmed me. I stood in awe of the sun's beauty as its rays poured over me and warmed my spirit. I felt connected. I felt whole.

I saw a glow on the horizon, unlike the sun and different from the moon and stars. An ember, the residue of a fire that had burned through the night, tirelessly, provided warmth. I was drawn to it. Unafraid that my branches might catch fire and burn, I reached for her abdomen. I searched. As my hands pressed on, I began to feel the Earth slipping from the sky. I reached upward, grasping for the restoration of harmonious interconnectedness, but in the sky, there is nothing to grab onto. You may grow into it, enjoy its beauty, bask in its breezes, and breathe in its life-giving oxygen, but you cannot hold on to it or possess it.

My arms grew weary, my leaves were wilted, so I drank from the spring beneath my foundation. My roots nourished me with courage, patience, trust, and humility. She reached for my hand. Her spirit filled me and strengthened me as she ascended toward the sky. I began to feel stronger and reached toward the sky, hoping to catch one last glimpse of her ember and saw her reflection in the sun. Her rays poured over me and warmed my spirit. I felt whole once again.

This nursing story is a reflection of a nursing situation grounded in caring. It demonstrates the perspective of enhancing other as one lives and grows in caring, which subsequently results in the enhancement of self as the nurse lives and grows in caring.

Ways of Knowing

I chose this story as the medium with which to share. Nursing as caring encourages nurses to choose various art forms as media for sharing and reflection. This is aesthetic knowing. It is the artful integration of all the ways of knowing to create a meaningful, caring moment that is born in a nursing situation.

Personal knowing is that which is known intuitively by encountering self and other. Authentic presence is a key component for my intuitive experiences when I just know. This patient trusted me and humbled herself to ask me to validate her concern that the mass in her belly was of grave concern. The patient knew, intuitively, before I laid my hands on her. There is a lot to be gained by learning to trust our intuition, and we can "know" more by engaging in authentic presence. Authentic presence, for me, removes all physical boundaries to my coming to know other. It is a spiritual connectedness that has no time limits or physical boundaries. It is a feeling of interconnectedness with the patient

that reverberates beyond the room, city, state, country, world, and galaxy. It brings with it the wisdom of the universe.

The first three basic assumptions inherent in nursing as caring facilitate the lived experience of authentic presence in this moment. The assumption that this person is a caring person by virtue of her humanness, complete in that moment, gave me the courage to enter into authentic presence to come to know her as a complete, caring person in that moment. As the moment unfolded, our mutual trust enhanced and supported who we were as we lived and grew in that caring encounter.

The patient's need to share with me a special gift was validation that she felt it, too. The fifth basic assumption of the theory of nursing as caring is personhood, which is enhanced through participation in nurturing relationships. As the patient demonstrated in the words of her song, she knew that her physical existence was coming to an end and she was not afraid. There was a mutual knowingness that was unspoken, even without the lab work or biopsies. Her lack of fear and her courage allowed her spirit to soar free in the open sky, giving me a glimpse of the spiritual existence.

This is not to devalue the importance of empirical knowledge. It, too, is an important part of coming to know other. Empirical knowledge is the information that is organized into laws and theories to describe, explain, or predict phenomena. This knowledge is acquired through the senses. Based in the sciences, it is our understanding of anatomy and physiology, diagnostic processes, and treatment regimens. For me, it is the concrete form of the foundation upon which my practice is built.

Empirical knowledge is essential to be recognized as a profession. The sixth assumption of nursing as caring is that nursing is both a discipline and a profession. The scientific evidence that lends theory-based knowledge to our profession gives us the diagnostic reasoning we need to address the physical needs that people have. In this particular situation, the

Continued

Practice Exemplar cont.

laboratory findings confirmed that which we knew personally. Often the bereaved loved ones need a diagnosis to help cope with the grief of losing a family member.

This brings us to ethical knowing—the patience and compassion to be with grieving family members when they are not ready to let go of a loved one who is ready to die. Ethical knowing is also the recognition that these family members are caring persons as well, coping in the only way they know how, through their experiences. Humility has allowed me to come to know and respect the family's perspective. Patience is needed to allow other to come to know hope in the moment a loved one is diagnosed with a terminal illness. Hope for a spiritual existence beyond this world was revealed to me in this nursing situation.

Each of the patterns of knowing—aesthetic, personal, empirical, and ethical—is borrowed from Carper (1978). They serve as conceptual tools to help us understand and implement the theory of nursing as caring.

Nursing as caring provides a theoretical perspective with an organizing framework that guides practice and allows for the generation of new knowledge. In addition, it lends a methodological process to define, explain, and verify this knowledge. This theory reaches beyond the received view of traditional science. Nursing as caring guides the use of nursing knowledge and information from other disciplines in ways appropriate to nursing. Through the application of this theory, I have come to know new possibilities for nursing practice.

I believe now more than ever that, with the advancing roles of nurses, we need to be clear on what it is that we do that is different from other practitioners. As advanced practice nurses (APNs) we assume more responsibilities and perform tasks that were traditionally reserved for those of the medical profession; the overlapping further blurs the boundaries of our professions. We need to maintain our nursing perspective. As nurse practitioners continue to be lumped into categories with other midlevel practitioners, we need to demonstrate to our patients that our profession was born of a need from society, a need that only nurses can fill. If there is no call to nursing, our profession will dissolve into the sea of midlevel practitioners.

Nursing theory sets apart what nurse practitioners do from any other profession. To ensure that our practice maintains its identity, the practice must be built upon research-based nursing theory. The theory of nursing as caring is one such theory.

References

Boykin, A. (Ed.). (1994). *Living a caring-based program.* New York: National League for Nursing Press.

Boykin, A., Bulfin, S., Baldwin, J., & Southern, B. (2004). Transforming care in the emergency department. *Topics in Emergency Medicine, 26*(4), 331–336.

Boykin, A., Parker, M. E., & Schoenhofer, S. O. (1994). Aesthetic knowing grounded in an explicit conception of nursing. *Nursing Science Quarterly, 7,* 158–161.

Boykin, A., & Raines, D. (2006). Design and structure: An expression of caring. *International Journal for Human Caring, 10*(4), 45–49.

Boykin, A., & Schoenhofer, S. O. (1990). Caring in nursing: Analysis of extant theory. *Nursing Science Quarterly, 3*(4), 149–155.

Boykin, A., & Schoenhofer, S. O. (1991). Story as link between nursing practice, ontology, epistemology. *Image, 23,* 245–248.

Boykin, A., & Schoenhofer, S. O. (1993). *Nursing as caring: A model for transforming practice.* New York: National League for Nursing Press.

Boykin, A., & Schoenhofer, S. O. (1997). Reframing nursing outcomes. *Advanced Practice Nursing Quarterly, 1*(3), 60–65.

Boykin, A., & Schoenhofer, S. O. (2000). Invest in yourself. Is there really time to care? *Nursing Forum, 35*(4), 36–38.

Boykin, A., & Schoenhofer, S. O. (2001a). *Nursing as caring: A model for transforming practice.* Sudbury, MA: Jones and Bartlett.

Boykin, A., & Schoenhofer, S. O. (2001b). The role of nursing leadership in creating caring environments in health care delivery systems. *Nursing Administration Quarterly, 25*(1), 1–7.

Boykin, A., Schoenhofer, S., Bulfin, S., Baldwin, J., & McCarthy, D. (2005). Living caring in practice: The transformative power of the theory of nursing as caring. *International Journal for Human Caring, 9*(3), 15–19.

Boykin, A., Schoenhofer, S. O., Smith, N., St. Jean, J., & Aleman, D. (2003). Transforming practice using a caring-based nursing model. *Nursing Administration Quarterly, 27*, 223–230.

Carper, B. A. (1978). Fundamental patterns of knowing in nursing. *Advances in Nursing Science, 1*(1), 13–24.

Collins, J. M. (1993). I care for him. *Nightingale Songs, 2*(4), 3. Retrieved from http://www.fau.edu/divdept/nursing/ngsongs/vol2num4.htm (Accessed March 28, 2004).

Gaut, D., & Boykin, A. (Eds.). (1994). *Caring as healing: Renewal through hope.* New York: National League for Nursing Press.

Guralnik, D. (1976). *Webster's new world dictionary of the American language.* Cleveland: William Collings & World.

King, A., & Brownell, J. (1976). *The curriculum and the disciplines of knowledge.* Huntington, NY: Robert E. Krieger.

Locsin, R. C. (1995). Machine technologies and caring in nursing. *Image, 27,* 201–203.

Locsin, R. C. (2001). *Advancing technology, caring and nursing.* Westport, CT: Auburn House.

Mayeroff, M. (1971). *On caring.* New York: Harper & Row.

Orlando, I. (1961). *The dynamic nurse-patient relationship: Function, process and principles.* New York: G. P. Putnam's Sons. Nursing as Caring Web site. www.nursingascaring.com

Paterson, J. G., & Zderad, L. T. (1988). *Humanistic nursing.* New York: National League for Nursing Press.

Roach, S. (1987/2002). *Caring, the human mode of being. A blueprint for the health professions.* Ottawa, Canada: CHA Press.

Schoenhofer, S. O. (1995). Rethinking primary care: Connections to nursing. *Advances in Nursing Science, 17*(4), 12–21.

Schoenhofer, S. O. (2001). A framework for caring in a technologically dependent nursing practice environment. In: R. C. Locsin (Ed.), *Advancing technology, caring and nursing* (pp. 3–11). Westport, CT: Auburn House.

Schoenhofer, S. O. (2002a). Choosing personhood: Intentionality and the theory of nursing as caring. *Holistic Nursing Practice, 16,* 36–40.

Schoenhofer, S. O. (2002b). Considering philosophical underpinnings of an emergent methodology for nursing as caring inquiry. *Nursing Science Quarterly, 15*(4), 275–281.

Schoenhofer, S. O., Bingham, V., & Hutchins, G. C. (1998). Giving of oneself on another's behalf: The phenomenology of everyday caring. *International Journal for Human Caring, 2*(1), 23–29.

Schoenhofer, S. O., & Boykin, A. (1993). Nursing as caring: An emerging general theory of nursing. In Parker, M. E. (Ed.), *Patterns of nursing theories in practice* (pp. 83–92). New York: National League for Nursing Press.

Schoenhofer, S. O., & Boykin, A. (1998a). The value of caring experienced in nursing. *International Journal for Human Caring, 2*(3), 9–15.

Schoenhofer, S. O., & Boykin, A. (1998b). Discovering the value of nursing in high-technology environments: Outcomes revisited. *Holistic Nursing Practice, 12*(4), 31–39.

Touhy, T., & Boykin, A. (2008). Caring as the central domain in nursing education. *International Journal for Human Caring, 12*(2), 8–15.

Touhy, T., Strews, W., & Brown, C. (2003). *Caring from the heart.* CD-ROM available from Dr. Theris Touhy, Christine E. Lynn College of Nursing, Florida Atlantic University, 777 Glades Rd., Boca Raton, FL 33431-0991.

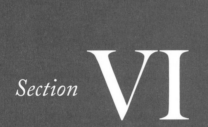

Section VI

Middle-Range Theories

Middle-Range Theories

Nine middle-range theories in nursing are presented in the final section. Each chapter is written by the scholars who developed the theory. Although we determine all to be at the middle range because of their more circumscribed focus on a phenomenon and more immediate relationship to practice and research, they still vary in level of abstraction. Comfort is an important concept to nursing practice. Kolcaba's middle-range theory of comfort is presented in Chapter 22. She defines comfort as "to strengthen greatly" and identifies relief, ease, and transcendence as types of comfort and physical, psychospiritual, environmental, and sociocultural as contexts in which comfort occurs. Duffy's Quality-Caring Model, described in Chapter 23, is a relatively new theory that is being used in many healthcare settings to address the issues of patient satisfaction and the lack of patients' feeling cared for in the acute care environment. In this model the goal of nursing is to engage in a caring relationship with self and others to engender feeling "cared for." Reed's Theory of Self-Transcendence is presented in Chapter 24. The focus of the theory is on facilitating self-transcendence for the purpose of enhancing well-being. Reed defines self-transcendence as the capacity to expand the self-boundary intrapersonally (toward greater awareness of one's beliefs, values, and dreams), interpersonally (to connect with others, nature, and surrounding environment), transpersonally (to relate in some way to dimensions beyond the ordinary and observable world), and temporally (to integrate one's past and future in a way that expands and gives meaning to the present). In Chapter 25 Swanson describes her trajectory and the process of developing of her middle-range theory of caring from research. The theory includes the concepts of knowing, being with, doing for, enabling, and maintaining belief. Smith and Liehr present story theory in Chapter 26. They posit that story is a narrative happening wherein a person connects with self-in-relation through nurse–person intentional dialogue to create ease. This theory has already been applied in a number of practice and research initiatives. Parker and Barry's Community Nursing Practice Model has guided nursing practice in community settings in several countries. The model is represented by concentric circles with the nursing situation as core and connected with the outer spheres of influence in the community and environment. Chapter 28 contains Locsin's Theory of Technological Competency-Caring. This theory dissolves the artificial and often assumed dichotomy between technology and caring, and asserts that technology is a way of coming to know the person as whole. Ray and Turkel authored Chapter 29 on Ray's Theory of Bureaucratic Caring. The theory uses a multidimensional, holographic model to facilitate the understanding of caring within the complex environment of healthcare systems. In Chapter 30 Smith presents her theory of unitary caring for the first time. The theory evolved from viewing caring through the lens of Rogers' Science of Unitary Human Beings.

Chapter 22

Katharine Kolcaba's Comfort Theory

KATHARINE KOLCABA

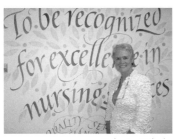

Katharine Kolcaba

Introducing the Theorist

Katharine Kolcaba was born and educated in Cleveland, Ohio. In 1965, she received a diploma in nursing and practiced part time for many years in the operating room, medical–surgical units, long-term care, and home care before returning to school. In 1987, she graduated with the first R.N. to M.S.N. class at the Frances Payne Bolton School of Nursing, Case Western Reserve University (CWRU), with a specialty in gerontology. While attending graduate school, Kolcaba maintained a head nurse position on a dementia unit. In the context of that unit, she began theorizing about comfort.

After graduating with her master's degree in nursing, Kolcaba joined the faculty at the University of Akron (UA) College of Nursing, where her clinical expertise was gerontology and dementia care. She returned to CWRU to pursue her doctorate in nursing on a part-time basis while teaching full time. Over the next 10 years, she used course work from her doctoral program to further develop her theory. During that time, Kolcaba published a framework for dementia care (1992a), diagrammed the aspects of comfort (1991), operationalized comfort as an outcome of care (1992b), contextualized comfort in a middle range theory (1994), tested the theory in several intervention studies (Kolcaba, 1999, 2003, 2004; Kolcaba, Tilton & Drouin, 2006; Dowd, Kolcaba, Steiner, & Fashinpaur, 2007), and further refined the theory to include hospital-based outcomes (2001). She has an extensive series of publications to document each step in the process, most of which have been compiled in her book *Comfort Theory and Practice*

(2003). Many publications and comfort assessments also are available on her web site at www.TheComfortLine.com.

Kolcaba taught nursing at UA for 22 years and is now an associate professor emeritus. Kolcaba still teaches her web-based theory course once a year and she represents her own company, The Comfort Line, as a consultant. In this capacity, she works with health care agencies and hospitals who choose to apply Comfort Theory on an institutional-wide basis. She also is founder and member of her local parish nurse program and is a member of ANA and Sigma Theta Tau. Kolcaba continues to work with students at all levels and with nurses who are conducting comfort studies. She resides in the Cleveland area with her husband, near her two daughters, their children, and her mother. One other daughter resides in Chicago.

Overview of the Theory

In Comfort Theory (CT), comfort is a noun or an adjective, and an outcome of intentional, patient/family focused, quality care. In spite of everyone's familiarity with the idea of comfort, it is a very complex term that has several meanings and usages in ordinary language. The use of comfort as a noun and an outcome is specific to CT and different from its alternative usages as a verb, adverb, and process (Kolcaba, 1995). From a search of the literature, Kolcaba learned that the original definition of comfort meant "to strengthen greatly." From other disciplines, she learned that (1) the need for comfort is basic, (2) persons experience comfort holistically, (3) self-comforting measures can be healthy or unhealthy, and (4) enhanced comfort (when achieved in healthy ways) leads to greater productivity.

Kolcaba used three nursing theories to describe three distinct types of comfort (Kolcaba, 2003). Relief was synthesized from the work of Orlando (1961/1990), who stated that nurses relieved the needs expressed by patients. Ease was synthesized from the work of Henderson (1978), who described 13 basic functions of humans that needed to be maintained for homeostasis. Transcendence was derived from Paterson and Zderad (1976), who believed that patients could rise above their difficulties with the help of nurses.

The four contexts in which comfort is experienced by patients are physical, psychospiritual, sociocultural, and environmental and came from a further review of literature regarding holism in nursing (Kolcaba, 1991, 2003). When these four contexts of experience are juxtaposed with the three types of comfort, a taxonomic structure (TS) or grid is created that covers the nursing meaning of comfort as a patient outcome. This TS, with definitions of each type and context of comfort, provides a map of the content of comfort so that nurses can use it to pattern their care for each patient and family member. Kolcaba's technical definition of the outcome of comfort is: The immediate experience of being strengthened when needs for relief, ease, and transcendence are addressed in four contexts of experience. Figure 22-1 contains the TS of comfort with the corresponding definitions of relief, ease, transcendence and the physical, psychospiritual, environmental and sociocultural contexts.

Other uses of the TS of comfort are (1) for determining the existence and extent of unmet comfort needs in patients or family members; (2) for designing comforting interventions, which often can be "bundled" in a single patient interaction; and (3) for creating measurements of holistic comfort for documentation in practice and research; such measurements would be conducted before and after comfort interventions and/or interactions. (A place to note the nature and time of the nursing intervention next to baseline and subsequent comfort measurements is essential in medical records. These strategies are discussed further in a later section of this chapter.)

One way to think about the grid is that comfort is an umbrella outcome that entails relief from discomforts such as anxiety, pain, environmental stressors, and/or social isolation. Because the TS represents a holistic definition of comfort, the cells on the grid are interrelated and as a whole, comfort

	Relief	Ease	Transcendence
Physical	Pain		
Psychospiritual	Anxiety		
Environmental			
Sociocultural			

Figure 22 · 1 Taxonomic structure of comfort.

interventions directed to one part of the grid have effects on all parts of the grid. Total comfort is also greater than the sum of its individual parts. Therefore, comfort interventions to treat anxiety also may reduce the dosage of analgesia needed for adequate pain relief. On a comfort continuum, the concept of Total Comfort (as much as can be expected given the circumstances) is at one extreme end, and Suffering is at the other end.

Propositions of Comfort Theory

CT contains three intuitive parts that can be applied or tested separately or as a whole. The first part states that comforting interventions, when effective, result in increased comfort for recipients (patients and families), compared to a pre-intervention baseline. Increased comfort is the immediate desired outcome for this kind of care. Comfort interventions address basic human needs, such as rest, homeostasis, therapeutic communication, and viewing patients holistically. These

comfort interventions are often nontechnical and complement delivery of technical care. Care providers, such as nurses, may also be considered recipients if the institution makes a commitment to improving comfort in its work setting (discussed later).

When comfort is not enhanced to the fullest extent possible, nurses consider intervening variables for as possible explanations as to why comfort interventions did not work. Abusive homes, lack of financial resources, devastating diagnoses, or cognitive/psychological impairments may render ineffective the most appropriate interventions and comforting actions. The aspect of transcendence, however, guides nurses to help patients "rise above" or be inspired to achieve mutually determined goals regardless of life circumstances. Nurses who practice CT never give up "being with" and inspiring their patients. Thus, this focus on comfort is proactive, energized, intentional, and longed for by recipients of care in all settings.

The second part states that increased comfort of recipients results in their being strengthened for their tasks ahead, which are called health-seeking behaviors (HSBs). HSBs are subsequent recipient goals and are negotiated between nurses and the recipients. In the practice of nursing administration, when the intended recipients are bedside nurses, HSBs are negotiated with nursing staff.

The third part states that increased engagement in HSBs results in increased Institutional Integrity (InI). Enhanced InI strengthens the institution and its ability to gather evidence for best practices and best policies. Best practices and policies lead to quality care, which, in many ways, benefits the "bottom" financial line of the institution.

Kolcaba believes that nurses already know how and want to practice comforting care, and that it can be easily incorporated into every nursing action. Many nurses deliver comforting care intuitively, but do not document its total effects of patients as enhanced comfort. The explicit focus on and documentation of this type of holistic care is called comfort management and, as shown in the

TS, includes more than relief of pain or anxiety. Thus, when nurses adopt CT as their personal philosophy for practice, they are utilizing a simple pattern for individualized care that is efficient, creative, and satisfying to themselves and recipients of their care. When enhanced comfort is documented, nurses can also demonstrate their real contributions to better institutional outcomes such as higher patient satisfaction, fewer readmissions, or shorter length of stay. The diagram of CT shows the relationships between the simple concepts (Fig. 22-2). Definitions of the concepts are below the diagram.

Theoretical Definitions for Diagram Concepts

In the context of comfort theory, **health care needs** are defined as needs for comfort, arising from stressful health care situations that cannot be met by recipients' traditional support systems. They include physical, psychospiritual, sociocultural, and environmental needs made apparent through monitoring and verbal or nonverbal reports, needs related to pathophysiological parameters, needs for education and

Conceptual framework for Comfort Theory

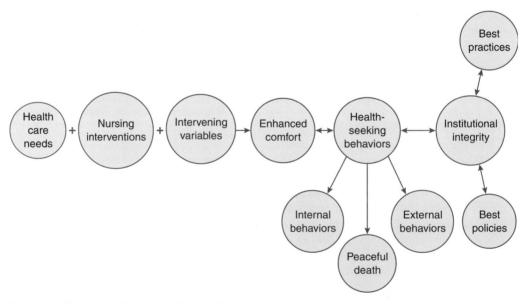

Figure 22 · 2 Conceptual framework for comfort theory.

support, and needs for financial counseling and intervention.

Comfort interventions are defined as intentional actions designed to address specific comfort needs of recipients, including physiological, social, cultural, financial, psychological, spiritual, environmental, and physical interventions. Within these contexts of experience, there are three types of comfort interventions described later: technical, coaching, and comfort food for the soul.

Intervening variables are defined as interacting forces that influence recipients' perceptions of total comfort. These consist of variables such as past experiences, age, attitude, emotional state, support system, prognosis, finances, education, cultural background, and the totality of elements in recipients' experience.

Comfort was defined technically earlier in this chapter. It is the state that is experienced immediately by recipients of comfort interventions. It entails the holistic experience of <u>being</u> *strengthened* through having comfort needs addressed.

The concept of **health-seeking behaviors** was developed by Dr. Rozella Schlotfeldt (1975) and represents the broad category of subsequent outcomes related to the pursuit of health. Schlotfeldt stated that HSBs could be internal or external. She was ahead of her time in thinking that a peaceful death could also be an HSB. Realistic HSBs are determined by recipients of care in collaboration with their health care team.

Institutional integrity is defined as those corporations, communities, schools, hospitals, regions, states, and countries that possess qualities of being complete, whole, sound, upright, appealing, ethical, and sincere. When an institution displays this type of integrity, it can produce valuable evidence for best practices and best policies. **Best practices** are health care interventions that produce the best possible patient and family outcomes based on empirical evidence. **Best policies** are institutional or regional policies ranging from basic protocols for procedures and medical conditions, to systems for access and delivery of health care. Best

policies are also determined from empirical evidence.

As stated previously, the diagram and specific definitions for the concepts in CT provide a pattern and practical rationale for practicing comfort management. This kind of care is individualized, efficient, holistic, and therapeutic. Importantly, the nurturing aspect of nursing provides the altruistic motivation for practicing comfort management. It is the traditional mission and passion of nursing (Kolcaba, 2003; Morse, 1992). But the practical rationale is important at the institutional level, because without administrative support for optimum staffing and employment practices, nurses often cannot give the kind of care to which they were born or for which they were educated.

For teaching and learning purposes, care plans based on CT are provided on Kolcaba's website and in her book (Kolcaba, 2003). One is for patients and one is for patients and family members, as defined by the patient. Note, for teaching and learning, it is not necessary to distinguish among relief, ease, and transcendence when assessing and intervening for unmet comfort needs. Institutional outcomes are not included in the care plans, because these data are not accessible to students and beginning nurses. An additional column can be added to the care plans, especially for the InI outcome of patient satisfaction so that learners can "see" the relationship between their comforting interventions and the broader integrity of the institution (Kolcaba, 1995). These care plans can also be applied in home care and in long-term care.

Application of the Theory in Practice

According to CT, there are three types of comforting interventions: technical, coaching, and comfort food for the soul. *Technical interventions* are those that are specified by other disciplines or by nursing protocols; they include medications, treatments, monitoring schedules, insertion of lines, and so forth. For patients, competency in the administration and documentation of technical interventions is the minimum expectation for nurses. *Coaching* consists of supportive nursing actions, active listening, referrals to other members of the health care team, advocacy, reassurance, and so forth. *Comfort Food for the Soul* are those extra special, holistic, and more time-consuming nursing interventions such as back or hand massage, guided imagery, music or art therapy, a walk outside, or special arrangements for family members. The latter two types of interventions require considerably more expertise and confidence by nurses and are what patients most remember. And they are what Benner (1984) would ascribe to "expert" nurses.

However, most nurses focus on technical interventions first, and when time permits, implement coaching techniques. Interestingly, charting usually accounts only for technical interventions and the effects of analgesia; there are no places in traditional hospital records to record the more important healing interventions. But, patients rarely remember the technical interventions; the important interventions to patients and their families are those that are not documented such as: coaching and comfort food for the soul, the most important work of expert nurses. Thus, there is a perpetual disconnect between legal charting and actions that patients want and need from their nurses, and which we claim to be the essence of nursing. It is no wonder that, when pressed, nurses cannot describe the impact they make with patients and their families—coaching and comfort food interventions are not valued by administrators and are not even visible in patient care records.

CT provides the language and rationale to once again claim and document essential nursing activities that are most beneficial to patients and family members in stressful health care situations. It is also important to remember that the outcome of enhanced comfort is a *value-added* outcome; that is, it is a positive measure of quality care rather than a measure of what is not quality care such as the currently measured outcomes of nosocomial infections, falls, decubitus ulcers, medication errors, and failure to rescue. (Note, would YOU want to go to a hospital which was looking only at their rates of medication errors or "failures to rescue?")

How to BE a Nurse

CT guides nurses to detect comfort needs of patients and families that are not being addressed and to develop interventions to meet those needs. Their caring actions are intuitive, but in this theory, caring is a comfort intervention in and of itself. CT describes how to care and how to BE a nurse, what is important to patients and families, and factors that facilitate healing. In addition, all technical nursing interventions are delivered in a comforting way.

Nurses and patients want to experience intentional and meaningful moments with each other and with family members, the kind that patients might call *wow moments.* ("Wow! I'll always remember that nurse.") Nurses usually sense when this happens, and these instances are sustaining, satisfying, and profound for them as well as for their patients. But nurses often fail to understand and share how the moment intentionally came to be created, especially if they practice without a theory. These special instances require appropriate theories to add both personal and disciplinary structure and meaning to such experiences (Chinn, 1997). When nurses are able to describe their "wow moments" in terms of CT, the nature of their interactions becomes purposeful and repeatable, and these transformative interactions become associated with the power of nursing in general, not just with one nurse. The cumulative power of these moments strengthens not only the recipients, but also nurses who create the moments, and the discipline that lays claim to them.

CT states that the process of comforting a patient entails the *intention* to comfort, to be present, and to deliver comforting interventions based on the patients' and loved ones' unmet comfort needs (Kolcaba, 2003; Kolcaba, on line). If the patient needs time to voice concerns and questions, the nurse listens attentively and provides culturally appropriate encouragement and body language (a comforting intervention).

The nurse knows exactly why and when to do this, because he or she is tuned into the whole person as patient and because the nurse wants to provide comfort, to soothe in times of distress and sorrow. Such an explanation of *how* to BE a nurse is lacking in most other theories.

Institutional Advocacy

It is not enough for institution administrators to state that they want nurses and other care providers to practice comforting care—they need to implement documentation and reinforcement strategies to ensure this is done and to show that they value this kind of care. If administrators do not take on this responsibility, practicing nurses can be self-advocates and begin to document comforting interventions and their effects in narrative charting. Whether top-down and/or from the grass roots, the institutional ideal is for health care institutions to provide ways in which comfort needs of patients and family members are routinely charted, beginning with baseline comfort levels. Comforting interventions are described and implemented, and comfort levels are reassessed and charted. Modifications to the interventions are made, until comfort levels are sufficiently increased. Preferences of patients and families are honored wherever possible. In appropriate settings, comfort contracts (Appendix A) can be instituted and followed throughout a defined clinical situation such as surgery, labor and delivery, or an acute psychiatric episode.

According to CT, technical interventions should be documented as usual (often on a checklist including times), but methods of intentional caring also should be documented – in the same way that administration of pain medication is noted in two places. There are many suggestions for documentation on the instrument section at Kolcaba's website, including a verbal rating scale, a numeric diagram, comfort daisies for children, a comfort behaviors checklist for nonverbal or unresponsive patients, and several questionnaires about patient comfort for different research settings. These instruments can be downloaded from the website and utilized in practice and/or

research, without permission, because the website is in the public domain. The address is www.TheComfortLine.com (Appendix B).

In addition to providing methods for documentation of comfort needs and comforting measures, there are other ways that institutions can demonstrate their commitment to comfort management. These include building comfort management into orientation, inservice programs, performance reviews, and methods for nursing assignments (based in part on comfort needs of patients and family members). An example of an institution that has implemented such strategies across all departments is The Mount Sinai Hospital, New York City (contact person: Carol Porter, chief nursing officer).

Institutional Awards

Institutions have adopted CT to enhance nurses' work environments, such as in the quest for national recognition including Magnet Status, the Baldrich Award, and the Beacon Award. Many institutions discover that the application process for these types of awards is simplified when a theoretical framework is adopted. The main benefit of doing so is that employees are on the "same page," in the case of CT, comforting patients and family members in their own personalized styles and capacities. Moreover, and perhaps most importantly, is that administrative commitment to a philosophy of comfort management includes sufficient staffing levels in all departments to support this type of holistic health care. A large hospital system that adopted CT to undergird their application for Magnet Status, and was successful in achieving Magnet Status shortly thereafter, is Southern New Hampshire Medical Center (SNHMC) (contact person, Collette Tilton, CNO) (Kolcaba, Tilton, & Drouin, 2006).

When SNHMC decided to apply for Magnet Status, nurses from middle management formed a committee and reviewed several nursing theories. They chose CT because it most accurately reflected their values and goals. Kolcaba was contacted to arrange a consultative visit, which occurred after a sufficient time to prepare the other departments, including upper administrative levels, for the visit.

As part of this consultation, Kolcaba and the CNO visited all departments. They requested suggestions from the staff for ideas that would increase their comfort at work. The many suggestions that were given came to be added to comfort "wish lists" on each unit. One astute young nurse asked where to send the items on the wish list. The CNO replied, "Most of your suggestions will not require additional funds, and you can implement those items on your own units. For items that do require more money, please send them to me."

Another strategy adopted during this visit consisted of brief instructions about designing and implementing small "comfort studies" specific to each unit and to common clinical problems. The diagram of CT (see Fig. 22-2) defines the research process when comfort studies are undertaken, often a requirement for national awards. Strategies for publicizing the results of these studies, as well as the institutional commitment to comfort management, were also suggested.

The Meaning of Comfort Theory for Practice

Kolcaba routinely asks nurses and students in her audiences about their experiences during past hospitalizations, either as a patient or a family member. She asks if they remember any of their nurses, and if so, what do they remember? The stories that emerge are usually about nurses who demonstrated small, nontechnical, but very comforting acts of compassion and understanding. Examples of these interventions are: a brief back massage, helping a child make a phone call, sitting beside an anxious patient, making eye contact during an interaction, gently encouraging ambulation, listening attentively to role change issues, holding a dying patient's hand, washing a patient's hair, making a family member comfortable during an overnight stay, and so forth. These types of interventions are remembered by patients for years after a stressful health care episode because emotions run high and kind encounters

are precious. Each is an example of a holistic comfort intervention that has greater positive effects on the patients' total comfort than could be imagined by the caregiver. These comforting interventions are examples of "wow moments" for receivers, and the exchange also renews the givers of such acts in existential ways. Moreover, such comforting interventions can be delivered by any member of the health care team or department within the context of their job description.

How Comfort Theory Lives in Practice

Best Practices

Currently, there is administrative interest in improving the "patient experience"—a factor that typically is measured by items on patient satisfaction instruments, the results of which are posted on public websites. The quality of the "patient experience," as rated by patients after a hospital stay, determines choices by insurance companies for future coverage of their enrollees. Often, these items are nursing sensitive, meaning that if nurses demonstrate simple comforting techniques, patients will respond favorably to those "patient experience" questions.

One administrative approach to enhancing the "patient experience" has been to implement scripting, whereby members of the health care team memorize specific prewritten statements to use during common patient encounters. An example is a standard script to be delivered on first introducing oneself to the patient such as, "Hello, I am Nurse Thomas and I will be in charge of your care for today. If you need anything at all, please let me know." This approach may negate individualized care, the special needs of the patient and family, and the particular communication skills of the team member. And most patients can determine when such statements are prescripted, especially when they hear the same statements several times from different caregivers over the course of a hospital stay.

A different approach is to undergird all patient interactions with principles of CT, which caregivers learn in orientation and in-service programs. Principles of CT that are relevant to the patient experience are that (1) each interaction entails therapeutic use of self; (2) caregivers assess for comfort needs of patients and family members and design their interaction to meet those needs; (3) caregivers approach each patient and family member with the intent to comfort and make a personal, culturally appropriate connection; and (4) caregivers regularly reassess comfort of patients and family members and document comfort levels routinely. Utilizing this approach facilitates individualized and efficient care and a more positive patient experience. Two examples of how CT is being used to enhance the patient experience are at the Mount Sinai Hospital, New York City (Carol Porter, CNO, contact person) and at Kaiser Permanente Hospital in San Francisco (Katy Kennedy, contact person).

Electronic Database

To support CT in practice, components have been incorporated into national electronic databases, such as the National Interventions Classification (NIC) and the National Outcomes Classification (NOC) systems (The Iowa Taxonomy) as well as the North American Nursing Diagnosis Association (NANDA). Comforting interventions, comfort outcomes, and comfort diagnoses are included in these data systems, meaning that individualized comfort needs and the effectiveness of interventions to meet those needs can be charted electronically and entered into larger databases by a hospital system, at the local, state, region, or country level. While there are at least 13 national databases for nursing, and others for medicine, when hospital systems select and contribute data to a mainstream system, documentation of patient care problems, interventions, and outcomes can be more widely compared, leading to more consistent and higher quality patient care practices. In this regard, an important feature of CT is the universality of its main concept, comfort. This is a word that is understood by all health-related disciplines and is translatable into most languages, as evident with the number of foreign language comfort instruments available on Kolcaba's website.

Best Policies

An example of how CT is used in practice is the creation of a policy for Comfort Management by the American Society of Peri-Anesthesia Nurses (ASPAN). This national association is composed of nurses who work in the following areas: ambulatory surgery, perioperative staging, operating room, postanesthesia recovery, and step-down. ASPAN decided collectively to apply CT in an explicit way throughout patients' surgical experiences. Kolcaba served as consultant and facilitator in this process.

First, they achieved national consensus about the development of Guidelines for Comfort Management that would complement their existing Guidelines for Pain Management. The process proceeded with a survey of its membership about providing comfort to patients, then with a report of findings, then the conference about components of Comfort Management, and finally the composition of the guidelines (Kolcaba & Wilson, 2002; Wilson & Kolcaba, 2004).

The guidelines contain information about how to (1) perform a comfort assessment, (2) create a comfort contract with patients before surgery, (3) discover the interventions that patients and families use at home for specific discomforts, (4) use a checklist for comfort common management strategies, (5) document changes in comfort, and (6) implement pre- and post-testing for contact hours in comfort management. The completed Guidelines for Comfort Management are available on ASPAN's website (www.ASPAN.org). This is an example of a grassroots change (within a national association of nurses) that was disseminated to all perianesthesia settings and soon became a practice expectation. This example could be followed by any nursing specialty, at the macro level, or any patient care unit, at the micro level. The important point is that the model was initiated by nurses and is now an expectation that the Joint Commission reviews on recertification.

Practice Exemplar

Nurse Smith worked for approximately 15 years in a single large hospital system. Because of her strong work ethic and creative ideas, she had been promoted over the years from staff nurse to positions in upper management. In addition to her BSN, she had her MBA and was also enrolled in a DNP program. While attending graduate school at the age of 45, she developed breast cancer and was a patient in her own system. She was full of anxiety about her prognosis, treatment, and role change and spent many days in various settings including in-patient, out-patient, surgery, radiation therapy, and chemotherapy. Her treatment spanned several months in close contact with the nurses from her own organization.

To her chagrin, during this time of high comfort needs, Nurse Smith received little or no comfort from the nurses with whom she came in contact. She recalled that no personal connections were made by these nurses, who delivered their interventions mechanically, with a noticeable lack of personalized eye contact. Nurse Smith felt lonely, scared, and in more objective moments, deeply concerned for her profession.

Shortly after her recovery from intensive therapies, Nurse Smith applied for the Chief Nursing Officer (CNO) position. As part of her interview, she told the administrators who would be choosing the next CNO about her experience as a patient in their organization. She knew from her own personal episode that the "patient experience" could be greatly improved and she had an idea about how to make that happen. Her vision was for her hospital to adopt CT for its multidisciplinary framework to undergird the patient experience. Every encounter with patients and families would be a comforting and connecting experience. There would be no need for scripting because each encounter would be based on comforting the patient and family in some way and would be individualized, sincere, and unique to the skills of the caregiver. She believed that such encounters would take the same amount of time, or less, than impersonal ones and indeed, they would help allay anxiety almost immediately. She was hired.

CT was officially adopted by this institution, integrating the following components: commitment by administration, retelling of the CNO's story, redefining quality care in terms of comfort for patients and families, orientation to CT for all personnel, an introduction of CT to the academic community including nursing students, small changes in the way care would be delivered, comfort rounds, comfort charting (electronic and paper based), performance review/clinical ladders, and marketing strategies—putting their commitment to comforting care "out there." Data are currently being collected regarding the extent to which the patient experience was improved following the "rollout" of CT.

References

Benner, P. (1984). *From novice to expert.* Menlo Park, CA: Addison Wesley.

Dowd, T., Kolcaba, K., & Steiner, R. (2003). The addition of coaching to cognitive strategies: Interventions for persons with compromised urinary bladder syndrome. *Journal of Ostomy and Wound Management, 30*(2), 90–99.

Dowd, T., Kolcaba, K., Steiner, R., & Fashinpaur, D. (2007). Comparison of healing touch and coaching on stress and comfort in young college students. *Holistic Nursing Practice, 21*(4), 194–202.

Henderson, V. (1978). *Principles and practice of nursing.* New York: Macmillan.

Kolcaba, K. (1991). A taxonomic structure for the concept comfort. *Image: The Journal of Nursing Scholarship, 23*(4), 237–240.

Kolcaba, K. (1992a). The concept of comfort in an environmental framework. *Journal of Gerontological Nursing, 18*(6), 33–38.

Kolcaba, K. (1992b). Holistic comfort: Operationalizing the construct as a nurse-sensitive outcome. *ANS Advances in Nursing Science, 15*(1), 1–10.

Kolcaba, K. (1994). A theory of holistic comfort for nursing. *Journal of Advanced Nursing, 19*, 1178–1184.

Kolcaba, K. (1995). The art of comfort care. *Image: The Journal of Nursing Scholarship, 27*(4), 287–289.

Kolcaba, K. (2001). Evolution of the midrange theory of comfort for outcomes research. *Nursing Outlook, 49*(2), 86–92.

Kolcaba, K. (2003). *Comfort theory and practice: A vision for holistic health care and research* (pp. 113–124). New York: Springer.

Kolcaba, K. (2008). *TheComfortLine.com* (Accessed July 15, 2008).

Kolcaba, K., Dowd, T., Steiner, R., & Mitzel, A. (2004). Efficacy of hand massage for enhancing comfort of hospice patients. *Journal of Hospice and Palliative Care, 6*(2), 91–101.

Kolcaba, K., & Fox, C. (1999). The effects of guided imagery on comfort of women with early-stage breast cancer going through radiation therapy. *Oncology Nursing Forum, 26*(1), 67–71.

Kolcaba, K., Schirm, V., & Steiner, R. (2006). Effects of hand massage on comfort of nursing home residents. *Geriatric Nursing, 27*(2), 85–91.

Kolcaba, K., Tilton, C., & Drouin, C. (2006). Comfort theory: A unifying framework to enhance the practice environment. *Journal of Nursing Administration, 36*(11), 538–544.

Kolcaba, K., & Wilson, L. (2002). The framework of comfort care for perianesthesia nursing. *Journal of Perianesthesia Nursing, 17*(2), 102–114. With post-test for 1.2 contact hours.

Morse, J. (1992) Comfort: The refocusing of nursing care. *Clinical Nursing Research. 1*(1), 91–106.

Orlando, I. (1961/1990). *The dynamic nurse-patient relationship.* New York: National League for Nursing Press.

Paterson, J., & Zderad, L. (1976/1988). *Humanistic nursing.* New York: National League for Nursing Press.

Schlotfeldt, R. (1975). The need for a conceptual framework. In: P. Verhonic (Ed.), *Nursing Research* (pp. 3–25). Boston: Little, Brown.

Wilson, L., & Kolcaba, K. (2004). Practical application of Comfort Theory in the perianesthesia setting. *Journal of PeriAnesthesia Nursing, 19*(3), 164–173.

Appendix A: Example of a Comfort Contract

Thank you for taking the time to complete the comfort contract. The purpose of this contract is to increase your comfort and pain management while you are hospitalized. Please rate your expectation of comfort from 0 to 10 (10 is highest) for each situation listed. Please use the comfort scale as directed for all items except when indicated otherwise and take your time and complete the following questions.

Use Comfort Scale as directed in figure 22-3.

Extreme discomfort		Comfort			Extreme comfort
1 2	3	4 5	6 7	8	9 10

Figure 22 · 3 Comfort scale.

The Comfort Experience

1. I expect a comfort level of:
   a. _____ when the anesthesia wears off.
   b. _____ on postoperative day 1
   c. _____ on postoperative day 3 (when ambulating)
   d. _____ on postoperative day 5 (study conclusion day)

2. These interventions might assist to increase my comfort:

   Warming blanket (recovery room)
   Pet visitation
   Family visits (when anesthesia wears off)
   Music
   Cold washcloth
   Pillows—location: _____
   Massage
   Other _____
   (*Circle All that Apply.*)

3. In the past, I have required (small, moderate, large) amounts of pain medication to keep me comfortable.

4. I have had success with the following medications during my previous admissions to the hospital _____

5. The following medications I had taken have resulted in undesirable outcomes
   _____
   The undesirable outcomes have included
   _____
   _____
   _____

Nursing Interventions

6. I prefer personal hygiene to be performed during the (morning, afternoon, evening).
7. I prefer my family to be present (all the time, occasionally, not at all) during my recovery.
8. I wish to have the following family member(s) present:_____.
9. I prefer to exclude the following persons from visiting my room_____.
10. I prefer to have a fan present in my room. (Yes/No)
11. I prefer updates regarding my status (only when asked, daily, not at all).

Appendix B

Comfort is a concept that has a strong association with nursing. Nurses traditionally provide comfort to patients and their families through interventions that can be called comfort measures. The intentional comforting actions of nurses strengthen patients and their families (who can be found in their own homes, in hospitals, agencies, communities, states, and nations). When patients and families are strengthened by actions of health care personnel (nurses!), they can better engage in *health-seeking behaviors.* The positive relationships between these deliberate nursing actions and comfort is entailed in the *first* part of Kolcaba's middle-range Theory of Comfort.

Enhanced comfort is an immediate desirable outcome of nursing care, according to Comfort Theory. In addition, it theoretically and positively correlates with desired health-seeking

Developed by students at The University of Akron and distributed with their permission: Robert Bearss, Brent Ferroni, Ryan Hartnett, Kristy Kuzmiak, Brittney Stover, Spring 2006.

behaviors (HSBs). The concept was first introduced by Schlotfeldt (1975). HSBs can be internal (healing, immune function, number of T cells, etc.), external (health-related activities, functional outcomes, etc.), or a peaceful death. The relationships between comfort and health-seeking behaviors are considered in the second part of Kolcaba's comfort theory.

Health-Seeking Behaviors (HSBs) are in reference to the small or large group of patients being analyzed. HSBs of patients or larger groups, in turn, are positively related to Institutional Integrity.

Institutional Integrity (InI) is NEWLY (Kolcaba, 2007) defined as the values, financial stability, and wholeness of health care organizations at local, regional, state, and national levels. In addition to hospital systems, the definition of "institutions" includes public health agencies, Medicare and Medicaid programs, home care agencies, and nursing home consortiums. Examples of variables related to this expanded definition of InI include cost savings, improved access, decreased morbidity rates, decreased hospitalizations and readmissions, improved health-related outcomes, efficiency of services and billing, and positive cost–benefit ratios. Relationships among comfort, HSBs, and InI constitute the third part of the theory. Tests of the theory can be on the first part, the second part, the third part, or the whole theory.

Types of comfort:

Relief: The state of having a specific comfort need met.

Ease: The state of calm or contentment.

Transcendence: The state in which one can rise above problems or pain.

Context in which comfort occurs:

Physical: Pertaining to bodily sensations and homeostatic mechanisms.

Psychospiritual: Pertaining to internal awareness of self, including esteem, concept, sexuality, meaning in one's life, and one's relationship to a higher order or being.

Environmental: Pertaining to the external background of human experience (temperature, light, sound, odor, color, furniture, landscape, etc.)

Sociocultural: Pertaining to interpersonal, family, and societal relationships (finances, teaching, health care personnel, etc.), as well as to family traditions, rituals, and religious practices.

Chapter 23

Joanne Duffy's Quality Caring Model

JOANNE R. DUFFY

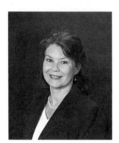

Joanne R. Duffy

Introducing the Theorist

Joanne R. Duffy, PhD, RN, FAAN, has more than 35 years of experience in clinical, administrative, and academic nursing. She is at present a professor at Indiana University School of Nursing where she teaches at the graduate level and conducts research in relationship-centered caring. Dr. Duffy graduated from St. Joseph's Hospital School of Nursing in Providence, RI, completed her BSN at Salve Regina College in Newport, RI and her master's and doctoral degrees at the Catholic University of America in Washington, DC. She is a Fellow of the American Academy of Nursing, a Magnet Hospital appraiser, and an international consultant.

Dr. Duffy has held associate director of nursing positions at two academic medical centers—George Washington University Medical Center and Georgetown University Medical Center—and has simultaneously served in academic appointments. She developed the Cardiovascular Center for Outcomes Analysis and administrated the Transplant Center at INOVA Fairfax Hospital in Virginia. She has special expertise in outcomes measurement, and the focus of her work has been on maximizing outcomes of health care recipients, particularly those with cardiovascular disease. She was a nursing consultant to the multidisciplinary study team for the national APACHE study of outcomes from intensive care and received the First Annual Health Care Research Award from the National Institute of Health Care Management for this work.

Dr. Duffy was the first to examine the link between nurse caring behaviors and patient outcomes and developed the caring assessment tool in multiple versions. She is especially interested in the hidden value of nursing's work. Dr. Duffy assisted the American Nurses Association in the development and implementation of acute care and community nursing-sensitive quality indicators and is leading a national demonstration project to ensure caring–healing–protective environments for hospitalized older adults and nurses. Dr. Duffy is an outspoken proponent of quality health care, particularly for hospitalized older adults. She has exposed the significance of nursing's work through the mid-range Quality-Caring Model© and employs innovative approaches to educate health care providers on relationship-building.

Introducing the Model

The Quality-Caring Model© was initially developed in 2003 to guide practice and research (Duffy & Hoskins, 2003). The seeds of the model were sown during discussions concerning nursing interventions, but it was informed from earlier work on caring (Duffy, 1992). While examining the outcomes variable of patient satisfaction, Dr. Duffy found that hospitalized patients who were dissatisfied often expressed, "nurses just don't seem to care." This concern was corroborated in the literature and represented a clinical problem that significantly impacted patient quality. Over time, Dr. Duffy continued to study human interactions during illness, developing tools to measure caring (Duffy, 2002; Duffy, Hoskins, & Seifert, 2007) and studying the linkage between nurse caring and selected health care outcomes (Duffy, 1992, 1993).

In 2002, it became apparent that there were few nursing theories that could guide the development of a caring-based nursing intervention while simultaneously speaking to the relationship between nurse caring and quality. As part of a research team, Drs. Duffy and Hoskins developed and tested the model in a group of heart failure patients (Duffy, Hoskins, & Dudley-Brown, 2005). Caring relationships were the core concept in this model, and were believed to be integrated, although often

hidden, in the daily work of nursing. This form of caring was considered different from the caring that occurs between family and friends because nurse caring requires specialized knowledge, attitudes, and behaviors that are directed toward health and healing. Through this specialized knowledge recipients feel "cared for," which was theorized to free them to take risks, to learn new healthy behaviors, or to participate effectively in decision-making based on evidence. This sense of "feeling cared for" was considered an antecedent necessary to influence improved intermediate and terminal outcomes, particularly nursing-sensitive outcomes such as knowledge (including self-knowledge), safety, comfort, anxiety, adherence, human dignity, health, and satisfaction. Furthermore, the model was considered supportive to professional nursing. Blending societal needs for measurable outcomes with the unique relationship-centered processes central to daily nursing practice represented a practical, postmodern approach.

The major purposes of the Quality-Caring Model© at that time were to:

- Guide professional practice
- Describe the conceptual–theoretical–empirical linkages between quality of care and human caring
- Propose a research agenda that would provide evidence of the value of nursing (Duffy & Hoskins, 2003).

Since 2003, the Quality-Caring Model© has been revised (Fig. 23-1) to meet the demands of a complex, interdependent, and global health care system that "requires a more sophisticated workforce, one that understands the significance of systems thinking, whose practice is based on knowledge, multiple and oftentimes competing connections, and one that values relationships as the basis for actions and decision-making" (Duffy, 2009, p.192). In this revised version, the link between caring relationships and quality care is even more explicit, challenging the nursing profession to use this knowledge in daily practice. The revised model is considered a middle-range

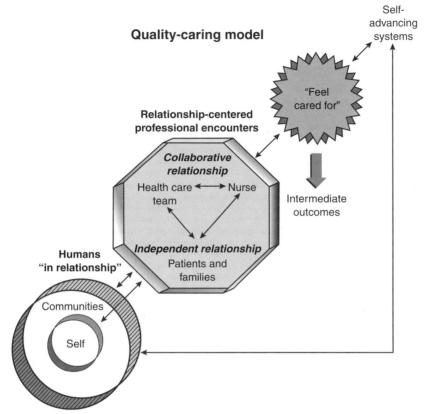

Figure 23 • 1 Revised Quality-Caring Model©. *(From Duffy, J. [2009]. Quality caring in nursing: Applying theory to clinical practice, education, and leadership [p. 198]. New York: Springer.)*

theory because it draws on others' work. It views quality as a dynamic, nonlinear characteristic that is influenced by caring relationships. When caring relationships are fully integrated aspects of nursing practice, human connections are formed that may influence future interactions with health care providers; such interactions may enhance health outcomes for patients and families. Nurses also benefit from practicing in congruence with their true nature, often deriving meaning from this work.

Concepts, Assumptions, and Propositions

In this revision of the Quality-Caring Model©, there are four main concepts. The first is *humans in relationship*. This idea refers to the notion that humans are multidimensional

beings with various characteristics that make them unique. Recognizing human characteristics, including how they differ and yet are the same, provides an understanding that influences human interactions and nursing interventions. Humans are also social beings connected to others through birth or in work, play, learning, worship, and local communities. It is through these connections that humans mature, enhance their communities, and advance.

Relationship-centered professional encounters consist of the independent relationship between the nurse and patient/family and the collaborative relationship that nurses establish with members of the health care team. When these relationships are of a caring nature, the intermediate outcome of "feeling cared for" is generated. Embedded in this concept are the caring factors that are discussed in the next section. *Feeling cared for* is a positive emotion that signifies to patients and families that they matter. It allows one to relax and feel secure about health care needs. It is an important antecedent to quality health outcomes, particularly those that are nursing-sensitive.

Patients and families who experience caring relationships with the health care team are more apt to concentrate on their health, focus on learning about it, modify lifestyles, adhere to the recommendations and regimens, and actively participate in health care decisions. They feel understood and more confident in their abilities. Over time, persons who experience caring interactions with health professionals progress to self-caring individuals. *Self-caring* is the final concept in this model. It is a human phenomenon that is stimulated by caring relationships. Self-caring is a capacity that cannot be controlled; it emerges over time driven by caring connections. Self-caring represents quality in that it is dynamic and enhances an individual's well-being. The overall purposes of the revised Quality-Caring Model© are to (1) guide professional practice and (2) provide a foundation for nursing research. It can also be used in nursing education (to guide curriculum development and facilitate caring student–teacher relationships) and in nursing leadership as a basis for human interactions and decision-making.

Assumptions of the revised Quality-Caring Model© include the following:

- Humans are multidimensional beings capable of growth and change.
- Humans exist in relationship to themselves, others, communities or groups, and nature.
- Humans evolve over time and in space.
- Humans are inherently worthy.
- Caring is embedded in the daily work of nursing.
- Caring is a tangible concept that can be measured.
- Caring relationships benefit both the one caring and the one being cared for.
- Caring relationships benefit society.
- Caring is done "in relationship."
- Feeling "cared for" is a positive emotion.

Propositions from the revised Quality-Caring Model© include:

- Human caring capacity can be developed.
- Caring relationships are composed of discrete factors.
- Caring relationships require intent, choice, specialized knowledge and skills, and time.
- Engagement in communities through caring relationships enhances self-caring.
- Independent caring relationships between patients and nurses influence feeling "cared for."
- Collaborative caring relationships among nurses and members of the health care team influence feeling "cared for."
- Feeling "cared for" is an antecedent to self-advancing systems.
- Feeling "cared for" influences the attainment of intermediate and terminal health outcomes.
- Self-advancement is a nonlinear, complex process that emerges over time and in space.
- Self-advancing systems are naturally self-caring or self-healing.
- Relationships characterized as caring contribute to individual, group, and system self-advancement (Duffy, 2009).

"**The overall role of the nurse in this model is to engage in caring relationships with self and others to engender feeling 'cared for'**" (Duffy, 2009, p. 199). Such actions positively influence intermediate and terminal health outcomes by easing anxieties and leveling the playing field for genuine reciprocal interactions. Feeling "cared for" leads the way to future interactions and may influence healing. Caring relationships also advantage nurses because sharing oneself with another authentically raises awareness and promotes self-knowing. Caring relationships enhance nursing-sensitive patient outcomes and may influence clinical autonomy (Weston, 2008).

The revised Quality-Caring Model© specifically emphasizes the following responsibilities of professional nurses:

- Attain and continuously advance knowledge and expertise in the caring factors.

- Initiate, cultivate, and sustain caring relationships with patients and families.
- Initiate, cultivate, and sustain caring relationships with other nurses and all members of the health care team.
- Maintain an awareness of the patient/family point of view.
- Carry on self-caring activities, including professional development.
- Integrate caring relationships with specific evidence-based nursing interventions to positively influence health.
- Advance quality health care through research and continuous improvement.
- Using the expertise of caring relationships embedded in nursing, actively participate in community groups.
- Contribute to the knowledge of caring and ultimately the profession of nursing, using varied approaches of inquiry.
- Maintain an open, flexible approach.

Caring Relationships

There are four caring relationships essential to quality caring (Fig. 23-2). The first is the relationship with self. Because humans are multidimensional (comprised of bio–psycho–social–cultural–spiritual components) that continuously interact in concert with the

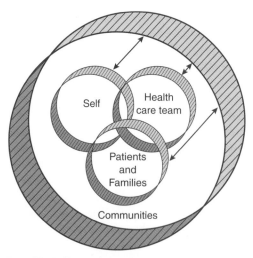

Figure 23 • 2 Four relationships necessary for quality caring.

universe, their fundamental nature is integrated or whole. The many seemingly different parts relate to and depend on each other, generating an orientation of the self that represents a source of understanding often lost in the business of life. Individuals tend to go about their day habitually moving from one task to another without noticing their internal bodily processes, feelings, or connections with others. This externally driven focus separates individuals from those internal forces that hold a special knowledge of self. In nursing, professionals care for others and their families with ease, frequently "forgetting" to connect with self. Yet, allowing oneself to slow down enough to access his or her own genuineness offers a clarity that is life-enhancing. Some would say such inner awareness is necessary for authentic interaction and health (Davidson et al., 2003), while others (Siegel, 2007) believe it is necessary to adequately care for others. As human beings, professional nurses who are regularly "in touch" with themselves set up the conditions for self-caring, a state that offers a rich supply of energy and renewal.

In nursing, remaining self aware is a necessary prerequisite for caring relationships because in knowing the self, it is possible to know others. Regular mindfulness activities such as prayer, meditation, quiet time, attention to physical health through regular exercise and proper nutrition, and creative activities, when performed in a conscious manner, promote insight. Likewise in the work environment, short pauses, consciously remembering to center on the person being cared for, attending to bodily needs such as nourishment and elimination, and even short time outs ensures that the caring focus of nursing remains the priority. Reflective awareness by actively soliciting feedback about one's performance is another method of attaining self-knowledge that may offer professional nurses a boost in self-confidence or specific learning opportunities. Reflective analysis in which thoughts are actually documented in written or taped format and then analyzed for their subjective meanings can be used to inform clinical practice. Professional nurses need to acknowledge and reflect on the important work they do in order to value themselves and nursing, a precondition for caring relationships (Foster, 2004).

As the primary focus of nursing, patients and families who are ill are vulnerable and dependent on nurses for caring. Initiating, cultivating, and sustaining caring relationships with patients and families is an independent function of professional nursing that involves intention, choice, specific knowledge and skills, and time (Duffy, 2009). Intending to care depends on one's attitudes and beliefs; it shapes a nurse's choice and resulting behaviors, specifically whether "to care" for another. Such choice is a conscious decision that is required for effective caring relationships. Deep awareness of the self enhances caring intention and consequential behaviors become more positively focused toward the patient/family.

Collaborative relationships with members of the health care team are essential to quality health care (Knaus, Draper, Wagner, & Zimmerman, 1986) and are depicted as an important relationship in the Quality-Caring Model.© Nurses are already connected to one another by the work they do, and with other members of the health team by the commonality of simultaneously providing services to patients and families. *But collaboration connotes mutual respect for the work of other health professionals and occurs "in relationship."* Ongoing interaction is key to collaboration to seek the other's point of view, validate the work, share responsibilities, and evaluate the care. The Quality-Caring Model© maintains that professional nurses have a responsibility for implementing collegial, caring interpersonal relationships with each other and members of the health care team. Discussing specific clinical issues pertinent to patients, participating in joint rounds, improving quality or research projects, holding family conferences, and discharging rounds are all examples of positive collaboration that benefit not only patients and families but the healthcare team as well. Affirming each others' unique contribution to patient care through genuine collaboration contributes to a healthy work environment that may increase work satisfaction.

Finally, caring for the communities nurses live and work in reflects a caring relationship essential to the revised Quality-Caring Model.© This relationship is predicated on the belief that humans interact with groups beyond the family to connect, share similar history and customs, and enhance the lives of each other. Engaging in communities provides professional nurses opportunities to use caring relationships as the basis for improving health or decreasing disease. Such activities contribute to the ongoing vitality of the community and enrich nurses' personal lives. The four relationships essential to quality caring when well-developed and practiced with knowledge of the caring factors meets the needs of patients and families for quality health care.

The Caring Factors

Caring is not just a mind-set or simple acts of kindness; rather, clinical caring requires knowledge (Mayerhoff, 1971) and skills. Many have theorized about the qualities necessary for therapeutic relationships (Rogers, 1961; Yalom, 1975), but Watson (1979, 1985) identified 10 factors necessary for human caring in the patient–nurse relationship. Through empirical testing, eight factors were identified in a sample of 557 medical–surgical patients that represented caring (Duffy, Hoskins, & Seifert, 2007). These factors point to the specific knowledge and skills necessary for caring relationships. The following represent the caring factors (as defined by this group of medical-surgical patients):

- Mutual problem-solving
- Attentive reassurance
- Human respect
- Encouraging manner
- Appreciation of unique meaning
- Healing environment
- Affiliation needs
- Basic human needs (Duffy, Hoskins, & Seifert, 2007)

The caring factors relate to Watson's original Carative Factors (Watson, 1979, 1985), but also are consistent with aspects of other nursing theorists' work (Swanson, 1991; Peplau, 1988; Roach, 1984; Boykin & Schoenhofer, 1993; Leininger, 1981; Nightingale, 1992; Johnson, 1990; King, 1981; Orem, 2001; Henderson, 1980; Roy, 1980) and empirical research (Cossette, Cote, Pepin, Ricard, & D'Aoust, 2006; Boudreaux, Francis, & Loyacano, 2002; Campbell & Rudisill, 2006; Mangurten et al., 2006; Paul, Hendry, & Cabrelli, 2004; Wolf, Zuzelo, Goldberg, Crothers, & Jacobson, 2006). *Mutual problemsolving* represents the largest factor and refers to assisting patients and families to learn about, question, and participate in their health or illness. This is accomplished reciprocally and requires professional interaction that is informed and engaging. This factor recognizes that patients and families are the decision-makers. Facilitating informed alternatives is crucial. *Attentive reassurance* refers to being available and offering a positive outlook to patients and families that helps them feel secure. Professional nurses who use this factor are able to "be with" their patients long enough to focus on their needs, listen, and present some cheerful dialog. *Human respect* implies valuing the person of the other by acting in such a way that demonstrates that value. For example, calling a patient by his or her preferred name, performing tasks in a gentle manner, and maintaining eye contact show regard for the other. Using an *encouraging manner* or a supportive demeanor during interactions conveys confidence in the patient and is expressed verbally and nonverbally. It is especially important to maintain uniformity between messages expressed and those implied by body language. *Appreciation of unique meanings* helps a patient feel understood because the nurse uses this factor to acknowledge what is significant to patients and families. In other words, nurses aim to see things from the patient's point of view including his or her sociocultural meanings. In this way, nurses tailor interventions in the patient's frame of reference. Cultivating a *healing environment*, including appealing surroundings, decreasing stressors (noise, lighting), ensuring patient privacy and confidentiality, and practicing in a safe manner are included in this factor. The particular norms and customs of a department to which a patient is admitted also have impact on the environment. This factor is receiving renewed interest today as professional nurses are being viewed as crucial to patient safety (Institute of Medicine, 2004). Ensuring that *basic human needs* are attended to during an illness (including the higher order needs [Maslow, 1954]) has been a major role of the professional nurse that today is often delegated to unlicensed assistive personnel. Often this factor is blended with other nursing activities such as assessments, teaching and learning, and emotional support. Providing for basic human needs is an opportunity to further the development of caring relationships. Finally, appreciating the significance of *affiliation needs* refers to making sure that patients are not only allowed access to their families, but also that families are included in care decisions. Being open and approachable to families and keeping them informed is important to patients' well-being and should be a normal part of nursing care.

The caring factors are used "in relationship" with others and comprise the "knowledge and skills" required for caring relationships. Using them is dependent on patient needs and the context of the situation. Not all factors are necessarily used at once; rather, the professional nurse uses his or her judgment to make use of them. When applied with expertise, these factors are theorized to positively impact recipients such that they feel "cared for." In fact, "feeling cared for" is calming to the patient, leaving him or her to concentrate on the meaning of illness and the requirements for health and healing. Feeling cared for also sets up the conditions for future interactions that eventually lead to outcomes of care. "In other words, the patient's ability to progress is mediated somewhat by the feelings generated as a consequence of caring relationships" (Duffy, 2009). Performing nursing in such a way that valuable time is spent predominantly in caring relationships with patients and families (i.e., using the caring factors) ensures that patients and families feel "cared for" and that health outcomes are positively impacted.

The caring factors are applicable to the other three relationships pertinent to the Quality-Caring Model©. For example, collaborative relationships founded on the caring factors enhance teamwork and cooperation. As experts in caring, professional nurses are in a unique position to profoundly benefit the health care system. Uniting caring knowledge and caring action/s in relationships with self, patients and families, coworkers, and the community provides opportunities for creative innovations, improvements in practice, and a source of energy for future interactions. Furthermore, some nurses who practice this way describe richer work experiences that are naturally renewing (D'Antonio, 2008).

Applications of the Model

The Quality-Caring Model© provides the clinician with a way of practicing nursing that is primarily relationship-centered. In doing so, it honors the interdependencies necessary for human advancement. It provides a "way of being with" patients and families through the caring factors that can be used to guide nursing interventions and ongoing learning about the self. The model offers a way to relate to and engage with other health care providers and the community. In addition, because caring relationships can be measured and their consequences assessed, the model affords an evaluation design for improvement of services. Specific nursing-sensitive outcomes are likely to be influenced through use of the model so it becomes useful as a foundation for research. Lastly, using the Quality-Caring Model© purports to benefit professional nurses as well as patients and families.

Practice Exemplar

Mr. N is a 56-year-old man with amyotrophic lateral sclerosis who lives at home with his wife. He has been living with the disease for several years and is a quadriplegic who is wheelchair bound. Mr. N and his wife invested in an expensive electronic wheelchair that can support his computer system, which he uses for communication and work activities. Mr. N is a computer programmer who still works at home through this system. He communicates a little verbally, but mostly he uses his eyes in a signaling system that his wife taught him. His secretions have been gradually getting worse (despite medications) and he had a gastrostomy tube placed 4 months ago because swallowing was becoming unbearable. His pulmonary function studies were normal and his neurologist suggested that he consider an elective tracheostomy to avert an emergency. Mr. N subsequently entered a large teaching magnet hospital at

7:30 A.M. to have this surgery performed. He arrived in his wheelchair accompanied by his wife. He was nervous about the procedure, not only related to the surgery itself, but also because he knew he would not be able to talk afterwards. The admitting office was busy so the technician took his time gathering insurance information and then wheeled Mr. N down to the preop area. He sat in the wheelchair for 45 minutes until a nurse, who was busy on the phone, arrived. She introduced herself and stated that he should undress and get in bed so she could begin her assessment. Mr. N's wife undressed him, as she always does at home, and then asked for help getting him in bed. A tech came to help and Mr. N was placed safely in the hospital bed. The nurse returned with a clipboard and began her assessment, collecting pertinent history. Then she began a physical assessment. Her resultant problem list consisted

Continued

Practice Exemplar cont.

of two problems: shortness of breath due to inadequate airway clearance and inadequate mobility. She told Mr. N a little about the upcoming surgery and asked his wife to sign the consent papers. The anesthesiologist arrived to start the anesthesia, so Mrs. N kissed her husband and he was wheeled into the OR. In an hour, he was in the recovery area and when Mrs. N saw her husband, he was swollen around the eyes, teary, and extremely anxious. He was attached to a ventilator, but he was able to take his own breath some of the time. He was looking around, eyes darting from person to person with obvious fright. Since he could not move on his own, his wife, who understood his anxiety, sat by his side and used their communication system to "talk" to him. He told her he felt like he couldn't breathe. Mrs. N, in turn, relayed this to the nurse who asked her to tell him that this was a normal feeling after a trach. Mr. N continued to experience anxiety, often coughing, and was eventually placed in the farthest bed so as to not disturb the other patients. Unfortunately, Mrs. N could not allay his concerns and he continued to feel anxious and distressed.

It was 5:00 P.M. and Mr. N was doing well according to the nurses in the post-anesthesia care unit (PACU); they began his discharge by searching for an ICU bed, but there were no available beds in this busy teaching hospital. Unfortunately, Mr. N had to stay in the PACU overnight until an ICU bed became available. Two other patients were also staying overnight. The PACU nurses were unhappy with this arrangement because it meant two of them would have to stay on call to staff the unit. They were overheard talking to each other, saying, "If I had wanted to work on a surgical floor, I wouldn't have applied to the PACU." Mr. N continued to display anxiety, often gagging and looking fearful with his eyes. His wife could not help him because she didn't know enough about the procedure to answer his questions. She thought maybe he was in pain, but he denied this. He continued to remain lying in the bed with his frightened

look. The wife asked the PACU nurses for help in figuring out what was wrong, but they saw that his vital signs, blood gasses, and dressing were normal. One nurse decided to suction him but there were few secretions. Her technique was rather rough, Mr. N grimaced with pain, and Mrs. N asked if it would always be this way. The nurse said it would get better with time and went over to talk to the other nurse. Mr. N remained anxious throughout the night while his wife sat by his side. Neither of them slept. He was taken to the intermediate care unit at 8:30 A.M.

On this unit, Mr. N was cared for by a young nurse named Molly who had graduated 2 years earlier. Molly stopped briefly to slow herself down and readjust her thoughts toward Mr. N before she entered his room. Taking a couple of slow deep breaths, Molly entered the room and quickly scanned the environment and the patient to notice anything significant. She introduced herself by name and then looked Mr. N in the eyes, smiled, and squeezed his hand lightly *(human respect)*. Then she asked what he would like to be called while he stayed with them and wrote that name on a board on the wall opposite his bed. Since he couldn't talk, Molly asked Mrs. N to explain the communication system they used at home and she tried it with Mr. N to better understand his needs. Using the Quality Caring Model© as a frame of reference, Molly completed a physical assessment that included physiological, emotional, sociocultural, and spiritual components. Her goal was to use this opportunity to initiate a caring relationship with Mr. N and his wife that could grow and be sustained throughout the hospitalization experience. Through this process, Molly came to know Mr. N as a software engineer who still worked from home, had a married adult daughter and two grandchildren, is an avid tennis fan (had been a player before his illness), and who was anxious and tired. She also learned he received his diagnosis 8 years earlier and had progressively become weaker and eventually wheelchair bound. His father had died of a heart attack at 63 years of age and his mother was alive and well, living in upstate New York. Mr. N was taking a diuretic and an angiotensin-converting enzyme (ACE) inhibitor for hypertension and medication to reduce his pulmonary secretions. His vital signs were good. Although he was slightly tachycardic with a heart rate of 112, his neck dressing was dry and his back showed evidence of a beginning pressure ulcer at the coccyx region. Mrs. N, who was all of 110 pounds, relayed her difficulty in caring for Mr. N while she worked full time as a security analyst. This couple regularly visited with a Lutheran minister who had been a family friend for years. This physical assessment time provided Molly the opportunity to understand the unique human being (Mr. N) in relationship to his family, his work, and life role *(appreciation of unique meanings)* and to begin a relationship-centered professional encounter that was based on these findings.

She documented the results of the assessment in the computer, looking frequently at Mr. N so he could see her. The problem list Molly came up with included issues such as airway maintenance, anxiety, impaired communication, altered family processes, impaired physical mobility, potential skin breakdown, inadequate knowledge, and hypertension. Then she sat down and using the caring factor, *mutual problem solving,* explained to Mr. and Mrs. N what would happen on this unit, including how long the couple might stay, and how and when to contact her. She engaged participation by inviting questions and asked them for guidance regarding Mr. N's normal routines. She relayed that she would be there all day and gave them her telephone number. Then she asked them what they knew about recovering from a trach and listened attentively to their responses. She sat a little toward the patient and looked at him as he "talked." This took longer than usual because he used the alphabet to spell out words *(encouraging manner)*. She explained a little about living with a trach, but together they decided to wait until after they had some sleep to review trach care. Molly

assured them that they had the capacity to live well with this chronic disease, using examples of what she had already observed about the couple *(attentive reassurance)*. Molly then asked Mrs. N if she wanted something to drink and made sure Mr. N was hydrated as well. Then she offered him mouth care and turned him slightly to the side with a pillow behind his back. Molly closed the blinds and offered Mrs. N a pillow and a reclining chair and let them sleep for 2 hours, as they had been up all night *(healing environment)*. She put a sign on the door reminding others that the patient was sleeping *(basic human needs and affiliation needs)*. For the first time in more than 24 hours, Mr. N was able to relax and shut his eyes, showing evidence of feeling "cared for."

Molly's professional encounter with this couple was relaxed, genuine, and distinguished by the caring factors. With only 2 years' experience, Molly was competent in their use. Molly's focus and knowledge of herself provided the strength to meet this couple's needs. During the time they were resting, Molly checked on the couple quietly and frequently *(healing environment)*. At one of these opportunities, Mrs. N sought out Molly to relay her anxieties about taking Mr. N home with the trach. Molly listened and encouraged Mrs. N to adjust first to this new environment while she (Molly) would come back later to help them understand how to live with a trach *(affiliation needs)*.

Molly also spent some time completing Mr. N's care plan. She listed his problems and developed some interventions based on her knowledge of his family situation, his own routines, and their joint interactions. When the surgeon came for rounds, Molly accompanied him and they conversed about Mr. N's vital signs, dressing, and secretions. Including Mr. N in the discussions, they asked how he was feeling and he communicated with Molly's help. During a conversation at the nurses' station, both professionals agreed that Mr. N could go home with support the next day. The surgeon relied on Molly's judgment about Nr. N's readiness for discharge because

Continued

he had come to know her these last 2 years as a competent and caring nurse. Molly trusted her recommendations; their encounter was collaborative and friendly.

Later that day, Molly returned with a written set of instructions about caring for trachs. She reviewed the instructions with both Mr. and Mrs. N, answering questions, allowing Mrs. N to "practice" with the suction catheters. She used a positive approach, reassuring Mrs. N that she could do this and that she would be there in a couple of hours to review the procedure again *(attentive reassurance and encouraging manner)*. Molly then called the social worker and the home care team to get things rolling for discharge. During report, Molly reviewed Mr. N's problem list and her recommended interventions to the oncoming nurse, including those she had initiated. She felt good that Mr. and Mrs. N were learning about the trach and pleased that she had relieved some of their anxiety. She said good-bye to all her patients and went to her weekly yoga class to unwind. The next morning, Molly had the same assignment and worked with Mr. and Mrs. N to ensure their self-caring needs were met.

Although this "case" is typical in many acute care facilities, Mr. N is a unique individual who experienced two different nursing encounters. In the first instance, one might say that his physical needs were met, yet he was not affirmed as the one being treated (the nurses talked to his wife about him), he was not adequately assessed by the preop nurse, he remained anxious for many hours postop, was isolated from others, didn't sleep, overheard professional nurses talking about not wanting to be there, was treated roughly, and was not turned for 12 hours despite the fact that he was paralyzed. On the intermediate care unit, the nurse used the caring factors to initiate and cultivate a caring relationship with him from admission. She used this relationship as the basis for care that included attention to his basic needs for sleep, comfort, and nutrition. Molly helped Mr. N understand his new situation and included his wife, who would be his caretaker. She was collaborative with the physician and positive in her demeanor. She referred to the patient as Mr. N and used her time appropriately to ensure that his transition to home would occur safely. In essence, this nurse saw the patient as a whole person, not a physical body with a trach, and used her caring knowledge and skills to build a relationship that generated trust and security. Through ongoing interaction, a connection developed between the nurse and patient that provided the insight necessary for effectively following the nursing process including specific interventions and evaluation. Although the tasks she performed were routine in nature, this nurse balanced doing with being caring. The caring relationship she established created a higher quality nursing care that benefited both the patient and the nurse.

Acknowledging the unique caring nature of nursing and demonstrating a professional commitment to it offers a way for nursing to help patients make sense of their illnesses. It also provides an opportunity for nursing to claim a unique place in the health care system by generating evidence of the value of caring through research.

Evaluating and Improving Caring Practice

The Quality-Caring Model© maintains that quality nursing care is based on the use of best evidence and asserts that it is a nursing responsibility to gather and use such evidence in daily practice. This means that professional nurses must be competent in evaluating their practice, critically appraising caring research in order to judge its trustworthiness and participate in ongoing evaluation and research concerning caring.

Evaluation of nursing practice is an ongoing process that is usually based on performance behaviors or competency statements. It is important to begin evaluation by first artic-ulating the caring factors because they provide the attitudes and behaviors required in caring relationships. The caring factors can be used to develop competency statements or per-formance expectations from which individual nurses can complete self-evaluations or gather peer evaluations that nursing leaders can use in annual evaluations. A more comprehensive approach using the 360 method (Edwards & Ewen, 1996; London & Smither, 1995) pro-vides assessments from the perspective of the one being evaluated (nurse self-evaluation), those being "cared for" (patients and families), the supervisor, and colleagues (other nurses, physicians, other members of the health care team). Using the perspective of the patient (the one being "cared for") directly points to ways nurses can improve their practice. The 360 approach to evaluating caring compe-tence is thorough and relationship centered; it takes advantage of multiple sources and per-spectives to provide important feedback about nursing practice.

Effectively appraising caring research informs nursing practice by providing evi-dence that can guide nursing interventions. Unit-based journal clubs, nursing rounds, or even quality improvement data can provide forums for such appraisal. Translating find-ings of such research into practice and evalu-ating the outcomes provide opportunities for improvement.

Because the model provides a set of con-cepts, assumptions, and propositions, ques-tions generated from these theoretical ideas can provide the basis for research. For example, the proposition, "feeling cared for influences the attainment of ...health outcomes" (Duffy, 2009, p. 199) could be tested by linking the results of an instrument measuring caring with a set of specific patient outcomes. In fact, nurse researchers have investigated this and found some evidence that caring is linked to patient satisfaction, postoperative recovery, and decreased anxiety (Burt, 2007; Swan, 1998; Wolf, Zuzelo, Goldberg, Crothers, & Jacobson, 1998). Others have developed car-ing nursing interventions and used them to study effects on specific patient outcomes (Duffy, Hoskins, & Dudley-Brown, 2005; Erci et al., 2003). Such research adds to the knowledge base and offers implications for the improvement of nursing practice. Study-ing caring through research is important to provide evidence of nursing's contribution to health care and to advance the profession. Such evidence provides policymakers with documentation of nursing's value that may impact important decisions such as funding, job descriptions, promotion and advance-ment, and staffing. To that end, the Quality-Caring Model© provides a foundation for research. Ensuring that results are disseminated quickly to the nursing community through publications and presentations is a nursing responsibility that can advance caring science.

At the systems level, assessing caring on a unit or organizational basis provides some evidence of how well professional practice models are integrated into practice and points to performance improvement recommenda-tions. Many tools exist that are available to assist this process (Watson, 2002). However, they vary in terms of how they define caring, the approach, how they are administered and scored, whose view they are obtaining (e.g., patients, nurses, or others), and validity and reliability. Only a few directly gather informa-tion from patients. This is an important component of assessment because the one being "cared for" is the direct source of knowl-edge and others' opinions may not be consis-tent. One instrument, the *Caring Assessment Tool*® (CAT) (Duffy, Hoskins, & Seifert, 2007), a 36-item instrument designed to cap-ture patients' perceptions of nurse caring, has been used with success in many health care institutions. This tool has established validity and reliability and is available in English, Spanish, and Japanese. Using this tool pro-vides an evaluation of nurse caring behaviors as perceived by patients that can be used for performance improvement and practice revi-sions. Another instrument that was adapted from the CAT© is the Caring Assessment Tool for Administration (Duffy, 2002). This tool is a 39-item questionnaire that assesses how nurses perceive nurse manager caring behaviors and has become important in the assessment of caring practice environments. Many other instruments exist to measure caring, however, ensuring that the conceptual base, population and setting, and perspective of the respondent are consistent with your own are vital to successful evaluation.

A recent innovative project that allows multiple institutions to benchmark their caring knowledge is the International Caring Comparative Database© (ICCD) (Duffy & Brewer, in press). This ongoing quality improvement initiative includes several acute care institutions that routinely (quarterly) collect patient level caring data. The participating institutions receive reports that allow clinicians and administrators to benchmark themselves with other institutions, monitor improvements in nursing practice, link caring processes with nursing-sensitive outcomes measures, and assess how structural indicators such as staffing patterns or nurse credentials affect caring processes.

Up until now, weaknesses in caring evaluation and research including the lag behind new caring theories, the vagueness between findings and components of theory, measurement issues, and poorly designed studies with small and/or nonprobability samples have created gaps in caring knowledge. Linking caring to nursing-sensitive patient outcomes, improving existing caring instruments, caring-based interventional research, educational caring, and cost–benefit analyses are urgently needed to provide evidence of nursing's value. Using rigorous methods, research that builds on the work of others and includes multiple patient populations and settings would test the validity of caring theories and advance nursing practice.

■ Summary

Practice-based knowledge is a hallmark of a profession; therefore, a strong alignment between a theory and the practice of it enhances its significance to society. Caring and quality in health care are implicitly tied together. Because humans exist in relation to others, caring relationships facilitate human advancement and the future interactions so necessary for excellent health care. Independent and collaborative caring relationships in health care contribute to patients' welfare in that they promote comfort, safety, consistent communication, and learning. Professional nurses who regularly relate to themselves and their communities are more equipped to engage in genuine independent and collaborative caring relationships with patients and families as well as advance their own self-caring. Spending time "in relationship" focuses attention on the patient versus the disease or task and generates a meaningful practice that is the basis for joy. In essence, the model benefits both patients and nurses, the profession, and the health care system. Theory-guided, evidence-based professional practice that is holistic and meaningful can make a profound impact on patient outcomes.

Implications of the revised Quality-Caring Model© exist for educators to help students learn caring. Using values-based methods with meaningful evaluation techniques and frequent caring student–teacher interactions, nurse educators can greatly enhance learning outcomes. Clinical courses in which caring behaviors are valued and role-modeled by faculty are essential. It is crucial that those nurses in leadership positions create caring–healing–protective environments for staff and patients in a cost-effective manner. Redesigning professional work so that its primary function is relationship centered and decisions are participative is paramount to quality caring. Finally, showing evidence of nursing's foremost professional purpose (caring) through ordinary everyday caring actions blended with a culture of continuous inquiry creates novel possibilities for advancing the profession.

Institutions Using the Quality–Caring Model© as the Foundation for Professional Practice

Holy Cross Hospital, Silver Spring, MD

St. Alphonsus Medical Center, Boise, ID

Children's Mercy Hospital, Kansas City, MO

St. Joseph's Medical Center, Towson, MD

Johns Hopkins–Bayview, Baltimore, MD

Virginia Hospital Center Emergency Department, Arlington, VA

Spectrum Health, Grand Rapids, MI

Nashoba Valley Hospital, Ayer, MA

Lowell General Hospital, Lowell, MA

Northern Michigan Medical Center, Petrosky, MI

Institutions Participating in the International Caring Comparative Database (ICCD)©

John C. Lincoln Memorial Hospital, Scottsdale, AZ

Scottsdale Healthcare, Scottsdale, AZ

St. Mary's Bon Secours Hospital, Richmond, VA

Memorial Regional Hospital, Mechanicsville, VA

St. Francis Hospital, Charleston, SC

Wake Forest Baptist Medical Center, Winston-Salem, NC

Mayo Hospitals and Clinics, Scottsdale, AZ

Miami Baptist Hospital, Miami, FL

Jacksonville Baptist Health System (five hospitals), Jacksonville, FL

References

Boudreaux, E. C., Francis, J. L., & Loyacano, T. (2002). Family presence during invasive procedures and resuscitations in the emergency department: A critical review and suggestions for future research. *Annals of Emergency Medicine, 40*, 193–205.

Boykin, A., & Schoenhofer, S. (1993). *Nursing as caring: A model for transforming practice.* New York: National League for Nursing Press.

Burt, K. (2007). The relationship between nurse caring and selected outcomes of care in hospitalized older adults. *Dissertation Abstracts International* (UMI No. 3257620).

Campbell, P., & Rudisill, P. (2006). Psychosocial needs of the critically ill obstetric patient: The nurse's role. *Critical Care Nursing Quarterly, 29*(10), 77–80.

Cossette, S., Cote, J. K., Pepin, J., Ricard, N., & D'Aoust, L. X. (2006). A dimensional structure of nurse–patient interactions from a caring perspective: refinement of the Caring Nurse–Patient Interaction Scale (CNPI-Short Scale). *Journal of Advanced Nursing 55*(2), 198–214.

D'Antonio, M. (2008). Why I almost quit nursing. *Johns Hopkins Nursing, 6*(2), 34–35.

Davidson, R. J., Kabat-Zinn, J., Schumaker, J., Rosenkranz, M., Muller, D., & Santorelli, S. F. (2003). Alterations in brain and immune function produced by mindfulness meditation. *Psychosomatic Medicine, 65*(4), 564–570.

Donabedian, A. (1966). Evaluating the quality of medical care. *Milbank Memorial Fund Quarterly: Health and Society, 44*(3, pt. 2),166–203.

Duffy, J. (1992). Impact of nurse caring on patient outcomes. In: D. A. Gaut (Ed.), *The presence of caring in Nursing* (pp. 113–136). New York: National League for Nursing Press.

Duffy, J. (1993). Caring behaviors of nurse managers: Relationships to staff nurse satisfaction and retention. In: D. Gaut (Ed.), *A global agenda for caring* (pp. 365–377). New York: National League for Nursing Press.

Duffy, J. (2002). The Caring Assessment Tool – Adm version. In: J. Watson (Ed.), *Instruments for assessing and measuring caring in nursing and health sciences.* New York: Springer.

Duffy, J. (2009). *Quality caring in nursing: Applying theory to clinical practice, education, and leadership.* New York: Springer.

Duffy, J., & Brewer, B. (in press). The International Caring Comparative Database (ICCD): Results from a pilot study of twelve hospitals. *JONA*

Duffy, J., & Hoskins, L. (2003). The Quality-Caring Model®: Blending dual paradigms, *Advances in Nursing Science, 26*(1), 77–88.

Duffy, J., Hoskins, L. M., & Dudley-Brown, S. (2005). Development and testing of a caring-based intervention for older adults with heart failure. *Journal of Cardiovascular Nursing, 20*(5), 325–333.

Duffy, J., Hoskins, L. M., & Seifert, R. F. (2007). Dimensions of caring: Psychometric properties of the caring assessment tool. *Advances in Nursing Science, 30*(3), 235–245.

Duffy, J., Larochelle, D., & Walsh, T. (in press). Externally benchmarking nurse caring: The International Caring Comparative Database.© *Journal of Nursing Care Quality.*

Duffy, J. (2009). *Quality Caring in Nursing: Applying Theory to Clinical Practice, Education, and Leadership.* New York: Springer Pubishing.

Edwards, M., & Ewen, A. J. (1996). *360 Degree feedback: The powerful new model for employee assessment &*

performance improvement. New York: American Management Association.

Erci, B., Sayan, A., Tortumluoag, G., Kilic, D., Sahin, O., & Gungurmus, A. (2003). The effectiveness of Watson's caring model on the quality of life and blood pressure on patients with hypertension. *Journal of Advanced Nursing, 41*(2), 130–139.

Foster, R. (2004). Self-care: Why is it so hard? *Journal of Specialists in Pediatric Nursing, 9*(4), 111–112.

Henderson, V. (1980). Nursing – yesterday and tomorrow. *Nursing Times, 76,* 905–907.

Institute of Medicine (2004). *Keeping patients safe: Transforming the work environment of nurses.* Washington, DC: author.

Johnson, D. E. (1990). The behavioral system model for nursing. In: M. E. Parker (Ed.), *Nursing theories in practice* (pp. 23–32). New York: National League for Nursing Press.

King, I. (1981). *A theory for nursing: Systems, concepts, process.* New York: John Wiley & Sons.

Knaus, W. A., Draper, E. A., Wagner, D. P., & Zimmerman, J. E. (1986). An evaluation of outcome from intensive care in major medical centers. *Annals of Internal Medicine, 104,* 410–418.

Leininger, M. M. (1981). The phenomenon of caring: Importance of research and theoretical considerations. In: M. M. Leininger (Ed.), *Caring: An essential human need.* Thorofare, NJ: Slack.

London, M., & Smither, J. W. (1995). Can multisource feedback change perceptions of goal accomplishments, self evaluations, and performance-related outcomes? Theory based applications and directions for research. *Personnel Psychology, 48,* 803–839.

Mangurten, J., Scott, S., Guzzetta, C., Clark, A. P., Vinson, L., Sperry, J., Hicks, B., Voelmeck, W. (2006). Effects of family presence during resuscitation and invasive procedures in a pediatric emergency department. *Journal of Emergency Nursing, 32*(3), 225–233.

Maslow, A. (1954). *Motivation and personality.* New York: Harper.

Mayerhoff, M. (1971). *On Caring.* New York: Harper & Row.

Nightingale, F. (1992). *Notes on nursing* (Com. Ed). Philadelphia: Lippincott.

Orem, D. (2001). *Nursing concepts of practice* (6th ed.). Wilkes Barre, PA: C. V. Mosby.

Paul, F., Hendry, C., & Cabrelli, L. (2004). Meeting patient and relatives' information needs upon transfer from an intensive care unit: The development and evaluation of an information booklet. *Journal of Clinical Nursing, 13,* 396–405.

Peplau, H. E. (1988). *Interpersonal relations in nursing.* New York: Springer.

Roach, S. (1984). *Caring: The human mode of being: Implications for nursing – perspectives in caring* (Monograph 1). Toronto, CA: Faculty of Nursing, University of Toronto.

Rogers, C. (1961). On becoming a person: A therapist's view of psychotherapy. *Archives of General Psychiatry, 62,* 1377–1384.

Roy, C. (1980). The Roy adaptation model. In: J. P. Riehl & C. Roy (Eds.), *Conceptual models for nursing practice* (2nd ed., pp. 179–188). New York: Appleton-Century-Crofts.

Siegel, D. J. (2007). *The mindful brain.* New York: W. W. Norton.

Swan, B. (1998). Postoperative nursing care contributions to symptom distress and functional status after ambulatory surgery. *MEDSURG Nursing, 7*(3), 148–158.

Swanson, K. (1991). Empirical development of a middle range theory of caring. *Nursing Research, 40,* 161–166.

Watson, J. (1979). *Nursing: The philosophy and science of caring.* Boston: Little, Brown (2nd printing 1985). Boulder, CO: Colorado University Press.

Watson, J. (1985). *Nursing: Human science and human care.* New York: National League for Nursing Press.

Watson, J. (2002). *Instruments for assessing and measuring caring in nursing and health sciences.* New York: Springer.

Weston, M. (2008). Defining control over nursing practice and autonomy. *Journal of Nursing Administration, 38*(9), 404–408.

Wolf, Z. R., Colahan, M., & Costello, A. (1998). Relationship between nurse caring and patient satisfaction. *MEDSURG Nursing, 72*(2), 99–105.

Wolf, Z. R., Zuzelo, P. R., Goldberg, E., Crothers, R., & Jacobson, N. (2006). The Caring Behaviors Inventory for Elders: Inventory for Elders: Development and psychometric characteristics. *International Journal for Human Caring, 10*(1), 49–59.

Yalom, I. D. (1975). *The theory and practice of group psychotherapy.* New York: Basic Books.

Chapter 24

Pamela Reed's Theory of Self-transcendence

PAMELA G. REED

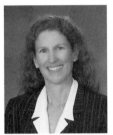

Pamela G. Reed

Introducing the Theorist

Pamela G. Reed is a professor at the University of Arizona College of Nursing in Tucson. She received her academic degrees from Wayne State University in Detroit, Michigan: a BSN and an MSN with a double major in Child & Adolescent Psychiatric–Mental Health Nursing and Nursing Education, which prepared her both as a clinical nurse specialist and nurse educator. In 1982, Dr. Reed received her PhD from Wayne State University, majoring in nursing research and theory with a minor in lifespan development and aging.

Dr. Reed was one of the first in the discipline to study spirituality as an area of scientific inquiry in nursing. She developed two widely used research instruments, the *Spiritual Perspective Scale* and the *Self-Transcendence Scale*. Her research in spirituality, mental health and well-being, and end of life has been strongly influenced by Martha Rogers' perspective of nursing and by lifespan development theories. She developed her nursing theory of self-transcendence based on her research and her developmental perspective of correlates of well-being. Her theory has been widely published and is used by many nursing students and researchers.

Dr. Reed is a fellow in the American Academy of Nursing and is a member of a number of professional organizations including Sigma Theta Tau International, the American Nurses Association, and the Society of Rogerian Scholars. She serves on editorial review boards of numerous journals and as contributing editor for a *Nursing Science Quarterly* column, Scholarly Dialogue. Reed is co-editor of a nursing theory text, *Perspectives on Nursing Theory*, now in its 5th edition.

Since January 1983 Dr. Reed has been on the University of Arizona faculty, where she teaches, writes, conducts research, and has served as Associate Dean for Academic Affairs for 7 years. She has received many teaching awards from faculty peers and students. In addition to her research publications, she frequently writes about the philosophical and theoretical dimensions of nursing with a focus on practice-based knowledge development. She lives with her husband and two daughters in the Tucson, Arizona desert.

Overview of the Theory

The theory of self-transcendence, like theories in general, is a compressed description of a phenomenon or process, which in this case is *self-transcendence*. The theory does not provide every instance and detail of self-transcendence. As it was once stated about Kepler's theory of planetary motion, the theory does not catalog "every position of every planet at every moment in time" (Kauffman, 1995, p. 22). Similarly, humans are too complex and unpredictable for a nursing theory to catalog all instances of self-transcendence. Rather, the theory consists of key concepts and propositions that describe the process of self-transcendence. In addition, theories are open systems that thrive in disequilibrium and need continued input to sustain their dynamic structure and usefulness. As such, I invite you to consider new ideas that *you* may have about how to apply, refine, or extend the theory of self-transcendence.

The focus of the theory of self-transcendence for nursing practice is on facilitating self-transcendence for the purpose of enhancing well-being. Theories from other sciences, such as psychology, may also address self-transcendence. However, what distinguishes this particular theory as a *nursing* theory is its inclusion of well-being of the whole person in the context of health experiences.

The theory proposes that when people face life-threatening illness or undergo health-related changes that intensify one's awareness of vulnerability, there may be a readiness or need to expand (or transcend) the self-boundary to integrate those changes in order to achieve a sense of well-being. Individuals often do this themselves, but in times of difficulty nurses and other health professionals can help in this process.

The original thinking for the theory of self-transcendence derived from a life-span developmental view of aging and mental health (Reed, 1983) coupled with Martha Rogers' (1970, 1980) conceptual system that describes the living processes of humans. When Reed's theory was first developed more than 15 years ago, it focused on self-transcendence as it emerges in later adulthood. However, the scope of the theory has been extended beyond this focus to address self-transcendence as a resource for well-being across the lifespan, particularly in times of serious health events where there is a heightened sense of vulnerability or mortality. This change in scope was suggested by findings of studies in which self-transcendence was measured in adolescents, young and middle-aged adults, as well as older adults. Chronological age is important in self-transcendence only insofar as advanced age, like health experiences at any age, may influence an expanded awareness of self in relation to human mortality and the greater environment and universe.

Assumptions

All theories are built upon various beliefs and philosophic ideas called *assumptions* that are considered to be generally true and accepted by the discipline. Unlike the *propositions* of a theory, *assumptions* are neither directly tested nor applied in research and practice. Instead, they support the development of ideas in a theory. Two key assumptions underlie the theory of self-transcendence and reflect ideas about humans as dynamic, open living systems. They derive from lifespan developmental theory and nursing theory.

Potential for Well-Being: A Nursing Process

The first major assumption of the self-transcendence theory is that humans possess an inner potential for healing, growth and well-being throughout the lifespan. This inner potential for well-being has been described most broadly as a *nursing process* (Reed, 1997), arguing that nurses focus their practice and study on *nursing* processes, much like chemists study chemical processes, sociologists study social processes, and developmentalists study developmental processes.

An underlying mechanism useful in explaining this inner potential for well-being is called *self-organization*, referring to a pattern in living systems of increasing complexity and organization over time (Kauffman, 1995; Reed, 1983). Self-organization occurs across living systems. According to the lifespan developmental perspective (Lerner, 2002), increasing complexity and organization is a fundamental pattern of change in *developmental* processes. Similarly, it is assumed that self-organization is fundamental in what I have called *nursing processes*, by which individuals and groups attain healing and well-being (Reed, 1997). What promotes human development is assumed to also facilitate a sense of well-being.

Martha Rogers' (1970, 1980) *principle of helicy* supports this idea of an inner nursing process of well-being: her principle proposes that human change is *innovative*, as well as irreversible and often unpredictable. This capacity for innovation is reflected in individuals' ability to undergo positive changes and experience well-being, even in difficult health experiences such as facing a terminal illness or end-of-life caregiving. Acknowledging an inner potential for well-being can be a source of hope in illness and end of life.

This idea of inherent nursing processes of well-being is related to familiar concepts like "inner healing" and "self-healing" described in other disciplines. But the nursing perspective emphasizes a potential for healing independent of biophysical perfection or medical cure. Biophysical health may play an important role in the process, but it is not essential. For example, sense of well-being may be experienced among dying or chronically ill individuals.

Although people possess this innovative capacity for well-being, the process may be difficult and require others' help. Serious health events as well as other crises tend to increase complexity in life that can diminish well-being unless the individual is able to integrate and organize the complexity. For example, serious health events confront the individual and family with new people and technology, new choices, lifestyle changes, new worries and fears, new decisions to be made, and new self-image. As health crises increase the complexity in persons' lives, a role of nursing is to help them organize and integrate this complexity by (1) providing critical information; (2) guiding them in ways to integrate the needed changes into their lives; and (3) supporting their efforts to find meaning in the situation by being a good listener, validating their feelings, and guiding them in identifying their strengths as well as areas where professional help may be needed.

To conclude, a basic assumption of the theory is that people possess a self-organizing potential that, when applied to nursing situations, is interpreted as a nursing process that promotes well-being. Self-transcendence is an example of humans' inherent nursing processes of well-being; it is one means of integrating and organizing complexity in life to promote well-being. Nurses in practice may discover other nursing processes by which healing and sense of well-being occur in patients. Ideas about other nursing processes can generate new nursing theories.

The Self-Boundary and Pandimensionality

Self-transcendence involves expanding the self-boundary. Underlying this idea is a second assumption that humans, as open systems, impose a conceptual boundary on their "openness" to define their reality and provide a sense of identity and security. This assumption is based on ideas from developmental psychology on the development of self-identity and from Rogers' (1970) early writings about human well-being and perceived boundaries.

In reference to *developmental* science, it is known that perceptions of self and the world change across the lifespan as persons become more differentiated, more complex, and define their identity. For example, theorists have identified the diffuse boundary between infant and parent: the increased sense of identity and self-consciousness in children and adolescents as they clarify their boundary between self and others; the increased differentiation of self and more secure sense of identity in middle adulthood; and the complex forms of self and connections to others in later adulthood and end of life.

In reference to *nursing* science, the theory of self-transcendence focuses on the perceived self-boundary that fluctuates during health-related events, which are like mini-developmental events in life. While developmental psychologists focus their theories and research on ontogenetic changes (change across decades), nurses focus their theories and practice on microgenetic change (changes that occur during health experiences in terms of hours, days, weeks, or months).

The self-boundary is reflected in perspectives regarding the inner-self: the relatedness of self to others, environment and nature, machines and technology; and the perceptions about relationships between body–mind–spirit, life, and death.

Rogers (1970, 1980, 1990) ideas challenged nurses' thinking about the usual boundaries between person and environment, and among past, present, and future. She proposed that humans were really infinite in space and time, extending beyond the "discernible mass" we identify as the human body, and without boundaries. She used the term *pandimensionality* (revised from the former terms *four-dimensionality* and *multidimensionality*) to express the unbounded nature of humans, even though she acknowledged that people perceive self-boundaries. Her principle of *integrality* emphasizes a fundamental connectedness between people and their environment. In addition, her concept of *relative present* challenged conventional distinctions among past, present, and future to emphasize instead the importance of the individual's own temporal perspective.

In summary, assumptions about pandimensionality and temporal perspective, which underlie the theory of self-transcendence, also may be considered in terms of how they are reflected in individuals' self-boundaries. For example, people may perceive death as a wall or a window. Dr. Rogers refrained from using the term *death* to describe the changes witnessed at end of life because the word *death* implied a boundary she thought was artificial and misrepresented the nature of human beings. Nevertheless, people impose boundaries on themselves in their journey through life in ways that can influence well-being. A person's self-boundary influences how she or he perceives self and the world and imagines the mysteries beyond this world.

From Assumptions to the Theory

The theory of self-transcendence is built on the assumption that humans possess an inner capacity—their own inner nursing processes—to integrate life's complexities in a way that facilitates well-being during health-related problems. This capacity is realized in part by expanding or adjusting one's self-boundary. The individual expands or alters the self-boundary by bringing in new perspectives, revising old beliefs, reaching out to others, and connecting to something greater than oneself. These perspectives help integrate and organize the complexity of life in a way that promotes well-being. A self-boundary can also be limiting or even destructive if it restrains a person's resources for innovation, organization, and ability to make meaning in a situation. The theory of self-transcendence acknowledges the human tendency to construct a self-boundary as well as the capacity to transcend limiting views of self and the world in ways that reflect the pandimensional nature of living systems. The theory is based on a pluralistic view of reality that accounts for multiple ways that people can expand their self-boundaries.

The Theory: Concepts and Relationships

Theories by definition consist of descriptions of concepts and proposals about how those concepts are related to each other. There are three major concepts in the theory: self-transcendence, well-being, and vulnerability (Fig. 24-1). The model below depicts the concepts and how they are related to each other.

Self-Transcendence

Self-transcendence is the core concept of the theory. It refers to the capacity to expand the self-boundary intrapersonally (toward greater awareness of one's beliefs, values and dreams), interpersonally (to connect with others, nature, and surrounding environment), transpersonally (to relate in some way to dimensions beyond the ordinary and observable world), and temporally (to integrate one's past and future in a way that expands and gives meaning to the present). Other dimensions may be identified.

Self-transcendence is evident in psychosocial and spiritual perspectives and practices regarding individuals' perceived self-boundaries: Do they have an awareness of their personal beliefs or dreams? Do they engage in meaningful relationships with others? Do they feel connected to their environment in

some way? Do they have a sense of relatedness to something greater than themselves? Do they dwell in the past, regret the past, fear the future, or live in the present? Self-transcendence provides for flexibility in one's self-boundary to extend the person beyond immediate and constricted views of self and the world. And it provides ways to organize and make meaning out of the increasing complexity that comes into one's life when faced with serious health-related events.

The term *self-transcendence* may evoke ideas about the mystical, supernatural, or other experiences that tend to disconnect self from others or from the present. However, spiritual meanings associated with this theory more often refer to terrestrial, everyday practices of spirituality in terms of reaching deeper within the self and reaching out to others, to nature, to one's God, or other means of adjusting the self-boundary to attain meaning in life and sense of connectedness. Self-transcendence embodies experiences that *connect* rather than *separate* a person from self, others, and the environment. The value of connecting with family and friends and

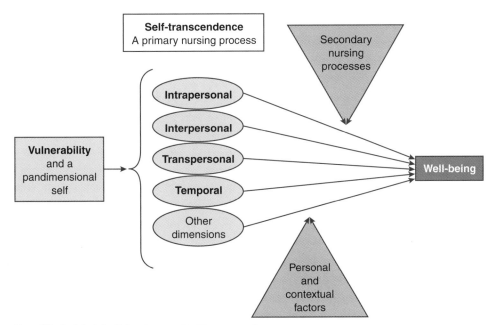

Figure 24 • 1 Model of the theory of self-transcendence.

having social support is well understood. Enjoyment found in being out in nature, taking in the beauty of the environment, appreciating the arts, caring for a pet, and feeling connected to society in some way are all recognized as important to one's well-being.

Nevertheless, relatedness to unseen or unobservable entities may be an important perspective within a person's self-boundary. Religious practices and beliefs are one common pathway to this experience. In society today, there is increasing acknowledgment of and opportunity to develop nonreligious spiritual perspectives that provide a sense of connection to something greater than the self. This reference to the unseen or the mystery in life blurs the traditional boundary in modern science between the conceptual and empirical, to allow for perspectives that may facilitate meaning and well-being.

Finally, expansion of the self-boundary may also involve connectedness with nonliving entities that influence well-being in profound ways. Objects can hold meaning and memories that are highly valued and included within the boundary of self. In addition, illness often confronts the individual with technology and machines that can be difficult to accept as a necessary part of one's life. However, as the contemporary philosopher Donna Haraway (1991) suggested, there can be liberating power in technologies if they are applied in an empowering rather than demeaning manner. People can expand their self-boundary by fusing "flesh and machine." It involves helping patients perceive fluid boundaries between biology and machine and rejecting societal pressure to accept one's limitations as 'natural' and unfortunate. Self-boundary expansion and well-being in the midst of serious illness involves the valorization of humans particularly in the contexts of disability and end of life.

The *Self-Transcendence Scale* (STS) was developed to measure self-transcendence. The STS is described at the end of this chapter. The instrument and the theory have evolved together to provide a reliable and valid approach to measuring self-transcendence. It is possible that self-transcendence may be measured by other means and instruments as well.

Vulnerability

Illness, disability, aging, bereavement, and end of life all mark times of vulnerability and increased awareness of mortality. A second key concept in the theory is vulnerability, which refers to an increased awareness of personal mortality. A wide variety of human experiences can increase this awareness, particularly health-related events that are life-threatening or that involve deep loss. From a developmental perspective, it has long been accepted that events that heighten one's sense of mortality can—if they do not crush the individual's inner self—trigger expansion of self and energize one's journey into life (Becker, 1973; Corless, Germino, & Pittman, 1994; Erikson, 1986; Frankl, 1963; Marshall, 1980). From a nursing perspective of a pandimensional self who has potential for innovative change (as described in the assumptions), it is theorized that vulnerability may lead to or be accompanied by increased self-transcendence.

Health experiences are major sources of increased vulnerability because they confront individuals and their families with issues or questions about mortality and immortality. A list of situations that may initiate or intensify this awareness of vulnerability include serious or life-limiting illness, disability, chronic illness, loss or anticipated loss, work with seriously ill patients, traumatic events, and catastrophic societal events. Self-transcendence may be a resource for well-being during these events by helping the person transform loss into a growth or healing experience. Vulnerability may be assessed in any number of ways that reflect a person's level of awareness or nearness of his or her mortality, or being at increased risk for illness, disability, or death.

Well-Being

The concept of self-transcendence is linked to the concept of well-being in that fluctuations in self-boundaries influence well-being and mental health. It is theorized that self-transcendence, as a nursing process, is linked logically with positive, health-promoting experiences. Self-transcendence is considered to be a correlate if not a predictor of well-being. Well-being is the third major concept in the theory. Well-being is defined broadly as a subjective feeling of health or wholeness as based on the person's own criteria at a given point in time. It involves an existential judgment by the individual, and is influenced by one's history, culture, values, family and other significant relationships, and biophysical factors.

There are many indicators of well-being that can be used in assessment. Nursing and other health and social sciences have identified a wide variety of measures of well-being, which reveal the diversity of values for wellness among individuals and health professionals. Examples of indicators of well-being that have been found to be significantly related to self-transcendence include life satisfaction, happiness, high morale in aging, self-care agency in chronic illness, sense of meaning in life, and specific indicators of mental health such as absence of depression and anxiety.

Dr. Martha Alligood, a scholar of nursing theory, suggested that the theory of self-transcendence could be called a *theory of well-being* (Reed, 2008). In a general sense, the theory of self-transcendence is indeed a *well-being theory*. The theory of self-transcendence provides an approach—specifically in reference to a person's self-boundary—to facilitating well-being in nursing practice. Other nursing theories, extant and still to be developed, can also be described as *well-being theories*, each proposing a unique focus on understanding and facilitating the person's healing potential and well-being in practice.

Additional Concepts in the Theory

One set of concepts that is important to consider in the theory refers to personal *and contextual* factors that may influence the relationship between self-transcendence and well-being. These concepts include the following as possibly significant in the theory: age, gender, ethnicity, years of education, illness intensity, life history, social support, and other factors concerning the person's social and physical environment. For example, the relationship between self-transcendence and well-being may be strengthened by advanced age, higher education, certain spiritual or religious or philosophical perspectives, and life experiences of significant loss. Family stress, caregiver stress, lack of social support or other resources that support self-transcendence may weaken the relationship between self-transcendence and well-being.

The other set of concepts in the theory are called *primary* and *secondary nursing processes* that support or enhance self-transcendence. As a *primary nursing process*, self-transcendence is accessed directly by and from within the individual or family without formal external intervention of a professional. When individuals acquire self-transcendent perspectives and behaviors on their own, self-transcendence functions as a *primary nursing process*. However, individuals often may require assistance or interventions of professional nurses or other health care providers. Nursing interventions function as *secondary nursing processes* in that they support and supplement individuals' and families' inner nursing processes of healing. *Secondary nursing processes* originate outside of the individual or family and are designed by professional nurses to facilitate well-being.

Note that the nursing processes (primary and secondary) addressed in this theory focus on self-transcendence. Other nursing theories have a different focus and inform nurses about other kinds of primary and secondary nursing processes that promote well-being. Self-transcendence is one of many nursing processes that promote healing and well-being. Nursing interventions can strengthen the relationship between a person's self-transcendence and well-being, as shown in the practice exemplar below.

Practice Exemplar

Several years ago, Rose was diagnosed with emphysema. In her youth and through young adulthood, Rose had been a professional dancer on Broadway. But she now found that what were once the strongest parts of her body—her legs—were no longer able to carry her around with grace and ease. Her illness had advanced to the point that she required supplemental oxygen and a walker at home. This made it difficult for her to get out of the house as often as she desired. She lived alone but her daughter, her family caregiver, visited her several times a week. Recently, Rose experienced a worsening of her physical symptoms and more difficulty breathing. Her daughter decided that it would be wise for Rose to move closer to her. Even though Rose's new apartment was more modern than her old house, and her daughter could visit more often, Rose wasn't as happy in her new surroundings. Her daughter was puzzled as to why Rose's mood seemed a little down during her frequent visits.

The nurse, Dr. N, who happened to have focused on the spiritual and psychosocial aspects of pulmonary health experiences for her doctoral studies, worked together with Rose and her family caregiver to better understand how to be of help. Rose's health and well-being required attention to various dimensions of her life. Together the three of them designed a plan of care that addressed Rose's needs regarding physical activity, nutrition, and medical aspects, along with discussing Rose's resources for maintaining a safe and clean home environment. But Dr. N also knew that facilitating Rose's well-being was more complex than addressing these physical aspects.

Theory as a Framework for Practice

Dr. N operated from basic assumptions and beliefs about human strengths and potential for transcending self-boundaries or limitations to attain a sense of well-being in the midst of vulnerability. She felt compassion, but not pity, for Rose and her caregiver.

The theory of self-transcendence provided a useful framework for Dr. N to enact her assumptions about healing in concrete ways to facilitate Rose's well-being. Dr. N was knowledgeable of four dimensions (intrapersonal, interpersonal, transpersonal, and temporal) to apply in her work with Rose and her family caregiver. The theory also allowed for the possibility that Dr. N. might discover another dimension of the self-boundary that could be significant to well-being in the unique realities of Rose's situation.

Vulnerability

The nurse first acknowledged the likelihood that Rose's worsening illness may be contributing to a heightened sense of vulnerability. The diagnosis of a serious illness necessitated relationships with new people (health care providers) and unfamiliar routines. It introduced strange, new information and terminology about the illness itself, medications, devices, treatments and self-care activities. Dr. N helped to demystify the health care regimen by clarifying information and teaching Rose and her daughter about procedures and available resources. The nurse also provided emotional support for their questions and concerns and helped them accept new elements of care into their life. Dr. N also worked to bolster hope and faith in themselves that they had the inner strength and ability to deal with the situation and perhaps even grow in some way from the difficult experience.

Intrapersonal

Rose explained that she was a private person and didn't like to depend on others; it surprised her to find out that it felt comforting to reach out and verbalize her concerns to another person. The nurse's open attitude and empathy gave Rose permission to express her inner feelings of anger and some of the regrets about her life now that she was facing its end. Rose said that the release of emotion made her feel better inside.

Reflecting on her feelings with Dr. N also helped Rose get more in touch with her beliefs about quality of life, values, goals for herself, and dreams for her daughter's future. This knowledge would prove useful later on in making decisions about treatments and the timing of hospice care. Their discussions also helped Rose expand her self-boundary inward, by acknowledging and integrating difficult feelings into her life. Whether she resolved all of her concerns was not as important as acknowledging them and accepting them so she could move on emotionally.

Interpersonal

Another area of difficulty for Rose was having to rely on a walker and oxygen on a daily basis. Besides the fact that these objects confronted her with her mortality, Rose found it embarrassing that she had to use a walker and oxygen wherever she went. She perceived these items as foreign and undignified objects that announced her aging and disability to the world.

In addition, Rose shared with the nurse that although the apartment was closer to her daughter and much nicer, she missed her friends in her former home and especially missed her "mailbox neighbor" who also carried an oxygen tank. They often chatted at the mailbox and shared ideas with one another regarding their disease and use of oxygen. When talking to the neighbor, Rose didn't feel so different.

Dr. N suggested that Rose participate in a pulmonary rehabilitation program. This program could help Rose get used to using her walker and oxygen, as well as meet new people who had similar problems. As part of the program, Rose attended a support group where she saw that everyone else not only had the same illness and experiences, but as she said, "they all looked like her too!" Rose no longer felt that she looked different and the support group became her friends. As Rose was able to expand her self-boundary to integrate these devices into her life, she became more accepting of her illness and herself overall. Attending the support group

also provided her opportunities to use her own experiences to help others. Sharing her wisdom with others was very gratifying and enhanced her well-being.

Transpersonal

Rose also admitted that she wasn't particularly religious but found herself praying each morning and evening. Dr. N was aware of research findings that suggested that religious beliefs once held in youth can become salient again at the end of life, even if they had been eschewed during adulthood. Regardless, Rose valued her own spiritual perspectives, which connected her to something beyond the ordinary that was greater than her self. Even though she had difficulty believing in a life after death, the idea of it as a possibility offered some comfort and helped Rose integrate the painful awareness about her own mortality and being separated from her family and friends. Dr. N supported Rose's transpersonal resources by guiding Rose through a spiritual history to help uncover other sources of strength that she could draw from as she struggled with her worsening illness.

Temporality

The illness initiated and intensified Rose's concerns about the future and fears about pain and mortality. Dr. N explored these concerns with Rose in a realistic yet empathetic manner. She guided Rose through a life review whereby Rose reflected on her past, made connections to the present, and discussed anticipating the unknown. The therapy helped Rose reflect on her life in a positive way and to use the past to enrich the present. The life review also helped Rose to recognize her strengths to deal with what may come in the future. Dr. N found that by simply reminding Rose to try to engage in positive self-talk was sometimes helpful in getting her through a difficult moment.

The nurse also facilitated Rose's fuller enjoyment in the present by encouraging positive experiences such as planning enjoyable activities, holding small celebrations, and taking pictures of important or memorable

Continued

events. These activities generated a legacy and a gift that connected Rose's present to her family's future. Expanding her self-boundary to incorporate other temporalities gave Rose access to meaningful experiences that often sustained her across the trajectory of her illness.

Rose's Self-Transcendence

Rose did not expect Dr. N or her daughter to create self-transcendent experiences for her. But their support and guidance buttressed her own inner healing potential for healing through the illness experience. Rose's openness to accepting help and guidance from the nurse was a first step in expanding her self-boundary. By nurturing connections to her beliefs and values, her God, her support group friends, and to her daughter and nurse, Rose was able to expand her self-boundaries in ways that enhanced her well-being within the context of her incurable illness.

The theory of self-transcendence was designed to provide a framework for assessing and studying how self-boundaries may be related to mental health and well-being. Transcending the self-boundary is not always easy and may require the support of another, even though the assumption is that self-transcendence is inherent. The theory can help inform nurses and patients of ways to adjust or expand self-boundaries to facilitate well-being.

■ Summary

The theory of self-transcendence comprises three key concepts: self-transcendence, well-being, and vulnerability. The concepts are defined broadly and fit many nursing situations where a person's health is challenged or limited. Three propositions are derived from the theory, which can be tested in a diversity of nursing care contexts. The propositions are stated using abstract terms such as "end-of-life issues," "well-being," and "personal factors." These general terms should be replaced with more specific, measurable terms to make the propositions applicable to a specific group of patients or clinical practice setting.

1. The first proposition of the theory, concerning vulnerability, is that self-transcendence is greater in persons facing end-of-life issues than in persons not facing such issues. End-of-life issues arise with life events, illness, aging, caregiving, and other experiences that increase awareness of personal mortality.
2. A second proposition is that self-transcendence is positively related to well-being. An increase in level of self-transcendence is related to an increase in level of well-being, however well-being is measured.
3. The third general proposition is that personal and contextual factors influence (positively or negatively) the relationship between self-transcendence and well-being.

In addition, a similar proposition can be added if a nursing intervention is under consideration. This proposition would propose that a given nursing intervention, for example, art-making, positively influences the relationship between self-transcendence and well-being.

The theory of self-transcendence, as displayed in Figure 24-1, is not too complex and is straightforward in its propositions. As nurses use the theory in research and practice, they may identify nuances to the three main propositions. For example, it is very possible that certain personal factors or nursing interventions may be found to relate *directly* to self-transcendence.

Overall, the concepts were designed to be clearly defined and easily measurable, yet to be broad enough in scope to allow nurses the flexibility in using the theory across a variety of the following components of the theory:

• Contexts of vulnerability
• Expressions of self-transcendence across the four (or more) dimensions
• Influential personal and contextual factors
• Interventions to promote self-transcendence
• Descriptions of well-being by patients and families

Practitioners as well as researchers both can use the theory to contribute new knowledge about facilitating human well-being across a variety of health experiences. The theory is dynamic and open to revision and further development. I invite nurses to participate in making self-transcendence a useful part of their practice with patients and to discover new dimensions and approaches to facilitating well-being.

References

Becker, E. (1973). *The denial of death*. New York: The Free Press.

Corless, I. B., Germino, B. B., & Pittman, M. (1994). *Dying, death, and bereavement: Theoretical perspectives and other ways of knowing*. Boston: Jones and Bartlett.

Erikson, E. H. (1986). *Vital involvement in old age*. New York: Norton.

Frankl, V. E. (1963). *Man's search for meaning*. New York: Pocket Books.

Haraway, D. (1991). *Simians, cyborgs and women*. New York: Routledge.

Kauffman, S. (1995). *At home in the universe: The search for laws of self-organization and complexity*. New York: Oxford University Press.

Lerner, R. M. (2002). *Concepts and theories of human development* (3rd ed.). New York: Random House.

Marshall, V. M. (1980). *Last chapter: A sociology of aging and dying*. Monterey, CA: Brooks-Cole.

Reed, P. G. (1983). Implications of the life-span developmental framework for well-being in adulthood and aging. *Advances in Nursing Science, 6*, 18–25.

Reed, P. G. (1986). Developmental resources and depression in the elderly. *Nursing Research, 35*(6), 368–374.

Reed, P. G. (1989). Mental health of older adults. *Western Journal of Nursing Research, 11*, 143–163.

Reed, P. G. (1991). Self-transcendence and mental health in the oldest-old adults. *Nursing Research, 40*(1), 5–11.

Reed, P. G. (1996). Transcendence: Formulating nursing perspectives. *Nursing Science Quarterly, 9*(1), 2-4.

Reed, P. G. (1997). Nursing: The ontology of the discipline. *Nursing Science Quarterly, 10*(2), 76–79.

Reed, P. G. (2008). Reed's theory of self-transcendence. *Nurse Theorists Portraits of Excellence Vol. 2*. Athens, OH: Fitne Video Productions.

Rogers, M. E. (1970). *An introduction to the theoretical basis of nursing*. Philadelphia: F. A. Davis.

Rogers, M. E. (1980). A science of unitary man. In: J. Riehl & C. Roy (Eds.), *Conceptual models for nursing practice* (2nd ed., pp. 329–338). New York: Appleton-Century-Crofts.

Rogers, M. E. (1990). Nursing: Science of unitary, irreducible, human beings: Update 1990. In: E. A. M. Barrett (Ed.), *Visions of Rogers' science based nursing* (pp. 5–12). New York: National League for Nursing Press.

Chapter 25

Kristen Swanson's Theory of Caring

KRISTEN M. SWANSON

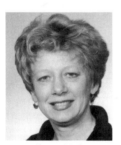

Kristen M. Swanson

The Journey of Theory Development Begins

In this revised chapter, I update answers to questions posed by students and practitioners who have wanted to know more about the origins and progress of my research and theorizing on caring. I have situated myself as a nurse and as a woman so that the context of my scholarship, particularly as it pertains to caring, may be understood. I consider myself to be a second-generation nursing scholar. I was taught by first-generation nurse scientists (that is, nurses who received their doctoral education in fields other than nursing). My struggles for identity as a woman, nurse, and academician were, like many women of my era (the baby boomers), a somewhat organic and reflective process of self-discovery during a rapidly changing social scene (witness the women's and civil rights movements). Third-generation nursing scholars (those taught by nurses whose doctoral preparation is in nursing) may find my "yearning" somewhat odd. To those who might offer critique about the egocentricity of my pondering, I offer the defense of having been brought up during an era in which nurses dealt with such struggles as, "Are we a profession? Have we a unique body of knowledge? Are we entitled to a space in the full (i.e., PhD-granting) academy?" I fully appreciate that questions of uniqueness and entitlement have not completely disappeared. Rather, they have faded as a backdrop to the weightier concerns of making a significant contribution to the health of all, keeping patients safe, educating and retaining a supply of nurses prepared to provide comprehensive patient-centered care to an aging population with increasingly complex and chronic health conditions, working collaboratively with consumers and other scientists and practitioners, practicing in a highly technological environment, embracing pluralism, and acknowledging the socially-constructed power differentials associated with gender, race, poverty, and class.

Turning Point

In September 1982, I had no intention of studying caring; my goal was to study what it was like for women to miscarry. It was my dissertation chair, Dr. Jean Watson, who guided me toward the need to examine caring in the context of miscarriage. I am forever grateful for her foresight and wisdom.

I believe that the key to my program of research is that I have studied human responses to a specific health problem (miscarriage) in a framework (caring) that assumed from the start that a clinical therapeutic had to be defined. So, hand in glove, the research has constantly gone back and forth between "what's wrong and what can be done about it," "what's right and how can it be strengthened," "what's real to women (and most recently their mates) who miscarry and how might care be customized to that reality," and "how can we measure the impact of caring-based interventions on couples' healing after miscarriage?" The back-and-forth nature of this line of inquiry has resulted in insights about the nature of miscarrying and caring that might otherwise have remained elusive.

Predoctoral Experiences

My preparation for studying caring-based therapeutics from a psychosocial perspective began, ironically, in a cardiac critical care unit. After receiving my BSN at the University of Rhode Island, I was wisely coached by Dean Barbara Tate to pursue a job at the brand-new University of Massachusetts Medical Center (U. Mass.) in Worcester, Massachusetts. I was drawn to that institution because of the nursing administration's clear articulation of how nursing could and should be. It was exciting to be there from day one. We were all part of

shaping the institutional vision for practice. It was phenomenal witnessing our collective capacity as nurses, physicians, respiratory therapists, and housekeepers to collaboratively make a profound difference in the lives of those we served. However, what I learned most from that experience came from the patients and their families. I realized that there was a powerful force that people could call upon to get themselves through incredibly difficult times. Watching patients move into a space of total dependency and come out the other side restored was like witnessing a miracle unfold. Sitting with spouses in the waiting room while they entrusted the hearts (and lives) of their partners to the surgical team was awe-inspiring. It was encouraging to observe the inner reserves family members could call upon in order to hand over that which they could not control. I felt so privileged, humbled, and grateful to be invited into the spaces that patients and families created in order to endure their transitions through illness, recovery, and, in some instances, death.

After a year and a half at the University of Massachusetts, I was still a fairly new nurse and was unclear what all of these emotional insights had to do with nursing. I saw them as something related to my spiritual beliefs and me, rather than about my profession. At that point, what mattered most to me as a nurse was my emerging technological savvy, understanding complex pathophysiological processes, and conveying that same information to other nurses. Hence, I applied to graduate schools with the intention of focusing on teaching and on the care of the acutely ill adult. Approximately 2 years after completing my baccalaureate degree, I enrolled in the Adult Health and Illness Nursing program at the University of Pennsylvania.

While at Penn, I served as the student representative to the graduate curriculum committee and, as such, was invited to attend a 2-day retreat to revise the master's program. I distinctly remember listening to Dr. Jacqueline Fawcett and listening in amazement as she spoke about health, environments, persons, and nursing; she claimed that these four concepts were the "stuff" that truly comprised nursing. I was hearing someone put voice to the inner stirrings I had kept to myself back in Massachusetts. It really impressed me that there were nurses who studied in such arenas. Shortly after the retreat, I received my MSN and was hired at Penn on a temporary basis to teach undergraduate medical–surgical nursing. I immediately enrolled as a postmaster's student in Dr. Fawcett's new course on the conceptual basis of nursing. It proved to be one of the best decisions I ever made, primarily because it helped me to figure out an answer to the constant question, "Why doesn't a smart girl like you enter medicine?" I finally knew that it was because nursing, a discipline that I was now starting to understand from an experiential, personal, and academic point of view, was more suited to my beliefs about serving people who were moving through the transitions of illness and wellness. It is safe to say that I was beginning to understand that my "gifts" lay not in the diagnosis and treatment of illness, but in the ability to understand and work with people going through transitions of health, illness, and healing.

Doctoral Studies

Such insights made me want more; hence, I applied for doctoral studies and was accepted into the graduate program at the University of Colorado. My area of study, psychosocial nursing, emphasized such concepts as loss, stress, coping, caring, transactions, and person–environment fit. Having been supported by a National Institute of Mental Health (NIMH) traineeship, one requirement of our program was a hands-on experience with the process of undergoing a health promotion activity. Our faculty offered us the opportunity to carry out the requirement by enrolling ourselves in some type of support or behavior-change program of our own choosing. Four weeks into the same semester in which I was required to complete that exercise, my first son was born. I decided to enroll in a cesarean birth support group as a way to deal

with the class assignment and the unexpected circumstances surrounding his birth. It so happened that an obstetrician had been invited to speak to the group about miscarriage at the first meeting I ever attended. I found his lecture informative with regard to the incidence, diagnosis, prognosis, and medical management of spontaneous abortion. However, when the physician sat down and the women began to talk about their personal experiences with miscarriage and other forms of pregnancy loss, I was suddenly overwhelmed with the realization that there had been a one-in-six chance that I could have miscarried my son. Up until that point, it had never occurred to me that anything could have gone wrong with something so central to my life. I was 29 years old and believed, quite naively, that anything was possible if you were only willing to work hard at it.

Two profound insights came to me from that meeting. First, I was acutely aware of the American Nurses' Association Social Policy Statement, that, "Nursing is the diagnosis and treatment of human responses to actual and potential health problems" (ANA, 1980, p. 9). It was clear to me that whereas the physician had talked about the health problem of spontaneously aborting, the women were living the human response to miscarrying. Second, being in my last semester of course work, I was desperately in need of a dissertation topic. From that point on it became clear to me that I wanted to understand what it was like to miscarry. The problem, of course, was that I was a critical care nurse and knew very little about anything related to childbearing. An additional concern was that during the early 1980s, there was a strong emphasis on epistemology, ontology, and the methodologies to support multiple ways of understanding nursing as a human science, however, our methods courses were traditionally quantitative. Luckily, two mentors came my way. Dr. Jody Glittenberg, a nurse anthropologist, agreed to guide me through a pre-dissertation pilot study of five women's experiences with miscarriage in order that I might learn about interpretive methods. Dr. Colleen Conway-Welch, a midwife, agreed to supervise my trek up the psychology-of-pregnancy learning curve.

Evolution of a Middle-Range Theory of Caring

Twenty women who had miscarried within 16 weeks of being interviewed agreed to participate in my phenomenological study of miscarriage and caring. These results have been published in greater depth elsewhere (Swanson, 1991; Swanson-Kauffman, 1985, 1986b).

Through that investigation, I proposed that caring consisted of five basic processes:

- Knowing
- Being with
- Doing for
- Enabling
- Maintaining belief

At that time, the definitions were fairly awkward and definitely tied to the context of miscarriage. In addition to naming those five categories, I also learned some important things about studying caring:

1. If you directly ask people to describe what caring means to them, you force them to speak so abstractly that it is hard to find any substance.
2. If you ask people to list behaviors or words that indicate that others care, you end up with a laundry list of "niceties."
3. If you ask people for detailed descriptions of what it was like for them to go through an event (i.e., miscarrying) and probe for their feelings and what the responses of others meant to them, it is much easier to unearth instances of people's caring and noncaring responses.
4. I learned that although my intentions were to gather data, many of my informants thanked me for what I did for them.

As it turned out, a side effect of gathering detailed accounts of the informants' experiences was that women felt heard, understood, and attended-to in a nonjudgmental fashion. In later years, this insight would become the grist for a series of caring-based intervention studies.

I have often been asked if my research was an application of Jean Watson's Theory of Human Caring (Watson, 1979/1985, 1985/1988). Neither Dr. Watson nor I have ever seen my research program as an application of her work per se, but we do agree that the compatibility of our scholarship lends credence to both of our claims about the nature of caring. I have come to view her work as having provided a research tradition that other scientists and I have followed. Watson's research tradition asserts that:

1. Caring is a central concept and way of relating in nursing.
2. Multiple methodologies are essential to understanding caring as a concept and way of relating.
3. It is important to study caring so that it may be better understood, consciously claimed, and intentionally acted upon to promote, maintain, and restore health and healing.

Refining the Theory Through Research
Postdoctoral Studies

Approximately 9 months after I completed the dissertation, my second son was born. He had a difficult start in life and spent a few days in the newborn intensive care unit (NICU). Through this event, I became aware that in my experience of childbearing loss (having a not-well child at birth), I, too, wished to receive the kinds of caring responses that my miscarriage informants had described. Hence, my next study, an individually awarded National Research Service Award postdoctoral fellowship (1989–1990), was inspired. Dr. Kathryn Barnard, at the University of Washington, agreed to sponsor this investigation and ended up opening doors for me that continue to open. With her guidance, I spent over a year "hanging out" in the NICU at the

University of Washington Medical Center (the staff gave me permission to acknowledge them and their practice site when discussing these findings).

The question I answered through the NICU phenomenological investigation was, "What is it like to be a provider of care to vulnerable infants?" In addition to my observational data, I did in-depth interviews with some of the mothers, fathers, physicians, nurses, and other health care professionals who were responsible for the care of five infants. The results of this investigation are published elsewhere (Swanson, 1990). With respect to understanding caring, there were three main findings:

1. Although the names of the caring categories were retained, they were grammatically edited and somewhat refined so as to be more generic.
2. It was evident that care in a complex context called upon providers to simultaneously balance *caring* (for self and other), *attaching* (to people and roles), *managing responsibilities* (self-, other-, and society-assigned), and *avoiding bad outcomes* (for self, other, and society).
3. What complicated everything was that each NICU provider (parent or professional) knew only a portion of the whole story surrounding the care of any one infant. Hence, there existed a strong potential for conflict stemming from misunderstanding others and second-guessing one another's motives.

While I was presenting the findings of the NICU study to a group of neonatologists, I received an interesting comment. One young physician told me that it was the caring and attaching parts of his vocation that brought him into medicine, yet he was primarily evaluated on and made accountable for the aspects of his job that dealt with managing responsibilities and avoiding bad outcomes. Such a schism in his role-performance expectations and evaluations had forced him to hold the caring and attaching parts of doing his job unexpressed. Unfortunately, it was his experience that those more person-centered aspects of his role could not be "stuffed" for too long and that they often came hauntingly into his consciousness at 3 A.M. His remarks left me to wonder if the true origin of burnout is the failure of professions and care delivery systems to adequately value, monitor, and reward practitioners whose comprehensive care embraces *caring, attaching, managing responsibilities,* and *avoiding bad outcomes*.

Caring for Socially At-Risk Mothers

While I was still a postdoctoral scholar, Dr. Barnard invited me to present my research on caring to a group of five master's-prepared public health nurses. They became quite excited and claimed that the early draft of the caring model captured what it had been like for them to care for a group of socially at-risk new mothers. About 4 years before our meeting, these five advanced practice nurses had participated in Dr. Barnard's Clinical Nursing Models Project (Barnard et al., 1988). They had provided care to 68 socially at-risk expectant mothers for approximately 18 months (from shortly after conception until their babies were 12 months old). The purpose of the intervention had been to help the mothers take care of themselves and control of their lives so they could ultimately take care of their babies. As I listened to these nurses endorsing the relevance of the caring model to their practice, I began to wonder what the mothers would have to say about the nurses. Would the mothers (1) remember the nurses and (2) describe the nurses as caring?

I was able to locate 8 of the original 68 mothers (a group of women with highly transient lifestyles). They agreed to participate in a study of what it had been like to receive an intensive long-term advanced practice nursing intervention. The result of this phenomenological inquiry was that the caring categories were further refined and a definition of caring was finally derived.

Hence, as a result of the miscarriage, NICU, and high-risk mothers studies, I began to call the caring model a middle-range theory of caring. I define caring as a "nurturing way of relating to a valued 'other' toward whom one feels a personal sense of commitment and responsibility" (Swanson, 1991, p. 162). "Knowing," striving to understand an event as it has meaning in the life of the other, involves avoiding assumptions, focusing on the one cared for, seeking cues, assessing thoroughly, and engaging the self of both the one caring and the one cared for. "Being with" means being emotionally present to the other. It includes being there, conveying availability, and sharing feelings while not burdening the one cared for. "Doing for" means doing for the other what he or she would do for him-or herself if it were at all possible. The therapeutic acts of doing for include anticipating needs, comforting, performing competently and skillfully, and protecting the other while preserving his or her dignity. "Enabling" means facilitating the other's passage through life transitions and unfamiliar events. It involves focusing on the event, informing, explaining, supporting, allowing and validating feelings, generating alternatives, thinking things through, and giving feedback. The last caring category is "maintaining belief," which means sustaining faith in the other's capacity to get through an event or transition and face a future with meaning. This means believing in the other and holding him or her in esteem, maintaining a hope-filled attitude, offering realistic optimism, helping find meaning, and going the distance or standing by the one cared for, no matter how his or her situation may unfold (Swanson, 1991, 1993, 1999b, 1999c).

Developing and Testing Theory-Guided Practice Applications

As my postdoctoral studies were coming to an end, Dr. Barnard challenged me and claimed, "I think you've described caring long enough. It's time you did something with it!" We discussed how data-gathering interviews were often perceived by study participants as caring.

Together we realized that, at the very least, open-ended interviews involved aspects of knowing, being with, and maintaining belief. We suspected that if doing-for and enabling interventions specifically focused on common human responses to health conditions were added, it would be possible to transform the techniques of phenomenological data gathering into a caring intervention. That conversation ultimately led to my design of a caring-based counseling intervention for women who miscarried.

Soon, I was writing a proposal for a Solomon four-group randomized experimental design (Swanson, 1999b, 1999c). It was funded by the National Institute of Nursing Research and the University of Washington Center for Women's Health Research. The primary purpose of the study was to examine the effects of three 1-hour-long, caring-based counseling sessions on the integration of loss (miscarriage impact) and women's emotional well-being (moods and self-esteem) in the first year after miscarrying. Additional aims of the study were to (1) examine the effects of early versus delayed measurement and the passage of time on women's healing in the first year after loss and (2) develop strategies to monitor caring as the intervention/process variable.

An assumption of the caring theory was that the recipient's well-being should be enhanced by receipt of caring from a provider informed about common human responses to a designated health problem (Swanson, 1993). Specifically, it was proposed that if women were guided through in-depth discussion of their experience and felt understood, informed, provided for, validated, and believed in, they would be better prepared to integrate miscarrying into their lives. The content for the three counseling sessions was derived from the miscarriage model—a phenomenologically derived model that summarized the common human responses to miscarriage (Swanson, 1999c; Swanson-Kauffman, 1983, 1985, 1986a, 1986b, 1988).

Women were randomly assigned to two levels of treatment (caring-based counseling and controls) and two levels of measurement ("early"—completion of outcome measures immediately, 6 weeks, 4 months, and 1 year postloss; or "delayed"—completion of outcome measures at 4 months and 1 year only). Counseling took place at 1, 5, and 11 weeks postloss. ANOVA was used to analyze treatment effects. Outcome measures included self-esteem (Rosenberg, 1965), overall emotional disturbance, anger, depression, anxiety, and confusion (McNair, Lorr, & Droppleman, 1981) and overall miscarriage impact, personal significance, devastating event, lost baby, and feeling of isolation (investigator-developed Impact of Miscarriage Scale).

A more detailed report of these findings is published elsewhere (Swanson, 1999b). There were 242 women enrolled, 185 of whom completed. Participants were within five weeks of loss at enrollment: 89 percent were partnered, 77 percent were employed, and 94 percent were Caucasian. Over one year, main effects included the following: (1) caring was effective in reducing overall emotional disturbance, anger, and depression and (2) with the passage of time, women attributed less personal significance to miscarrying and realized increased self-esteem and decreased anxiety, depression, anger, and confusion.

In summary, the Miscarriage Caring Project provided evidence that, although time had a healing effect on women after miscarrying, caring did make a difference in the amount of anger, depression, and overall disturbed moods that women experienced after miscarriage. This study was unique in that it employed a clinical research model to determine whether or not caring made a difference. I believe that its greatest strength lies in the fact that the intervention was based both on an empirically derived understanding of what it is like to miscarry and on a conscientious attempt to enact caring in counseling women through their loss. The greatest limitation of that study is that I derived the caring theory (developed from the intervention) and conducted most of the counseling sessions. Hence, it is unknown whether similar results would be derived under different

circumstances. My work is further limited by the lack of diversity in my research participants. Over the years, I have predominantly worked with middle-class, married, educated, Caucasian women. I am currently making a concerted effort to rectify this situation and to examine what it is like for diverse groups of women to experience both miscarriage and caring.

Monitoring caring as an intervention variable was the second specific aim of the Miscarriage Caring Project. Three strategies were employed to document that, as claimed, caring had occurred. First, approximately 10 percent of the intervention sessions were transcribed. Analysis was done by research associate Katherine Klaich, RN, PhD. As one of the counselors in the study, she found she could not approach analysis of the transcripts naively—that is, with no preconceived notions, as would be expected in the conduct of phenomenologic analysis. Hence, she employed both deductive and inductive content analytic techniques to render the transcribed counseling sessions meaningful. She began with the broad question, "Is there evidence of caring as defined by Swanson [1991] on the part of the nurse counselors?" The unit of analysis was each emic phrase that was used by the nurse counselor. Phrases were coded for which (if any) of the five caring processes were represented by the emic utterances. Each counselor statement was then further coded for which subcategory of the five processes was represented by the phrase. Twenty-nine subcategories of the five major processes were defined. With few exceptions (social chitchat), every therapeutic utterance of the nurse counselor could be accounted for by one of the subcategories.

The second way in which caring was monitored was through the completion of paper-and-pencil measures. Before each session, the counselor completed a Profile of Mood States (McNair, Lorr, & Droppleman, 1981) in order to document her pre-session moods (thus enabling examination of the association between counselor pre-session mood and self or client post-session ratings of caring). After each session, women were asked to complete Swanson's Caring Professional Scale (2002). Having been left alone to complete the measure, women were asked to place the evaluations in a sealed envelope. In the meantime, in another room, the counselor wrote out her counseling notes and completed the Counselor Rating Scale, a brief five-item rating of how well the session went.

The Caring Professional Scale (2002) originally consisted of 18 items on a 5-point Likert-type scale. It was developed through the Miscarriage Caring Project and was completed by participants in order to rate the nurse counselors who conducted the intervention and to evaluate the nurses, physicians, or midwives who took care of the women at the time of their miscarriage. The items included the following: "Was the health-care provider that just took care of you understanding, informative, aware of your feelings, centered on you?" The response set ranged from 1 ("yes, definitely") to 5 ("not at all"). The items were derived from the caring theory. Three negatively worded items (abrupt, emotionally distant, and insulting) were dropped due to minimal variability across all of the data sets. For the counselors at 1, 5, and 11 weeks post-loss, Cronbach alphas were .80, .95, and .90 (sample sizes for the counselor reliability estimates were 80, 87, and 76). The lower reliability estimates were because the counselors' caring professional scores were consistently high and lacked variability (mean item scores ranged from 4.52 to 5.0).

Noteworthy findings include the following:

1. Each counselor had a full range of pre-session feelings, and those feelings/moods were, as might be expected, highly intercorrelated.
2. For the most part, counselor pre-session mood was not associated with post-session evaluations.
3. The caring professional scores were extremely high for both counselors, indicating that, overall, the clients were pleased with what they received and, as claimed, caring was "delivered" and "received."

4. One of the counselors was a psychiatric nurse by background. She knew very little about miscarriage before participating in this study and had recently experienced a death in her family. The only time her pre-session moods (in this case, depression and confusion) were significantly associated ($p \le .05$) with any of the post-session ratings (both client caring professional score and counselor self-rating) was in Session I. During Session I, women discussed in-depth what the actual events of miscarrying felt like. It is possible that the counselor was so touched by and caught up in the sadness of the stories that her own vulnerabilities were a bit less veiled.
5. Session II, in which the two topics addressed were relationship oriented (who the woman could share her loss with and what it felt like to go out in public as a woman who had miscarried), was the only session in which the other counselor's vulnerabilities came through. This counselor had just gone through a divorce. Her post-session self-evaluation was significantly associated with her pre-session moods: depression ($p \le .05$) and low vigor, confusion, fatigue, and tension (all at $p \le .01$). Also, most notably, there was an association between this counselor's pre-session tension and clients' post-session Caring Professional scores ($p \le .05$).

Clarifying Caring Through Literary Meta-analysis

I also conducted an in-depth review of the literature. This literary meta-analysis is published elsewhere (Swanson, 1999a). Approximately 130 data-based publications on caring were reviewed for that state-of-the-science paper. Through it I developed a framework for discourse about caring knowledge in nursing. Proposed were five domains (or levels) of knowledge about caring in nursing. I believe that these domains are hierarchical and that studies conducted at any one domain (e.g., Level III) assume the presence of all previous domains (e.g., Levels I and II). The first domain includes descriptions of the capacities or characteristics of caring persons. Level II deals with the concerns and/or commitments that lead to caring actions. These are the values nurses hold that lead them to practice in a caring manner. Level III describes the conditions (nurse, patient, and organizational factors) that enhance or diminish the likelihood of caring occurring. Level IV summarizes caring actions. This summary consisted of two parts. In the first part, a meta-analysis of 18 quantitative studies of caring actions was performed. It was demonstrated that the top five caring behaviors valued by patients were that the nurse (1) helps the patient to feel confident that adequate care was provided; (2) knows how to give shots and manage equipment; (3) gets to know the patient as a person; (4) treats the patient with respect; and (5) puts the patient first, no matter what. By contrast, the top five caring behaviors valued by nurses were: (1) listens to the patient, (2) allows expression of feelings, (3) touches when comforting is needed, (4) perceives the patient's needs, and (5) realizes the patient knows him- or herself best. The second part of the caring actions summary was a review of 67 interpretive studies of how caring is expressed (the total number of participants was 2,314). These qualitative studies were classified under Swanson's caring processes, thus lending credibility to caring theory. The last domain was labeled "consequences." These are the intentional and unintentional outcomes of caring and noncaring for patient and provider. In summary, this literary meta-analysis clarified what "caring" means, as the term is used in nursing, and validated the generalizability or transferability of Swanson's caring theory beyond the perinatal contexts from which it was originally derived.

From Theory and Research Back to Practice

In 2004, I was honored to be named a Robert Wood Johnson Foundation (RWJF) Executive Nurse Fellow. When I wrote the application,

I set the goal to "leave the comfort of academia" and to make myself learn more about the world of nursing practice. I realized that if my work on caring was going to have relevance to nursing I needed to understand better what it was like to practice as a nurse in today's health care environment. I was delighted that Susan Grant (at that time Vice President for Patient Care at the University of Washington Medical Center) agreed to mentor me. My personal mantra was that I wanted to "help create the conditions that enable nurses to work in accordance with their core values of caring, healing, and keeping their patients safe." The journey I took as an Executive Nurse Fellow was extremely rewarding and, at the same time, daunting. The world of health care is undergoing rapid change. The vocabulary, pace, politics, technologies, locations, and challenges of health care are changing at warp speed. I learned that in the healthiest practice settings caring must take place at the organizational level and at the point of care. Institutional caring practices take the form of continuous quality improvements that strive to achieve the Institute of Medicine's (2001) call for health care that is delivered in a safe, efficient, effective, timely, equitable, and patient-centered manner. Providers experience the rewards of knowing their work matters when they practice in organizations that are driven to constantly enhance safe, effective, and compassionate care for patients, families, and employees. As a result of lessons learned through the RWJF fellowship I now routinely consult with health care facilities where the mission is to create and sustain a culture of caring.

The Journey Continues: The Couple's Miscarriage Project

I recently completed an NIH-NINR-funded randomized controlled trial of three caring-based interventions against a control condition to see if we can make a difference in men and women's healing after miscarriage. The purpose of this randomized trial was to compare the effects of nurse caring (three nurse counseling sessions), self-caring (three home-delivered videotapes and journals), combined caring (one nurse counseling plus three videotapes and journals), and no intervention (control) on the emotional healing, integration of loss, and couple well-being of women and their partners (husbands or male mates) in the first year after miscarrying. All intervention materials were developed based on the Miscarriage Model and the Caring Theory. We enrolled 341 couples. Intervention findings are currently under review for publication. Similar to the Miscarriage Caring Project we also focused on measuring caring as an intervention variable; those findings are soon to be submitted for publication.

■ Summary

Caring, to be effective, must be sensitive to those involved in caring transactions to the cultural contexts in which caring occurs, and to the common responses that individuals, families, groups, and communities experience when living with conditions of wellness and illness. Globally, we are living at a time where some people are living longer and with chronic health challenges; others are dying prematurely due to genetics, poverty, or war; and still others are committed to living healthy life practices that limit their "footprint" on Earth. Stepping back and asking what an ecological perspective on caring and health might look like, it is clear that the work that lies ahead must focus on the political, economic, social, institutional, spiritual, and personal practices necessary to promote a world where a healthy human ecology is possible.

References

American Nurses' Association (ANA). (1980). Nursing: A social policy statement. Kansas City, MO: American Nurses' Association.

Barnard, K. E., Magyary, D., Sumner, G., Booth, C. L., Mitchell, S. K., & Spieker, S. (1988). Prevention of parenting alterations for women with low social support. *Psychiatry, 51,* 248–253.

Institute of Medicine of the National Academies. (2001). Crossing the quality chasm: A new health system for the 21st century. Report Brief. Retrieved from http://www.iom.edu/CMS/8089/5432/27184. aspx (Accessed January 29, 2008).

McNair, D. M., Lorr, M., & Droppleman, L. F. (1981). *Profile of mood states: Manual.* San Diego: Educational and Industrial Testing Service.

Rosenberg, M. (1965). *Society and the adolescent self-image.* Princeton, NJ: Princeton University Press.

Swanson, K. M. (1990). Providing care in the NICU: Sometimes an act of love. *Advances in Nursing Science, 13*(1), 60–73.

Swanson, K. M. (1991). Empirical development of a middle-range theory of caring. *Nursing Research, 40,* 161–166.

Swanson, K. M. (1993). Nursing as informed caring for the well-being of others. *Image, 25,* 352–357.

Swanson, K. M. (1999a). What's known about caring in nursing science: A literary meta-analysis. In:

A. S. Hinshaw, S. Feetham, & J. Shaver (Eds.), *Handbook of clinical nursing research.* Thousand Oaks, CA: Sage.

Swanson, K. M. (1999b). The effects of caring, measurement, and time on miscarriage impact and women's well-being in the first year subsequent to loss. *Nursing Research, 48,* 6, 288–298.

Swanson, K. M. (1999c). Research-based practice with women who miscarry. *Image: Journal of Nursing Scholarship, 31,* 4, 339–345.

Swanson, K. M. (2002). Caring Profession Scale. In: J. Watson (Ed.), *Assessing and measuring caring in nursing and health science.* New York: Springer.

Swanson-Kauffman, K. M. (1983). The unborn one: The human experience of miscarriage (Doctoral dissertation, University of Colorado Health Sciences Center, 1983). *Dissertation Abstracts International, 43,* AAT8404456.

Swanson-Kauffman, K. M. (1985). Miscarriage: A new understanding of the mother's experience. *Proceedings of the 50th anniversary celebration of the University of Pennsylvania School of Nursing,* 63–78.

Swanson-Kauffman, K. M. (1986a). A combined qualitative methodology for nursing research. *Advances in Nursing Science, 8*(3), 58–69.

Swanson-Kauffman, K. M. (1986b). Caring in the instance of unexpected early pregnancy loss. *Topics in Clinical Nursing, 8*(2), 37–46.

Swanson-Kauffman, K. M. (1988). The caring needs of women who miscarry. In M. M. Leininger (Ed.), *Care: Discovery and uses in clinical and community nursing.* Detroit: Wayne State University Press.

Watson, M. J. (1979/1985). *Nursing: The philosophy and science of caring.* Boulder, CO: Colorado Associated Press.

Watson, M. J. (1985/1988). *Nursing: Human science and human care.* New York: National League for Nursing Press.

Chapter 26

Mary Jane Smith and Patricia Liehr's Story Theory

MARY JANE SMITH AND PATRICIA LIEHR

Introducing the Theorists
Overview of the Theory
Practice Exemplar: Advancing Practice
Scholarship Through Story Theory
Summary
References

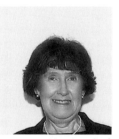

Mary Jane Smith

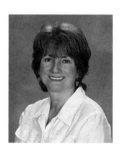

Patricia Liehr

Introducing the Theorists

Patricia R. Liehr, PhD, RN, graduated from Ohio Valley Hospital, School of Nursing in Pittsburgh, Pennsylvania. She completed her baccalaureate degree in nursing at Villa Maria College, her master's in family health nursing at Duquesne University, and her doctorate at the University of Maryland–Baltimore, School of Nursing, with an emphasis on psychophysiology. She completed postdoctoral studies at the University of Pennsylvania as a Robert Wood Johnson scholar. Dr. Liehr is currently the Associate Dean for Nursing Research and Scholarship at the Christine E. Lynn College of Nursing at Florida Atlantic University. She has taught nursing theory to master's and doctoral students for nearly two decades.

Mary Jane Smith, PhD, RN, earned her bachelor's and master's degrees from the University of Pittsburgh and her doctorate from New York University. She has held faculty positions at the following nursing schools: University of Pittsburgh, Duquesne University, Cornell University-New York Hospital, and Ohio State University; and she is currently Professor and Associate Dean for Graduate Academic Affairs at West Virginia University School of Nursing. She has been teaching theory to nursing students for nearly three decades.

Overview of the Theory

Stories are integral to nursing practice. Practice decisions are informed by both physiological bodily responses and the stories that infuse bodily responses with unique personal meaning. To focus on one without attention to the other contributes to less than the best

439

nursing care. There are times when one, either physiological bodily responses or stories, is foreground while the other is background; this foreground/background interplay dynamically emerges over the course of each nurse–person caring interaction. For instance, when a person, comes into the emergency room with crushing chest pain and then suddenly becomes unconsciousness, numbers are in the foreground. Heart rate, blood pressure, and respiratory rate guide critical immediate action. Within a short time, the nurse will want to begin to gather the story, including dimensions such as what the person was doing when the chest pain began, whether this has ever happened before, and what other life/health circumstances could have contributed to the chest pain. Stories are essential to even the most technology-driven nursing practice, and in some ways, the more technology-driven the practice, the more important the place of relevant health stories.

Our linear-thinking culture often places greater value on physiological bodily responses than stories. In fact, precious stories shared during nursing practice may be heard and disregarded or heard and acted upon without another thought about the practice-evidence generated. Practice stories are seldom heard and chronicled becoming part of the foundation of nursing practice evidence. The overall intent of this chapter is to describe Story Theory as a framework informing story-gathering and story analysis, thereby positioning story as a major thread of nursing practice evidence, contributing to substantive nursing knowledge.

This chapter first addresses the emergence of story or narrative as a topic of interest for health care providers, including nurses. Then, Story Theory is summarized, including the essential theory concepts (intentional dialogue, connecting with self-in-relation, creating ease) and discussion of ways that the theory comes alive in practice. Bringing the theory to life is described in the context of the theory method dimensions (complicating health challenges, developing story plot, movement toward resolving) aligned respectively with each theory concept. We discuss a seven-phase inquiry

process for using the evidence from practice stories to grow the substantive knowledge of the discipline. Finally, an exemplar is used to highlight use of the theory in practice through application of the seven-phase inquiry process.

Emergence of Story as a Topic of Interest

Story is not new to nursing. Nurse theorists (Boykin & Schoenhofer, 1991, 2001; Newman, 1999; Parse, 1981; Peplau, 1991; Watson, 1997) have called attention to the importance of listening to what matters since the time of Nightingale, who implored nurses to stop chattering and begin listening (Nightingale, 1969). Others (Benner, 1984; Chinn & Kramer, 1999; Ford & Turner, 2001) have used the stories of practicing nurses to understand both the challenge and the essence of nursing practice. In a discussion of the importance of story for research with minority populations, Banks-Wallace (2002) discussed the therapeutic value of storytelling. Story-sharing has also had a prominent place in research with elders (Heliker, 2007; Sierpina & Cole, 2004). It is often used by nurse researchers focused on the art of caring for people who have dementia (Crichton & Koch, 2007; Holm, Lepp, & Ringsberg, 2005; Keady, Williams, & Hughes-Roberts, 2007).

Recently, physicians have emphasized narrative medicine as both a way of learning clinical practice essentials and a way of approaching patients (Charon & Montello, 2002; Charon, 2006; Mehl-Medrona, 2007). Diamond, a psychotherapist, addressed the long history of using narrative, in forms such as personal testimony and letter-writing, to treat alcoholism and addiction. In his book, entitled *Narrative means to sober ends* (Diamond, 2000), he describes the spirit of narrative therapy: "Stories, not atoms, are the stuff that hold our lives – and our world together" (p. 5). This view of stories resonates with the foundational assumptions of Story theory and with a valuing of the important place of stories for health promotion. In *Narrative medicine: The use of history and story in the healing process,* Mehl-Madrona (2007) approached the topic of narrative from a Native American perspective, distinguishing narrative medicine from conventional medicine and proceeding to share Native American stories that he described as maps for healing. These writings and others "confirm our beliefs about the significance of story and remind us that this core dimension of nursing practice is now being recognized by other disciplines" (Liehr & Smith, 2008, p. 208). Although we, the authors, do not equate story with narrative, we accept the place of narrative within the context of story. Story moves beyond narrative, intricately weaving remembered events, personal interpretations of the moment and hopes and dreams to create the "now" moment, guiding choices in-the-moment.

Story Theory is one way to conceptualize an idea that has a long history in nursing and recently escalated attention from other disciplines. The authors believe that the structure of Story Theory creates possibilities for application and evaluation that are critical to the endeavor of building substantive disciplinary knowledge.

Foundations of the Theory

Story Theory proposes that story is a narrative happening wherein a person connects with self-in-relation through nurse–person intentional dialogue to create ease (Liehr & Smith, 2008). Ease emerges in the midst of accepting the whole story as one's own—a process of attentive embracing the complexity of one's situation. All nursing encounters occur within the context of story. The stories of the nurse, patient, family, and other health care providers are woven together to create the tapestry of the moment—this is the whole story in the moment. Each time a nurse engages a patient about what matters most regarding a health challenge, Story Theory is applicable. By abandoning preexisting assumptions, respecting the storyteller as the expert, and querying vague story directions, the nurse intentionally engages the other, enabling connecting with self-in-relation to create ease.

The theory is based on three assumptions that underpin the framework. The assumptions are that people (1) change as they interrelate with their world in a vast array of flowing connected dimensions; (2) live in an expanded present moment where past and future events are transformed in the here and now; and (3) experience meaning as a resonating awareness in the creative unfolding of human potential (Liehr & Smith, 2008). These assumptions are consistent with a unitary–transformative "view of the world," an inherently complex view (Newman, Sime, & Corcoran-Perry, 1991), establishing a value structure that creates a foundation for the theory concepts.

The three concepts of the theory are intentional dialogue, connecting with self-in-relation, and creating ease (Fig. 26-1). The related method dimensions are complicating health challenge, developing story plot, and movement toward resolving. The nurse engages a person through intentional dialogue about a complicating health challenge, where connecting with self-in-relation ensues as the developing story plot surfaces through story-sharing. As the storyteller makes explicit what may have been tacit (Polanyi, 1958), moments of ease accompany movement toward resolving the health challenge. Figure 26-1 depicts the theory model, indicating relationships among the theory concepts and related method dimensions.

The current theory model spreads a "wave" across all concepts in the theory, expressive of the energy essential to story-sharing through

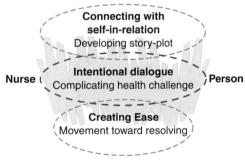

Figure 26 • 1 Story Theory with method.

intentional dialogue. The heavy dotted ellipse between nurse and person highlights nurse–person intentional dialogue, the core activity enabling connecting with self-in-relation and creating ease. There are three ellipses in the design of the model, mapping a vortex of a continually evolving process, encompassing all the theory concepts and associated method dimensions. The links between the essential elements of the model map the theory phenomenon as an energy-laden integrated whole.

Intentional Dialogue About a Complicating Health Challenge

Intentional dialogue is the central activity between nurse and person that brings story to life; it is querying emergence of a health challenge story in true presence (Smith & Liehr, 1999). This purposeful engagement with another creates potential for embracing the whole story in the moment as the nurse summons the storytellers' narrative focusing on what matters most about a complicating health challenge (Liehr & Smith, 2008). The complicating health challenge is a life circumstance wherein life change generates uneasiness. Understanding the uneasiness refines the health challenge to enable meaningful nurse–person interaction. For instance, getting married could be both a joyful and an uneasy transition. In this case, the complicating health challenge may be articulated as the transition from being single to being married. What matters most to the anticipatory bride may be the uncertainty she is feeling in the midst of excited planning. This joyful–uneasy paradox will become the focus for the nurse using Story Theory to guide practice; the nurse will listen to the bride's complaint of stomach pain within the context of joy–uneasiness emerging in the transition to married life.

In another example, for a woman facing the complicating health challenge of a breast cancer diagnosis, it is possible that the thought of losing her breast matters most, or it could be the threat imposed by the cancer, or the response of her husband to her changing body, or concern about who will care for her puppy while she is in the hospital. There is an endless list of possibilities known only to the person who is living the health challenge. The nurse can never assume to know what matters most about a health challenge regardless of the extent of experience in a particular practice environment. The nurse knows how to proceed only by querying what matters most about a complicating health challenge.

Connecting with Self-in-Relation Through Developing Story Plot

Connecting with self-in-relation occurs as reflective awareness on personal history (Smith & Liehr, 1999). It is an active process of recognizing self as related with others in a developing story-plot uncovered through intentional dialogue (Liehr & Smith, 2008). To connect with self-in-relation, people see themselves not as isolated individuals but as existing and growing in a context, which includes awareness of other people and times, sensitivity to bodily expression, and a sense of history and future in the present moment. "In following the story path, the nurse encourages reckoning with a personal history by traveling to the past to arrive at the story beginning, moving through the middle, and into the future all in the present, thus going into the depths of the story to find unique meanings that often lie hidden in the ambiguity of puzzling dilemmas" (Smith & Liehr, 2003, p. 171).

The story path is an expression of a developing story plot with high points, low points, and turning points. High points are times when things are going well by the storyteller's evaluation; low points are times when they are not going so well; and turning points are times when the story twists, sometimes subtly, sometimes dramatically, creating a shift in the forward view. Often, we and our colleagues have used a story path approach to gather stories (Hain, 2007, 2008; Williams, 2007) for research. The story path links present, past, and future (Liehr & Smith, 2000), beginning with the question, "What matters most to you right now about (the health challenge you are facing)?" This question is followed by one that queries the past, asking how it contributes to the present. Finally, hopes and dreams are elicited.

Figure 26-2 depicts a story path for Mary, a 29-year-old woman who has come to see the nurse practitioner for hypertension. Her blood pressure was recorded as 180/110 mm Hg on the primary care visit. The nurse has drawn a line on a sheet of paper and asked Mary to tell her where she is in her life path by marking the "present" on the line. Then, she asks Mary what matters most in this present moment. Mary talks about her discomfort with her elevated blood pressure at her young age. She adds detail about her job as a project director for a research study while having just finished full-time study for her master's degree and now beginning work on her doctoral degree in psychology. Mary's home situation is "stabilized" by her husband John, who she describes as mellow and the strongest supporter for "considering lifestyle changes to lower her high blood pressure." She tells the nurse that the only time her blood pressure is normal is on weekends, when she is away from work. She provides great detail about her work situation on this visit, describing work as an "out-of-control stress" environment aggravated by people who "seem to enjoy her stressful frenzy." Mary believes that work-related stress is the strongest contributor to her hypertension. The nurse clarifies

with Mary, "so...are you saying that stress-induced high blood pressure is your pressing concern right now?" Mary says "yes." What matters most to Mary about the health challenge of hypertension on this visit is her stressful work life, which she feels unable to control. The nurse then moves to the past and asks Mary to identify situations and events on her story path that contributed to her current health challenge of stress-induced high blood pressure, and then to the future, asking her to note hopes and dreams related to the health challenge. Mary notes story path events related to her father and identifies her desire to have a baby within the next 5 years. Each of these markings along the story path is discussed with the storyteller leading the way. The nurse makes notes on the story path so that both participants are engaged in the process, infusing the physiological indicator, a blood pressure of 180/110 mm Hg, with Mary's unique personal story.

Before ending any visit where story has been pulled into the foreground, it is important that the nurse ask if there is "anything else" about the health challenge that the storyteller wants to share to enhance understanding. What matters most about a health challenge may change from visit to visit and any single visit may encompass more than one issue that matters the most. Detailed story

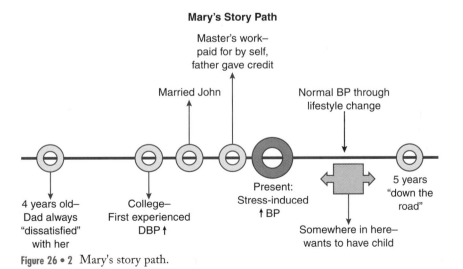

Figure 26 • 2 Mary's story path.

paths include bits of practice evidence gleaned from what the storyteller emphasized. This practice evidence has the potential to guide the next steps the nurse will take during this and upcoming visits.

Story path is just one approach to gathering the story in a practice setting. We have suggested others such as photographs, family trees, and pain diaries (Liehr & Smith, 2008). There seems to be value in eliciting a story through a collaborative creation that enhances the telling and takes the story to a structure such as story path. The possible approaches for story-gathering are limitless. The creative nurse will identify other unique approaches for querying what matters most about a health challenge. "Coming to grips" with what matters most is a process of embracing story, where paradoxically, embracing releases a person from story confines, engendering a sense of ease.

Creating Ease While Moving Toward Resolving

Creating ease is remembering disjointed story moments to experience flow in the midst of anchoring (Smith & Liehr, 1999). As a person anchors even for a moment, embracing the comprehensible whole, flow ensues as easiness-with-self situated in a complex context. Ease is neither assured nor pervasive during story-sharing. Sometimes it is elusive; sometimes it is experienced as only a moment in time. When story moments come together in a meaningful way for the person sharing a story, there is often some movement toward resolving the health challenge. Movement may be minuscule or it may be a leap; it enables a shift in one's perspective usually accompanied by action to address what matters most about the health challenge.

Practice Exemplar

Advancing Practice Scholarship Through Story Theory

We have proposed seven phases of inquiry for practicing nurses who want to develop practice evidence as a base for knowledge development (Smith & Liehr, 2005). The phases are: (1) gather a story about what matters most about a complicating health challenge; (2) compose a reconstructed story; (3) connect existing literature to the health challenge; (4) refine the name of the complicating health challenge; (5) describe the developing story plot with high points, low points, and turning points; (6) identify movement toward resolving; and (7) collect additional stories about the health challenge (Liehr & Smith, 2008). For the purposes of this chapter, we address all phases of the inquiry process except the last, which takes the nurse back to the practice environment to substantiate what emerged while completing the first six phases.

Phase one asks the practicing nurse to gather a story of what matters most about a complicating health challenge. Querying what matters most about the health challenge is coming to know the unique perspective of the person sharing the story. To gather the story, the nurse could use a structured approach such as story path or story-gathering could occur over time through attentive presence with another. Irrespective of how the nurse gathers the story, coming to know the other in this way culminates in a reconstructed story. The nurse in the forthcoming story queried the health challenge of transitioning to a nursing home environment for elders who had been living independently.

Phase two requires that the nurse compose a reconstructed story. A reconstructed story is a narrative creation with a beginning, a middle, and an end that weaves together the nurse's and the storyteller's perspective of the health challenge; the reconstructed story naturally incorporates what matters most about the health challenge. The reconstructed story shared in this chapter was written by a nurse who cared for Elizabeth during the last months of her life in a nursing home. The nurse had practiced in this nursing home for 10 years, often witnessing the health challenge of transitioning from independent to nursing home living. The story-gathering occurred over time and story moments are synthesized as a reconstructed story to serve as an evidence base for understanding the independent living to nursing home living transition.

Elizabeth was an 88-year-old woman who enjoyed independent living in her "bungalow" with her husband of 65 years. She and her husband resided in the independent living component of a continuing care community. Elizabeth had a long history of atrial fibrillation, chronic heart failure, and diabetes, but she managed to remain "independent," using a walker to get around. She attributed her independence to the devotion of her husband who watched over her medication routine, diet, and the balance between her activity/rest patterns. At the end of January, Elizabeth began having difficulty moving her left leg, especially when she awoke in the morning. It seemed to her that her leg had "fallen asleep" due to positioning during the night. Then, one February morning, Elizabeth's lower leg was painful, cool to touch, and slightly discolored. Her husband called the community nurse, who immediately sent Elizabeth to the hospital, where a popliteal clot was found to be occluding the artery. Amputation was considered but rejected due to the complexity of Elizabeth's health situation. "Clot-buster" was dripped directly into Elizabeth's clot for 7 hours while she lay on her back and the clot dissolved. Elizabeth was relieved because she had always feared "losing her leg" after witnessing her grandmother's double amputation as a result of long-standing diabetes.

After 10 days in the hospital, Elizabeth returned to the nursing home component of her continuing care community, planning to begin rehabilitation. Shortly after admission, she was diagnosed with the flu, delaying the start of rehabilitation. Once she began, the physical therapists referred to her as their "energizer bunny" because of her spirited approach to therapy. Throughout this time, it was very hard for Elizabeth to lift her left leg. No matter how hard she tried, she couldn't move it like she could move her right leg. Still, she was anticipating return to the bungalow to get on with everyday living with her husband. While Elizabeth was in the nursing home, her husband visited every day at mealtimes and when she was ready to go to sleep. She referred to these visits as the "best times of her day."

As part of the discharge plan, the physical therapists took Elizabeth to her bungalow to "try out" everyday activities. The difficulty moving her leg was magnified when she was in her usual environment and the therapists began to think that she may not be able to return home. About the same time, Elizabeth began to have dramatic blood sugar swings that were accompanied by confusion and twitching that engaged all parts of her body. Her husband was anxious and looking for answers while she was consistently questioning: "What's going to happen to me now?" Her health challenge at this time was an arduous struggle to resume normal "independent" living in her bungalow with her husband, and what mattered most at this point was the unfamiliar, uncontrollable bodily experience, and the uncertainty that ensued from unfamiliarity. The question, "What's going to happen to me now?" was one the nurse had heard repeatedly over her years of nursing home practice as residents began to understand that they may not return home. She had begun to view the question as a marker of transition that demanded her concentrated attention to what mattered most for the resident.

Elizabeth didn't understand why her leg wouldn't move even though she worked so hard in therapy; she tried to hide the twitching, which she had never experienced before. The twitching and her attempts to move her leg took a lot of energy and she often said that she was tired. She never stopped saying that she wanted to "go home," but at some point the nurse suspected that the meaning of "going home" had changed for Elizabeth.

Continued

The nurse asked her "Where is home?" and Elizabeth responded that she wasn't sure. Shortly thereafter, Elizabeth stopped asking to go to the bungalow and she expressed wishes for a peaceful death.

It became clear that Elizabeth was not getting better as her heart failure became more debilitating and blood sugar swings continued in spite of precise insulin dosing and measured carbohydrate intake. At this time, the doctor suggested hospice. Elizabeth and her husband listened to the description of hospice services, and she signed the hospice papers. While under hospice care, she stopped troubling over her failed effort to move her left leg, continued to have blood sugar swings, and never stopped trying to hide the twitching.

Appearances mattered to Elizabeth, and she continued to care about how she looked. One time she told the nurse that she wore her pink shirt as often as she could because her husband liked it. She asked to have her "roots" done, and the nurse took her to the beauty shop one floor away. When she returned, her husband took her picture. She was wearing her pink shirt and her husband later included the picture in a memorial collage that was created when she died. The long loving relationship between Elizabeth and her husband was most important to both of them in her last days. She giggled with him while recalling fun times they had over the years and she asked for hugs, an uncharacteristic request that became increasingly familiar to her husband during this time.

Elizabeth and her roommate told each other stories, shared chocolates, and looked out for each other as well as they could. Her roommate called her "sweet pea." On the day Elizabeth died, the roommate asked Elizabeth's husband and the nurse if she could pray with them.

Elizabeth had been in the nursing home about 3 months before she died. The course of her story shifted from one of expectation for familiar normalcy in her bungalow with her husband to one of peaceful going home. The nurse in this situation of caring for

Elizabeth was attentively present to the shifting story, following Elizabeth's lead to pursue meaning during the last months of her life.

Phase three of the story inquiry process requires that the nurse become familiar with the existing literature about the complicating health challenge—in this case, transitioning from independent to nursing home living. For the purposes of this chapter, only the beginnings of a literature review are reported. However, the practicing nurse interested in a particular health challenge will stay abreast of related literature and eventually develop a broad literature base informing ongoing interpretation of stories and physiological bodily responses. To begin this literature search, the phrases "nursing home transition" and "elder" were searched together.

Brandburg (2007) conducted an integrated literature review intended to synthesize the state of the science regarding transition to a nursing home for older adults. The 13 articles that met the inclusion criteria led to the creation of a "transition process framework" with the foundational concepts of initial reaction, transitional influences, adjustment, and acceptance. Brandburg (2007) reported that the initial reaction and adjustment phases of the process require approximately 6 months. During that time, people move from disorganization to reorganization and relationship building. They also move from a sense of homelessness to recognition of a new home where new relationships are developed and old ones are cultivated. She describes the "final" or acceptance phase as one where "reflecting on the transition experience in light of personal values helped many older adults accept their new home because they could find meaning in their present situation" (p. 55).

The theme of home that was noted by Brandburg (2007) was strongly described by Heliker and Scholler-Jaquish (2006) in a study of 10 newly admitted nursing home residents who were interviewed multiple times over their first 3 months of residency. Residents responded to the directive: "Tell me a story about what it is like for you to come here and live." Data from 32 interviews lasting from 15 to 60 minutes were analyzed using a hermeneutical phenomenological approach. Three themes emerged: becoming homeless, getting settled, learning the ropes, and creating a place. The first theme, becoming homeless, contributed to the researchers' conclusion that "...one cannot separate home, memories, and friends from one's very identity. Each continuously shapes and is shaped by the other" (p. 41). Getting settled and learning the ropes was a theme characterized by residents' shift from unknown to known, invisible to visible. Creating a place was a theme related to creating meaning in this new life situation. In their conclusion, the authors note the important place of story: "The challenge for nursing home staff is to create situations, a clearing for sharing stories.....that facilitate the co-creation of new meanings....A staff that listens to what matters to residents can interpret a plan of care that is meaningful" (p. 41).

Listening was the major theme in a brief by Maynes (2004). She shared the story of a patient she met on a short hospitalization, during which his cancer diagnosis was confirmed and he was evaluated as having a "poor prognosis." The nurse listened to the quiet man and honored his wish to return "home" to the farm country where he was raised. On the day he was to be transferred, the nurse went to his bedside to say good-bye, thankful that he would be returning to the place he loved. When she approached the bed, she realized that he had died. "I sat next to him, put his hand in mine, and whispered 'good-bye'" (p. 32).

Elizabeth's short nursing home stay fits most clearly with the initial reaction phase described by Brandburg (2007) and the becoming homeless theme described by Heliker and Scholler-Jaquish (2006), both of whom call attention to the meaning of home. The idea of "home" emerges strongly from the literature and story sources. Both Elizabeth and the man in Maynes' (2004) brief feel the pull of "home" as they approach death.

Merging Elizabeth's story with the relevant literature prepared the stage for the next step of the story inquiry process, refining the name of the complicating health challenge.

Phase four suggests that the nurse refine the name of the complicating health challenge, if necessary. There may be some times when the original name is confirmed as adequately expressive of the challenge and there are other times when the convergence of the reconstructed story with the existing literature demands that the health challenge name be refined. We believe that "naming" is most important for the continuing work and we advocate that the health challenge name be neither "too high" nor "too low" in level of abstraction. Names that are too high may be difficult to apply to practice situations and names that are too low may be meaningful for only a very few people. Considering Elizabeth's story and the existing literature, the name of the complicating health challenge was changed to "struggling to go home." This complicating health challenge name is consistent with the original name of transitioning from independent to nursing home living, but it captures more clearly what matters most about the transition. It is neither "so high" that it cannot be applied in practice nor "so low" that it applies on only a narrow subset of people. Because it is "in the middle," it may also have applicability to other populations, such as people who have been evacuated from their homes due to natural disasters or families of premature newborns who demand extended hospital stays.

Phase five of the story inquiry process focuses on the developing story plot through identification of high points, low points, and turning points. Turning points are shifts in what is happening to create a revision in the storyteller's forward view. These are situations or events that move the story along. High and low points note times when things are going well or not so well. Table 26-1 records the turning points, high points, and low points in Elizabeth's reconstructed story. Turning points may also be high points or low points, but this is not always the case. Sometimes

Continued

Practice Exemplar cont.

Table 26 · 1   Turning Points, High Points, and Low Points in Elizabeth's Story

Story Event	TP	HP	LP
Difficulty moving leg beginning in January			x
Change in leg pain, temperature, and color—leading to hospitalization	x		x
Decision not to amputate	x	x	
Clot was dissolved	x	x	
Return to nursing home for rehabilitation	x		
Diagnosed with flu	x		x
Couldn't move leg though she tried			x
Husband's four-times-daily visits		x	
Inability to perform usual activities with physical therapist in bungalow—aware she may not return	x		x
Blood sugar swings, confusion, and twitching			x
"What's going to happen to me now?"			x
Stopped asking about going to bungalow and began talking about peaceful death	x		
Signed hospice papers	x		
Getting "roots" done, giggling with husband, sharing chocolate with roommate		x	

TP = turning point; HP = high point; LP = low point.

turning points exist with no particular value assigned by the person living the story. In Elizabeth's story, turning points can be summarized as: (1) diagnosed health issues, (2) treatment milestones, and (3) the hospice decision. High points are: (1) "favorable" (according to Elizabeth) treatment milestones and (2) relationship-centered moments of joy. Low points are: (1) limitations in physical movement, (2) unfamiliar bodily experiences with and without diagnoses, and (3) uncertainty. As the practicing nurse collected more stories of this nature, comparison, contrast, and synthesis of turning points, high points, and low points would be possible and the evidence from stories could contribute to the knowledge base guiding practice with people who are transitioning into a nursing home. One last phase of analysis considers the evidence from stories to identify how people get through the health challenge.

Phase six asks that the practicing nurse identify how an individual moved toward resolving the health challenge. This phase of practice inquiry may be most instructive for the nurse's continuing work with a particular population because it taps the inherent wisdom of people living the challenge to understand how they got by. The question facing the nurse analyzing Elizabeth's reconstructed story is: How does Elizabeth move toward resolving the complicating health challenge of struggling to go home? Elizabeth put all her effort into her recovery so that her therapists called her their "energizer bunny." When her efforts failed and her bodily experience indicated that she was on a different path, she signed the hospice papers. Finally, Elizabeth enjoyed moments with her husband and her roommate and chose to do things that kept her appearance as she liked. Movement toward resolving recounted in the reconstructed story included the approaches of (1) devoting energy to recovery, (2) accepting hospice, (3) experiencing the joy of relationship, and (4) attending to self through personal appearance. The range of ways Elizabeth moved toward resolving reflects the dynamic and complex nature of story. What is characterized as movement toward resolving emerges as the story unfolds. The four approaches extracted from the reconstructed story have implications for people who are struggling to go home, regardless of the context of their situation. The story describes how one person created ease and offers an invitation to consider how others in similar situations may create ease as they move toward resolving a health challenge of struggling to go home. Once again, there is guidance for nursing practice in the wisdom of people living health challenges. The nurse could use what is learned from this story analysis to guide current practice and frame further inquiry.

■ Summary

This chapter has introduced the reader to story as an essential element of practice evidence. In the story of Elizabeth, story theory and its related method dimensions were addressed. The authors hope that practicing nurses can use the story inquiry process to mine story evidence for the precious contribution it can make to nursing knowledge. Each nurse at the bedside, in the clinic, or in the office is uniquely positioned to gather and analyze practice stories. The middle-range Story Theory is proposed as a framework for structuring story-gathering and analysis.

References

Banks-Wallace, J. (2002). Talk the talk: Storytelling and analysis rooted in African-American oral tradition. *Qualitative Health Research, 12*(3), 410–426.

Benner, P. (1984). *From novice to expert.* Menlo Park, CA: Addison-Wesley.

Boykin, A., & Schoenhofer, S. (1991). Story as a link between nursing practice, ontology and epistemology. *IMAGE: Journal of Nursing Scholarship, 23,* 245–248.

Boykin, A., & Schoenhofer, S. (2001). The role of nursing leadership in creating caring environments in health care delivery systems. *Nursing Administration Quarterly, 25*(3), 1–7.

Brandburg, G. (2007). Making the transition to nursing home life: A framework to help older adults adapt to the long-term care environment. *Journal of Gerontological Nursing, 33*(6), 50–56.

Charon, R. (2006). *Narrative medicine: Honoring the stories of illness.* New York: Oxford University Press.

Charon, R., & Montello, M. (2002). *Stories matter: The role of narrative in medical ethics.* New York: Routledge.

Chinn, P. L., & Kramer, M. K. (1999). *Theory and nursing integrated knowledge development.* St. Louis, MO: C. V. Mosby.

Crichton, J., & Koch, T. (2007). Living with dementia: Curating self-identity. *Dementia, 6*(3), 365–381.

Diamond, J. (2000). *Narrative means to sober ends: Treating addiction and its aftermath.* New York: Guilford.

Ford, K., & Turner, D. (2001). Stories seldom told: Pediatric nurses' experiences of caring for hospitalized children with special needs and their families. *Journal of Advanced Nursing, 33,* 288–295.

Hain, D. (2007). What matters most?: Promoting adherence by understanding health challenges faced by hemodialysis patients. *American Kidney Fund: Professional Advocate, 7*(1), 3.

Hain, E. (2008). Cognitive function and adherence of older adults undergoing hemodialysis. *Nephrology Nursing Journal, 35*(1), 23–29.

Heliker, D. (2007). Story sharing: Restoring the reciprocity of caring in long-term care. *Journal of Psychosocial Nursing and Mental Health Services, 45*(7), 20–23.

Heliker, D., & Scholler-Jaquish, A. (2006). Transition of new residents: Basing practice on resident's perspective. *Journal of Gerontological Nursing, 32*(9), 34–42.

Holm, A-K., Lepp, M., & Ringsberg, K. C. (2005). Dementia: Involving patients in storytelling—a caring intervention. A pilot study. *Journal of Clinical Nursing, 14,* 256–263.

Keady, J., Williams, S., & Hughes-Roberts, J. (2007). Making mistakes: Using co-constructed inquiry to illuminate meaning and relationships in the early adjustment to Alzheimer's disease – a single case study approach. *Dementia, 6*(3), 343–364.

Liehr, P., & Smith, M. J. (2000). Using story theory to guide nursing practice. *International Journal of Human Caring, 4,* 13–18.

Liehr, P., & Smith, M. J. (2008). Story theory. In: *Middle range theory for nursing* (2nd ed.). New York: Springer.

Maynes, R. (2004). Going home again. *Nursing 2004, 34*(4), 32.

Mehl-Madrona, L. (2007). *Narrative medicine: The use of history and story in the healing process.* Rochester, VT: Bear & Company.

Newman, M. A. (1999). The rhythm of relating in a paradigm of wholeness. *Image: Journal of Nursing Scholarship, 31,* 227–230.

Newman, M. A., Sime, A. M., & Corcoran-Perry, S. A. (1991). The focus of the discipline of nursing. *Advances in Nursing Science, 14*(1), 1–6.

Nightingale, F. (1969). *Notes on Nursing.* New York: Dover.

Parse, R. R. (1981). *Man-living-health: A theory of nursing.* New York: John Wiley & Sons.

Peplau, H. (1991). *Interpersonal relations in nursing.* New York: Springer.

Polanyi, M. (1958). *The study of man.* Chicago: The University of Chicago Press.

Sierpina, M., & Cole, T. R. (2004). *Care Management Journals, 5*(3), 175–182.

Smith, M. J., & Liehr, P. (1999). Attentively embracing story: A middle-range theory with practice and research implications. *Scholarly Inquiry for Nursing. Practice: An International Journal, 13,* 187–204.

Smith, M. J., & Liehr, P. (2003). The theory of attentively embracing story. In: *Middle range theory for nursing.* New York: Springer.

Smith, M. J., & Liehr, P. (2005). Story theory: Advancing nursing practice scholarship. *Holistic Nursing Practice, 19*(6), 272–276.

Watson, J. (1997). The theory of human caring: Retrospective and prospective. *Nursing Science Quarterly, 10,* 49–52.

Williams, L. (2007). Whatever it takes: Informal caregiving dynamics in blood and marrow transplantation. *Oncology Nursing Forum, 34*(2), 379–387.

Chapter *27*

The Community Nursing Practice Model

MARILYN E. PARKER AND
CHARLOTTE D. BARRY

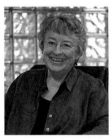

Marilyn E. Parker

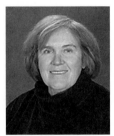

Charlotte D. Barry

Introducing the Theorists

Marilyn E. Parker is a professor at the Christine E. Lynn College of Nursing at Florida Atlantic University, where she is founding director of the Quantum Foundation Center for Innovation in School and Community Well-Being. She earned degrees from Incarnate Word College (BSN), the Catholic University of America (MSN), and Kansas State University (PhD). Her overall career mission is to enhance nursing practice, scholarship, and education through nursing theory, using both innovative and traditional means to improve care and advance the discipline.

As principal investigator for a program of grants to create and use a new Community Nursing Practice Model, Dr. Parker has provided leadership to develop transdisciplinary school-based wellness centers devoted to health and social services for children and families from underserved multicultural communities, teaching university students from several disciplines, and developing research and policy to promote community well-being.

Dr. Parker's active participation in nursing education and health care in several countries led to her 2001 Fulbright Scholar Award to Thailand where she continues collaboration with Thai colleagues. Her commitment to caring for underserved populations and to health policy evaluation led to being named a National Public Health Leadership Institute Fellow and to being elected a distinguished practitioner in the National Academies of Practice—Nursing. Dr. Parker is a fellow in the American Academy of Nursing.

Charlotte D. Barry is an associate professor and associate director at the Quantum Foundation Center for Innovation in School and Community Well-Being at the Florida Atlantic University Christine E. Lynn College of Nursing. Dr. Barry graduated from Brooklyn College, where she earned an associate degree in nursing; she holds a bachelor's degree in health administration, a master's degree in nursing from Florida Atlantic University in Boca Raton, and a PhD from the University of Miami, Florida. She is nationally certified in school nursing.

The focus of Dr. Barry's scholarship and teaching has been caring for persons in schools and communities. Current research includes the usefulness of the Community Nursing Practice Model to guide practice in the United States and Africa and school nursing practice issues including values, research, and delegation.

Dr. Barry provides leadership roles in many organizations, including the International Association of Human Caring (IAHC), the National Association of School Nursing (NASN), and the Florida Association of School Nurses (FASN). She serves on the Board of the NASN and is chair of the school nursing education special interest group. Active in FASN, she has served as president, treasurer, and board member.

Overview of the Model

The Community Nursing Practice Model (CNPM) described herein began with, and continues to be a blend of, the ideal and the practical. The ideal was the commitment to develop and use nursing concepts to guide nursing practice, education, and scholarship, and of a desire to develop a nursing practice as an essential component of a nursing college. The practical was the effort to bring this model to life within the context and structures of a community existing health care system. The model reflects the concept of nursing held by the faculty of nursing, *nursing is nurturing the wholeness of persons and environments through caring*, and the mission of the Christine E. Lynn College of Nursing

(Florida Atlantic University College of Nursing Philosophy and Mission, 1994/2003).

The concepts and relationships of the model are the guiding force for community practice. Through various participatory-action approaches, including ongoing shared reflection, intuitive insights, and discoveries, the Community Nursing Practice Model has evolved and continues to develop. The education of university students and the conduct of student and faculty research are integrated with nursing and social work practice. Throughout the early development and ongoing refinement of the model, there has been nurturing of collaborative community partnerships, evaluation and development of school and community health policy, and development of enriched community.

The model has been used as a framework for curriculum development for a master's program in advanced community nursing at Naresuan University, Phitsanulok, Thailand. The faculty of nursing at Mbarara University of Science and Technology, Mbarara, Uganda, has used the model to develop study of advanced community nursing and to design and operate the first school-based community nursing center in Uganda. The Community Nursing Practice Model guides a diverse, complex, and transdisciplinary practice of nursing and social work in school-based community wellness centers serving children and families from diverse multicultural communities and is accepted by local communities and providers as essential to the health care system. The model is featured in a major community nursing text (Clark, 2003). The practice received the 2001 award for Outstanding Faculty Practice from the National Organization of Nurse Practitioner Faculties.

Foundations of the Model

Essential values that form the basis of the model are (1) respect for person; (2) persons are caring, and caring is understood as the essence of nursing; and (3) persons are whole and always connected with one another in families and communities. These essential or transcendent values are always present in nursing situations, while other actualizing values guide practice in certain situations.

The principles of primary health care from the World Health Organization (1978) are the actualizing values. These additional concepts of the model are (1) access, (2) essentiality, (3) community participation, (4) empowerment, and (5) intersectoral collaboration. These also guide health care and social service practice. Concepts of practice that have emerged include transitional care and enhancing care. The model illuminates these values and each of the concepts in four interrelated themes: nursing, person, community, and environment, along with a structure of interconnecting services, activities, and community partnerships (Parker & Barry, 1999). An inquiry group method has been designed and is the primary means of ongoing assessment and evaluation (Parker, Barry, & King, 2000; Ryan, Hawkins, Parker, & Hawkins, 2004).

Nursing

The unique focus of nursing is nurturing the wholeness of persons and environments through caring (Florida Atlantic University [FAU], 1994/2003). Nursing practice, education, and scholarship require creative integration of multiple ways of knowing and understanding through knowledge synthesis within a context of value and meaning. Nursing knowledge is embedded in the nursing situation, the lived experience of caring between the nurse and the one receiving care. The nurse is authentically present for the other, to hear calls for caring and to create dynamic nursing responses. The school-based community wellness centers and satellite sites in the community become places for persons and families to access nursing and social services where they are: in homes, work camps, schools, or under trees in a community gathering spot. Nursing is dynamic and portable; there is no predetermined nursing and often no predetermined access place (Parker, 1997; Parker & Barry, 1999).

Nursing practice is further described within the context of transitional care and enhancing care. Transitional care is that in which clients and families are provided essential health care while being enrolled in a local insurance plan that will partially support that care. Over several weeks, clients are assisted to enroll in long-term forms of health care insurance and related benefits and are referred to a more permanent source of health care in the community. Transitional care, an ideal for nursing and social work practice, is sometimes not possible owing to immigration status, a complex and confounding application process, or other issues of the family.

Enhancing care describes nursing and social work that is intended to assist the client and family who need care in addition to that provided by a local health care provider.

Person

Respect for person is present in all aspects of nursing, with clients, community members, and colleagues. Respect includes a stance of humility that the nurse does not know all that can be known about a person and a situation, acknowledging that the person is the expert in his/her own care and knowing his/her experience. Respect carries with it an openness to learn and grow. Values and beliefs of various cultures are reflected in expressions of respect and caring. The person as whole and connected with others, not the disease or problem, is the focus of nursing.

Persons are empowered by understanding choices, how to choose, and how to live daily with choices made. The person defines what is necessary to well-being and what priorities exist in daily life of the family. Nursing and social work practice based on practical, sound, culturally acceptable, and cost-effective methods are necessary for well-being and wholeness of persons, families, and communities.

Early on, Swadener and Lubeck's (1995) work on deconstructing the discourse of risk was a major influence on practice. "At risk" connotes a deficiency that needs fixing; a doing to rather than collaborating with. Thinking about children and families "at promise" instead of "at risk" inspires an approach to knowing the other as whole and filled with potential.

Respect and caring in nursing require full participation of persons, families, and communities in assessment, design, and evaluation of services. Based on this concept, an inquiry group method is used for ongoing appraisal of services. This method is defined as a "route of knowing" and "a route to other questions." Each person is a coparticipant, an expert knower in their experience; the facilitator is expert knower of the process. The facilitator's role is to encourage expressions of knowing so calls for nursing and guidance for nursing responses can be heard. In this way, the essential care for persons and families can be known, and care designed, offered, and evaluated (Barry, 1998; Parker, Barry, & King, 2000).

Community

Community, as understood within the model, was formed from the classical definition offered by Smith and Maurer (1995) and from Peck's existential, relational view (1987). According to Smith and Maurer, a community is defined by its members and is characterized by shared values. This expanded notion of community moves away from a locale as a defining characteristic and includes self-defined groups who share common interests and concerns and who interact with one another.

Community, offered by Peck (1987), is a safe place for members and ensures the security of being included and honored. His work focuses on building community through a web of relationships grounded in acceptance of individual and cultural differences among faculty and staff and acceptance of others in the widening circles, including colleagues within the practice and discipline, other health care colleagues from varied disciplines, grant funders, and other collaborators. The notion of a transdisciplinary care is an exemplar of this approach to community. Another defining characteristic of community, according to Peck, is willingness to risk and tolerate a certain lack of structure. The practice guided by the model reflects this in fostering a creative approach to program development, implementation, evaluation, and research.

Practice in the model, whether unfolding in a clinic or under a tree where persons have gathered, provides a welcoming and safe place for sharing stories of caring. The intention to know others as experts in their self-care while listening to their hopes and dreams for well-being creates a communion between the client and provider that guides the development of a nurturing relationship. Knowing the other in relationship to their communities, such as family, school, work, worship, or play, honors the complexity of the context of persons' lives and offers the opportunity to understand and participate with them.

Environment

The notion of environment within this model provides the context for understanding the wholeness of interconnected lives. The environment, one of the oldest concepts in nursing described by Nightingale (1859/1992), is not only immediate effects of air, odors, noise, and warmth on the reparative powers of the patient, but also indicates the social settings that contribute to health and illness. Another nursing visionary, Lillian Wald, witnessed the hardships of poverty and disenfranchisement on the residents of the lower Manhattan immigrant communities. She developed the Henry Street Settlement House to provide a broad range of care that included direct physical care up to and including finding jobs, housing, and influencing the creation of child labor laws (Barry, 2003).

Chooporian (1986) re-inspired nurses to expand the notion of environment to include not only the immediate context of patients' lives, but also to think of the relationship between health and social issues that "influence human beings and hence create conditions for heath and illness" (p. 53). Reflecting on earth caring, Schuster (1990) urged another look at the environment, inviting nurses to consider a broader view that included nonhuman species and the nonhuman world. Acknowledging the interrelatedness of all living things energizes caring from this broader perspective into a wider circle. Kleffel (1996) described this as "an ecocentric approach grounded in the cosmos. The whole environment, including inanimate elements such as rocks and minerals, along with animate animals and plants, is assigned an intrinsic value" (p. 4). This directs thinking about the interconnectedness of all elements, both animate and inanimate. Teaching, practice, and scholarship require a caring context that respects, explores, nurtures, and celebrates the interconnectedness of all living things and inanimate objects throughout the global environment.

Structure of Services and Activities

The model is envisioned as three concentric circles around a core. Envisioning the model as a water color representation, one can appreciate the vibrancy of practice within the model, the amorphous interconnectedness of the core and the circles, and the "certain lack of structure" draws attention to the beauty in

creating, as well as the beauty in differences. The model calls into the circles others to create programs and environments to nurtured well being (Fig. 27-1).

Core Services

Core services are provided at each practice site and illuminate the focus of nursing: nurturing the wholeness of persons and environments through caring. The unique experiences of staff and faculty with those receiving care create the substance of the core: respecting self-care practice, honoring lay and indigenous care, inviting participation and listening to clients' stories of health and well-being, providing care that is essential for the other, supporting caring for self, family and community, providing care that is culturally competent, and collaborating with others for care. These services, provided to children, students, school staff, and families from the community, occur in the following and frequently overlapping categories of

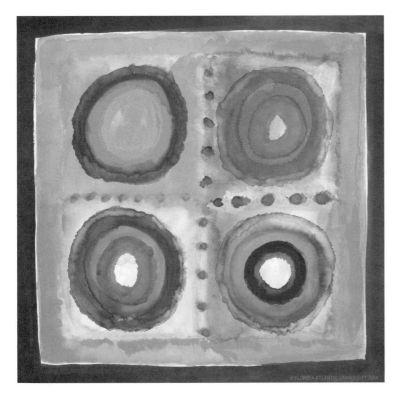

Figure 27 • 1 Community nursing practice model.

care: (1) *design and coordinate care:* examples are making and receiving referrals, navigation to other health services, and insurance enrollment, home visits, and programs such as the Celebrity Chef Cooking Club, Senior Health Program, or Yoga for Children; the concepts of transitional and enhancing care are illuminated here through the development of collaborative relationships; (2) *primary prevention and health education:* examples include child-development milestones, pre- and postnatal wellness, breast health, testicular examination, stress reduction, chronic illness management, car safety, and administration of immunizations; (3) *secondary prevention/health screening/early intervention:* examples include hearing and vision, height/weight/BMI, cholesterol, blood sugar, blood pressure, clinical breast exams, lead levels, assessment, and early management of health issues; (4) *tertiary prevention/primary care:* assessment, diagnosis, treatment, and care management for chronic health issues, crisis intervention and behavioral support, and collaborating with others for transitional and enhancing care.

First Circle

The first circle of the model depicts a widening circle of concern and support for well being of persons and communities. This circle includes persons and groups in each school and community who share concern for the well-being of persons served at the centers. This includes participants in inquiry groups, parents/guardians, school faculty, and noninstructional staff, after-school groups, parent/teacher organizations, and school advisory councils. The services provided within this circle might include: (1) *consultation and collaboration:* building relationships and community, answering inquiries on matters of health and well-being, providing in-service and health education, serving on school committees, reviewing policies and procedures; (2) *appraisal and evaluation:* conducting community assessments, appraising care provided, evaluating outcomes, and promoting programs that enhance well-being for individuals and communities.

Second Circle

The second circle draws attention to the wider context of concern and influence for well being and includes structured and organized groups whose members also share concern for the education and well-being of the persons served at the centers but within a wider range or jurisdiction such as a district or county. Examples of these policy-making or advising groups include the school district and county public health department, the county health-care district, Children's Service Council, American Lung Association, and the American Red Cross. Local funders who offer support for use of the model include the Health Care District of Palm Beach County, which offered initial support, and the Quantum Foundation, the ongoing sustaining funder. The services provided in this circle include (1) *consultation and collaboration:* building relationships and community with members of these groups, contributing to policy appraisal, development, and evaluation, leading and serving on teams and committees responsible for overseeing the care of students and families, and providing school nurse education; and (2) *research and evaluation:* assessing school health services, describing research findings for best practices related to school and community health, and designing research projects focused on school/community health issues, and/or school/community nursing practice.

Third Circle

The third circle includes state, regional, national, and international organizations with whom we are related in various ways. Services within this circle are focused on (1) *consultation and collaboration:* building relationships and community with members and collaborating about scholarship, policy, outcomes, practice, research, educational needs of school nurses and advanced practice nurses, and sustainability through ongoing and additional funding; (2) *appraisal and evaluation:* school nursing and advanced practice faculty organizations offer a milieu for discussion and appraisal of the services provided at the centers. Organizations in this circle include Florida Department of Health: Office of School Health, Florida Association of School Nurses, Florida Association of School Health, National Association of School Nurses, National Assembly of School-Based Health Centers, and the National Nursing Centers Consortium.

Connection of Core to Concentric Circles

Connections of the core to the concentric circles of services illuminate the appreciation of the complexity of the practice within the Community Nursing Practice Model. The core service of *consultation and collaboration* is a primary focus of practice, beginning with nursing and social work colleagues and extending to participating clients, families, policy makers, funders, and legislators. This value-laden service has been essential to the viability and sustainability of this model. It promotes the stance of humility that guides the respectful question throughout the circles: How can we be helpful to you? The answer directs the creation of respectful individualized care and program development. Essential health-care services are created within the core and extend into the first circle.

Connections to the second circle unfold from the collaborating relationships with colleagues in the health department, school district, health care district, and other groups taking the lead with school and community health. Committees on which center administrators and staff serve meet regularly to discuss school and community health issues and to seek consensus on possible solutions. These committees include the School Health Task Force and Advisory Groups and the Access Palm Beach County collaboration. The health department provides consultation on health and practice matters; the school district provides the physical space for the centers, and through a collaborative agreement with the health-care district, many of our clients without health insurance can be enrolled in a safety-net program of health services. Physicians are consultants for medical questions and referrals. School nurse education is also provided for nurses in the local county and in surrounding areas of this state.

Like the other circles, the third circle depicts the breadth of relationships developed at meetings, and through publications and presentations at local, regional, national, and international conferences. Administration and faculty have been recognized for the contribution made to the health and well-being of children and families. Faculty, staff, and students participate on panels, sharing their experiences in caring for underinsured and uninsured persons.

Practice Exemplar

A nursing situation titled *The Clothes Line* is offered as an exemplar from practice illuminating the core values and concepts of the CNPM, as well as collaborations developed in response to a call for nursing.

Cut-outs of cotton dresses, shirts, pants and socks strung on a clothes line are an aesthetic representation of a nursing situation grounded in the community nursing practice model. A group of nursing students studying community nursing at a homeless shelter asked the residents "How can we be helpful to you?" And they heard "We need to find jobs but don't have the right clothes, can you help us?" The students reflected, conferred and decided to try. They gathered clothes from their closets and their friends' closets that looked like a good fit and brought them to the shelter for the residents. Next they explored the neighborhood for resources and found a clothes cleaner nearby the shelter. After explaining to the manager the residents' need for clothes, a decision was made to set up a clothing collection box in the shop.

Continued

Practice Exemplar cont.

The students hoped that the prominently displayed collection box would attract others to leave clothes and also be accessible for the residents of the shelter to come pick out clothes for job hunting. The students returned to the shelter and explained the community clothing collection box. The residents expressed their gratitude to the students for listening to their hopes and dreams and for creating a way for them to "dress for success" and to get back on their feet. The students felt they had responded to a call for nursing; they connected to community resources, left behind a viable community project, and nurtured the wholeness of the persons living at the shelter.

Summary

The fundamental beliefs and commitment to the discipline and unique practice of nursing provided for both creating and sustaining this Community Nursing Practice Model. This model provides the environment in which nursing is practiced from the core beliefs of respect, caring, and wholeness. School-based wellness centers, developed and managed by nurses, have demonstrated the integration of the mission and philosophy of the College of Nursing. Members of the faculty and center staff are encouraged to practice from these beliefs and to reach out and through the concentric circles, strengthening and widening the web of relationships with colleagues, clients, and community members. Through use of this model, the ideals of the discipline are brought into reality of care for wholeness and well being of persons and families in multicultural communities.

References

Barry, C. (1994). Face painting as metaphor. In E. Schuster, & C. Brown (Eds.), *Exploring our environmental connections* (pp. 279–286). New York: National League for Nursing Press.

Barry, C. (1998). The celebrity chef cooking club: A peer involvement feeding program promoting cooperation and community building. *Florida Journal of School Health, 9*(1), 17–20.

Barry, C. (2003). *A retrospective: Looking back on Linda Rogers and the history of school nursing.* Paper presented at the 8th annual Florida Association of School Nurses Conference: Past, Present and Future: Continuing the Vision. Orlando, Florida, January 2003.

Barry, C. D., Blum, C. A., Eggenberger, T. L., Palmer-Hickman, C., & Mosley, R. (July/August 2009). Understanding homelessness using a simulated nursing experience. *Journal of Holistic Nursing Practice, 23*(4), 230–237.

Barry, C., Blum, C. A., & Purnell, M. (2007). Caring for Individuals Displaced by Hurricanes Katrina and Wilma: The Lived Experience of Student Nurses. *International Journal for Human Caring, 11(2)*, 67-73.

Barry, C., Bozas, L., Carswell, J., Hurtado, M., Keller, M., Lewis, E., Poole, K., & Tipton, B. (1998). Nursing a school-aged child provides an insight to the Guatemalan culture. *Florida Journal of School Health, 9*(1), 29–36.

Barry, C., & Gordon, S. (2006a). Theories and models of school nursing. In J. Selekman (Ed.), *Comprehensive Textbook of School Nursing.* Scarborough, ME: National Association of School Nursing.

Barry, C. D., & Gordon, S. C. (2006b). Caring for students in school using a community nursing practice model. *International Journal for Human Caring, 9*(3), 38-42.

Barry, C. D., & Gordon, S. C. (2009). Coming to know the community: Going to the mountain. In: R. C. Locsin & M. J. Purnell (Eds.), *A contemporary process of nursing: The (un)bearable weight of knowing in nursing.* New York: Springer.

Barry, C. D., Gordon, S. C., & Lange, B. (2007). The usefulness of the Community Nursing Model in school based community wellness centers: Voices from the U.S. and Africa. *Research and Theory for Nursing Practice: An International Journal, 21*(3), 174–184.

Chooporian, T. (1986). Reconceptualizing the environment. In: P. Mocia (Ed.), *New approaches to theory development* (pp. 39–54). New York: National League for Nursing Press.

Clark, M. J. (2003). *Community health nursing: Caring for populations.* Upper Saddle River, NJ: Prentice-Hall.

Florida Atlantic University Christine E. Lynn College of Nursing. (1994/2003). Mission and philosophy. In: *Faculty handbook.* Boca Raton, FL: Florida Atlantic University Christine E. Lynn College of Nursing.

Kleffel, D. (1996). Environmental paradigms: Moving toward an ecocentric perspective. *Advances in Nursing Science, 18*(4), 1–10.

Nightingale, F. (1859/1992). *Notes on nursing: Commemorative edition with commentaries by contemporary nursing leaders.* Philadelphia: J. B. Lippincott.

Parker, M. E. (1996). Designing a nursing model of primary health care and early intervention. Proposal funded by the health care district of Palm Beach County, FL.

Parker, M. E. (1997). Emerging innovations: Caring in action. *International Journal for Human Caring, 1*(2), 9–10.

Parker, M. E., & Barry, C. D. (1997). Love and suffering at the margins. Paper presented at the International Association of Human Caring Research Conference, the Primacy of Love and Existential Suffering, Helsinki, Finland.

Parker, M. E., & Barry, C. D. (1999). Community practice guided by a nursing model. *Nursing Science Quarterly, 12*(2), 125–131.

Parker, M. E., Barry, C. D., & King, B. (2000). Use of inquiry method for assessment and evaluation in a school-based community nursing project. *Family and Community Health, 23*(2), 54–61.

Parker, M. E., Pandya, A., Hsu, S., Noell, D., & Newlin, K. (2007), Assuring Nursing's Voice in the Electronic Health Record. In: *IEEE International Conference on Natural Language and Knowledge Development Engineering, Beijing, China. Proceedings.* Institute of Electrical and Electronics Engineers, NLP-KE 107.

Peck, S. (1987). *The different drum: Community making and peace.* New York: Simon & Schuster.

Ryan, E., Hawkins, W., Parker, M. E., & Hawkins, M. (2004). Perceptions of access to U. S. health care of Haitian immigrants in South Florida. *Florida Public Health Review, 1,* 36–43.

Schuster, E. (1990). Earth caring. *Advances in Nursing Science, 13*(1), 25–30.

Smith, C., & Mauer, F. (1995). *Community health nursing: Theory and practice.* Philadelphia: W.B. Saunders.

Swadener, B., & Lubeck, S. (1995). *Children and families "at promise." Deconstructing the discourse on risk.* Albany: State University of New York Press.

World Health Organization, Alma-Ata. (1978). *Primary health care.* Geneva, Switzerland: World Health Organization.

Chapter 28

Rozzano Locsin's Technological Competency as Caring and the Practice of Knowing Persons in Nursing

ROZZANO C. LOCSIN

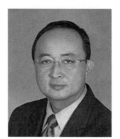

Rozzano C. Locsin

Introducing the Theorist

Rozzano C. Locsin is Professor of Nursing at Florida Atlantic University's Christine E. Lynn College of Nursing. "Life transitions in the health-illness experience" defines his program of research in which the model of "Technological competence as caring in nursing" is illustrated as the practice of "knowing persons" through technologies in nursing. Dr. Locsin was a Fulbright Scholar to Uganda in 2000, a recipient of the 2004–2006 Fulbright Alumni Initiative Award to Uganda, and Fulbright Senior Specialist in Global and Public Health and International Development. He received the prestigious Edith Moore Copeland Excellence in Creativity Award from Sigma Theta Tau International Honor Society of Nursing, and two lifetime achievement awards from premier schools of nursing in the Philippines. His edited book *Advancing Technology, Caring, and Nursing* was published in 2001. His middle-range nursing theory, *Technological Competency as Caring in Nursing: A Model for Practice*, was released in March 2005. He co-edited the book *Technology and Nursing: Practice, Process and Issues*, published in 2007. A fourth book, *A Contemporary Process of Nursing: The (Unbearable) Weight of Knowing in Nursing*, was published in 2009. His interest in global nursing and care initiatives enhances his appreciation of the dynamic nature of humans, and of nursing as the practice of continuous knowing of persons through contemporary technologies within a caring in nursing framework. He holds baccalaureate and masters degrees in Nursing from Silliman University in the Philippines, and a PhD in Nursing from the University of the Philippines. He was inducted as a Fellow of the American Academy of Nursing in 2006.

Overview of the Theory

There is a great demand for a practice of nursing based on an authentic intention to know humans fully as persons rather than as objects of care. Nurses want to use creative, imaginative, and innovative ways of affirming, appreciating, and celebrating humans as whole persons. Often the best way to realize these intentions is through expert, competent use of nursing technologies (Locsin, 1998).

Frequently perceived as the practice of using machines in nursing (Locsin, 1995), technological competency as caring in nursing is the practice of knowing persons as whole (Locsin, 2001), frequently with the use of health-care technologies. Contemporary definitions of technology include a means to an end, an instrument, a tool, or a human activity that increases or enhances efficiency (Heidegger, 1977). Conceptualizing technology and caring in nursing practice is problematic. Viewing them in harmonious coexistence is crucial to understanding technological competency as an expression of caring (Locsin, 2005).

The purpose of this chapter is to explain "knowing persons through technological competency as a practice of nursing," a framework of nursing that guides its practice, grounded in the theoretical construct of *technology competency as caring in nursing* (Locsin, 2005). This model of practice illuminates the harmonious relationship between technological competency and caring in nursing. In this model, the focus of nursing is the person, a human being whose hopes, dreams, and aspirations are focused on living life fully as a caring person (Boykin & Schoenhofer, 2001).

As a model of practice, *technological competency as caring in nursing* (Locsin, 2005) is as valuable today as it has been and will continue to be in the future. Advancing technologies in

health care demand expertise with technologies. Often, such expertise is perceived as non-caring in situations where the focus of knowing is on the technology, rather than on the person. It is the premise of this chapter, however, that being technologically competent is being caring. For the purposes of this theory, the following assumptions are posited:

- Persons are whole or complete in the moment (Boykin & Schoenhofer, 2001).
- Knowing persons is a practice process of nursing that allows for continuous appreciation of persons moment to moment (Locsin, 2005).
- Nursing is a discipline and a professional practice (Boykin & Schoenhofer, 2001)
- Technology is used to know persons fully in the moment (Locsin, 2005).

The ultimate purpose of technological competency in nursing is to acknowledge the person as a focus of nursing and that various technological means can and should be used in the practice of knowing persons in nursing.

This acknowledgment of persons brings together the relatively abstract concept of wholeness of person with the more concrete concept of technology. Such acknowledgment compels the redesigning of nursing processes—ways of expressing, celebrating, and appreciating the practice of nursing as continuously knowing persons as whole moment to moment. In this practice of nursing, technology is used not to know "what is the person?" but rather to know "who is the person?" Appropriately, answers to the former question allude to an expectation of knowing empirical aspects and facts about the composite person; the latter question requires the understanding of an unpredictable, irreducible person who is more than and different from the sum of his or her empirical self. The former question alludes to the idea of persons as objects; the latter addresses the uniqueness and individuality of persons as humans who continuously unfold and who therefore require continuous knowing (Locsin, 2005).

Persons as Whole and Complete in the Moment

One of the earlier definitions of the word *person* was evident in Hudson's 1988 publication claiming that the "emphasis on inclusive rather than sexist language has brought into prominence the use of the word 'person'" (p. 12). The origin of the word *person* is from the Greek word *prosopon*, which means the actor's mask of Greek tragedy; in Roman origin, *persona* indicated the role played by the individual in social or legal relationships. Hudson (1988) also declares that "an individual in isolation is contrary to an understanding of 'person'" (p. 15). A necessary appreciation of persons is the view that humans are whole or complete in the moment. As such, there is no need to fix them or to make them complete again (Boykin & Schoenhofer, 2001). There is nothing missing that requires nurses' intervening to make persons "whole or complete" again, or for nurses to assist in this completion. Persons are complete in the moment. Their varying situations of care call for creativity, innovation, and imagination from nurses so that they may come to know the nursed as "whole" person. The uniqueness of the person emerges in the response called forth in particular situations.

Inherent in humans as unpredictable, dynamic, and living beings is the regard for self-as-person. This appreciation is like the human concern for security, safety, self-esteem, and actualization popularized by Maslow (1943) in his quintessential theoretical model on the "hierarchy of needs." More important, however, is the understanding that being human is being a person, regardless of biophysical parts or technological enhancements.

Because the future may require relative appreciation of persons, if the ultimate criterion of being human today is that humans are only those who are all natural, organic, and functional, being human may not be so easy to determine. The purely natural human being may be rare. The understanding that technology-supported life is artificial and therefore is not natural stimulates discussions among practitioners of nursing (Locsin & Campling, 2005), particularly when the subject of concern is technology-dependent care and technology competency as an expression of caring in nursing. Hudson (1988) suggests that "false comfort may be offered whenever it is implied that this life and this body are significantly less important than the 'spiritual body' and the 'next life'... the time has come to enhance an awareness of the post human or spiritual future" (p. 13). What structural requirements will the post human possess? Today, some humans have anatomic and/or physiologic components that are already electronic and/or mechanical, such as mechanical cardiac valves, self-injecting insulin pumps, cardiac pacemakers, or artificial limbs, all appearing as excellent facsimiles of the real. Yet the idea of a "whole person" and being natural continues to persist as a requirement of what a human being should be (Fig. 28-1).

How Are Persons Known?

Often, questioning in order to know the person is limited to inquiry about body parts. For example, "How are your knees?" instead of "How are you doing with your knees?" Of what purpose is the question? Is it to know the person, or to know the condition of the specific composite part? Perhaps inadvertently, unconsciously, or both, one consciously inquires about the body part because of a culturally founded reason, or the customary focus on another's bodily features that defines the person!

How are persons as human beings known? Historically, humans were depicted through drawings and paintings. Art works using colors represented the human being in imaginative ways as conceptualized by painters and illustrators. Through colors, aesthetic representations provided vivid depictions of the human being. Artists and their works became commodities, and Leonardo DaVinci topped this list as, perhaps, the most popular of illustrators and painters. Studying the human being as object allowed him to illustrate the composite of the human being through dissected remains. Illustrations such as these may have influenced Michelangelo in his creation

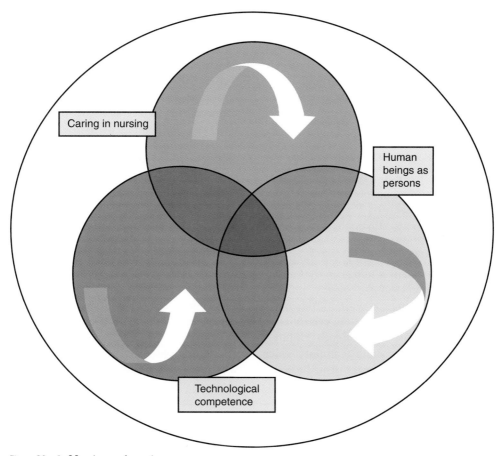

Figure 28 • 1 Nursing as knowing persons.

of masterful artworks such as David and Moses. The clarity, definition, and fidelity of the representation provided the utmost appreciation of the human being. Yet the question remains: does the human being become a person, or is he a person always? Is the composition of the human being the ultimate descriptor, characteristic, and quality of a whole and complete person? What happens when the human being has no limbs—or at the least has limbs which are not functional? Is this human being a person?

Consider the case of a baby born without limbs but was alive and well. When the baby became ill, he was rushed to a hospital. To the chagrin of the nurses and physicians, they were at first unable to care for the baby. Their main question was "How can we initiate IVs

when there are no extremities?" They may also have wondered, "On growing up, will this baby be concerned about what it is like to have no limbs, or will he wish he had limbs so he could 'go' places like others?" (Barnard & Locsin, 2007, p. 17).

Consider also the "Girl with Eight Limbs" from a province in India, who was subjected to intense surgical intervention to remove the other "non-functional" limbs which were putting her life in a precarious situation. What do you think this girl thinks now? "Am I complete or incomplete? Am I normal or abnormal, just because I am like everyone else – with two upper limbs and two lower limbs?" (PBS).

In an episode of the television series *The Twilight Zone*, a woman so hideous she was thought unworthy to be seen, had to hide her face behind a veil. She was shunned and denied by her family. It was an unbearable life for her and for her family as well. In the end, the revelation focused on the adage "beauty is in the eye of the beholder" (Serling, 1960). The people who shunned the woman had faces like those of pigs, while she had more "human-like" features. In fact, she was a beautiful human woman whom everyone found to be ugly, embarrassing, pitiful, and a misfit, and was advised to move to a distant colony with a small population of people like her.

In a recent Associated Press news article, "The Androgynous Pharoah? Akhenated Had Feminine Physique" (*USA Today*, May 2, 2008), writer Alex Dominguez presented Dr. Irwin Braverman's findings on the controversial "feminine" features of the pharaoh Akhenaten. Dominguez wrote, "Akhenaten wasn't the most manly pharaoh, even though he fathered at least a half-dozen children. In fact, his form was quite feminine, which has puzzled experts for years. And he was a bit of an egghead." The pharaoh had "an androgynous appearance. He had a female physique with wide hips and breasts, but he was male and he was fertile and he had six daughters," Braverman is quoted as saying. "But nevertheless, he looked like he had a female physique." Apparently, what constitutes "knowing" whether a human being is a man or a woman is the physical appearance. This makes Braverman's study of the Pharoah Akhenaten most meaningful.

An example of person as object, known as a composite of physical elements, is the legendary Frankenstein monster, an entity assembled from various human parts. The monster was created and made human in the sense of being a composite of parts, but also in the sense of his essence being energy (electricity).

The Process of Knowing Persons

Persons possess the prerogative and the choice whether or not to allow nurses to know them fully. Entering the world of the other is a critical requisite to knowing as a process of nursing. Establishing rapport, trust, confidence, commitment, and the compassion to know

others fully as persons is integral to this crucial positioning.

Wholeness is the idealized condition or situation of the one who is nursed. This idealization is held within the nurse's understanding of persons as complete human beings "in the moment." Expressions of this completeness vary from moment to moment. These expressions are human illustrations of living and growing. Using technology alone and focusing on the received technological data rather than on continually "knowing" the other fully as person can lead to the nurse thinking of the person as an object who needs to be completed and made whole again. Paradoxically, because of the idea that humans are unpredictable, it is not entirely possible for the nurse to fully know another human being—except in the moment and only if the person allows the nurse to know him or her by entering into the other's world.

In this perspective, the condition in which the nurse and the other allow knowing each other exists as the nursing situation, the shared lived experience between the nurse and nursed (Boykin & Schoenhofer, 2001).

In this relationship, trust is established that the nurse will know the other fully as person; the trust that the nurse will not judge the person or categorize the person as just another human being or experience, but rather as a unique person who has hopes and aspirations that are singularly his or her own.

It is the nurse's responsibility to know the person's hopes and aspirations. Technological competency as caring allows for this understanding. In doing so, the nurse also sanctions the other (the nursed) to know him or her as person. The expectation is that the nurse is to use multiple ways of knowing competently in using technologies in order to know the other fully as person. The nurse's responsibility is immeasurable in creating conditions that demand technological competency and care, much like the wish to create a computerized human facsimile. In creating a nursing situation of care, there is a requisite competency to know persons fully, to understand, and to appreciate the important nuances of the person's dreams and desires.

There are many ways of interpreting the concept of "person as whole." Three of the popular interpretations are derivations of the concept of person from dominant perspectives, those views that shape the popular understanding of the concept. One of these interpretations is the mind–body dualism popularly ascribed to Descartes, which supplies the continuing citation of the connection between mind and body. At least in nursing, the mind–body–spirit connection is popularized by Jean Watson (1985) in her theory of transpersonal caring. The simultaneity paradigm (Parse, 1998) categorizes the human–environmental mutual connection as the relationship that best serves the human science nursing perspective and grounds theoretical frameworks and models of practice, including those of the caring sciences. These contemporary and popular elucidations create conceptions of humans as the focus of nursing and of knowing persons in their wholeness as the practice of nursing.

The process of nursing is a dynamic unfolding of situations encompassing knowledgeable practices. The meaning of the process is characterized by listening, knowing, being with, enabling, and maintaining belief (Swanson, 1991). The following occurrences exemplify the process:

- Knowing and appreciating uniqueness of persons
- Designing participation in caring
- Implementing and evaluating (a simultaneous illustration and exercise of conjoining relationships crucial to knowing persons by using nursing technologies)
- Verifying knowledge of person through continuous knowing

In this model of practice, knowing is the primary process. "Knowing nursing means knowing in the realms of personal, ethical, empirical, and aesthetic—all at once" (Boykin & Schoenhofer, 2001, p. 6). The continuous, circular process demonstrates the ever-changing, dynamic, cyclical nature of knowing

in nursing. Knowledge about the person that is derived from assessing, intervening, evaluating, and further assessing additionally informs the nurse that in knowing persons, one comes to understand the condition of more knowing about the person and about his or her being, in order to affirm, support, and celebrate his or her dreams and aspirations in the moment. Supporting this process of knowing is the understanding that persons are unpredictable and simultaneously conceal and reveal themselves as persons from one moment to the next (Parse, 1998).

The nurse can know the person fully only in the moment.

This knowing occurs only when the person allows the nurse to enter his or her world. When this happens, the nurse and nursed become vulnerable as they move toward further continuous knowing.

Vulnerability allows participation, so that the nurse and nursed continue knowing each other moment to moment. In such situations, Daniels (1998) explains that "nurse's work is to ameliorate vulnerability" (p. 191). The embodiment of vulnerability in caring situations enables its recognition in others, participating in mutual vulnerability conditions, and sharing in the humanness of being vulnerable. Further, Daniels declares that "vulnerable individuals seek nursing care, and nurses seek those who are vulnerable" (p. 192). Allowing the nurse to enter the world of the one nursed is the mutual engagement of "power with" rather than having "power over" through a created hierarchy (Daniels, 1998). The nurse does not know more about the person than the person knows about him- or herself. No one knows the experience better than the person who encounters the situation.

Nonetheless, there is the possibility that the nurse will be able to predict and prescribe for the one nursed. When this occurs, these situations forcibly lead the nurse to appreciate persons more as object than as person. Such a situation can occur only when the nurse has assumed to "have known" the one nursed. While it can be assumed that with the process of "knowing persons as whole," opportunities to continuously know the other become limitless, there is also a much greater likelihood that having "already known" the one nursed, the nurse will predict and prescribe activities or ways for the one nursed, ultimately causing objectification of person (Fig. 28-2).

To Know and Knowing

It is interesting to read the 10 common definitions of the word "know" as a verb listed in the 1987 *Reader's Digest Illustrated Encyclopedic Dictionary* (p. 932). Of these, nine appropriately describe the intended use of the word in nursing, facilitating its understanding for the purpose and process of competently using technologies in nursing. These descriptions are:

• To perceive directly with the senses or mind
• To be certain of, regard, or accept as true beyond doubt
• To be capable of, have the skills to
• To have thorough or practical understanding of, as through experience of
• To be subjected to or limited by
• To recognize the character or quality of
• To be able to distinguish, recognize
• To be acquainted or familiar with
• To see, hear, or experience

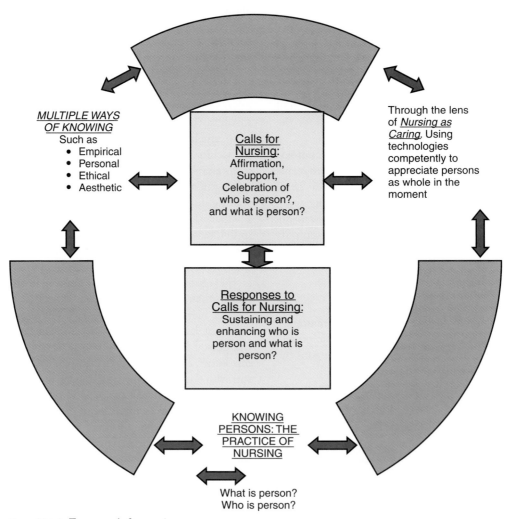

Figure 28 • 2 Framework for nursing.

While the action word "know" sustains the notion that nursing is concerned with activity and that the one who acts is knowledgeable (in the sense of understanding the rationales behind the activities), the word "knowing" is a key concept that alludes to the focus of an action from a cognitive perspective requiring description. "Knowing" perfectly describes the ways of nursing—transpiring continuously as explicated from the framework of "knowing persons." It is the use of the word "knowing" in which the process of nursing as "knowing persons" is lived. The framework for practice clearly shows the circuitous and continuous process of knowing persons as a practice of nursing.

It is appreciated that nurses practice nursing from a theoretical perspective rather than from tradition or from blind obedience to instructions and directions. Nevertheless, processes of nursing that are derived from extant theories of nursing continue to dictate and prescribe how a nurse should nurse. Contrary to this popular conception, "knowing persons" as a model of practice using technologies of nursing achieves for the nurse an appreciation of expertise and the knowledge of persons in the moment. Technologies allow nurses to know about the person only as much as the person permits the nurse to know. It can be true that technologies detect the anatomical, physiological, chemical, and/or biological conditions of a person. This identifies the person as a living human being. However, with knowing persons, the nurse is allowed to understand and anticipate the ever-changing person from moment to moment.

The purpose of knowing the person is derived from the nurse's intention to nurse (Purnell & Locsin, 2000)—a continuing appreciation of the person as ever-changing and never static: one who is a dynamic human being. The information derived from knowing the person is only relevant for the moment, for the person's "state" can change moment to moment. Importantly, knowing the "who or what" of persons helps nurses realize that a person is more than simply the physiochemical and anatomical being. Knowing persons allows the nurse to know "who and what" is the person.

Knowing When Using Technology

From such a view, it may seem that the process of knowing is possible only when using technologies in nursing. This perception, which is not necessarily true, is supported by the idea that nursing is technology when technology is appreciated as anything that creates efficiency, be this an instrument or a tool, such as machines, or the activity of nurses when nursing. Sandelowski (1993) has argued about the metaphorical depiction of nursing as technology, or with technology as nursing, and the semiotic relationship of these concepts. Locsin and Purnell (2007) have declared that accompanying the rapture of technologies in nursing is the consequent suffering or the price of advancing dependency on technologies that critically influence contemporary human lives. With increased use of technologies and ensuing technological dependency experienced by recipients of care, the imperative is to provide technological competency as caring in nursing (Locsin, 2005).

Regardless, the idea of knowing persons guiding nursing practice is novel in the sense that there is no ideal prescription; rather there is the wholesome appreciation of an informed practice that allows the use of multiple ways of knowing such as described by Phenix (1964) and expanded by Carper (1978). These ways of knowing involve the empirical, ethical, personal, and aesthetic. Aesthetic expressions document, communicate, and perpetuate the appreciation of nursing as transpiring moment to moment. Popular aesthetic expressions include storytelling; poetry; visual expressions as in drawings, illustrations, and paintings; and aural renditions such as music. Encountering aesthetic expressions again allows the nurse and the nursed to relive the occasion anew. Reflecting on these experiences using the fundamental patterns of knowing (Carper, 1978) enhances learning, motivates the furtherance of knowledgeable practice, and increases the valuing of nursing as a professional practice grounded in a legitimate theoretical perspective of nursing.

The use of technologies in nursing is consequent to the contemporary demands for nursing actions requiring technological knowing (Locsin, 2009). Technological knowing is demanded for the ultimate purpose of knowing the real person. The concept of technological knowing is construed as the practice process of using technologies of care to acknowledge the value of knowing the one nursed through contemporary technological advancements. Important along with technology use in nursing is the condition that the one nursed allows him- or herself to be known as person.

Technological competency in nursing fosters the recognition and realization of persons as participants in their care rather than objects of care. The idea of "participation in their care" stems from active engagement, in which the nurse enters the world of the one nursed through available appropriate technologies, attempting to know the nursed more fully in the moment. In this practice, the assumption is understood that the one nursed allows the nurse to enter his or her world so that together they may mutually support, affirm, and celebrate each other's being. In this relationship of the knower and the one known, technology provides the efficiency and the valuing that marks their mutual and momentary reality (Locsin, 2009).

There is no letting up, because advancing technology currently encompasses the bulk of functional activities that nurses are expected to perform, particularly when the practice is in a clinical setting. Clinical nursing is firmly rooted in the clinical health model (Smith, 1983) in which the organismic and mechanistic views of humans as persons convincingly dictate the practice of nursing. Nevertheless, the process of knowing persons will prevail, for the model of technological competency as caring in nursing provides the nurse the fitting stimulation and motivation (and the prospective autonomy to judge critically) a mode of action that desires an appreciation of persons as whole.

The model articulates continuous knowing. **Continuing to know persons deters objectification, a process that ultimately regards human beings as "stuff" to care about, rather than as knowledgeable participants in their care.**

Participating in his or her care frees the person from having to be "assigned" a care that he or she may not want or need. This relationship signifies responsiveness (Hudson, 1988). Continuous knowing results from the contention that findings through consequent knowing further inform the desire to know "who is" and "what is" the person. Doing so inhibits substantiation as the ultimate reason for nursing. Continuous knowing overpowers the motivation to prescribe and direct the person's life. Rather, it affirms, supports, and celebrates his or her hopes, dreams, and aspirations as a participating human being.

Calls and Responses for Nursing

Calls for nursing are illuminations of the persons' hopes, dreams, and aspirations. Calls for nursing are individual expressions by persons who seek ways toward affirmation, support, and celebration as person. The nurse appreciates the uniqueness of persons in his or her nursing. In doing so, the nurse sustains and enhances the wholeness of the human being, while facilitating the realization of the persons' completeness through "acting for or with" the person. This is a way of affirming, supporting, and celebrating the person's wholeness.

The nurse relies on the person for calls for nursing. These calls are specific mechanisms that persons use while allowing the nurse to respond with authentic intentions to know them fully as persons in the moment. Calls for nursing may be expressed in various ways, often as hopes and dreams, such as the hope to be with friends while recuperating in the hospital, or the desire to play the piano when fingers are well enough to function effectively, or simply the ultimate desire to go home, or the wish to die peacefully. As uniquely as these calls for nursing are expressed, the nurse knows the person continuously moment to moment. One way of communicating created nursing responses may be as patterns of information, such as those derived from machines like the EKG monitor, in order to know the physiological status of the person in the moment or to administer life-saving medications, institute transfer plans, or refer patients for services to other health-care professionals.

The entirety of nursing is to direct, focus, attain, sustain, and maintain the person. In doing so, hearing calls for nursing is continuous and momentarily complete. Knowing persons allows the nurse to use technologies in articulating calls for nursing. The empirical, personal, ethical, and aesthetic ways of knowing that are fundamental to understanding persons as whole increase the likelihood of knowing persons in the moment.

As unpredictable and dynamic, human beings are ever changing moment to moment. This characteristic challenges the nurse to know persons continuously as whole, rejecting the traditional conception of possibly knowing persons completely at once, in order to prescribe and predict their expressions of wholeness. In continuously knowing persons as whole through articulated technologies in nursing, the nurse can perhaps intervene to facilitate patients' recognition of their wholeness in the moment.

Applications of the Theory

Locsin's theory is relatively new. Applications of the theory of *Technological Competency as Caring in Nursing* has been elusive although anecdotal references as to its utility exist. Through these anecdotes received in various occasions especially after presentations and conversations and through personal communications via electronic mails, these positive declarations continue to provide the confirmation that the theory is useful particularly in nursing practice. Often during class presentations and in scholarly/academic conferences, students and participants express their claims that the theory resonates well in their practice, affirming their understanding of nursing, and confirming their appreciation of knowing persons through technologies as practice. However, there has been an absence of comments from practitioners who have signified that the theory has guided their practice, or of any researcher who has claimed that he or she has used the theory as framework in any study. Nevertheless, the claims that the theory has affirmed one's practice exist.

Practice Exemplar

In one South Florida migrant camp during the time of the harvest, a beautiful infant child—a firstborn son—was born to two proud parents. The child was healthy but he was born without arms and legs. Two weeks after birth, the infant caught an infection suddenly and was rushed to an area hospital for help. Physicians and nurses were stunned: How could they perform the needed technology-based care such as drawing blood for laboratory tests, and placing a cuff on the arm or leg to measure blood pressure? Their ability to care for the infant was limited by the technological design of available medical devices and the assumed presentation of human completeness. The technology available required a focus on the usual anatomical and physiological composition of a human being; that is the design required a person to have both torso and limbs intact (Locsin & Barnard, 2007).

The technological challenges expressed by the health care personnel, especially nurses, focused on how they can monitor the infant's vital signs when the technologies required "limbs" which were missing? The challenge was directed towards their views on knowing of persons as whole—responding to the essentiality of technological competency as caring in nursing. The understanding of wholeness of persons departs from the traditional view of

Continued

humans as composites of human parts, and that human wholeness is the complete human with the standard parts. What about those born without these composite human parts, like the infant born without all four limbs? What about those with technological parts as replacements for lost or missing parts, those individuals with artificial limbs, electronic/mechanical devices that make them live? They continue to be human, to be whole, and through technological marvels, the nurse is able to know these persons more fully as persons. As with the infant without limbs, the technologies could not be used, deterring the nurse from knowing the infant's physiological responses. The ultimate question raised is focused on how much "fullness" can be known of the person, when technologies cannot be used? This is an example of the realization that machine technologies (Locsin, 1995) allow the nurse (rather than limits) to know the person more fully as person. Knowing person as process of nursing is synonymous with everyday approaches to theory-based nursing practice; that is, nursing practice guided by theories of nursing.

■ Summary

The purpose of this chapter is to describe and explain "knowing persons as whole," a framework of nursing guiding a practice grounded in the theoretical construct of *technological competency as caring in nursing* (Locsin, 2005). This framework of practice illuminates the harmonious relationship between technological competency and caring in nursing. In this model, the focus of nursing is the person.

Critical to understanding the phenomenon of technological competency as caring in nursing are the conceptual descriptions of technology, caring, and nursing. Assumptions about human beings as persons, nursing as caring, and technological competency are presented as foundational to the process of knowing persons as whole in the moment—a process of nursing grounded in the perspective of technological competency as caring in nursing.

The process of knowing persons as whole is explicated as technological efficiency in nursing practice. The model of practice is illustrated through the understanding of technology and caring as coexisting in nursing. The process of knowing persons is continuous. In this process of nursing, with calls and responses, the nurse and nursed come to know each other more fully as persons in the moment. Grounding the process is the appreciation of persons as whole and complete in the moment, of human beings as unpredictable, of technological competency as an expression of caring in nursing, and of nursing as critical to health care.

References

Barnard, A., & Locsin, R. (2007). Technology and nursing: Concepts, practice, and issues. London, UK, Palgrave-Macmillan, Co.

Boykin, A., & Schoenhofer, S. (2001). Nursing as caring: A model for transforming practice. Boston: Jones and Bartlett and New York: National League for Nursing Press.

Carper, B. (1978). Fundamental patterns of knowing in nursing. *Advances in Nursing Science, 1*(1), 13–24.

Daniels, L. (1998). Vulnerability as a key to authenticity. *Image: Journal of Nursing Scholarship, 30*(2), 191–192.

Heidegger, M. (1977). *The question concerning technology.* New York: Harper and Row.

Hudson, R. (1988). Whole or parts—a theological perspective on "person." *The Australian Journal of Advanced Nursing, 6*(1), 12–20.

Hudson, G. (1993). Empathy and technology in the coronary care unit. *Intensive Critical Care Nursing, 9*(1), 55–61.

Locsin, R. (1995). Machine technologies and caring in nursing. *Image: Journal of Nursing Scholarship, 27*(3), 201–203.

Locsin, R. (1998). Technologic competence as expression of caring in critical care settings. *Holistic Nursing Practice, 12*(4), 50–56.

Locsin, R. (2001). Practicing nursing: Technological competency as an expression of caring in nursing. In: *Advancing technology, caring, and nursing.* Westport, CT: Auburn House, Greenwood Publishing Group.

Locsin, R. (2005). *Technological competency as caring in nursing: A model for practice.* Indianapolis, IN: Sigma Theta Tau International.

Locsin, R. (2009). Painting a clear picture: The technological knowing of persons as contemporary process of nursing. In: R. Locsin & M. Purnell (Eds.), *A contemporary process of nursing: The (un)bearable weight of knowing persons in nursing.* New York: Springer.

Locsin, R., & Campling, A. (2005). Techno sapiens and posthumans: Nursing, caring and technology. In: R. Locsin (Ed.), *Technological competency as caring in nursing: A model for practice.* Indianapolis, IN: Sigma Theta Tau International.

Locsin, R., & Purnell, M. J. (2007). Rapture and suffering with technology in nursing. *International Journal for Human Caring, 11*(1), 38–43.

Maslow, A. H. (1943). A theory of human motivation. *Psychological Review, 50,* 370–396.

Parse, R. R. (1998). *The human becoming school of thought.* Thousand Oaks, CA: Sage.

Phenix, P. H. (1964). *Realms of meaning.* New York: McGraw-Hill.

Purnell, M., & Locsin, R. (2000). Intentionality: Unification in nursing. Unpublished manuscript. Florida Atlantic University College of Nursing, Boca Raton, Florida.

Reader's Digest Association. (1987). *Reader's Digest illustrated encyclopedic dictionary* (p. 932). Pleasantville, NY: The Reader's Digest Association.

Sandelowski, M. (1993). Toward a theory of technology dependency. *Nursing Outlook, 41*(1), 36–42.

Serling, R. (1960). Season 2, Episode 6 of *The Twilight Zone,* "Eye of the Beholder." CBS.

Smith, J. (1983). *The idea of health: Implications for the nursing professional.* New York: Teachers College Press.

Swanson, M. (1991). Dimensions of caring interventions. *Nursing Research, 40,* 161–166.

Watson, J. (1985). *Nursing: Human science and human care.* East Norwalk, CT: Appleton-Century-Crofts.

Chapter 29

Marilyn Anne Ray's Theory of Bureaucratic Caring

MARILYN ANNE RAY AND
MARIAN C. TURKEL

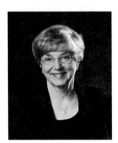

Marilyn Anne Ray

Introducing the Theorist

Marilyn Anne (Dee) Ray, RN, PhD, CTN is a Professor Emeritus at Florida Atlantic University, The Christine E. Lynn College of Nursing, in Boca Raton, Florida. She holds a bachelor of science and a master of science in nursing from the University of Colorado in Denver, Colorado, a master of arts in cultural anthropology from McMaster University in Hamilton, Canada, and a doctorate from the University of Utah in Transcultural Nursing. She retired as a colonel in 1999 after 30 years of service with the United States Air Force Reserve Nurse Corps. As a certified transcultural nurse (CTN), she has published widely on the subjects of caring in organizational cultures, caring theory and inquiry development, transcultural caring, and transcultural ethics. She has held faculty positions at the University of California San Francisco, University of San Francisco, McMaster University, University of Colorado and Florida Atlantic University, and Scholar positions at Florida Atlantic University and Virginia Commonwealth University. Ray has enjoyed many diverse teaching and learning assignments around the world. She is a review board member of the *Journal of Transcultural Nursing*. Ray has conducted phenomenological, ethnographic, and grounded theory research on different topics related to nursing administration and practice, and the United States military. Ray's research has revolved around cultural, technological, political, and economic issues related to caring in complex organizations. Her latest research conducted with Dr. Marian Turkel used both qualitative and quantitative research methods to study the complex nurse–patient relational caring process and its impact on economic and patient outcomes in hospitals. In her role as professor emeritus, Ray is actively engaged in mentoring new faculty members and guiding doctoral students, both in the United States and abroad, whose studies focus on the research of administrative and clinical practice, including the clinical nurse leader role, patient safety, and the ethical practice of nursing, and transcultural nursing.

Overview of the Theory

This chapter presents a discussion of contemporary nursing culture and shares theoretical views in nursing and those related to the author's theoretical vision and development of professional nursing. The Theory of Bureaucratic Caring is discussed first as a grounded theory (both substantive and formal) and then as a holographic theory. Within this chapter, Dr. Marian Turkel, Director of Professional Nursing Practice, Albert Einstein Healthcare Network, Philadelphia, Pennsylvania integrates the relevance of the theory in administrative and clinical practice.

The Generation of Bureaucratic Caring Theory

The Theory of Bureaucratic Caring was generated in a hospital organization from a qualitative research study using three research approaches 30 years ago (Ray, 1981). Data analysis involved the description of the hospital as a culture (*ethnography*), the meaning of caring in the life world (*phenomenology*), and the discovery of conceptual categories and subcategories and theories of the structure and process of caring in the complex organization (*grounded theory method*). Substantive theory called Differential Caring was generated from the diversity and dominant meanings of caring expressed by participants on different units in the hospital. The formal theory was developed from interpretation of the initial qualitative data and data related to complex systems, such as bureaucracy. The culture of the hospital was a dynamic unity

illustrating caring as not only humanistic (physical), ethical, spiritual/religious, social-cultural, and educational, but also as part of the structural—political, economic, legal, and technological—characteristics of a complex organization. These co-determining processes related to the thesis of caring and the antithesis of bureaucracy were synthesized into the Theory of Bureaucratic Caring (Fig. 29-1). After additional research and continued reflection on what was occurring in science and in nursing science, Ray revisited the theory, and discovered that the theory itself incorporated many concepts from the new sciences of complexity (the science of change and wholeness). The theory, as shown in Figure 29-2, was then revealed as holographic (Coffman, 2006; Ray, 2006; Turkel, 2007).

Theory in Nursing

Theory is the intellectual life of nursing (Levine, 1995). Scientific theories in the discipline of nursing have developed out of the choices and assumptions a particular theorist believes about nursing, what the basis of nursing's knowledge is, the state of the science, the results of research, and what nurses do or how they practice in the real world (Ray, 1998a).

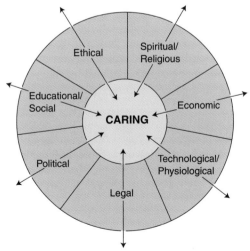

Figure 29 • 1 Grounded Theory of Bureaucratic Caring (Differential Caring and Bureaucratic Caring theories).

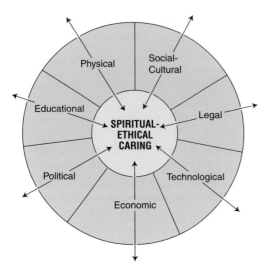

Figure 29 • 2 Holographic Theory of Bureaucratic Caring.

Van Manen (1982) refers to theory as "wakefulness of mind," awareness or the 'pure' viewing of truth. *Truth* in this sense is from the Greek view which is not the property of consensus among concepts or the consensus among theorists but the disclosure of the essential nature or the 'good' of things. Therefore, theoretical truth refers to 'contemplating the good' (van Manen, 1982). Collectively, theories in nursing have focused on the 'good of nursing'—what nursing is and what it does or should do. Based on the assumption of nursing as 'serving the good,' the locus of the discipline centers on wholeness and the dynamics of unity (body, mind, and spirit), caring for others in the human health experience, the human-environment integral relationship, energy patterns, human becoming, transcultural care, organizational caring, and facilitating health and well-being through choice and social justice (Davidson & Ray, 1991; Leininger, 1991; Newman, 1992; Newman, Sime, & Corcoran-Perry, 1991; Newman, Smith, Pharris, & Jones, 2008; Ray, 1989a,b, 2006; Roach, 2002; Rogers, 1970; Watson, 1988, 2005). Theories in nursing are ethical, spiritual and contextual. Theories of nursing thus direct or enlighten the good.

Theories such as the classical grand theories in nursing of Rogers, Leininger, Newman, Watson, and Parse demonstrate a diversity of integrated approaches to nursing based on the worldview, education, and research of an individual theorist. Ongoing research through testing and evaluation supports the validity and reliability of the theories. Many grounded or middle-range theories also have been generated (Liehr & Smith, 1999). They focus on particular aspects of nursing practice and are commonly discovered as substantive theories in and from nursing practice. As such, some scholars view middle-range theories as more relevant and useful to nursing than the application of grand theories (Cody, 1996). However, rather than show partiality for one theory over another, the diversity of nursing theories that emphasize particular and holistic points of view actually support the new picture of reality in science that there is more than one lens from which a phenomenon can be viewed and studied.

Complexity and Nursing Theory

"Complexity theory is a scientific theory of dynamical systems collectively referred to as the sciences of complexity" (Ray, 1998a, p. 91). They illuminate the nature and creativity of science itself. Revolutionary approaches to new scientific theory development have transpired, such as quantum theory, the science of wholeness, holographic and chaos theories, fractals or the idea of self-similarity, networks of relationships and complex information systems, and the concepts of choice and self-organization (Bar-Yam, 2004; Bassingthwaighte, Liebovitch, & West, 1994; Battista, 1982; Briggs & Peat, 1989, 1999; Davidson & Ray, 1991; Harmon, 1998; Lindberg, Nash, & Lindberg, 2008; Peat, 2003; Ray, 1998a; Wheatley, 1999; Wilbur, 1982).

Complexity theory is replacing other theories, such as Newtonian physics and even Einstein's beliefs and those of other scientists as well, that the physical world is governed by laws and order. New scientific views state that phenomena that are antithetical actually coexist—determinism with uncertainty and reversibility with irreversibility (Nicolis & Prigogine, 1989). "Opposing things can happen at the same time, in the same space, without contradicting each other" (Thoma, 2003, p. 17). Thus, both linear and nonlinear and simple (e.g., gravity) and complex (economic and cultural) systems exist together. One of the tools or metaphors in the studies of complexity is chaos theory. Chaos deals with life at the edge, or the notion that the concept of order exists within disorder at the system communication or choice point phases where old patterns disintegrate or new patterns emerge (Davidson & Ray, 1991; Lindberg et al., 2008; Newman et al., 2008; Ray, 1994a, 1998b; Ray et al., 1995). This new science, which signifies interrelationship of mind and matter, interconnectedness and choice, carries with it a moral responsibility and the quest toward wisdom, which includes awareness, information systems, networks of relationships, patterns of energy and creativity, information about the environment, and emergence (Davidson & Ray, 1991; Fox, 1994). The conception of the interconnectedness and relational reality of all things, the interdependence of all human–environmental phenomena, and the discovery of order in a chaotic world demonstrate the pioneering story of twentieth century science and how the insightful idea of belongingness and relationality (a powerful nursing concept) is shaping the science of the 21st century.

Within nursing, certain nursing theorists have embraced the notion of nursing as complexity in which consciousness, human–environmental mutual relationship, caring, and choice-making are central concepts (Davidson & Ray, 1991; Lindberg et al., 2008; Newman, 1986, 1992; Newman et al., 2008; Ray, 1994a, 1998a; Rogers, 1970). Given the nature of nursing as unitary, holistic, relational, and caring, and health as expanded consciousness (Pharris, in Parker, 2006; Newman et al., 2008), there is a coherent link between the importance of theory as wakefulness and professional practice. This author holds the position that nurses do need to be exposed to ideas and need diverse nursing theories to stimulate thinking. The only way that nursing can critique itself is by understanding the intellectual views of scholars in the complex world of nursing science, research, education, and practice. Theories, as the integration of knowledge, research, and experience, highlight the way in which scholars and practitioners of nursing interpret their world and the context where nursing is lived. Theories in this sense are also philosophies or ideologies that serve a practical purpose. Thus, the idea that theories are the pure viewing of truth (wakefulness or awareness) and that they can be judged in light of their practical consequences (Bohman, 2005) underscores the importance of nursing theory as both a scholarly enterprise and a wise practice that identifies and participates in the complexities of inquiry about relationships, knowledgeable caring, health, and the universe.

The Theory of Bureaucratic Caring illuminated in this chapter is a holistic theory with a practical purpose. Substantive and formal theories (Differential Caring and the Theory of Bureaucratic Caring respectively) emerged from researching the values, beliefs, attitudes and behaviors of health professionals and patients in the complex organization of the hospital (Coffman, 2006; Ray, 1981, 1984, 1989a, 2006; Turkel, 2007). The Bureaucratic Caring Theory was illustrated first as grounded theory. As stated, after reflection and further research in the organizational culture, the theory was illustrated as a holographic theory showing the growth and development of the nature of nursing over time. In the holographic model, caring (the center of the model) is highlighted as spiritual and ethical in relation to the physical (humanistic), the social–cultural and educational, and the more structural dimensions of a complex organization: the political, economic, legal, and technological. Thus, spiritual–ethical caring honors the good of caring, commits to the moral position of caring, respects creativity, and integrates the networks of complex organizational or bureaucratic systems. This chapter invites us to increase our awareness of theory generation and application in practice situations. The Theory of Bureaucratic Caring as a holographic model will facilitate and increase our understanding of the practice of nursing in complex contemporary health care environments.

Contemporary Nursing Practice as Complex, Dynamic and Emergent

The practice of nursing is dynamic, always changing, and emerging with new possibilities as people relate to each other. Contemporary nursing practice, however, continues to occur in organizations that are generally bureaucratic or systematic in nature. Although there has been much discussion about the "end of bureaucracy" to cope better with 21st-century innovation and work life within complex systems (Perrow, 1986; Pinchot & Pinchot, 1994; Sorbello, 2008a,b), bureaucracy remains a valuable tool to identify and understand the fundamentally different structural principles that undergird coordinated and relational organizational systems. Bureaucracies are organizational systems that can be viewed as cultures. Organizational cultures have a rich heritage and have been studied as both formal and informal systems since the 1930s in the United States (Bolman, 2008; Brenton & Driskill, 2005; Morgan, 1997; Pensky, 2005; Porter-O'Grady & Malloch, 2003, 2007; Ray, 1981, 1984, 1989a, 2006; Ray in Coffman, 2006; Smircich, 1985; Swinderman, 2005; Turkel & Ray, 2000, 2001). Informal organizational culture integrates codes of ethics and conduct encompassing commitment, identity, character, coherence, and a sense of community in social interaction and the social environment. The informal organizational culture is considered essential to the successful functioning or the administering of the formal organization: political power and authority, technological computation, and economic and legal exchange. The formal organization thus comprises political, economic, legal, and technical systems (the typical phenomena of bureaucracies). Bureaucracies themselves create their own cultural orientations, patterns, goals, rituals, languages, and norms within the structural elements of the political, economic, legal, and technological dimensions (Britain & Cohen, 1980).

What distinguishes "organizations as cultures" from other paradigms, such as organizations as machines, brains, or other images (Morgan, 1997), is its foundation in anthropology or the study of how people *act* in communities or formalized structures and the *significance or meaning* of work life (Brenton & Driskill, 2005; Cuilla, 2000; Louis, 1985). Organizational cultures, therefore, are viewed as social constructions, symbolically formed and reproduced through interaction (Smircich, 1985).

The beliefs about work emerge in organizations through relationships, and organizational mission and policy statements. A nation's prevailing tenets and expectations about the nature of work, leisure, and employment are pivotal to the work life of people; hence, there is an interplay between the macrocosm of a national/global culture and the microcosm of specific organizations (Eisenberg & Goodall, 1993; Schein, 2004). In recent years, organizational cultures have emerged as globalizing corporate systems with multiple descriptions of meaning. However, economics or the "bottom line" is the potent equalizer of most macro- and microcultures (Eisler, 2007; Henderson, 2006). There is an ever greater concentration of economic and political power in a handful of corporations, which separate their interests (usually profit-driven) from the interests of humans, which are life-centered (Eisler, 2007; Henderson, 2006; Korten, 1995; Turkel & Ray, 2000, 2001).

Health care and its activities are tightly interwoven into the social and economic fabric of nations. Values that drive a nation are experienced in the health care arena. For example, for the most part, "cost and profit" have transformed health care in the United States. As health care organizations continually are affected by issues of cost and profit, health-care systems undergo immense change. Over recent years, confidence in major health-care institutions and their leaders have fallen so low as to put the legitimacy of executives who manage health care systems at risk. Trust is a major issue (Ray, Turkel, &

Marino, 2002). Old rules of loyalty and commitment to employees, investment in the worker, fairness in pay, and the need to provide good benefits are in jeopardy. Health-care systems have fallen victim to the corporatization of the human enterprise. Consequently, the conflict between health care as a business and caring as a human need has resulted in a crisis in nursing in terms of shortages of professional nurses, and the quality of care provided by health-care organizations (Anderson & McDaniel, 2008; Begun & White, 2008; Eisler, 2007; Page, 2004; Satterly, 2004; Sorbello, 2008b).

The actual work of nurses, while undervalued in terms of both cost and worth (Ray, 1987a; Turkel & Ray, 2000, 2001), currently is being evaluated in terms of issues of patient safety and clinical nurse leadership (Page, 2004). Since the Institute of Medicine report (Page, 2004), a resurgence of interest is taking place in the meaningfulness of work and patient safety in many hospitals. Nursing education and the clinical nurse leader role are highlighted as bridges to quality (Long, 2003; Stanley, 2006). The language of trust and morally worthy work (Cuilla, 2000; Ray, Turkel, & Marino, 2002; Wiggins, 2006) is beginning to replace the language of downsizing and restructuring at the same time that mergers and acquisitions still hold sway in contemporary corporate environments. Cuilla (2000) stated that "[t]he most meaningful jobs are those in which people directly help others [provide care] or create products that make life better for people" (p. 225). Although the traditional work of nurses is defined as directly helping others through *knowledgable* caring (Watson, 2005), contemporary nurses' work and its meaning is also defined by and in the organizational context—the structural dimensions of political, economic, legal, and technological systems (Ray, 1989a, 2006; Turkel, 2007). Urging nurses, physicians, and administrators to find cohesion among these dimensions in organizations and the dynamics of unity of human beings (body, mind, and spirit integration) call for the reinvention of work (Fox, 1994).

Incorporating business principles and creativity of caring, the "work of the soul" or relational self-organization (Ray, 1994a, 1998; Ray, Turkel, & Marino, 2002) means leading in a new way (Porter-O'Grady & Malloch, 2007; Turkel & Ray, 2004). It is a witness to the power and depth of transformation: reseeing the good of nursing, searching for meaning in life, creating caring organizations, and finding new meaning in the complexities of work itself.

Organizational Cultures as Transformational Bureaucracies

The transformation of nursing toward a greater understanding of relational self-organization and creativity (work of the soul—spiritual–ethical caring) is not necessarily a new pursuit for the profession: what it reveals is a movement from invisibility to visibility. Identifying professional nurse caring work as having value and an expression of one's soul or one's creative self at work replaces the notion of nursing as performing only machinelike tasks.

Bureaucracy, still considered by some as a machinelike metaphor, as we have identified, continues to play a significant role in the meanings and symbols of organizations (Coffman, 2006; Perrow, 1986; Ray, 1981, 1989a, 2006). The social theorist Weber (1999) actually predicted that the future belonged to the bureaucracy and not to the working class. Weber, who saw bureaucracy as an efficient and superior form of organizational arrangement, predicted that the bureaucratization of enterprise would dominate the world (Bell, 1974; Weber, 1999). This, of course, is witnessed by the current globalization of commerce and technical information systems. In terms of global commerce, recent acquisitions and mergers of industrial firms and even health-care systems, especially in the United States, are larger and hold more power than some world governments. (Yet, to maintain the integrity of large scale, for-profit corporations, often governments have to step in with increased regulation and infuse systems with monetary guarantees.) Information technology systems often are in the hands of a few who direct and guide knowledge. We can see this happening with the development of informatics in hospitals and other health care systems (Swinderman, 2005). The concept of bureaucratization is thus a worldwide phenomenon (Ray, 1989). Although they considered it less effective than other forms of organization, Britain and Cohen (1980) stated that, "Like it or not, humankind is being driven to a bureaucratized world whose forms and functions, whose authority and power must be understood if they are ever to be even partially controlled" (p. 27). "The study of bureaucracies is, in effect, the study of the most salient and powerful organizations of the contemporary world" (p. 27). As bureaucracies grow, so too will the importance of family, kin, community, organizational life, culture, ethnicity, and what is now termed, panethnicity, an understanding of diversity within wholeness (Britain & Cohen, 1989; Tuan, 1998).

The characteristics of bureaucracies are as follows:

- A division of labor based on departments, leadership, and authority
- A hierarchy of offices [bureaus or units] with diverse cultural orientations
- A set of general policies and rules that govern performances
- A separation of the personal from the official
- A selection of personnel on the basis of technical/professional qualifications
- Equal treatment of all employees or standards of fairness and reimbursement
- Employment viewed as a career by participants
- Protection of dismissal by tenure or evaluation (from Perrow, 1986; Eisenberg & Goodall, 1993).

Bureaucracy thus incorporates within the human and ethical dimension the political (power and authority), legal (policies and rules), economic (cost systems), and technical (professional, informational, and computational) dimensions. At the same time, bureaucracies integrate the whole social and cultural system. Bureaucracy, while condemned by some as associated with red tape and inflexibility, continues to provide the most reasonable way in which to view systems and facilitate the preservation and understanding of organizations. In the past two decades, there has been a call for decentralization and the "flattening" of organizational structures—to become less bureaucratic and more participative or heterarchical (Porter-O'Grady & Malloch, 2005, 2007). Many firms have begun to hold to new principles that honor creativity and imagination (Morgan, 1997). Even nursing has advanced in a more collaborative or decentralized manner by its focus on patient-centered nursing and a movement from more centralized control and administration to more decentralized self-governance (Long, 2003; Nyberg, 1998). But creative views still need to be marked with understanding of structural systems of bureaucracy as globalization, information, and economics sweep the world.

Leadership models, which are fundamentally hierarchical because of the need for order, continue to head the short-lived participative movement toward decentralization. Even the new Clinical Nurse Leader role sets a nursing leader apart from his or her peers in terms of knowledge and authority. Power is still in the hands of a few. As local and global economic markets rule, there is a call for creating a "caring economics" and a need to be creative and ethical in terms of the worldwide technological and economic transformation taking place (Eisler, 2007; Ray, 1987a). We have to look at the social, psychological, and spiritual factors that shape our societies and organizations. As a result, the concept of bureaucracy does not seem as bad as was once thought because it addresses human, and in many respects, humane action. It can be considered as a much less radical paradigm than the business paradigm that focuses only on competition and response to market forces, subsequently eradicating standards of fairness or social justice for humans in the workplace.

Caring as the Unifying Focus of Nursing

Caring in nursing speaks of relationships, compassion, human dignity, ethics, justice, and competent and knowledgeable caring practice (Ray, 1981, 1989b; Roach 2002; Watson, 2005). It is holistic, humane, and dynamic; thus, it facilitates growth and development of human persons and helps to make things work in health care agencies. As such, caring is considered by many nurse scholars to be the essence of nursing (Boykin & Schoenhofer, 2001; Leininger, 1981b, 1991, 1997; Morse, Solberg, Neander, Bottorff, & Johnson, 1990; Ray, 1989a,b, 1994a,b; Swanson, 1991; Watson, 1985, 1988, 1997, 2005). Although not uniformly accepted, Newman, Sime, and Corcoran-Perry (1991) and Newman (1992) characterized the social mandate of the discipline of nursing as caring in the human health experience. Newman et al. (2008) further emphasized her initial idea that health is the focus, the rhythmic fluctuations of the life process, as well as caring, consciousness, mutual process, patterning, presence, and meaning (Newman et al., 2008). Caring and health thus are influential concepts. The expression "caring" in the human health experience emphasizes the social mandate to which nursing has responded throughout its history and encompasses the scope of the discipline (Roach, 2002; Watson, 2005). Caring, with multiple meanings, however, is manifested in different and complex ways in the nursing discipline and profession (Morse et al., 1990; Newman, 1992; Ray, 1981, 1989a,b).

Various paradigms that enfold the care and caring ideal exist in nursing. The totality (Fawcett, 1993), the simultaneity (Parse, 1987), and the unitary–transformative (Newman, 1992; Newman et al., 2008) paradigms have been the prevailing worldviews in nursing and have directed nursing theories. The *totality* paradigm demonstrates that nursing, person, society, environment, and health characterize the nature of nursing. The *simultaneity* paradigm illuminates the human–environmental integral nature of nursing. The *unitary–transformative* paradigm states that what constitutes nursing's reality is the view that the human being is unitary and evolving as a self-organizing field embedded in a larger self-organizing field identified by pattern and interaction with the larger whole. Health is considered expanded consciousness (Newman et al., 2008). "Health in the face of illness [prevention of disease or dis-ease] derives meaning through a caring nurse–patient relationship" (Newman et al., 2008, p. E17–18). Many caring theories correspond to one or all of these paradigms (Morse et al., 1990). The Theory of Bureaucratic Caring has its roots in all these paradigms and most specifically in the unitary–transformative paradigm by its synthesis of caring and the organizational (bureaucratic) context, holism, and the dynamics and relational self-organizing emergent process of the human–environmental integral relationship.

Description of Bureaucratic Caring Theory

The Theory of Bureaucratic Caring, as reported, originated as a grounded theory from a qualitative study using phenomenology, ethnography, and grounded theory methods of caring in the organizational culture, and appeared first as the author's dissertation in 1981 and as a chapter and article in 1984 and 1989, respectively. In the qualitative study of caring in the organizational context, the research revealed that nurses and other professionals struggled with the paradox of serving the bureaucracy and serving humans, especially patients, through caring. Caring, however, had multiple meanings and was expressed differently in terms of the way a particular unit was organized. The system phenomena of political, economic, legal, and technological became integrated into the meaning system of caring just as the humanistic, social, educational, ethical, and spiritual. The discovery of bureaucratic caring resulted in both substantive theory (grounded in the context of meaning) and formal theory (integrated from the substantive theory and general understanding of dimensions of complex bureaucracies) (Ray, 1981, 1984, 1989a).

The bureaucracy represented a living system. Caring was portrayed not only as the more interpersonal relational patterns of humanness and compassion, but also as how the official structures of the bureaucracy, especially the political and economic, were infused into the meaning system of professionals. Even patients saw the "system" as affecting how they understood caring in their own health care experiences (Ray, 1981, 1989a; Ray & Turkel, 2001–2004). The substantive theory (grounded) emerged as Differential Caring Theory and showed that caring in the complex organization of the hospital was complex and differentiated itself in terms of meaning by its specific context—dominant caring dimensions related to areas of practice or units wherein professionals worked and clients resided. Differential Caring Theory showed that professionals and patients on different units espoused different and dominant caring meanings based on their personal and organizational goals and values. For example, participants in the oncology unit espoused caring as intimate and spiritual; in contrast, participants in the Intensive Care Unit espoused caring as more technological; in the administration, participants espoused caring as maintaining economic viability. The formal Theory of Bureaucratic Caring symbolized a dynamic structure of caring, which was synthesized from a dialectic using the tenets of the philosophy of Hegel (*thesis, antithesis, and synthesis*); the dialectic between the thesis of caring as humanistic, social, educational, ethical, and religious/spiritual (dimensions of humanism, morality, and spirituality), and the antithesis of caring as economic, political, legal, and technological (dimensions of bureaucracy) (Coffman, 2006; Ray, 1981, 1989a, 2006; Turkel, 2007).

Although the later depictions of the model demonstrate that the dimensions are equal, the initial research revealed that economic and political patterns of meaning were more dominant followed by the technical and legal dimensions, and then the social and ethical/spiritual dimensions. Subsequently, the model was pictured with co-equal dimensions. The current holographic model shows the primacy of caring as spiritual–ethical and the other dimension as equal, indicating the holistic nature of the interface between the spiritual and ethical and the bureaucratic dimensions.

Subsequently, the theory was revealed as holographic, showing that caring is complex, holistic, and dynamic. Interactions and symbolic systems of meaning by nurses and others are formed and reproduced from the constructions or dominant values held and evolving within the organization. In some respect, "we are the organization."

The theory has been embraced by educators, researchers, technologists, nursing administrators, and clinicians who, after witnessing changes in health care policy in the past decade, have begun to appreciate how the context—micro- and macro-cultures—influences nursing. Moving away from just centering on patient care to the economic justification of nursing and health care systems has prompted professionals to desire a fuller understanding of how to preserve humanistic caring within the business or corporate (economic and political) culture (Miller, 1989; Nyberg, 1989, 1991, 1998; Turkel, 2007). The theory also has been used as a foundation for additional research and observational studies of the nurse–patient caring relationship and system issues, such as in public health administration, curriculum development, correctional facility health care, technology and information technology, economics of caring, the clinical nurse leader role, ethics and the moral community, legal caring, pediatric pain, and medication errors in complex organizations (Al-Ayed, 2008; Coffman, 2006; Gomez, 2008; Gibson, 2008; Manworren, 2008; McCray-Stewart, 2008; O'Brien, 2008; Ray, 1987b, 1993, 1997a, 1998a,b; Ray, Turkel & Marino, 2002; Sorbello, 2008a; Swinderman, 2005; Turkel, 1997, 2007; Turkel & Ray, 2000, 2001, 2009).

Evolution of Theory Development

Facing the challenge of the economic and patient safety crises in health care and nursing, disillusionment of registered nurses about the disregard for their caring services, and the concern of the nursing profession and the public about the effects of the shortage of nurses (Page, 2004), working for the good of the profession and preservation of the nurse–patient caring relationship is imperative. Running away from the chaos of hospitals or misunderstanding the meaning of work life cannot become the norm. Wherever nurses go, they will be "haunted" by bureaucracies, some functional, many problematic. What, then, is the deeper reality of nursing practice? Why are theories in practice important? The following is a presentation of theoretical views that relate to Bureaucratic Caring Theory, culminating in a vision for understanding the deeper significance of nursing life as holistic, the dynamics of unity.

Substantive Theory and Formal Theory

Glaser and Strauss (1967; Glaser, 1978; Strauss & Corbin, 1998) were the first sociologists to present the perspective of social theory, both substantive and formal, discovered from inductive research processes. Substantive and formal theories emerge from in-depth qualitative studies of social–cultural processes— action and interaction associated with the social world. The researcher considers evidence about how one event affects another and explains the things observed and recorded by developing theoretical relationships about the data. Theoretical sampling (Glaser, 1978) refines, elaborates, and exhausts conceptual categories so that an actual integration of descriptors and categories about a phenomenon or social process can facilitate the discovery of substantive theory. The discovery of a basic social process is the foundation for substantive theory. The formal theory is generated from both the inductive process, based on substantive knowledge/theory, and deductive approaches, which draw upon cumulative knowledge from the social world to examine the initial propositions advanced. A formal theory reflects the structure of both processes.

Formal Theory Analysis

The Theory of Bureaucratic Caring integrated knowledge from data that are associated with researching the meaning and action of caring in the bureaucratic, organizational or institutional culture of a hospital, which resulted in a substantive Theory of Differential Caring. Narrative responses to the meaning of caring reported by different health-care professionals and patients produced varied beliefs and values, ranging from humanistic definitions, such as empathy, love, and ethical and religious delineations, to technological (patient-assist machines or other technologies), legal (policies and rules), political (power and control), and economic (money, budget) descriptions. The formal theory evolved as a result of using the Hegelian *dialectical* process of thesis, antithesis, synthesis, as an analytic tool. In this research caring was the thesis, bureaucracy was the antithesis of caring, and Bureaucratic Caring Theory was the synthesis. The laws of the dialectic include:

- Examining and connecting co-determining *polar* opposites (thesis and antithesis)
- Negation of each of the *separate* yet co-determining opposites (thesis and antithesis)
- Synthesis of the polar opposites into a new conceptualization (change and spiral transformation) (Moccia, 1986; Ray, 1981).

Thus, in this research, the co-determining opposites were the *thesis* of caring which included the humanistic, social, ethical, educational, and religious/spiritual dimensions, and the *antithesis*, which included the structural dimensions of economics, politics, law, and technology of the bureaucracy. Negation of both the co-determining polar opposites became a *synthesis*, the dialectical, formal Theory of Bureaucratic Caring indicating change and transformation. The meaning of caring in the organizational/ institutional culture was illuminated as the Theory of Bureaucratic Caring, which is simply a representation of caring's integral nature (meaning) in contemporary organizational culture. The theory shows that caring reached its completeness through the process of its own relevance in practice (Ray, 1981, 1989a, 2006).

The Relationship Between Middle-Range and Formal Theory

Middle-range theory deals with a relatively broad scope of phenomena but does not cover the full range of phenomena of a discipline, as do grand theories that encompass the fullest range or the most global phenomena in the discipline (Chinn & Kramer, 1995; Liehr & Smith, 1999). As such, middle-range theories are generally considered narrower in scope than grand theories, and to some extent not as broad as formal theory within the grounded theory tradition. Middle range theories include the following: intermediate in scope; testable; grounded in research; neither too broad nor too narrow; less concrete than practice theory; substantively specific; consisting of a limited number of variables; focused on limited aspects of reality; and can be built on the work of other middle range theories (Liehr & Smith, 1999, pp. 82–83).

There is a paradox in viewing caring or the study of caring *only* as middle-range theory. Caring in nursing, for example, may be considered by some scholars in the discipline as having a narrow scope or a foundation for a middle-range theory from nursing practice situations. However, others who have adopted the unitary–transformative paradigmatic view of the discipline of nursing as health and caring, see caring manifesting consciousness, belongingness, intentionality, seeing the self, other and environment as interconnected, dynamic flow, pattern appreciation, the infinite (the quality of caring as love or divine energy), and complexity where creative emergence unfolds through intrinsic properties of living what matters and choice. Caring in this view is specific and universal, human and transcendent (Newman, 1992; Newman et al., 2008; Smith, 2004; Ray, 1997b). Moreover, those who have studied caring in the human health experience in complex organizations see caring as a broad enough ideal to embrace and capture the holistic nature of nursing (body, mind, spirit, and coexistent with the context or environment).

Is the Theory of Bureaucratic Caring a middle-range theory as well as a grounded substantive and formal theory? Middle-range theories, especially substantive theories are abstract enough to extend beyond data generated in a specific space, place, and time, but specific enough to allow for testing the theory in different arenas or permitting interventions for practice to transform nursing practice (Moody, 1990). Middle-range theory embodies the perspective that these theories fall between the concrete world of practice and the grand theories that guide nursing research and practice (Moody, 1990; Liehr & Smith, 1999). The initial dialectical theory showed that "the meaning of living caring in organizational life" with the meaning and symbols in an institutional/organizational culture reflects not only the microculture of a personal–health care organization connection, but also a connection that reflects the macro or dominant culture of a nation-state. The meaning of "caring" in the organization showed that meaning was constituted interpersonally but within a larger pattern of significance. Organizations or bureaucracies are representations of our humanity and the social order (Bolman & Dial, 2008; Smircich, 1985; Schein, 2004). They are living systems. Social forms and social arrangements reflect the interplay among cultural systems of thought, language, communication, organizations, nations and in the modern era, the globe. Bureaucratic Caring Theory reflected the symbols of the spiritual, ethical and psychodynamics of caring in human experience, and the political and economic power and authority, technology and the law in complex human systems. However, within the concrete world of human experience, caring was illuminated as a universal ideal, that is, not only unique *in* nursing but universal *to* what it means to be human (Boykin & Schoenhofer, 2001; Roach, 2002). Therefore, the Theory of Bureaucratic Caring is a grounded theory and a middle-range theory. Furthermore, the theory may be considered a grand or holographic theory because of the nature of caring and culture as holistic and ubiquitous.

Holographic Emergence in Bureaucratic Caring Theory

The holographic paradigm in science recognizes that the ontology or "what is" of the universe or creation is the interconnectedness of all things, that the epistemology or knowledge that exists is *in* the relationship rather than in the objective world or subjective experience, that uncertainty is inherent in the relationship because everything is in process, and that information and choice hold the key to grasping the holistic and complex nature of the meaning of holography or the whole (Battista, 1982; Harmon, 1998). *Holography* means that the implicate order (the whole) and explicate order (the part) are interconnected, that everything is a holon, including humans, in the sense that everything is a whole in one context and a part in another—each part being in the whole and the whole being in the part (Cannato, 2006; Harmon, 1998; Peat, 2003; Wilber, 1982). For example, "The molecule depends on the atom, the cell depends on the molecule, and all depend on the stability of the interconnected system in order to thrive" (Cannato, 2006, p. 98). All cycles of activities are linked coherently together; the more energy is stored within systems, the more subcycles there are. It is the relational and reciprocal aspect of relationship itself, information and choice that makes it holistic rather than mechanistic, which subsequently opens all systems to diversity and emergence (integrated sets of possibilities) (Davidson & Ray, 1991; Ray, 1998,b; Thoma, 2003). Holistic science is a human–environmental mutual process, and a dynamic unity, and a transformative process. Holistic science (and art) thus captures the idea that all systems, including health care systems, are living systems, are both wholes and parts, and depend on networks of relationships, information, and communication flow.

The human–environmental mutual process is not a new idea to nursing. It was a central theoretical perspective of Martha Rogers (1970), and central to beliefs in anthropology and transcultural nursing advanced by Leininger (1991), and was a foundation for other theories, such as those of Parse, Newman, and Reed (Marriner Tomey & Alligood, 2006). This notion is seen again at a different time and through a different lens. In the author's work, the focus is on the caring patterns of the nurse–patient relationship within the bureaucratic context of a hospital. The Bureaucratic Caring Theory already considered paradoxical (bureaucratic caring), identified the linkage between caring as humanistic, social–cultural, educational, and spiritual–ethical, *and* the organizational hospital system as structural: political, economic, legal, and technological. Caring is a relational pattern; it is the flow of nurses' and others' own experiences in the structural context of the organization. This simultaneous process illuminates the idea that the whole and parts are one and the same; all cycles of activities are linked coherently together but each may be doing different things at different paces; all the parts are participating in the whole and the whole is participating as a part in different contexts of meaning (Davidson & Ray, 1991; Rogers, 1970; Thoma, 2003). Information (caring and system data) unfolds and emerges at the same time, in the same space without contradicting each other. Bureaucratic Caring Theory as a holographic theory furthers the vision of nursing and organizations as complex, dynamic, relational, integral, informational, and emergent—open to sets of possibilities because of the synchronicity of interacting parts and the whole. Everything interconnects; we are all creative manifestations of the oneness of the environment (context), moving in relationship and continually transforming (emerging—growing and developing) (Thoma, 2003). Because of the knowledge of complexity as holography (holistic science and art), we all need to become more aware of the meaning of participatory life and ways of relating to the reality of complex organizations or bureaucracies. Rather than continuing mechanistic approaches of prediction and control that may have worked to some extent to gain precise knowledge in the past, we must now give way to new understanding. Nurses and other professionals must be open to change, to the integral nature of the dynamic unity of the human and environment, and to phenomena that are coherent and emergent wholes (body, mind, spirit and context) that make up our world of caring, health, healing, and well-being (Davidson & Ray, 1991; Rogers, 1970).

The Theory of Bureaucratic Caring as Holographic Theory

How can the Theory of Bureaucratic Caring be viewed as a holographic theory? As presented, the theory arose initially from interpretations and choices that were made about the meaning and structure of caring in organizational life. The process parallels ideas from complexity sciences and specifically holography: consciousness or awareness, intentionality of the mutual human–environmental caring relationships, quality of the caring transactions, and the effective ability to analyze, negotiate, make choices, and reconcile paradoxes between caring and the system demands. The humanistic nurse–patient care needs and professional responsibilities in terms of the structural considerations of the system (political, economic, legal, and technological dimensions) were always emerging from sets of caring possibilities. Awareness of belongingness, the mutual human–environmental relationship, the implicate (the whole) and explicate (the part) order—the whole is reflected in the part, and part reveals the whole, respect for the good of all things, and communication, choice and emergence are central to holistic science. Similarly, these concepts were central to the interpretation of caring as a whole in the complex organization. The dialectic of caring (the thesis, the implicit order or the whole) in relation to the various structures (the antithesis of the system, explicit order or part) is reconciled and transformed by a synthesis of the polar opposites into the Theory of Bureaucratic Caring. The synthesis of Bureaucratic Caring Theory shows that everything is interconnected—humanistic spiritual–ethical caring and the organizational system—the whole is in the part and the part is in the whole, therefore, nursing in the system is a holon.

Transforming the Organization

How can knowledge of holistic caring interconnectedness motivate nursing to help nurses to continue to embrace the human dimension within the current political, economic, legal, and technologic environment of health care? Can higher ground be reclaimed for the 21st century? Higher ground requires that we make excellent choices at the "edge of chaos" where possibilities exist to either transform or disintegrate. Understanding of spiritual-ethical caring in the holographic Theory of Bureaucratic Caring helps us to connect at our deepest level. Nursing and others in complex systems can reclaim higher ground by doing the "work of the soul" (understanding and engaging creatively, and taking ethical responsibility for the other and the organizational system). The model (see Fig. 29-2) presents a vision of nursing but it is based on the reality of practice through continuous research and observation. The model emphasizes a direction toward the unity of experience. Spirituality involves creativity and choice and refers to genuineness, vitality, and depth. It is revealed in attachment, love, and community and comprehended within as intimacy and spirit (Harmon, 1998; Secretan, 1997). Ethics deals with our moral responsibility to one another and to the organizations within which we work. Secretan (p. 27) states: "Most of us have an innate understanding of soul, even though each of us might define it in a very different and personal way."

Fox (1994) calls for the theology of work—a redefinition of work. Because of the crisis of our relationship to work, we are challenged to reinvent it. For nursing, this is important because work puts us in touch with others, not only in terms of personal gain, but also at the level of service to humanity or the community of patients/clients and other professionals. Work must be spiritual and ethical, with recognition of the creative spirit at work in us. Nurses must be the "custodians of the human spirit" (Secretan, 1997, p. 27).

The ethical imperatives of caring that join with the spiritual relate to questions or issues about our moral obligations to others. The ethics of caring as edifying the good through communication and interaction involve never treating people simply as a means to an end or as ends in themselves, but rather as beings that have the capacity to make choices about the meaning of life, health, and caring. Ethical content—as principles of doing good, doing no harm, allowing choice, being fair, and promise-keeping—functions as the compass in our decisions to sustain humanity in the context of political, economic, and technological situations within organizations. Roach (2002) pointed out that ethical caring is operative at the level of discernment of principles, in the commitment needed to carry them out, and in the decisions or choices to uphold human dignity through love and compassion. Furthermore, Roach (2002) remarked that health is a community responsibility, an idea that is rooted in ancient Hebrew ethics. The expression of human caring as an ethical act is inspired by spiritual traditions that emphasize charity. For nursing, spiritual/ethical caring does not question whether or not to care in complex systems but intimates how sincere deliberations and ultimately the facilitation of choices for the good of others can or should be accomplished. By integrating knowledgeable caring creatively, by staying intentional and conscious of dynamic movements within the circle of life and relationships, and by leading in a new way in complex systems, nurses are engaging in new and exciting work (Eisler, 2007; O'Grady & Malloch, 2007; Ray, Turkel, & Marino, 2002; Turkel & Ray, 2004). Holistic science and art is a witness to the power and depth of transformation: to reseeing the good of nursing as spiritual and ethical, to believing in human potential, to continually searching for meaning in life, to creating caring organizations, to co-creating new possibilites, and to finding new meaning in the complexities of work life itself.

The scientist Sheldrake (1991, p. 207) remarked: The recognition that we need to change the way we live [work] is gaining ground. It is like waking up from a dream. It brings with it a spirit of repentence, seeing in a new way, a change of heart. This conversion is intensified by the sense that the end of the age of oppression is at hand.

Summary

The values of nursing are deepening, and as a discipline and profession, nursing is expanding its consciousness. Nursing is being shaped by the historical revolution occurring in science, social sciences, and theology as well as the revolution of its own commitment to caring, health and understanding holism and complex systems (Davidson & Ray, 1991; Lindberg et al., 2008; Newman et al., 2008; Ray, 1998a, 2006; Reed, 1997; Watson, 2005). Freeman (in Appell & Triloki, 1988) pointed out that human values are a function of the capacity to make choices, and called for a paradigm giving recognition to awareness and choice. As noted, a revision toward this end is taking place in science based upon a new holographic scientific worldview. Nursing has the capacity to make creative and moral choices for a preferred future. Constructs of consciousness and choice are central and demonstrate that phenomena of the universe, including society and what happens in nursing, arise from the choices that are or are not made (Davidson & Ray, 1991; Harmon, 1998; Newman et al., 2008). As the Theory of Bureaucratic Caring has reinforced, caring is the primordial construct and consciousness of nursing. Nursing theory focuses on the capacity to direct the good. In nursing, the critical task is to comprehend the meaning of the networks and complexity of relationship, between what is given in culture (the norms), and what is chosen (the moral and spiritual). In nursing, the unitary-transformative paradigm and the various theories of Newman, Leininger, Parse, Rogers, and the holographic Theory of Bureaucratic Caring are challenging nursing to become aware and understand their future. The unitary-transformative paradigm of nursing and its holographic tenets are consistent with the changing images of the new science despite the reality that nursing continues to be threatened by the business model over its long-term human interests for facilitating health and well-being (Davidson & Ray, 1991; Lindberg et al., 2008; Ray, 1994a, 1998; Reed, 1997; Smith, 2004; Vicenzi, White, & Begun, 1997). The creative, intuitive, ethical, and spiritual mind is unlimited, however. Through "authentic conscience" (Harmon, 1998), we must find hope in our creative powers.

The latest presentation of Bureaucratic Caring Theory is a creative enterprise. The theory reflects incorporation of tenets of the new sciences of complexity highlighting holography. Holographic theory illuminates holistic science and art, the interconnectedness of all things, human-environment integral relationships, scientific chaos, holographic patterning (the whole is in the part and the part in the whole), informational networks, relational self-organization, transformation, change, choice, and emergence (Bar-Yam, 2004; Davidson & Ray, 1991; Lindberg et al., 2008; Ray, 1991, 1994, 1998a; Turkel & Ray, 2000, 2001; Thoma, 2003). In the revised model of the Theory of Bureaucratic Caring, everything is infused with spiritual/ethical caring (the center of the model) by its integrative and relational connection to the structures of organizational life (relational self-organization). Spiritual/ethical caring is both a part and a whole, and every part secures its purpose and meaning from each of the parts that can also be considered wholes. In other words, the theoretical model shows how spiritual/ethical caring is involved with qualitatively different processes or systems; for example, political, economic, technological, and legal. The systems, when integrated and presented as open and interactive, are a whole and must operate as such by conscious choice, especially by the choice making of nursing, which always has, or should have, the interest of humanity at heart.

Envisioning the theory as holographic from its initial substantive and formal grounded theories shows that through creativity and imagination, nursing can build the profession it wants. Nurses are calling for expression of their own spiritual and ethical existence. Nurses are also calling for understanding of the nurse-patient caring relationship in complex organizations. The new scientific, spiritual and experiential approach to nursing theory as holographic will have positive effects. The union of science, ethics, and spirit will

engender a new sense of hope for transformation in the work world. This transformation toward relational caring organizations can occur in the economic and politically driven atmosphere of today. The deep values that underlie choice to do good for the many will be felt both inside and outside organizations. We must awaken our consciences and act on this awareness and no longer surrender to injustices and oppressiveness of systems that focus primarily on the good of a few. "Healing a sick society [work world] is a part of the ministry of making whole" (Fox, 1994, p. 305). The holographic Theory of Bureaucratic Caring—idealistic, yet practical; visionary, yet real—can give direction and impetus to lead the way.

Application of the Theory

Ray (1989a, p. 31) warned that the "transformation of America and other health care systems to corporate enterprises emphasizing competitive management and economic gain seriously challenges nursing's humanistic philosophies and theories, and nursing's administrative and clinical policies." Approximately 20 years later, in the current health care environment, there is an intense focus on operating costs and the bottom line, and caring is often not valued within the organizational culture. However, nurse researchers, nurse administrators, and nurses in practice can use the Theory of Bureaucratic Caring as a framework to guide practice and decision making.

As the United States is in the midst of debate concerning the future of health care access and coverage the focus is on the concept of economics. From an economic perspective, health-care organizations and insurance companies are businesses. The competition for survival among organizations is becoming stronger, cost controls are becoming tighter, and reimbursement is declining. However, the human dimension of health care is missing from the economic discussion.

In the economic debate, the belief in caring for the patients as the goal of health-care organizations and insurance companies has been lost. Ray (1987a, 1989a) questioned how economic caring decisions are made related to patient care in order to enhance the human perspective within a corporate culture. When patients are hospitalized, it is the caring and compassion of the registered nurse that the patients perceive as quality care and what makes a difference in their recovery (Turkel, 1997).

Historically, nursing care delivery has not been financed or costed out in terms of reimbursement as a single entity. In the United States, the prospective payment system of diagnostic related groups (DRGs) connected nursing services to the bed rate for patients (Shaffer, 1985). The current reimbursement systems, including health maintenance organizations (HMOs), managed care, Medicare, Medicaid, and private insurers, are reimbursing hospitals at a flat capitated rate. Subsequently, it is hospital administrators who must determine how these dollars will be allocated within their institutions. Thus, it is necessary for caring nursing interactions to be viewed as having value as an economic resource. When professional nursing salary dollars are viewed as an economic liability that limits the potential profit margins of organizations they are examined closely. It is imperative to the future of professional nursing practice that we study and document the economic value of caring, so that human caring is not subsumed by the economics of health care. Nurses, who understand the economics of as well as the politics and technical complexities of health care organizations, will be able to synthesize this knowledge into a framework for practice that integrates the dimensions of the Theory of Bureaucratic Caring. Although caring and economics may seem paradoxical, contemporary health-care concerns emphasize the importance of understanding the cost of caring in relation to quality.

Ray (1981, 1987a,b, 1989a, 1998a,b); Ray and Turkel (1999, 2000–2004, 2001, 2003); Turkel and Ray (2003); Ray, Turkel, and Marino (2002); and Turkel (1997, 2001), have used dimensions of the Theory of Bureaucratic Caring to examine the paradox between the concept of human caring and political, economic, legal and technological dimensions in complex organizations. Moreover, recently, Al-Ayed (2008), Gibson (2008), Gomez (2008), McCray-Stewart (2008), O'Brien (2008) and Swinderman (2005) have used the theory to evaluate medication errors, interviews in the justice system, nursing education and practice, health care in correctional facilities and public health nursing, and informatics respectively. For additional information, please visit DavisPlus at http://davisplus.fadavis.com. It was a challenge for nurses to combine the science and art of caring within the complex health-care environment. However, any efforts to reshape the health-care system in the United States and other countries must take into account the *value* of caring within bureaucracies.

Relevance of the Theory of Bureaucratic Caring to Nursing Education

The theory is relevant to nursing education because of the focus on caring in nursing practice and the conceptualization of the health care system (Coffman, 2006). When developing the curriculum for a baccalaureate program, the faculty at Nevada State College combined Ray's Theory of Bureaucratic Caring with theoretical constructs from Watson (1985) and Johns (2000) as a conceptaul framework. According to this framework, the holographic theory of caring recognizes the interconnectedness of all things and that everything is a whole in one context and a part of the whole in another context. Spiritual-ethical caring, the focus for communication, infuses all nursing phenomena including physical, social–cultural, legal, technological, economic, political, and educational forces (Nevada State College, 2003, p. 2).

Turkel (2001) used the theory to guide curriculum development in the master's of science program in nursing administration at Florida Atlantic University. Dimensions from the theory, including ethical, spiritual, economic, technological, legal, political, and social, served as a framework for the exploration of current health care issues. The economic dimension of the theory was a central component in several courses. Students were challenged to analyze the current economic and reimbursement structure of health care from the perspective of a caring lens.

Practice Exemplar

The following exemplar from the practice setting was previously published by Turkel (2007). The situation reflects the lived experiences of how the Theory of Bureaucratic Caring serves as a framework for nursing practice and guides decision-making.

Megan Smith, RN, MSN, was recently hired as the Chief Nurse Executive (CNE) for a 500-bed inner city hospital. The payer mix for this patient population was once private insurance but now it is approximately 75% Medicare and Medicaid. When Megan met with the nursing staff, they stated, "We are not valued or treated with respect. The administrators only see us as numbers. We are implementing a new computerized documentation system, getting new monitors, being told that patient safety is important and getting ready for a survey from The Joint Commission. With all the rules and regulations, it is stressful to find time to actually care for our patients. Plus we need more help."

Megan was committed to being an advocate for nursing while realizing the professional accountabilty of considering the economic, political, and technological perspectives of her decision-making. Megan promised the nurses that she would review the budget and follow-up with their concerns. She explained to the nurses that providing safe, high quality patient care in a caring and compassionate manner was the top priority for the organization.

Later that week, Megan met with the Chief Executive Officer (CEO) to share the concerns of the nursing staff. Her first priority was to increase the number of registered nurses and to hire two additional clinical nurse specialists. The CEO was reluctant to spend the additional financial resources. Megan explained that increasing the number of registered nurses would decrease the number of falls and pressure ulcers and increase compliance related to patient safety. Additional registered nurses would increase satisfaction for both nurses and patients as the nurses would have more time to focus on developing caring relationships with patients and their families. In addition, the registered nurses would have time to focus on providing patient teaching and discharge planning. Megan presented the CEO with quantitative data to demonstrate the costs associated with falls, pressure ulcers, and patients returning to the emergency department (ED) within 48 hours post-discharge because of inadequate education or discharge planning. The request for additional registered nurses and clinical nurse specialists was approved. Six months later the number of falls, pressure ulcers, medication errors, and return visits to the ED had decreased. Scores on the patient satisfaction survey related to nurses informing patients, showing concern, and checking patient identification bands increased.

The additional clinical nurse specialists served as mentors to increase the technical skills of the inexperienced graduate nurses and to demonstrate how the use of technology in terms of cardiac monitoring would enhance the caring interactions between the registered nurse and patient. Customized programing of the new clinical documentation system afforded nurses the opportunity to document interventions related to specific dimensions of the Bureaucratic Caring Theory.

Dimensions of the Theory of Bureaucratic Caring

The economic, political, technological, and spiritual dimensions of bureaucratic caring can be used to guide practice. Now is the time for professional nurses to become proactive and use theory-based practice to shape their future instead of having the future dictated by others outside the discipline. Staff nurses can hold close their core value that caring is the essence of nursing and can still retain a focus on meeting the bottom line. Empirical studies have firmly established a link between caring and positive patient outcomes. Positive patient outcomes are needed for organizational survival in this competitive era of health care. Given this, professional nursing practice must embrace and illuminate the caring philosophy in relation to complex organizational phenomena.

Staff nurses value the caring relationship between nurse and patient. However, nurses are practicing in an environment where the economics and costs of health care permeate discussions and clinical decisions. The focus on costs is not a transient response to shrinking reimbursement; instead, it has become the catalyst for change within health care organizations.

Nurses are continuing to struggle not only with economic changes, but also with political and technological changes. With a system goal of decreasing length of stay and increasing staffing ratios, nurses need to establish trust and initiate a relationship during their first encounter with a patient. As this relationship is being established, nurses need to focus on "being, knowing, and doing all at once" (Turkel, 1997). From a patient perspective, being there means completing a task while simultaneously engaging with a patient. This holistic approach to practice means not only viewing the patient as a person in all of his or her complexity, but also viewing the patient and the needs of professional nursing within the complex organizational environment.

Changes that incorporated the human caring dimension and the critical nature that human relationships play in hospital organizations were identified by Ray more than two decades ago. Ray (1987a) described the problems associated with economic changes in health care and the negative impact economics would have on nurse caring. Current research (Turkel & Ray, 2000, 2001, 2003) on the economics of the nurse–patient relationship showed that the preservation of this relationship and humanistic caring was continuing to grow despite the heavy emphasis by administrators and insurance companies on cost control. The researchers recommend that administrators recognize and respect the contributions nursing could make in developing hospital organizations as politically moral, caring organizations.

Application of Theory to Contemporary Nursing Practice

The American Nurses Credentialing Center (ANCC) Magnet Recognition Program® recognizes excellence in professional nursing practice. Organizations need to provide written narratives and sources of evidence related to the development, dissemination, and enculturation of best practices, quality care, technical skill, and patient preference. This emphasis on *professional* nursing practice within the Magnet Recognition Program has resulted in organizations integrating nursing research and professional models of care delivery using nursing theory into the practice setting.

In the past, organizations provided sources of evidence and written narratives illustrating the dissemination, enculturation, and sustainability of the Fourteen Forces of Magnetism across the organization (ANCC, 2005). Recently, a new model was developed (ANCC, 2008). The new model has five components that contain the Forces of Magnetism. The five components include transformational leadership; structural empowerment; exemplary professional nursing practice; new knowledge, innovation and improvements; and empirical quality results. The Theory of Bureaucratic Caring can be integrated into each of these components.

Transformational leadership represents quality of nursing leadership and management style. Under quality of nursing leadership reference can be made to the nursing strategic plan and the goal of balancing caring and economics in clinical decision making. For management style, reference can be made as to why the direct care registered nurses selected the theory for practice and how they use the theory in everyday nursing situations.

Structural empowerment represents organizational structure, personnel policies and programs, community and the healthcare organization, image of nursing and professional development. For organizational structure, an example can be a direct care registered nurse making a presentation to the board of trustees on how caring makes a difference in practice. Caring attributes as part of the professional evaluation and job descriptions can be used as evidence under personnel polices and programs. As part of community and the health care organization, registered nurses are involved in community caring. Being in the community requires integration of the social, political, and cultural dimensions of the theory. Having a formal practice theory supports the professional image of nursing within the organization. On-going education including interactive dialogue and reflective practice related to the theory can be referenced under professional development.

Exemplary professional practice includes professional models of care, consultation and resources, autonomy, nurses as teachers, and interdisciplinary relations. Nursing situations reflecting clinical decision making and staffing patterns balancing caring and economics are examples of evidence to support a professional model of care. For consultation and resources, reference can be made to external consultation with nursing scholars and how attendance at professional conferences makes a difference in nursing practice and patient outcomes. Under autonomy, the component of spiritual-ethical caring illustrates how nurses serve as advocates for patients and families. The educational dimension of the theory supports nurses as teachers as the professional nurse develops innovative, individualized, evidence-based patient education initiatives. If an organization is truly focused on transformation and excellence, the theory can be interdisciplinary beyond nursing and serve as the plan of care for the healthcare team.

The component of new knowledge, innovation, and improvements includes quality improvement. Unit-based patient care projects and evidence-based best practice related to the theory is included under this component.

The fifth component, empirical quality, incorporates quality of care. Examples of education related to spiritual ethical caring and research projects documenting the difference in patient outcomes serve as evidence for this component.

Summary

The foundation for professional caring is the blending of the humanistic and empirical aspects of care as well as understanding caring in complex organizations. In today's environment, the nurse needs to integrate caring, knowledge, and skills all at once. Given political and economic constraints, the art of caring cannot occur in isolation from meeting the physical needs of patients and incorporating the dimensions of the economic, political, technological, spiritual-ethical caring dimensions. When caring is defined solely as science *or* as art, empirical or aesthetic nursing respectively, neither is adequate to reflect the reality of current practice. Nurses must be able to understand and articulate the politics and the economics of nursing practice and health care. Classes that examine the environment of practice generally, and the politics and the economics of health care in relation to caring, must be integrated into nursing education and staff development curricula.

Nurses need to search continually for different approaches to professional practice that will incorporate caring in an increasingly political, technical, and cost-driven environment. Doing more with less no longer works; nurses must move outside of the box to create innovative practice models based on nursing theory.

Administrative nursing research needs to continue to focus on the relationship among staff nursing, caring, patient outcomes, and complex organizational economic outcomes. Ongoing research is required to firmly establish the nurse–patient relationship as an economic resource in the new paradigm of evidence-based practice of health care delivery (Ray & Turkel, 2008). Findings from additional research studies may continue to support the Theory of Bureaucratic Caring as both a middle-range and holographic practice theory.

Nurses need repeated exposure to the economics and costs associated with health care as well as knowledge of complex technological organizational environments. Lack of knowledge in these areas means that others outside of nursing will continue to make the political and economic decisions concerning the practice of nursing. Having an in-depth knowledge of the politics and economics of health care will allow nurses to challenge and change the system. A new theory-based model can be created for nursing practice that supports human caring in relation to the organization's economic, technical, and political values. The multiple dimensions of Bureaucratic Caring Theory serve as a philosophical/theoretical framework to guide both contemporary and futuristic research and theory-based nursing practice. Thus, having this in-depth knowledge will allow nurses to continually challenge and transform the system.

References

Al-Ayed, B. (2008). Applying Bureaucratic Caring Theory in medication errors phenomena. University of Jordan, Amman, Jordan.

American Nurses Credentialing Center (ANCC). (2005). *Magnet recognition program: Application manual.* Silver Spring, MD: American Nurses Credentialing Center.

American Nurses Credentialing Center (ANCC). (2008). *Magnet recognition program: Application manual.* Silver Spring, MD: American Nurses Credentialing Center.

Anderson, R., & McDaniel, R. (2008). Taking complexity science seriously: New research, new methods. In: C. Lindberg, S. Nash, & C. Lindberg (Eds.), *On the edge: Nursing in the age of complexity.* Bordentown, NJ: Plexus Press.

Appell, G., & Triloki, N. (Eds.). (1988). *Choice and morality in anthropological perspective.* Albany: State University of New York Press.

Bar-Yam, Y. (2004). *Making things work: Solving complex problems in a complex world.* NECSI: Boston: Knowledge Press.

Bassingthwaighte, J., Liebovitch, L., & West, B. (1994). *Fractal physiology.* New York: Oxford University Press.

Battista, J. (1982). The holographic model, holistic paradigm, information theory, and consciousness. In: K. Wilber (Ed.), *The holographic paradigm and other paradoxes* (pp. 143–150). Boulder, CO: Shambhala.

Begun, J., & White, K. (2008). The challenge of change: Inspiring leadership. In: C. Lindberg, S. Nash, & C. Lindberg (Eds.), *On the edge: Nursing in the age of complexity.* Bordentown, NJ: Plexus Press.

Bell, D. (1974). *The coming of post-industrial society.* New York: Basic Books.

Bohman, J. (2005). Toward a critical theory of globalization: Democratic practice and multiperspectival inquiry. In: M. Pensky (Ed.), *Globalizing critical theory.* Lanham: Rowman & Littlefield.

Bolman, L., & Dial, T. (2008). *Reframing organizations: Artistry, choice, and leadership* (4th ed.). San Francisco: Jossey-Bass.

Boykin, A., & Schoenhofer, S. (2001). *Nursing as caring: A model for transforming practice* (2nd ed.). Sudbury, MA: Jones and Bartlett.

Brenton, A., & Driskill, G. (Eds.). (2005). *Organizational culture in action.* Thousand Oaks, CA: Sage.

Briggs, J. & Peat, F. (1989). *Turbulent mirror.* New York: Harper & Row.

Briggs, J., & Peat, F. (1999). *Seven lessons of chaos.* New York: HarperCollins.

Britain, G., & Cohen, R. (1980). *Hierarchy and society: Anthropological perspectives on bureaucracy.* Philadelphia: ISHI.

Cannato, J. (2006). *Radical amazement.* Notre Dame, IN: Sorin Books.

Chinn, P., & Kramer, M. (1995). *Theory and nursing: A systematic approach* (4th ed.). St. Louis: C. V. Mosby.

Cody, W. (1996). Drowning in eclecticism. *Nursing Science Quarterly, 9,* 96–98.

Coffman, S. (2006). Ray's theory of bureaucratic caring. In: A. M. Tomey & M. Alligood (Eds.), *Nursing theorists and their work* (6th ed.). St. Louis: C. V. Mosby.

Cuilla, J. (2000). *The working life: The promise and betrayal of modern work.* New York: Times Books/Random House.

Davidson, A., & Ray, M. (1991). Studying the human-environment phenomenon using the science of complexity. *Advances in Nursing Science, 14*(2), 73–87.

Dolan, J. (1985). *Nursing in society: A historical perspective.* Philadelphia: W. B. Saunders.

Eisenberg, E., & Goodall, H. (1993). *Organizational communication.* New York: St. Martin's Press.

Eisler, R. (2007). *The real wealth of nations.* San Francisco: Berrett-Koehler.

Fawcett, J. (1993). From a plethora of paradigms to parsimony in worldviews. *Nursing Science Quarterly, 6,* 56–58.

Fox, M. (1994). *The reinvention of work.* San Francisco: Harper.

Gibson, S. (2008). Legal caring: Preventing re-traumatization of abused children through the caring nursing interview using Roach's Six Cs. *International Journal for Human Caring, 12*(4), 32–37.

Glaser, B. (1978). *Theoretical sensitivity.* Mill Valley, CA: The Sociology Press.

Glaser, B., & Strauss, A. (1967). *The discovery of grounded theory: Strategies for qualitative research.* Hawthorne, NY: Aldine de Gruyter.

Gomez, O. (2008). *Application of Bureaucratic Caring Theory.* Professor of Research Group in Management Nursing, National University, Bogata, Colombia.

Harmon, W. (1998). *Global mind change* (2nd ed.). San Francisco: Berrett-Koehler.

Henderson, H. (2006). *Ethical markets: Growing the green economy.* White River Junction, VT: Chelsea Green.

Johns, C. (2000). *Becoming a reflective practitioner.* Oxford: Blackwell Science.

Ketter, J. (1995). Re-engineering the workforce. *The American Nurse, 27*(3), 1, 14.

Korten, D. (1995). *When corporations rule the world.* San Francisco: Berrett-Koehler.

Leininger, M. (1981a). The phenomenon of caring: Importance, research questions and theoretical considerations. In M. Leininger (Ed.), *Caring: An essential human need* (pp. 3–15). Thorofare, NJ: Slack.

Leininger, M. (Ed.). (1981b). *Caring: An essential human need.* Thorofare, NJ: Slack.

Leininger, M. (1991). *Culture care diversity and universality: A theory of nursing.* New York: National League for Nursing Press.

Leininger, M. (1997). Transcultural nursing research to transform nursing education and practice: 40 years. *Image: Journal of Nursing Scholarship, 29,* 341–354.

Leininger, M., & McFarland, M. (Eds.). (1996). *Culture care diversity and universality: A theory of nursing* (2nd ed.). Sudbury, MA; Jones and Bartlett.

Levine, M. (1995). The rhetoric of nursing theory. *Image: Journal of Nursing Scholarship, 27,* 11–14.

Liehr, P., & Smith, M. J. (1999). Middle range theory: Spinning research and practice to create knowledge for the new millennium. *Advances in Nursing Science, 21*(4), 81–91.

Lindberg, C., Nash, S., & Lindberg, C. (Eds.). (2008). *On the edge: Nursing in the age of complexity.* Bordentown, NJ: PlexusPress.

Long, K. (2003). The Institute of Medicine Report, health profession education: A bridge to quality. *Policy, Politics & Nursing, 4*(4), 259–262.

Louis, M. (1985). An investigator's guide to workplace culture. In P. Frost, L. Moore, M. Louis, C. Lundberg, & J. Martin (Eds.), *Organizational culture.* Beverly Hills: Sage.

Manworren, R. (2008). *A pilot study to test the feasibility of using human factors engineering methods to measure factors that compete or influence nurses' abilities to relieve acute pediatric pain* (Application of the Bureaucratic Caring Theory). The University of Texas at Arlington, School of Nursing, Arlington, Texas.

Marriner Tomey, A., & Alligood, M. (2006). *Nursing theorists and their work* (6th ed.). St. Louis, MO: C. V. Mosby.

McCray-Stewart, D. (2008). *Application of bureaucratic caring theory.* Administrator, State of Georgia Correctional Facility (Prison System).

Miller, K. (1989). The human care perspective on nursing administration. *Journal of Nursing Administration, 25*(11), 29–32.

Miller, K. (1995). Keeping the care in nursing care. *Journal of Nursing Administration, 25*(11), 29–32.

Minyard, K., Wall, J., & Turner, R. (1986). RNs may cost less than you think. *Journal of Nursing Administration, 16*(5), 29–34.

Moccia, P. (Ed.). (1986). *New approaches to theory development.* New York: National League for Nursing Press.

Moody, L. (1990). *Advancing nursing science through research.* Newbury Park, CA: Sage.

Morgan, G. (1997). *Images of organization* (2nd ed.). Thousand Oaks, CA: Sage.

Morse, J., Solberg, S., Neander, W., Bottorff, J., & Johnson, J. (1990). Concepts of caring and caring as a concept. *Advances in Nursing Science, 13,* 1–14.

Nevada State College. (2003, August 19). *Nursing organizing framework.* Henderson, NV: Author.

Newman, M. (1986). *Health as expanding consciousness.* St. Louis: C. V. Mosby.

Newman, M. (1992). Prevailing paradigms in nursing. *Nursing Outlook, 40,* 10–14.

Newman, M., Sime, A., & Corcoran-Perry, S. (1991). The focus of the discipline of nursing. *Advances in Nursing Science, 14*(1), 1–6.

Newman, M., Smith, M., Pharris, M., & Jones, D. (2008). The focus of the discipline revisited. *Advances in Nursing Science, 31*(1), E16–27.

Nicolis, G., & Prigogine, I. (1989). *Explaining complexity.* New York: W. H. Freeman.

Nightingale, F. (1860/1969). *Notes on nursing: What it is and what it is not.* New York: Dover.

Nyberg, J. (1989). The element of caring in nursing administration. *Nursing Administration Quarterly, 13,* 9–16.

Nyberg, J. (1991). Theoretical explanations of human care and economics: Foundations of nursing administration practice. *Advances in Nursing Science, 13*(1), 74–84.

Nyberg, J. (1998). A caring approach in nursing administration. Niwot, CO: University Press of Colorado.

O'Brien, K. (2008). *Application of Bureaucratic Caring Theory in Public Health Nursing.* Director of Public Health Nursing, State of Colorado, Denver, CO.

Page, A. (Ed.). (2004). *Keeping patients safe: Transforming the work environment of nurses.* (Institute of Medicine Report). Washington, DC: The National Academies Press.

Parse, R. (1987). *Nursing science: Maps, paradigms, theories, and critiques.* Philadelphia: W. B. Saunders.

Peat, F. (2003). *From certainty to uncertainty: The story of science and ideas in the twentieth century.* Washington, DC: Joseph Henry Press.

Pensky, M. (Ed.). (2005). *Globalizing critical theory.* Lanham: Rowman & Littlefield.

Perrow, C. (1986). *Complex organizations: A critical essay* (3rd ed.). New York: McGraw-Hill.

Pharris, M. (2006). Margaret A. Newman's theory of health as expanding consciousness and its applications. In: M. Parker (Ed.), *Nursing theories & nursing practice* (2nd ed., pp. 217–234). Philadelphia: F. A. Davis.

Pinchot, G., & Pinchot, E. (1994). *The end of bureaucracy & the rise of the intelligent organization.* San Francisco: Berrett-Koehler.

Porter-O'Grady, T. (1979). Financial planning: Budgeting for nurses, part I. *Supervisor Nurse, 10,* 35–38.

Porter-O'Grady, T., & Malloch, K. (2005). *Introduction to evidence-based practice in nursing and health care.* Sudbury, MA: Jones and Bartlett.

Porter-O'Grady, T., & Malloch, K. (2007). *Quantum leadership* (2nd ed.). Sudbury, MA: Jones and Bartlett.

Ray, M. (1981). *A study of caring within the institutional culture.* Unpublished doctoral dissertation. Salt Lake City, UT: University of Utah.

Ray, M. (1984). The development of a nursing classification system of caring. In M. Leininger (Ed.), *Care, the essence of nursing and health* (pp. 95–112). Thorofare, NJ: Slack.

Ray, M. (1987a). Health care economics and human caring: Why the moral conflict must be resolved. *Family and Community Health, 10*(1), 35–43.

Ray, M. (1987b). Technological caring: A new model in critical care. *Dimensions of Critical Care Nursing, 2*(3), 166–173.

Ray, M. (1989a). The Theory of Bureaucratic Caring for nursing practice in the organizational culture. *Nursing Administration Quarterly, 13*(2), 31–42.

Ray, M. (1989b). Transcultural caring: Political and economic caring visions. *Journal of Transcultural Nursing, 1*(1), 17–21.

Ray, M. (1993). A study of care processes using Total Quality Management as a framework in a USAF regional hospital emergency service and related services. *Military Medicine, 158*(6), 396–403.

Ray, M. (1994a). Complex caring dynamics: A unifying model of nursing inquiry. *Theoretic and Applied Chaos in Nursing, 1*(1), 23–32.

Ray, M. (1994b). Communal moral experience as the starting point for research in health care ethics. *Nursing Outlook, 41,* 104–109.

Ray, M. (1997a). The ethical theory of Existential Authenticity. *Canadian Journal of Nursing Research, 22*(1), 111–126.

Ray, M. (1997b). Illuminating the meaning of caring: unfolding the sacred art of divine love. In: M. Roach (Ed.), *Caring from the heart: The convergence of caring and spirituality* (pp. 163–178). New York: Paulist Press.

Ray, M. (1998a). Complexity and nursing science. *Nursing Science Quarterly, 11,* 91–93.

Ray, M. (1998b). The interface of caring and technology: A new reflexive ethics in intermediate care. *Holistic Nursing Practice, 12*(4), 71–79.

Ray, M. (2006). Marilyn Anne Ray's Theory of Bureaucratic Caring. In: M. Parker (Ed.), *Nursing theories, nursing practice* (2nd ed.). Philadelphia: F. A. Davis.

Ray, M. (2010). *Transcultural caring dynamics in nursing and health care.* Philadelphia: F. A. Davis.

Ray, M., DiDominic, V., Dittman, P., Hurst, P., Seaver, J., Sorbello, B., & Ross, M. (1995). The edge of chaos: Caring and the bottom line. *Nursing Management, 26*(9), 48–50.

Ray, M., & Turkel, M. (1999). *Econometric analysis of the nurse–patient relationship.* Qualitative Data Analysis, Grant funded by Department of Defense, TriService Nursing Research Program, Bethesda, MD.

Ray, M., & Turkel, M. (2000–2004). *Economic and patient outcomes of the nursepatient relationship.* Grant funded by the Department of Defense, Tri-Service Nursing Research Program, Bethesda, MD.

Ray, M., & Turkel, M. (2001). Impact of TRICARE/Managed Care on Total Force Readiness. *Military Medicine, 166*(4), 281–289.

Ray, M., & Turkel, M. (2008). Relational caring questionnaires. In: J. Watson (Ed.), *Assessing and measuring caring in nursing and health science* (2nd ed.). New York: Springer.

Ray, M., Turkel, M., & Marino, F. (2002). The transformative process for nursing in workforce redevelopment. *Nursing Administration Quarterly, 26*(2), 1–14.

Reed, P. (1997). Nursing: The ontology of the discipline. *Nursing Science Quarterly, 10,* 76–79.

Roach, M. S. (2002). *The human act of caring* (rev. ed.). Ottawa, Canada: Canadian Hospital Association Press.

Rogers, M. (1970). *An introduction to the theoretical basis of nursing.* Philadelphia: F. A. Davis.

Satterly, F. (2004). *Where have all the nurses gone?: The impact of the nursing shortage on American healthcare.* New York: Prometheus Books.

Schein, E. (2004). *Organizational culture and leadership* (3rd ed). San Franscisco: Jossey-Bass.

Secretan, L. (1997). *Reclaiming higher ground.* New York: McGraw-Hill.

Shaffer, F. (1985). *Costing out nursing: Pricing our product.* New York: National League for Nursing Press.

Sheldrake, R. (1991). *The rebirth of nature.* New York: Bantam.

Smircich, L. (1985). Is the concept of culture a paradigm for understanding organizations and ourselves? In: P. Frost, L. Moore, M. Louis, C. Lundberg, & J. Martin (Eds.), *Organizational culture.* Beverly Hills: Sage.

Smith, M. (2004). Review of research related to Watson's theory of caring. *Nursing Science Quarterly, 17*(1), 13–25.

Sorbello, B. (2008a). *Clinical nurse leader (SM) stories: A phenomenological study about the meaning of leadership at the bedside.* Ph.D. Proposal. Florida Atlantic University, The Christine E. Lynn College of Nursing, Boca Raton, Florida.

Sorbello, B. (2008b). Finance: It's not a dirty word. *American Nurse Today, 3*(8), 32–35.

Stanley, J. (2006). In command of care: Clinical nurse leadership explored. *Journal of Research in Nursing, 11*(91), 20–39.

Strauss, A., & Corbin, J. (1998). *Basics of qualitative research* (2nd ed.). Newbury Park, CA: Sage.

Swanson, K. (1991). Empirical development of a middle-range theory of caring. *Nursing Research, 40*, 161–166.

Swinderman, T. (2005). The magnetic appeal of nurse informaticians: Caring attractor for emergence. PhD dissertation, Florida Atlantic University.

Thoma, H. (2003). Holistic science: All at the same time. *Resurgence, 1*(216), 15–17.

Trossman, S. (1998). The human connection: Nurses and their patients. *The American Nurse, 30*(5), 1, 8.

Tuan, M. (1998). *Forever foreigners or honorary whites?* New Brunswick, NJ: Rutgers University Press.

Turkel, M. (1993). *Nurse–patient interactions in the critical-care setting.* Unpublished research findings.

Turkel, M. (1997). *Struggling to find a balance: A grounded theory study of the nurse-patient relationship in the changing health care environment.* Unpublished doctoral dissertation, University of Miami, Florida. Microfilm #9805958.

Turkel, M. (2001). Struggling to find a balance: The paradox between caring and economics. *Nursing Administration Quarterly, 26*(1), 67–82.

Turkel, M., & Ray, M. (2000). Relational complexity: A theory of the nurse-patient relationship within an economic context. *Nursing Science Quarterly, 13*(4), 307–313.

Turkel, M. (2006). What is evidence-based practice? Integration of evidence-based practice in nursing. In: S. Bayea & M. Slattery (Eds.), *Evidence-based practice in nursing.* Marblehead, MA: HcPro.

Turkel, M. (2007). Dr. Marilyn Ray's Theory of Bureaucratic Caring. *International Journal for Human Caring, 11*(4), 57–74.

Turkel, M., & Ray, M. (2001). Relational complexity: From grounded theory to instrument development and theoretical testing. *Nursing Science Quarterly, 14*(4), 281–287.

Turkel, M., & Ray, M. (2003). A process model for policy analysis within the context of political caring. *International Journal for Human Caring, 7*(3), 26–34.

Turkel, M., & Ray, M. (2004). Creating a caring practice environment through self-renewal. *Nursing Administration Quarterly, 28*(4), 249–254.

Turkel, M., & Ray, M. (2009). Caring for "Not so picture perfect patients": Ethical caring in the moral community of nursing. In: R. Locsin & M. Purnell (Eds.), *A contemporary nursing process: The (un)bearable weight of knowing persons* (pp. 225–249). New York: Springer.

U.S. DHHS (2000). The registered nurse population: Findings from the national sample survey of registered nurses. U.S. DHHS/Division of Nursing. Washington, DC. Retrieved from www.bhpr.hrsa.gov/healthworkforce/reports/rnproject

Van Manen, M. (1982). Edifying theory: Serving the good. *Theory into Practice, 31*, 45–49.

Vicenzi, A., White, K., & Begun, J. (1997). Chaos in nursing: Make it work for you. *American Journal of Nursing, 97*, 26–32.

Watson, J. (1985). *Human science, human care: A theory of nursing.* East Norwalk, CT: Appleton & Lange.

Watson, J. (1988). New dimensions of human caring theory. *Nursing Science Quarterly, 1*, 175–181.

Watson, J. (1997). The theory of human caring: Retrospective and prospective. *Nursing Science Quarterly, 10*(1), 175–181.

Watson, J. (2005). *Caring science as sacred science.* Philadelphia: F. A. Davis.

Weber, M. (1999). The ideal bureaucracy. In: M. Matteson & J. Ivancevich (Eds.), *Management and organizational behavior classics* (7th ed.). Chicago: Irwin McGraw-Hill.

Wheatley, M. (1999). *Leadership and the new science* (2nd ed.). San Francisco: Berrett-Koehler.

Wiggins, M. (2006). Clinical nurse leader. Evolution of a revolution. The partnership care delivery model. *Journal of Nursing Administration, 36*(7/8), 341–345.

Wilbur, K. (Ed.). (1982). *The holographic paradigm and other paradoxes.* Boulder, CO: Shambhala.

Chapter 30

Marlaine Smith's Theory of Unitary Caring

MARLAINE C. SMITH

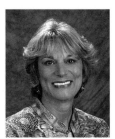

Marlaine C. Smith

Introducing the Theorist

Marlaine C. Smith is currently the Helen K. Persson Eminent Scholar and Associate Dean for Academic Programs at the Christine E. Lynn College of Nursing at Florida Atlantic University. Dr. Smith has been a nurse since 1972, and has practiced in acute care and public health settings in large metropolitan areas and a rural small town. She graduated from Duquesne University with a BSN, the University of Pittsburgh with two master's degrees in public health and nursing with a specialty in oncology and nursing education, and New York University with a PhD in Nursing. Dr. Smith held faculty and academic administrative positions at Duquesne University, Penn State University, LaRoche College, and University of Colorado before her current position.

Dr. Smith is known for her work in two areas: metatheory, or the study of nursing theories and theoretical issues, and research related to healing through touch therapies. She has studied, written about, and conducted research related to Rogers' Science of Unitary Human Beings, Parse's Man-Living-Health (now humanbecoming), Watson's Theory of Transpersonal Caring, and Newman's Health as Expanding Consciousness, and has written many commentaries on issues related to nursing theory development. She conducted five studies examining how the touch therapies of massage, therapeutic touch, hand massage, and simple touch can affect pain, symptom distress, quality of life, sleep, and other important outcomes for persons in acute and longterm care settings. The last completed study was funded by the National Institutes of Health, Center for Complementary and Alternative Medicine.

Dr. Smith has been interested in transtheoretical work, that is, looking across nursing theories for points of convergence. The unitary theory of caring developed while studying the literature on caring in nursing, and then analyzing this literature through the theoretical lens of the Science of Unitary Human Beings. Dr. Smith was the recipient of the National League for Nursing's Martha E. Rogers Award for the Advancement of Nursing Science, is a Distinguished Alumna of New York University Division of Nursing, and is a fellow in the American Academy of Nursing.

Overview of the Theory

There has been a significant body of literature in nursing explicating caring as a phenomenon that is central to nursing's focus as a discipline and profession (Boykin & Schoenhofer, 1993, 2001; Leininger, 1977; Roach, 1987; Stevenson & Tripp-Reimer, 1990; Watson, 1979, 1985). At the same time, there has been a corresponding body of literature critiquing the assertion that caring is an identifying concept for the discipline, and that the existing literature related to caring is ambiguous and provides no direction for meaningful inquiry (Morse, Solberg, Neander, Bottorf, & Johnson, 1990; Rogers in Smith, 1988; Paley, 2001; Smith, 1990). After an analysis of the caring literature, I agreed that caring was a multidimensional concept that assumed multiple meanings depending on the framework within which it was situated or the lens from which it was viewed (Smith, 1999). Paley (1996) argued that a concept acquires its meaning within the context of the theory within which it resides. Concepts are theoretical niches, and to understand a concept fully, the theory in which the concept lives and derives its meaning must be clearly explicated. This chapter is the explication of a middle range theory of caring within the perspective of the unitary–transformative paradigm. For this reason, it is called a unitary theory of caring. This chapter contains a description of the theory development process, the assumptions underpinning the theory, the

concepts of the theory, the empirical referents of the theory, and a practice exemplar that illustrates the major concepts.

Process of Theory Development

This process of developing a middle-range theory was guided by the question: "What is the substantive domain of caring knowledge from a unitary perspective?" Through a unitary lens the question was framed as: What is the quality of being in mutual process that is called "caring" within other theoretical contexts? This question was answered through a process of concept clarification that evolved from Paley's assertion that concepts were niches within theories. This concept clarification involved the following processes: (1) identifying the existing meanings of the concept in context, (2) identifying theoretical niches, (3) synthesis of the concept through identifying constitutive meanings, and (4) instantiation of the concept (Smith, 1999). Identification of the existing meanings of the concept occurred through reviewing the literature on caring that described it as a way of being. Exemplar sources (Boykin & Schoenhofer, 1993; Eriksson, 1997; Gadow, 1980, 1985, 1989; Gaut, 1983; Gendron, 1988; Leininger, 1990; Mayeroff, 1971; Montgomery, 1990; Rawnsley, 1990; Ray, 1981, 1997; Roach, 1987; Sherwood, 1997; Swanson, 1991; Watson, 1979, 1985) were reviewed in this process. From these sources semantic expressions, or phrases that captured the essential meaning of caring as a way of being, were listed. Next, the literature written by unitary scholars (Barrett, 1990; Cowling, 1990, 1993a, 1997; Krieger, 1979; Madrid, 1997; Madrid & Barrett, 1992; Newman, 1994; Quinn, 1992; Rogers, 1994) was examined for existing concepts that corresponded to the semantic expressions of caring. These were identified as theoretical niches in the unitary literature. Constitutive meanings, phrases that captured the meaning of a cluster of semantic expressions, were named using language consistent with a unitary perspective. Five constitutive meanings were developed (Smith, 1999). Since the initial publication, the work was expanded with assumptions and empirical referents (Cowling, Smith, & Watson, 2008) to form a middle range theory. The theory is connected philosophically to the unitary–transformative paradigm, has five concepts that describe the phenomenon of caring from a unitary perspective, and can guide practice behaviors and research questions at the empirical level (Smith & Liehr, 2008).

Assumptions

Assumptions of the unitary theory of caring come from Rogers' Science of Unitary Human Beings (1970, 1994), Newman's Theory of Health as Expanding Consciousness (1994, 2008), and Watson's Theory of Transpersonal Caring (1985, 2002, 2005). To fully understand the meaning of the theory, readers will benefit from studying these sources.

1. Human beings are unitary or irreducible, in mutual process with an environment that is coextensive with the Universe, participating knowingly in patterning, and ever-evolving through expanding consciousness (Newman, 1994; Rogers, 1992).
2. Caring is a quality of participating knowingly in human–environmental field patterning (Smith, 1999).
3. Caring is the process through which human wholeness is affirmed, and which potentiates the emergence of innovative patterning and possibilities (Cowling, Smith, & Watson, 2008, E44).
4. Caring accompanies expanding consciousness potentiating greater meaning, insight, and transformative ways of relating to self and others (Cowling, Smith, & Watson, 2008).
5. Caring consciousness is resonating with the pan-dimensional Universe (Watson, 2005; Rogers, 1994; Watson & Smith, 2002).

Concepts

After establishing the theoretical linkages to the unitary-transformative paradigm, the five concepts of this theory are explicated. The five concepts were developed from an analysis of literature on caring and similar concepts described by unitary scholars. The theoretical concepts have their underpinnings in each of the assumptions.

Manifesting Intentions

Manifesting intentions is the first concept in the unitary theory of caring; it was originally defined as "creating, holding, and expressing thoughts, images, beliefs, hopes, and actions that affirm possibilities for human betterment and well-being" (Smith, 1999, p. 21). From this point of view, the nurse is a healing environment, creating sacred space through her thoughts, feelings, intentions, and actions (Quinn, 1992). Understanding intentionality in this way comes with an assumption that underlying the world of form that is accessed by sensory perception, there is the primary reality that is pandimensional (Rogers, 1994) and beyond access through the five senses alone. David Bohm's (1980) concept of the holographic Universe with implicate/explicate orders of reality is consistent with this point of view. The implicate order is the primary, unseen pattern, while the explicate order is the manifestation of this underlying pattern that is accessible through the senses. Caring is engaging with both orders of reality, holding intentions through affirmations and images, and expressing these intentions through actions. Thoughts, feelings, perceptions, and images are as potent as our words and actions. Intentions are meaningful energetic blueprints for transformation (Smith, 1999). What we hold in our hearts matters. (Cowling, Smith, & Watson, 2008, p. E46). Manifesting intentions encompasses actions that create healing environments, preserve dignity, humanity, and reverence for personhood, focus attention to and concern for the other, and facilitate authentic presence.

Appreciating Pattern

Appreciating pattern is the second concept in this theory. This concept was referenced by both Dolores Krieger (1979) and Richard Cowling (1990, 1993a, 1993b, 1997), and defined by Cowling (1997) as "seeing underneath all that is fragmented to the real existence of wholeness and acknowledging that with awe" (p. 136). Cowling (1997) describes the process of approaching knowing the other with gratitude and enjoyment. This contrasts with a clinical problem-solving approach. While appreciating pattern is an existing concept in unitary theory, it corresponds to many important meanings within caring theories including valuing and celebrating the wholeness and uniqueness of persons, acknowledging pattern without attempting to change it, recognizing the person as perfect in the moment, being sensitive to the unfolding pattern of the whole, and coming to know the other. Pattern is reflected in meaning, so finding out what is meaningful to the other becomes primary in knowing pattern (Newman, 2008). Appreciating pattern is coming to know the uniqueness of the other. It is grasping the wholeness of the other (individual, family, and community), not through analysis, but through sensing, co-exploring experiences, and listening to the other's story. This happens through letting go of preconceptions and the need to categorize, classify, diagnose, or judge. When we resist labeling and diagnosing we can glimpse the dynamic being that is sharing this moment with us. Appreciating pattern is being-with in wonder at this work of art before us, this life that reflects the diversity of creation.

Attuning to Dynamic Flow

Attuning to dynamic flow is the third concept in this unitary theory of caring. Attuning to dynamic flow was originally defined as "dancing to the rhythms within continuous mutual process" (Smith, 1999, p. 23). Caring is flowing with the co-created rhythms of relating in the moment. It happens by being truly present in the moment and is a back and forth movement of relationship building through a "vibrational sensing of where to place focus and attention" (Smith, 1999, p. 23). This includes expressions of caring and unitary relating from the literature such as: attuning to the subtle cues in the moment (Montgomery, 1990), shifting perspectives and patterns of response (Mayeroff, 1971), relating in a

complex synchronized integration (Gendron, 1988), and experiencing energetic resonance (Quinn, 1992). It is hearing the call that may be spoken or unspoken. Newman (2008) describes the process of resonance as a way of knowing that presents itself through intuitive insights and feelings. Intellectualization can actually break this resonant field that is created through true presence. Caring is not taking the lead and telling the person what he/she needs to do. It is understanding where the other wants to go and moving with him/her in the struggle to get there. It is going to the relationship without an agenda, a plan, a bag of tricks, but trusting in the transformative power of healing presence.

Experiencing the Infinite

The next concept in the theory is experiencing the infinite. This concept was defined as "pandimensional awareness of coextensiveness with the universe occurring in the context of human relating" (Smith, 1999, p. 24). This is described by many caring theorists as spiritual union (Watson, 1985), Divine Love (Ray, 1997), or an actual caring occasion (Watson, 1985). Experiencing the Infinite is the recognition that the nurse-person relationship is sacred, we meet the Holy in it, and when we are with others in this way, there are no limits to the possibilities. Miracles happen! There are miracles of healing that happen with our patients every day that can be potentiated through love and caring. This can be recognizing who one really is, appreciating the Oneness of Being with all there is, and finding hope in the darkest of hours. All of this is mediated by our outlook, how we view our world, and what we entertain as possibilities. William Blake said, "The tree which moves some to tears of joy is in the eyes of others only a green thing that stands in the way." Experiencing the infinite occurs in moments of grace, experiencing the presence of God in relationship with others. In those moments there is an experience of connectedness to all-that-is extending beyond space-time boundaries that defies description in ordinary language.

Inviting Creative Emergence

The final concept in this theory of unitary caring is inviting creative emergence. This concept was taken from Quinn's (1992) description of healing and Newman's (1994, 2008) descriptions of transforming presence. Descriptions of caring in the literature that correspond to this concept are a "transformative experience wherein the constant birthing of love in caring actions is the growth of spiritual life within" (Roach, 1987), allowing a person to grow in his/her own time and way (Mayeroff, 1971), and calling to a deeper life, the spiritual life, of each person (Ray, 1997). Caring is inspiring the other to birth oneself anew in the moment. It might be through an activity, realization, decision, a new role, a new life pattern. The nurse creates a safe space for this new life to emerge through supporting, coaching, and providing confidence when it is lacking. This concept relates caring to healing. Caring is the vehicle through which healing occurs. Caring takes trust and patience. People change and grow in their own ways and in their own time. They know their way and we journey with them. This invitation for creative emergence is gentle and encouraging. Quinn (1992) calls it being a midwife to healing.

Empirical Indicators

An empirical indicator is a "concrete and specific real world proxy for a middle range theory concept..." (Fawcett, 2000, p. 20). It is taking a conceptual abstraction and moving it to a place where it lives...where it can be seen, heard, felt, experienced, or measured. There are empirical indicators for both practice and research. Those for practice are useful in translating the theoretical concept to guides for nursing practice. Those for research can be used to generate research questions, develop measures of the concept, or develop paths of inquiry where the concept might be explicated through experiences. Each of the concepts is discussed at the empirical level.

Manifesting Intentions

As far as the concept of *manifesting intentions*, nurses enter a caring relationship with intention, through preparing to become the energetic environment that potentiates healing. Nurses prepare by centering or connecting to the True Self, going to that place within where it is possible to hear the still small voice. Nurses prepare by focusing on the present moment, leaving behind the thoughts racing in their heads that interfere with being truly present with those they serve. Nurses prepare for caring by holding intentions that change the vibratory pattern of the energy field. Marcus Aurelius said, "The soul becomes dyed by the color of its thoughts." The soul of our practice is dyed by our pattern of thinking. If we cultivate the habit of focusing, centering, and setting intentions before any patient encounter; we can create the space for caring and healing. This way of being-with can be developed through self reflection, expressing intentions through touch and energy work, centering exercises, spiritual practices such as meditation and prayer, mantram repetition, and experiences in nature (Cowling, Smith, & Watson, 2008). The development of an inner life is critical for the full expression of caring in nursing. If caring is a way of being, nurses must develop these competencies as much as any other in order to evolve as caring beings. Rituals can structure the process of setting intentions that are manifest in the nursing situation. Watson (2008) gives an example of creating a handwashing ritual where nurses use this daily practice as a way of centering and leaving behind any thoughts that might interrupt presence. Morning huddles are used in some settings as a ritual to come together as a team and set the intentions for the day. Nurses can develop rituals related to giving report that signify the duty to care (Cowling, Smith, & Watson, 2008).

The concept of manifesting intentions can be studied. Activities such as centering, setting an intention, affirmations, meditations, prayers, values-based decision making, and use of mantrams could be tested using any variety of outcomes associated with nurses or their clients. One could explore how nurse centering before care influences outcomes related to patient safety or how the handwashing ritual described above might improve patient satisfaction. One could study if there were healing outcomes associated with Reiki, therapeutic touch, or prayer since these express intentionality. Does our growing intention of healing the planet result in actions and outcomes that reflect a healthier environment for all?

Appreciating Pattern

In a unitary theory of caring, nurses would approach coming to know their patients in an entirely different way. The nursing process, or the problem-solving process, would not be consistent with caring from this point of view. It would involve knowing the other through using the sensory and extrasensory abilities to grasp wholeness. Nursing assessments would include exploring the unique life patterns of the person, exploring what is most important in the moment, and hearing the person's story. Perhaps the first questions that we ask our patients should be "What is important to you right now?" and "What matters most in this moment?" (Boykin & Schoenhofer, 2006). Cowling (1997) and Newman (1994, 2008) have both developed clear praxis methods that focus on pattern appreciation and pattern recognition. Nurses need to develop their abilities to appreciate pattern. Skills of pattern seeing, listening, grasping the essence, and art and music appreciation correspond to this ability of appreciating pattern (Cowling, Smith, & Watson, 2008). In interdisciplinary team conferences, nursing is the voice that represents the wholeness of the person; no other discipline does this. Instead of describing a community by its census and health statistics, we come to know it by asking its members to describe the essence of the community. We can use bulletin boards in patient rooms as places that persons and families can display their uniqueness and what is most important to them.

Research related to pattern appreciation already exists. Cowling's unitary pattern appreciation is a praxis method (combines research and practice) in which he and the participant/client explore patterning together; this is then captured and shared through aesthetic expressions. Through using Newman's praxis method, nurses engage persons in an exploration of the meaningful events and relationships in their lives toward recognizing pattern and making choices about those patterns.

Attuning to Dynamic Flow

Attuning to dynamic flow is lived in practice through sensing the readiness to begin to talk about sensitive issues or the willingness to take on a major life change. It might be staying engaged with a person and family members as they struggle together with the decision to move to hospice care. It might be knowing when a person needs the nurse to be tough, urging him to get out of bed and walk after surgery or to be soft, facilitating some quiet space for a person to be alone for awhile. Nurses need to cultivate their abilities related to this through sensing, hearing and moving with rhythms, presencing, and focusing. Learning to listen for shifts and pauses and learning to listen to and trust intuitive insights is important. There are hospital myths about the nurse who walks by a patient's room and knows that the patient is going to code. This may be an example of being sensitive to changes and shifts within a situation, attuning to the information that is embedded in the field of consciousness.

There are research possibilities related to this concept. It would be interesting to study how nurses attune to the dynamic flow of relationship with an unconscious person or a neonate. What are the cues that they pick up and act on? What are the ways that they sense beyond the senses to understand what is happening or what is being communicated to them? The study of intuition in practice is an example of an empirical indicator of this concept.

Experiencing the infinite. One example of experiencing the infinite is seeing the sacred in mundane activities. It is recognizing the extraordinary in the ordinariness of our activities. This might be made concrete by practice rituals that can help us to recognize and celebrate the work of nursing. One such ritual that has been used is the "blessing of the hands." Another way to experience the infinite in practice is to validate its existence through nursing practice stories. We don't take the time to really appreciate the incredible moments experienced in caring with others. The sensitivity to experience the infinite in our practice may be developed through spiritual practice or a practice that fosters deep reflection. This could be meditation, prayer, centering, being in nature, or walking a labyrinth (Cowling, Smith, & Watson, 2008, p. E48).

The research questions that are related to this concept might be studying nurses' and patients' stories of the extraordinary moments experienced in nursing practice.

Inviting Creative Emergence

There are many examples in nursing practice that can illustrate how caring can invite creative emergence. This can happen when we help women become mothers through teaching them the necessary skills to care for their babies and help them to grow, or when we connect people to resources in the community that allow them to live with greater ease in the midst of a family crisis. It is helping others live their lives differently and discover new ways of becoming.

The empirical indicators for research might be developing an instrument to measure satisfaction or pride associated with life changes. Studies could be structured to explore differences in outcomes when lifestyle change is approached with a nondirective model suggested by this concept, rather than a structured directive approach to lifestyle change.

Practice Exemplar

Sue is a family nurse practitioner working in a community-based family practice with a physician colleague. She practices from a nursing model, using theories in the unitary-transformative paradigm as a guide for her practice. Beth is a 55-year-old attorney who has been seeing Sue for her primary care for some time. She is waiting in the examining room.

Sue has had a busy morning with time pressures and some difficult patient encounters. She is "backed up" with two patients waiting for her. She approaches the examining room and pulls out the chart. She smiles as she sees Beth's name. In front of the door, she pauses, closes her eyes, takes several deep breaths and centers herself, repeating her mantram. She sets an intention to be fully and authentically present with Beth in this encounter and to enter a relationship with her that facilitates their mutual well-being.

Sue opens the door and finds Beth sitting on the chair fully clothed. Sue approaches her warmly, holding out her hand and touching her on the shoulder. She pulls up her chair and puts the chart aside. "OK, Beth, what's going on? How are you?"

Beth talks rapidly, wringing her hands and tugging on her sleeve. "I was on vacation last week in North Carolina with my friends. We were having a relaxing time, and as I was getting out of the car I felt myself go into atrial fibrillation. My heart rate went way up like it does to about 270, and I felt just awful, like I couldn't breathe, lightheaded....I thought I was going to die."

"Oh, how scary....that's awful."

"I know. I ended up in the Emergency Room of this tiny hospital where they treated me with IV anti-arrhythmic drugs, and finally my heart rate went down, and I converted to sinus rhythm in about three hours. But this is the third time that this has happened to me, and the second time when I've been away from home. I just need to get to the bottom of this. I'm frustrated and scared."

"Of course you are," Sue continues. "OK tell me how things are going with you generally and anything unusual that you were doing on vacation that might have precipitated this episode."

"Well, you know I had that episode of diverticulitis before I left for vacation, and

Continued

you prescribed the Cipro for me. Well, I was not feeling great on vacation, the pain was better, but I had constipation, but took the Miralax and the fiber that I always take. We went on a boat trip the day before and I took some Dramamine, too. Also, my friends and I were drinking wine every night. That's all I can think of."

"What about home and work?"

Beth looks down at her hands. "Well, Bob still can't find a job, and things have been crazy at work. I just can't seem to get ahead of it. I have a major brief due in a couple of weeks...It was hard to leave for vacation. I love being with my friends, but I was torn about taking the time."

Sue pauses then says, "Tell me more about this feeling of being torn between what you love and what you have to do."

"I guess I'm in that space a lot lately, Sue." Beth begins crying. "I don't think I'm doing what I love to do...I feel like I'm not in control of my life."

Sue hands Beth some tissues and sits quietly with her, gently touching her arm as Beth sobs. In the moment Beth sobs for the loss of joy in her life now, and at the memory of her mother telling her she had to go into a practical career like law, not fiction writing. In the moment Sue imagines holding and rocking Beth in the space between them. In her mind's eye she whispers comforting words. In silence, they both experience an intimacy that is beyond language.

When Beth stops crying she looks up and asks, "What do I do now?"

"Let's take care of the A-fib issue first, Beth. Are you still on the same dose of the beta blocker that your cardiologist prescribed?"

"Yes, Toprol 25 mg."

"OK. I want you to get in to see the cardiologist as soon as possible and discuss this with him. You have some options with ablation or other anti-arrhythmics. You might want to talk with an electrophysiologist as well. I'll make a referral. Also, I just checked the side effects of Cipro, and atrial fibrillation is a rare side effect. So taking the Cipro could

have triggered this event given your history. And of course Dramamine and alcohol could have contributed. And at the time this happened you were just getting over diverticulitis and weren't feeling great. But, we also need to focus on this distress that you are experiencing related to your work. I'd like you to do some journaling for a period of two weeks. Write down the things that you love, your passions, what makes your heart sing? Don't over-think it, Beth. If you have images or messages that come to you, jot them down. Make an appointment in two weeks, and we'll talk about what you discovered. OK?"

"Yes, OK." Beth nods tentatively.

"Before you leave I'm going to listen to your heart and check your blood pressure again. Hop up on the table." Sue auscultates Beth's heart sounds and measures her blood pressure. "Everything is fine. Your heart rate is regular at 60, and your blood pressure is OK, but a bit higher than we'd like it to be: 130/82. I know you experience some "white coat hypertension." We'll check it again next week. You check it too at the machine in the grocery store and keep track. Bring that back in two weeks too."

Sue puts two hands on Beth's shoulders. "I'm in this with you. You'll figure this out. Change can be hard, but it's how we grow. Anything else that we need to talk about today?"

"No, I feel better....thanks, Sue."

"Thank you! I'll see you in two weeks."

(The encounter took 15 minutes).

The five concepts of the unitary theory of caring were evident. First, *manifesting intention* was visible in the preparation before Sue entered the room. She was aware that she, as nurse, is an environment for healing (Quinn, 1992). Sue set an intention and entered the nursing situation being fully present to Beth. She shared her intentions with Beth when she said, "I'm in this with you," and in her use of touch and eye contact to communicate her desire to be present and in partnership with Beth. *Appreciating pattern* was evident as Sue asks Beth about what was going on with her, how she was, and if there was anything different about the time that led up to the episode of atrial fibrillation. Sue values the uniqueness of Beth's experience and Beth's own insights about events that led up to the episode, affirming that Beth's knowledge of her own pattern had validity. Intuitively, Sue asked the questions, "What about home and work?" and "Tell me more about this feeling of being torn between what you love to do and what you have to do." This second question emerged from Sue's tuning into meaning and resonating with the whole, illustrating the concept of *attuning to dynamic flow*. This led to the revelation of Beth's life pattern that could have remained undisclosed had Sue not attended to the intuitive flash. As Sue silently sat with Beth as she sobbed, they both experienced an intimacy beyond words, and a pandimensional awareness of past–present–future in the moment. This is an example of the concept of *experiencing the infinite*. Finally, when Beth expresses that she is not doing what she loves, Sue is *inviting creative emergence* by asking her to attend to any cues she may receive about what she would love to do and to record this in a journal. She asks her to return for a follow-up visit in 2 weeks.

Often, the argument is advanced that "there is no time to care in this way," but this encounter took 15 minutes, no longer than a conventional, medically-focused primary care visit. It isn't the time we have; it is what we do with that time that counts.

Summary

The unitary theory of caring provides a constellation of concepts that describe caring from a unitary perspective. The theory is constituted with five concepts: manifesting intentions, appreciating pattern, attuning to dynamic flow, experiencing the Infinite, and inviting creative emergence. Assumptions of the theory were explication, each concept was described, and examples of empirical indicators for practice and research were offered. The unitary theory of caring is new; it can grow through those who invest in it through testing it in practice and research.

References

Barrett, E. A. M. (1990). *Visions of Rogers' science-based nursing*. New York: National League for Nursing Press.

Bohm, D. (1980). *Wholeness and the implicate order*. London: Routledge & Kegan Paul.

Boykin, A., & Schoenhofer, S. (1993). *Nursing as caring: A model for transforming practice*. New York: National League for Nursing Press.

Boykin, A., & Schoenhofer, S. (2001). *Nursing as caring: A model for transforming practice* (2nd ed.). Sudbury, MA: Jones and Bartlett.

Boykin, A., & Schoenhofer, S. (2006). Anne Boykin and Savina Schoenhofer's Nursing as Caring theory. In: M. Parker (Ed.), *Nursing theories and nursing practice* (pp. 334–348). Philadelphia: F. A. Davis.

Cowling, W. R. (1990). A template for unitary pattern-based practice. In: E. A. M. Barrett (Ed.), *Visions of Rogers' science-based nursing* (pp. 45-65). New York: National League for Nursing Press.

Cowling, W. R. (1993a). Unitary knowing in nursing practice. *Nursing Science Quarterly, 6*, 201–207.

Cowling, W. R. (1993b). Unitary practice: revisionary assumptions. In: M. Parker (Ed.), *Patterns of nursing theories in practice*. New York: National League for Nursing Press.

Cowling, W. R. (1997). Pattern appreciation: The unitary science/practice of reaching for essence. In: M. Madrid (Ed.), *Patterns of Rogerian knowing*. New York: National League for Nursing Press.

Cowling, W. R., Smith, M. C., & Watson, J. (2008). The power of wholeness, consciousness and caring: A dialogue on nursing science, art and healing. *Advances in Nursing Science, 31*(1), E41–E51.

Eriksson, K. (1997). Understanding the world of the patient, the suffering human being: The new clinical paradigm from nursing to caring. *Advanced Practice Nursing Quarterly, 3*(1), 8–13.

Fawcett, J. (2000). *Analysis and evaluation of contemporary nursing knowledge: Nursing models and theories.* Philadelphia: F. A. Davis.

Gadow, S. (1980). Existential advocacy: Philosophical foundations of nursing. In: S. Spicker & S. Gadow (Eds.), *Nursing images and ideals.* New York: Springer.

Gadow, S. A. (1985). Nurse and patient: the caring relationship. In: A. Bishop & J. Scudder (Eds.), *Caring, curing, coping: Nurse, physician, patient relationships.* Tuscaloosa, AL: University of Alabama Press.

Gadow, S. A. (1989). Clinical subjectivity: Advocacy with silent patients. *Nursing Clinics of North America, 24,* 535–541.

Gaut, D. A. (1983). Development of a theoretically adequate description of caring. *Western Journal of Nursing Research, 5,* 313–324.

Gendron, D. (1988). The expressive form of caring. *Perspectives in caring monograph 2.* Toronto: University of Toronto Faculty of Nursing.

Krieger, D. (1979). *The therapeutic touch: How to use your hands to help or heal.* Englewood Cliffs, NJ: Prentice-Hall.

Leininger, M. (1977). *Caring: The essence and central focus of nursing.* American Nurses' Foundation. Nursing Research Report.

Leininger, M. M. (1990). Historic and epistemologic dimensions of care and caring with future directions. In: J. S. Stevenson & T. Tripp-Reimer (Eds.), *Knowledge about care and caring: State of the art and future developments.* Kansas City, MO: American Academy of Nursing.

Madrid, M. (1997). *Patterns of Rogerian knowing.* New York: National League for Nursing Press.

Madrid, M., & Barrett, E. A. M. (Eds.). (1992). *Rogers' scientific art of nursing practice.* New York: National League for Nursing Press.

Mayeroff, M. (1971). *On caring.* New York: Harper & Row.

Montgomery, C. (1990). *Healing through communication: The practice of caring.* Newbury Park: CA: Sage.

Morse, J. M., Solberg, S. M., Neander, W. L., Bottorff, J. L., & Johnson, J. L. (1990). Concepts of caring and caring as a concept. *Advances in Nursing Science, 13,* 1–14.

Newman, M. A. (1994). *Health as expanding consciousness.* New York: National League for Nursing Press.

Newman, M. A. (2008). *Transforming presence: The difference that nursing makes.* Philadelphia: F. A. Davis.

Paley, J. (1996). How not to clarify concepts in nursing. *Journal of Advanced Nursing, 24,* 572–578.

Paley, J. (2001). An archaeology of caring knowledge. *Journal of Advanced Nursing, 36*(2), 188–198.

Quinn, J. F. (1992). Holding sacred space: the nurse as healing environment. *Holistic Nursing Practice, 6,* 26–36.

Rawnsley, M. (1990). Of human bonding: The context of nursing as caring. *Advances in Nursing Science, 13*(2), 41–48.

Ray, M. A. (1981). A philosophical analysis of caring within nursing. In: M. M. Leininger (Ed.), *Caring: An essential human need.* Thorofare, NJ: Slack.

Ray, M. A. (1997). Illuminating the meaning of caring: Unfolding the sacred art of divine love. In: M. S. Roach (Ed.), *Caring from the heart: The convergence of caring and spirituality.* New York: Paulist Press.

Roach, S. (1987). *The human act of caring.* Ottawa: The Canadian Hospital Association.

Rogers, M. E. (1970). *An introduction to the theoretical basis of nursing.* Philadelphia: F. A. Davis.

Rogers, M. E. In: M. J. Smith (1988). Perspectives on nursing science. *Nursing Science Quarterly, 1,* 80–85.

Rogers, M. E. (1994). The science of unitary human beings: Current perspectives. *Nursing Science Quarterly, 7,* 33–35.

Sherwood, G. D. (1997). Metasynthesis of qualitative analysis of caring: Defining a therapeutic model of nursing. *Advanced Practice Nursing Quarterly, 3*(1), 32–42.

Smith, M. C. (1999). Caring and the science of unitary human beings. *Advances in Nursing Science, 21*(4), 14–28.

Smith, M. J. (1990). Caring: Ubiquitous or unique. *Nursing Science Quarterly, 3,* 54.

Smith, M. J., & Liehr, P. R. (2008). *Middle range theory for nursing* (2nd ed.). New York: Springer.

Swanson, K. M. (1991). Empirical development of a middle range theory of caring. *Nursing Research, 40,* 161–165.

Stevenson, J., & Tripp-Reimer, T. (Eds.). (1990). *Knowledge about care and caring: Proceedings of a Wingspread Conference.* February 1–3. Kansas City, MO: American Academy of Nursing.

Watson, J. (1979). *Nursing: The philosophy and science of caring.* Boston: Little, Brown & Co.

Watson, J. (2008). *Nursing: The philosophy and science of caring.* Boulder: University Press of Colorado.

Watson, J. (1985). *Nursing: Human science and human care: A theory of nursing.* East Norwalk, CT: Appleton-Century-Crofts.

Watson, J. (2005). *Caring science as sacred science.* Philadelphia: F. A. Davis.

Watson, J., & Smith, M. C. (2002). Caring science and the science of unitary human beings: a transtheoretical discourse for nursing knowledge development. *Journal of Advanced Nursing, 37*(5), 452–461.

Index

Note: Page numbers followed by *f* refer to figures; page numbers followed by *t* refer to tables; page numbers followed by *b* refer to boxes.